Atlas of Pediatric Vascular Anomalies

Amr Abdelhamid AbouZeid
Shaimaa AbdelSattar Mohammad
Iman Ahmed Ragab

Atlas of Pediatric Vascular Anomalies

Clinical and Pathological Diversity

Springer

Amr Abdelhamid AbouZeid
Department of Pediatric Surgery
Ain Shams University, Faculty of Medicine
Cairo, Egypt

Iman Ahmed Ragab
Department of Pediatrics, Hematology-Oncology Unit
Ain Shams University, Faculty of Medicine
Cairo, Egypt

Shaimaa AbdelSattar Mohammad
Department of Diagnostic and Interventional Radiology and Molecular Imaging
Ain Shams University, Faculty of Medicine
Cairo, Egypt

ISBN 978-3-032-30865-8 ISBN 978-3-032-30866-5 (eBook)
https://doi.org/10.1007/978-3-032-30866-5

This Springer imprint is published by the registered company Springer Nature Switzerland AG
The registered company address is: Gewerbestrasse 11, 6330 Cham, Switzerland

To all the parents, doctors, nurses, and all those who strive to improve the quality of life of individuals born with vascular anomalies.
In appreciation of Dr. J. Leonel Villavicencio, whose lifelong work in the management of vascular malformations has inspired generations of clinicians and researchers; he so beautifully captured the essence of our mission in this challenging and often misunderstood field of medicine when he wrote:
"We are here to care for those who cannot care for themselves and who, in desperation, turn their eyes to us hoping to find relief."

Preface

The field of vascular anomalies occupies a unique and complex position within medicine. The remarkable pathological diversity—encompassing tumors, malformations, and overgrowth conditions—combined with their occurrence across different regions and organ systems, places the subject well beyond the scope of any single specialty. Indeed, some authors have aptly described vascular anomalies as "orphans" in the medical universe.

For decades, progress in this field was hindered by a confusing and inconsistent terminology, often compounded by the use of multiple eponyms that reflected the limited understanding of these conditions at the time. A turning point came in 1982, when Mullikan and Young introduced a modern binary classification of vascular anomalies. This breakthrough not only brought clarity but also paved the way for subsequent advances in genetics and pharmacotherapy.

Building on this foundation, the International Society for the Study of Vascular Anomalies (ISSVA) was officially founded in 1992 to unify global efforts in research, foster collaboration across specialties, and publish updated editions of the classification system. These initiatives coincided with the development of dedicated multidisciplinary clinics, which have since become exemplary models of collaborative medical practice.

The progress achieved to date is the outcome of decades of dedicated work by experts from diverse specialties—including surgery, radiology, and pediatrics—in leading centers around the world. Their contributions have shaped the modern approach to diagnosing and managing vascular anomalies. In preparing this volume, we have drawn extensively upon their scholarship and clinical experience, and we gratefully acknowledge this indebtedness in the list of references provided at the end of each chapter.

In this atlas, we aimed to provide a concise yet comprehensive resource that relies primarily on a rich collection of figures rather than extensive text. The illustrations encompass various aspects of vascular anomalies, including clinical and operative photographs, as well as diverse imaging modalities that reveal the intricate details of these complex and heterogeneous conditions. Our goal is for this volume to serve as a valuable reference for physicians across various specialties involved in the care of patients with vascular anomalies.

Cairo, Egypt

Amr Abdelhamid AbouZeid
Shaimaa AbdelSattar Mohammad
Iman Ahmed Ragab

Competing Interests The authors have no competing interests to declare that are relevant to the content of this manuscript.

Contents

Part I

Introduction

Classification and Molecular Basis of Vascular Anomalies

1

Introduction

Vascular anomalies represent a diverse group of disorders involving abnormal development or growth of blood and lymphatic vessels. They are broadly categorized into two main groups: vascular tumors and vascular malformations, based on their biological behavior and cellular characteristics (Fig. 1.1).

Vascular tumors—the most common example being infantile hemangiomas—are proliferative lesions characterized by active endothelial cell division and growth. These lesions typically appear shortly after birth, undergo a phase of rapid proliferation, and then gradually involute overtime. Their dynamic nature reflects a true neoplastic process, although usually benign.

In contrast, vascular malformations are structural anomalies of blood vessels that arise from errors during vascular morphogenesis. Unlike vascular tumors, they are not characterized by endothelial proliferation but rather by abnormally formed and persistently dilated vascular channels. These lesions are present at birth, although they may become more apparent later, and they enlarge proportionally with the individual's growth or may expand due to trauma, hormonal changes, or infection. Vascular malformations are further subdivided into slow-flow lesions, such as venous, lymphatic, capillary malformations; and fast-flow lesions, such as arteriovenous malformations and arteriovenous fistula [1, 2].

The International Society for the Study of Vascular Anomalies (ISSVA) provided a classification system for these anomalies, which was most recently updated in 2025. Under this system, vascular anomalies are divided into three principal categories: vascular tumors, vascular malformations, and a newer category called Potentially Unique Vascular Anomalies (PUVA)—replacing the older concept of "provisionally unclassified" lesions [1].

A. A. AbouZeid et al., *Atlas of Pediatric Vascular Anomalies*, https://doi.org/10.1007/978-3-032-30866-5_1

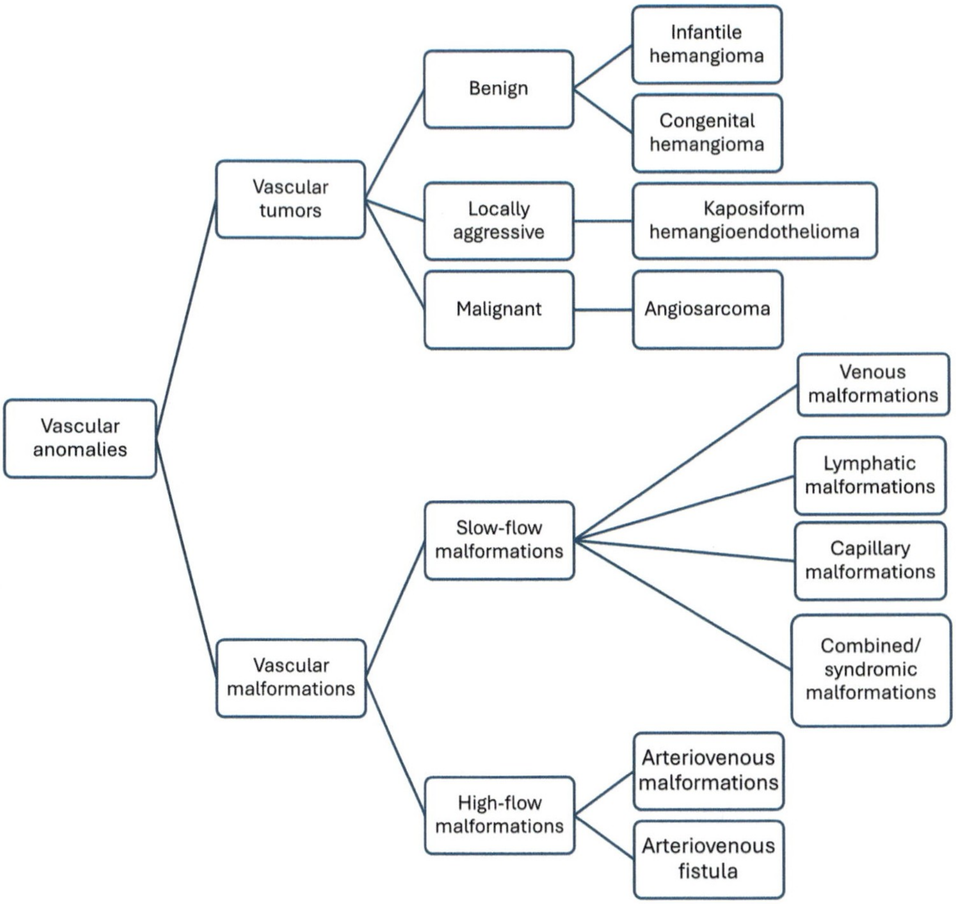

Fig. 1.1 Classification of the main types of vascular anomalies

Vascular Tumors

Vascular tumors are classified into three main categories: benign, borderline, and malignant. The benign group includes several types of hemangiomas, with infantile hemangiomas being the most common. These lesions are typically absent at birth but emerge within the first days of life, exhibiting a characteristic triphasic evolution consisting of a proliferative phase, a plateau phase, and a gradual involutional phase, with spontaneous regression generally achieved by 5–9 years of age (for additional information, please refer to Chap. 3). Another benign type is the congenital hemangioma (Chap. 5), which is fully developed at birth and demonstrates one of three growth behaviors: rapidly involuting congenital hemangioma (RICH), non-involuting congenital hemangioma (NICH), or partially involuting (PICH). These are primarily linked to GNA spectrum variants (GNAQ/GNA11). Other less common benign vascular tumors include tufted angioma, cherry angioma, pyogenic granuloma, and various other hemangioma subtypes.

The borderline group encompasses lesions with intermediate biological behavior, including kaposiform hemangioendothelioma (KHE), retiform hemangioendothelioma, papillary intralymphatic angioendothelioma, pseudomyogenic hemangioendothelioma, Kaposi sarcoma, and multifocal lymphangioendotheliomatosis with thrombocytopenia. Among these, KHE is the most common and is associated with dysregulation of both angiogenesis and lymphangiogenesis (for additional information, please refer to Chap. 7) [3].

The malignant group comprises angiosarcoma and epithelioid hemangioendothelioma, both of which exhibit aggressive clinical behavior and require careful pathological and molecular characterization [1].

Vascular Malformations

Most vascular malformations are either present at birth or become noticeable shortly afterward. They generally increase in size gradually over a person's lifetime, although new lesions can occasionally appear later. Among these, venous malformations (VMs) are among the most frequently encountered types in clinical practice, with an estimated incidence of 1–2 per 10,000 births [4] and a prevalence of approximately 1% [5]. They are typically classified as slow-flow lesions [6] and are most commonly found in the skin or mucous membranes. Clinically, VMs present as bluish, soft, and compressible lesions, while histologically, they consist of dilated, irregular venous channels lined by a single layer of endothelial cells, surrounded by a disorganized extracellular matrix and smooth muscle layer (for additional information, please refer to Chaps. 13, 14, 15, and 16).

Lymphatic anomalies are broadly classified into lymphatic malformations (LMs) and lymphedema. LMs may occur as isolated lesions or as part of a complex, multifocal disease (for additional information, please refer to Chaps. 9, 10, 11, and 12). The latter constitute the group of complex lymphatic anomalies, which encompass generalized lymphatic anomaly (GLA), Gorham–Stout disease (GSD), kaposiform lymphangiomatosis (KLA), and central conducting lymphatic anomalies [7].

Capillary malformations (CMs) typically present as flat, red-to-purple lesions, and approximately 0.3% of newborns are affected at birth, most commonly with what is known as a port-wine stain (for additional information, please refer to Chap. 18) [8]. The high-flow vascular malformations, mainly arteriovenous malformations (AVMs), represent the most aggressive type, as their progressive enlargement can lead to destruction of adjacent tissues and structures (for additional information, please refer to Chap. 17) [9].

Understanding the Molecular Basis of Vascular Anomalies

Vascular anomalies can vary widely in their clinical presentation—from simple capillary malformations to complex lesions involving arteries, veins, and lymphatics. In recent years, remarkable advances in molecular genetics have transformed our understanding of these anomalies, revealing that they often arise from specific genetic mutations that disrupt normal signaling pathways controlling vascular development and maintenance. Broadly, vascular anomalies result from either inherited (germline) or acquired (somatic) mutations [10].

- In inherited forms, individuals are born with a genetic alteration that typically causes a loss of function in a protein crucial for vascular stability. The actual vascular lesion often appears later, after a "second-hit" mutation occurs in affected cells.
- In sporadic forms, which are more common, the lesions arise from gain-of-function somatic mutations that occur during development or postnatally in a subset of endothelial cells.

The genes most commonly implicated in vascular anomalies are components of pathways regulating angiogenesis, lymphangiogenesis, vascular cell growth, and apoptosis [11]. The principal molecular pathways involved include the angiopoietin/TIE2 (angiopoietin-1 receptor) pathway, the PI3K (phosphoinositide 3-kinase)/AKT (protein kinase B)/mTOR (mammalian target of rapamycin) pathway, the EPHB4 (Ephrin B4)/Ras/MEK/ERK signaling cascade, as well as TGF-β (transforming growth factor beta) and G protein–coupled receptor signaling molecules such as GNAQ, GNA11, and GNA14 [9].

Understanding these molecular mechanisms has not only clarified why certain vascular anomalies develop but has also paved the way for targeted therapies. Drugs that inhibit overactive pathways—such as mTOR inhibitors for PIK3CA-related malformations or MEK inhibitors for RAS-driven lesions—are emerging as promising treatments that address the root molecular cause rather than just the symptoms. In the following sections, we will explore in detail the two major signaling networks most commonly involved in vascular malformations:

1. The PI3K/AKT/mTOR pathway, which plays a central role in venous and lymphatic malformations.
2. The RAS/RAF/MEK/ERK pathway, which contributes to several fast-flow and capillary malformations.

First: Vascular Anomalies and PI3K/AKT/mTOR Signaling Pathway

This signaling pathway is activated when a ligand binds to its receptor tyrosine kinase (RTK)—for instance, epidermal growth factor (EGF) binding to the epidermal growth factor receptor (EGFR) or angiopoietin binding to TIE2—thereby initiating the regulation of cell proliferation [12]. Upon activation, phosphoinositide 3-kinase (PI3K) phosphorylates phosphatidylinositol-4,5-bisphosphate (PIP_2) to form phosphatidylinositol-3,4,5-trisphosphate (PIP_3), which in turn activates its downstream effector, AKT [13]. The enzyme PTEN (phosphatase and tensin homolog) serves as a negative regulator of this pathway by dephosphorylating PIP_3, thereby counteracting PI3K activity and maintaining signaling balance [11].

PI3K in Venous Malformations Most venous malformations (VMs) are associated with gain-of-function mutations in the TEK gene, which is located on chromosome 9p21 and encodes the endothelial receptor tyrosine kinase TIE2. Binding of angiopoietin-1 (ANGPT1) to TIE2 induces receptor activation, which in turn stimulates the PI3K/AKT/mTOR signaling pathway [14]. A significant proportion of sporadic unifocal and multifocal VMs, as well as blue rubber bleb nevus syndrome and inherited cutaneo-mucosal VMs, are linked to gain-of-function TEK mutations [15]. The most frequent mutation in sporadic VMs is L914F [16], whereas the R849W mutation is most commonly associated with autosomal-dominant cutaneo-mucosal VMs [11]. Blue rubber bleb nevus syndrome is characterized by numerous cutaneous and gastrointestinal VMs, sometimes numbering in the hundreds, which can lead to consumptive coagulopathy and chronic anemia. The number of lesions often increases with age. This syndrome is most commonly associated with a carboxy-terminal double mutation (T1105N–T1106P), although other variants such as Y897F–R915L have also been identified [17]. Additionally, sporadic VMs may carry somatic mutations in PIK3CA (phosphatidylinositol-4,5-bisphosphate 3-kinase catalytic subunit alpha), further contributing to aberrant PI3K/AKT pathway activation [18].

PI3K in Isolated Lymphatic Malformations or with PIK3CA Related Overgrowth The majority of lymphatic malformations (LMs) contain somatic hotspot mutations in PIK3CA, similar to those identified in venous malformations (VMs). Two main categories of PIK3CA mutations have been described in PIK3CA-mutated vascular anomalies. The first group, known as hotspot mutations, are frequently observed in cancer and include p.Glu542Lys, p.Glu545Lys (helical domain), and p.His1047Arg (kinase domain) [18, 19]. These variants are strongly associated with PIK3CA-related overgrowth syndromes (PROS) [20]. The second group, comprising non-hotspot mutations, occurs less commonly and is linked to specific PROS phenotypes, such as megalencephaly–capillary malformation (CM) syndrome and congenital lipomatous overgrowth with vascular anomalies, epidermal nevi, and scoliosis (CLOVES) syndrome [9].

PTEN Hamartoma Tumor Syndrome PTEN Hamartoma Tumor Syndrome (PHTS) is caused by autosomal dominant loss-of-function mutations in the PTEN gene [21]. Affected individuals typically present with macrocephaly, lipomas, and papillomas or trichilemmomas, along with fast-flow vascular lesions. In addition to these features, patients with PHTS are predisposed to developing multiple types of cancer [11].

Hereditary Hemorrhagic Telangiectasia Hereditary Hemorrhagic Telangiectasia (HHT), also called Osler–Weber–Rendu syndrome, is an autosomal dominant disorder clinically marked by multiple cutaneous telangiectasias affecting the face, oral mucosa, and hands, along with arteriovenous malformations (AVMs) in internal organs such as the central nervous system, lungs, and liver [22]. Genetically, HHT is linked to several loss-of-function mutations, including those in the Endoglin (ENG) gene associated with HHT1 [23], the activin receptor-like kinase 1 (ACVRL1) gene implicated in HHT2 [24], and the MADH4 gene encoding SMAD4, found in the juvenile polyposis/HHT overlap syndrome [25]. Endoglin is a critical component of the BMP9/BMP10/ALK1 signaling pathway, which activates the transcription factors R-SMAD1/5/8 and SMAD4, thereby suppressing endothelial cell migration and proliferation [26]. Moreover, AKT pathway activation occurs through PTEN inhibition, a process that can be counteracted by PI3K inhibition [27].

Glomuvenous Malformation Glomuvenous malformation (GVM) is an autosomal dominant disorder resulting from loss-of-function mutations in the glomulin (GLMN/FAP68) gene [28]. Normally, glomulin is released from the c-MET receptor, initiating PI3K-dependent downstream signaling. In GVM, the lack of functional glomulin allows FK-binding protein 12 (FKBP12) to bind to the transforming growth factor beta 1 (TGF-β1) receptor, thereby inhibiting TGF-β signaling and disrupting vascular smooth muscle cell (vSMC) differentiation [29]. This dysregulation ultimately leads to increased mTOR pathway activity [30].

Second: Vascular Anomalies and RAS/RAF/MEK/ERK Signaling

RASopathies encompass a group of vascular anomalies resulting from disturbances in the RAS/RAF/MEK/ERK signaling cascade. This pathway is normally activated by various growth factors, cytokines, and G protein–coupled receptor (GPCR) ligands, which stimulate RAS through the exchange of GDP for GTP. Once activated, RAS binds to RAF, initiating a phosphorylation cascade in which RAF activates MEK, and MEK subsequently activates ERK. The activated ERK proteins then dimerize and translocate to the nucleus, where they regulate the expression and activity of multiple target proteins involved in cell growth and differentiation [31]. Vascular malformations associated with aberrant activation of the RAS signaling pathway include verrucous venous malformations, kaposiform lymphangiomatosis (KLA), capillary malformation–arteriovenous malformation (CM-AVM) syndromes, and arteriovenous malformations (AVMs) (Fig. 1.2).

Ras Pathway in Venous Malformations Verrucous venous malformations (VVMs) are characterized by raised, deep red lesions that gradually become hyperkeratotic over time. These lesions are caused by somatic activating mutations in the mitogen-activated protein kinase 3 (MAP3K3) gene, a member of the MAP3K family of serine/threonine kinases [32]. Other vascular lesions linked to RAS pathway abnormalities include hyperkeratotic cutaneous capillary venous malformations (VMs). These lesions appear as crimson-colored plaques with a hyperkeratotic dermis and are often associated with cerebral cavernous malformations. They result from inherited loss-of-function mutations in the Krev interaction trapped 1 (KRIT1) gene, which forms a complex with CCM2 and CCM3 proteins to inhibit MAP3K3 activity [33].

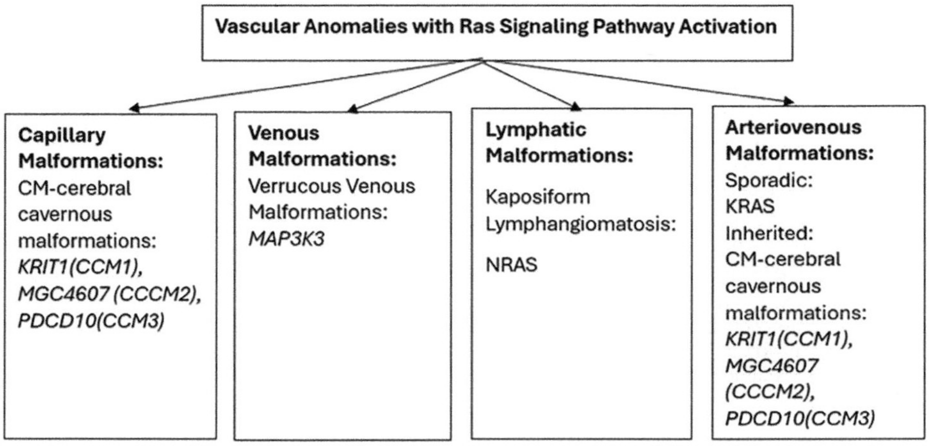

Fig. 1.2 The main vascular anomalies associated with activation of RAS signaling pathway

Ras Pathway in Capillary Malformations and Arteriovenous Malformations Capillary malformation–arteriovenous malformation (CM-AVM) is an autosomal dominant vascular malformation syndrome. Two genetic subtypes have been identified. CM-AVM1 results from mutations in the RASA1 gene, which encodes RAS p21 protein activator 1 (p120Ras-GAP). This protein negatively regulates the RAS/MAPK/ERK signaling pathway, thereby controlling cell growth, differentiation, proliferation, and endothelial cell (EC) network organization [11]. In contrast, CM-AVM2 is caused by loss-of-function mutations in the EPHB4 gene, which also modulates the RAS/MAPK/ERK pathway. Clinically, affected patients often present with small telangiectasias around the lips and upper thorax, as well as intracerebral fast-flow lesions [34]. Moreover, somatic activating mutations in MAP2K1 (encoding MEK1) have been identified in peripheral extracranial arteriovenous malformations (AVMs), leading to increased RAS/MAPK pathway activity [35]. Similarly, somatic mutations in KRAS have been detected in intracranial AVMs, further supporting the role of RAS pathway dysregulation in these lesions [36].

Ras Pathway in Lymphatic Malformations Another type of vascular anomalies associated with RAS pathway abnormalities is Kaposiform lymphangiomatosis (KLA), where a somatic activating in NRAS p.Q61R was identified [37].

GNAQ and GNA11 Mutations

Capillary malformations (CM) either sporadic or in association with Sturge Weber Syndrome (SWS) are caused by somatic variants in *GNAQ* [38, 39] . *GNAQ* variants in CM and SWS involve a single-nucleotide variant at codon 183 (R183Q) in *GNAQ*, which activates the extracellular signal-regulated kinase (ERK) pathway [40]. In congenital hemangiomas, mosaic missense mutations in GNAQ and GNA11 could be detected at position glutamine 209 which differ from those found in CMs [41].

References

1. Goldenberg DC, Vikkula M, Penington A, Blei F, Schultze-Kool L, Wassef M, et al. Updated classification of vascular anomalies: a living document from the International Society for the Study of Vascular Anomalies Classification Group. J Vasc Anom. 2025;6(2):e113.
2. Nguyen HL, Boon LM, Vikkula M. Genetics of vascular anomalies. Semin Pediatr Surg. 2020;29(5):150967.
3. Ji Y, Chen S, Yang K, Xia C, Li L. Kaposiform hemangioendothelioma: current knowledge and future perspectives. Orphanet J Rare Dis. 2020;15(1):39.
4. Vikkula M, Boon LM, Mulliken JB. Molecular genetics of vascular malformations. Matrix Biol. 2001;20(5–6):327–35.
5. Puig S, Casati B, Staudenherz A, Paya K. Vascular low-flow malformations in children: current concepts for classification, diagnosis and therapy. Eur J Radiol. 2005;53(1):35–45.
6. Legiehn GM, Heran MKS. Venous malformations: classification, development, diagnosis, and interventional radiologic management. Radiol Clin North Am. 2008;46(3):545–97, vi.
7. Mäkinen T, Boon LM, Vikkula M, Alitalo K. Lymphatic malformations: genetics, mechanisms and therapeutic strategies. Circ Res. 2021;129(1):136–54.
8. Lorenz S, Maier C, Segerer H, Landthaler M, Hohenleutner U. Skin changes in newborn infants in the first 5 days of life. Hautarzt. 2000;51(6):396–400.
9. Queisser A, Seront E, Boon LM, Vikkula M. Genetic basis and therapies for vascular anomalies. Circ Res. 2021;129(1):155–73.
10. Dekeuleneer V, Seront E, Van Damme A, Boon LM, Vikkula M. Theranostic advances in vascular malformations. J Invest Dermatol. 2020;140(4):756–63.
11. Queisser A, Boon LM, Vikkula M. Etiology and genetics of congenital vascular lesions. Otolaryngol Clin N Am. 2018;51(1):41–53.
12. Karar J, Maity A. PI3K/AKT/mTOR pathway in angiogenesis. Front Mol Neurosci. 2011;4:4.
13. Pang C, Lim CS, Brookes J, Tsui J, Hamilton G. Emerging importance of molecular pathogenesis of vascular malformations in clinical practice and classifications. Vasc Med. 2020;25(4):364–77.

14. Kangas J, Nätynki M, Eklund L. Development of molecular therapies for venous malformations. Basic Clin Pharmacol Toxicol. 2018;123(S5):6–19.
15. Limaye N, Wouters V, Uebelhoer M, Tuominen M, Wirkkala R, Mulliken JB, et al. Somatic mutations in angiopoietin receptor gene TEK cause solitary and multiple sporadic venous malformations. Nat Genet. 2009;41(1):118–24.
16. Soblet J, Limaye N, Uebelhoer M, Boon LM, Vikkula M. Variable somatic TIE2 mutations in half of sporadic venous malformations. Mol Syndromol. 2013;4(4):179–83.
17. Soblet J, Kangas J, Nätynki M, Mendola A, Helaers R, Uebelhoer M, et al. Blue rubber bleb nevus (BRBN) syndrome is caused by somatic TEK (TIE2) mutations. J Invest Dermatol. 2017;137(1):207–16.
18. Limaye N, Kangas J, Mendola A, Godfraind C, Schlögel MJ, Helaers R, et al. Somatic activating PIK3CA mutations cause venous malformation. Am J Hum Genet. 2015;97(6):914–21.
19. Castillo SD, Baselga E, Graupera M. PIK3CA mutations in vascular malformations. Curr Opin Hematol. 2019;26(3):170–8.
20. Kurek KC, Luks VL, Ayturk UM, Alomari AI, Fishman SJ, Spencer SA, et al. Somatic mosaic activating mutations in PIK3CA cause CLOVES syndrome. Am J Hum Genet. 2012;90(6):1108–15.
21. Liaw D, Marsh DJ, Li J, Dahia PLM, Wang SI, Zheng Z, et al. Germline mutations of the PTEN gene in Cowden disease, an inherited breast and thyroid cancer syndrome. Nat Genet. 1997;16(1):64–7.
22. Chung MG. Hereditary hemorrhagic telangiectasia. Handb Clin Neurol. 2015;132:185-97. https://doi.org/10.1016/B978-0-444-62702-5.00013-5. PMID: 26564080.
23. McAllister KA, Grogg KM, Johnson DW, Gallione CJ, Baldwin MA, Jackson CE, et al. Endoglin, a TGF-β binding protein of endothelial cells, is the gene for hereditary haemorrhagic telangiectasia type 1. Nat Genet. 1994;8(4):345–51.
24. Johnson DW, Berg JN, Baldwin MA, Gallione CJ, Marondel I, Yoon SJ, et al. Mutations in the activin receptor–like kinase 1 gene in hereditary haemorrhagic telangiectasia type 2. Nat Genet. 1996;13(2):189–95.
25. Gallione CJ, Repetto GM, Legius E, Rustgi AK, Schelley SL, Tejpar S, et al. A combined syndrome of juvenile polyposis and hereditary haemorrhagic telangiectasia associated with mutations in MADH4 (SMAD4). Lancet. 2004;363(9412):852–9.
26. Tillet E, Bailly S. Emerging roles of BMP9 and BMP10 in hereditary hemorrhagic telangiectasia. Front Genet. 2015;5
27. Ola R, Dubrac A, Han J, Zhang F, Fang JS, Larrivée B, et al. PI3 kinase inhibition improves vascular malformations in mouse models of hereditary haemorrhagic telangiectasia. Nat Commun. 2016;7(1):13650.
28. Brouillard P, Boon LM, Revencu N, Berg J, Dompmartin A, Dubois J, et al. Genotypes and phenotypes of 162 families with a glomulin mutation. Mol Syndromol. 2013;4(4):157–64.
29. Grisendi S, Chambraud B, Gout I, Comoglio PM, Crepaldi T. Ligand-regulated binding of FAP68 to the hepatocyte growth factor receptor. J Biol Chem. 2001;276(49):46632–8.
30. Uebelhoer M, Boon LM, Vikkula M. Vascular anomalies: from genetics toward models for therapeutic trials. Cold Spring Harb Perspect Med. 2012;2(8)
31. CC MC. Update on classification and diagnosis of vascular malformations. Curr Opin Pediatr. 2017;29(4):448–54.
32. Colmenero I, Knöpfel N. Venous malformations in childhood: clinical, histopathological and genetics update. Dermatopathology (Basel). 2021;8(4):477–93.
33. Eerola I. KRIT1 is mutated in hyperkeratotic cutaneous capillary-venous malformation associated with cerebral capillary malformation. Hum Mol Genet. 2000;9(9):1351–5.
34. Amyere M, Revencu N, Helaers R, Pairet E, Baselga E, Cordisco M, et al. Germline loss-of-function mutations in EPHB4 cause a second form of capillary malformation-arteriovenous malformation (CM-AVM2) deregulating RAS-MAPK Signaling. Circulation. 2017;136(11):1037–48.
35. Couto JA, Huang AY, Konczyk DJ, Goss JA, Fishman SJ, Mulliken JB, et al. Somatic MAP2K1 mutations are associated with extracranial arteriovenous malformation. Am J Hum Genet. 2017;100(3):546–54.
36. Nikolaev SI, Vetiska S, Bonilla X, Boudreau E, Jauhiainen S, Rezai Jahromi B, et al. Somatic activating *KRAS* mutations in arteriovenous malformations of the brain. N Engl J Med. 2018;378(3):250–61.
37. Nozawa A, Abe T, Niihori T, Ozeki M, Aoki Y, Ohnishi H. Lymphatic endothelial cell-specific NRAS p.Q61R mutant embryos show abnormal lymphatic vessel morphogenesis. Hum Mol Genet. 2024;33(16):1420–8.
38. Couto JA, Huang L, Vivero MP, Kamitaki N, Maclellan RA, Mulliken JB, et al. Endothelial cells from capillary malformations are enriched for somatic GNAQ mutations. Plast Reconstr Surg. 2016;137(1):77e–82e.
39. Lian CG, Sholl LM, Zakka LR, TM O, Liu C, Xu S, et al. Novel genetic mutations in a sporadic port-wine stain. JAMA Dermatol. 2014;150(12):1336–40.
40. Wellman RJ, Cho SB, Singh P, Tune M, Pardo CA, Comi AM, et al. Gαq and hyper-phosphorylated ERK expression in Sturge-weber syndrome leptomeningeal blood vessel endothelial cells. Vasc Med. 2019;24(1):72–5.
41. Ayturk UM, Couto JA, Hann S, Mulliken JB, Williams KL, Huang AY, et al. Somatic activating mutations in GNAQ and GNA11 are associated with congenital hemangioma. Am J Hum Genet. 2016;98(6):1271.

Imaging of Vascular Anomalies

2

Introduction

Vascular anomalies comprise a diverse set of disorders with variable degrees of complexity necessitating coordinated care through a multidisciplinary team. Radiologists play an essential role in this collaborative effort, significantly influencing both diagnosis and treatment planning. The careful selection of the appropriate imaging techniques is fundamental for precise diagnosis and guiding appropriate therapeutic strategies [1]. Additionally, engaging directly with patients in a vascular anomalies clinic or during ultrasound imaging allows radiologists to move beyond the images and connect on a personal level, putting a compassionate face to the profession and reinforcing their vital role in the patient's journey [2, 3]. In our experience, parents and guardians often show a sincere desire to understand their loved one's condition and view their imaging studies. This engagement not only fosters trust but also empowers them to participate more confidently in informed decision-making.

Clinical Toolkit

A brief clinical history taken by the radiologist can serve as a valuable diagnostic tool. Key questions include: When was the lesion first noticed by the patient, parent, or guardian? Was it present at birth? Has the lesion been growing? If so, is the growth proportional to the patient's overall growth or is it disproportionate? Are there any siblings or family members with similar findings? These questions can provide crucial insight into the nature and progression of the vascular anomaly (Fig. 2.1) [3].

Supplementary Information The online version contains supplementary material available at https://doi.org/10.1007/978-3-032-30866-5_2.

A. A. AbouZeid et al., *Atlas of Pediatric Vascular Anomalies*, https://doi.org/10.1007/978-3-032-30866-5_2

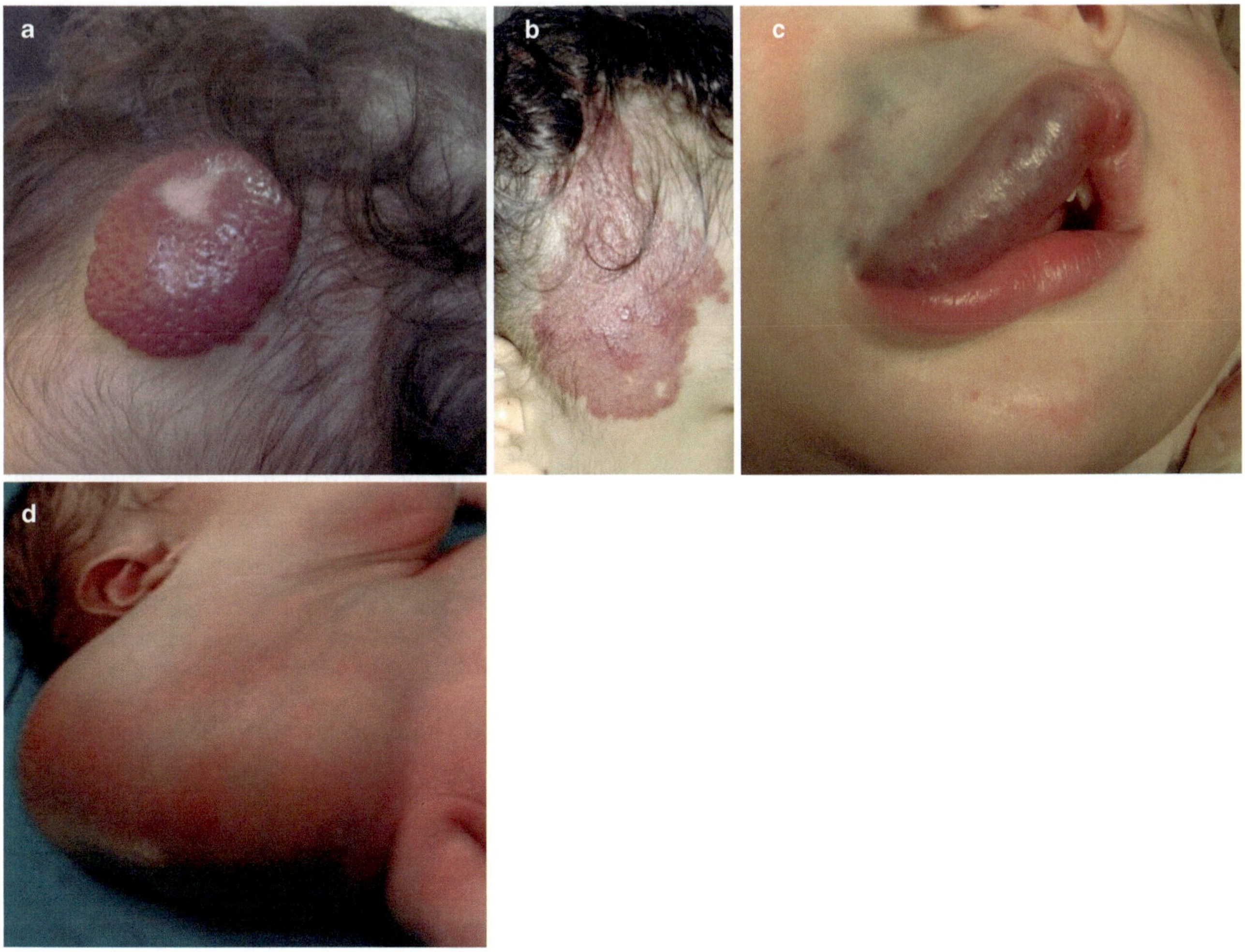

Fig. 2.1 Clinical photographs of vascular anomalies (**a**) Infantile hemangioma in an infant, presenting as a reddish swelling with rapid early growth. (**b**) Capillary malformation (port-wine stain) overlying an arteriovenous malformation, present since birth and associated with a palpable thrill. (**c**) Venous malformation, manifesting as bluish discoloration with swelling, present since birth. (**d**) Lymphatic malformation in a neonate, appearing as a large cystic swelling

Indication of Imaging and Selection of the Imaging Modality

Most of vascular anomalies are diagnosed on clinical basis. Nevertheless, ultrasound and MRI are the mainstay imaging modalities for detailed evaluation of these cases. American College of Radiology (ACR) developed appropriateness criteria for imaging soft tissue vascular malformation and infantile vascular anomalies focused on five main clinical variants [4]:

Variant 1 *Infant. Clinical signs or symptoms of infantile hemangioma. Initial imaging*

Although most infantile hemangioma are diagnosed on clinical bases, imaging may be required for superficial lesions with atypical features or for deep lesions that are difficult to be assessed clinically. Ultrasound and duplex Doppler are the main stay in the initial evaluation of infants with clinical signs or symptoms of infantile hemangioma. Further imaging is also required when the hemangioma has segmental distribution in the face or in the midline in the lumbosacral region. Hemangioma in these locations may be part of PHACE syndrome (posterior fossa malformations, hemangioma, arterial anomalies, coarctation of the aorta/cardiac defects, and eye abnormalities) and LUMBAR syndromes (Lower body hemangioma, Urogenital anomalies/ulceration, Myelopathy, Bony deformities, Anorectal malformations/arterial anomalies, and Renal anomalies) respectively. Hemangioma of the orbit, ears and breast may require further imaging [5]. Hemangioma of the beard distribution requires imaging to investigate the possibility of air way involvement. MRI without and with contrast enhancement and MR angiography may be appropriate in the evaluation of these lesions. MRI is essential to diagnose cord tethering and other spinal anomalies. CT with IV contrast may be appropriate when evaluation of the airway is indicated as hemangioma of the beard distribution [6].

***Variant** 2 Infant. Multiple cutaneous infantile hemangiomas, screening for infantile hepatic hemangiomas. Initial imaging*

Multiple cutaneous hemangioma (equal or more than 5) may indicate the presence of visceral or liver hemangioma, necessitating abdominal ultrasound and duplex Doppler. If the diagnosis is not confident by ultrasound, non-contrast MRI of the abdomen and dynamic contrast-enhanced MRI may be required for further characterization [7].

***Variant** 3 Child. Clinical signs or symptoms of vascular anomaly (tumor or malformation) not suggesting infantile hemangioma. Initial imaging*

Ultrasound and duplex Doppler are usually appropriate as the initial imaging modality in the initial evaluation of clinically suspected vascular anomaly. Ultrasound and duplex can differentiate vascular tumor with its soft tissue component and increased vascularity from other high flow lesions as arteriovenous malformation or arteriovenous fistula. Additionally, ultrasound can characterize venous and lymphatic malformation [8]. Noncontrast MRI can serve as a primary imaging technique alongside ultrasound. If the lesion has already been characterized clinically or via ultrasound, non-contrast imaging may be sufficient when the sole aim is to assess its deep extension. Additionally, non-contrast MR angiography is useful for initial mapping of the vascular anatomy, while dynamic contrast-enhanced angiography is employed to evaluate the lesion's flow dynamics and further define its characteristics [9].

***Variant** 4 Child. Ultrasound features raise suspicion for vascular malformation. Next imaging study*

In pediatric patients with ultrasound findings suggestive of a vascular malformation, MRI with and without contrast, along with dynamic MR angiography, is usually appropriate for lesion characterization, assessment of flow dynamics, and evaluation of deep tissue extension. Contrast-enhanced CT as well as CT angiography and venography may be appropriate, particularly for identifying bone involvement, such as erosion or abnormalities to overgrowth syndromes. CT is effective in detecting phleboliths, and CT angiography offers superior spatial resolution compared to MRI and ultrasound for detailed mapping of vascular structures, especially in the upper extremities and in cases of pulmonary arteriovenous malformations [10, 11].

***Variant** 5 Child. Established diagnosis of vascular malformation presenting with new or persistent signs or symptoms. Initial imaging*

During the management of vascular malformations in children, multiple sessions of sclerotherapy or embolization may be necessary. As a result, new or persistent symptoms can arise, warranting follow-up imaging to monitor the lesion and guide ongoing treatment. In this instance, ultrasound and duplex are usually appropriate for initial evaluation. Ultrasound may detect intervention-related soft tissue swelling or post-embolization occlusion. However, the presence of extensive embolization material may limit the performance of ultrasound. MRI and MR angiography and venography before and after contrast administration are usually appropriate as well [12, 13]. MRI can demonstrate post-therapy changes as well as therapy related complication as cellulitis, abscess, or vascular thrombosis. Also, MRI can reveal the site of new nidus in patients with arteriovenous malformation. Ultrasound with intravenous contrast can serve as a valuable addition to conventional ultrasound and duplex imaging by generating time-intensity curves that help evaluate blood flow dynamics before and after an intervention [14].

Technique of Different Imaging Modalities

Ultrasound

Following the initial clinical evaluation, ultrasound serves as the first-line imaging modality for assessing vascular anomalies due to its rapid, non-invasive nature. A key advantage of ultrasound is that it can be performed without requiring sedation. Ideally, the infant should be comfortably positioned on the mother's/guardian's lap during the examination. For anxious infants, imaging may be performed while the baby is asleep following feeding or during nursing to ensure cooperation and minimize distress.

Transducer Selection

Ultrasound is a valuable tool for assessing lesion morphology and detecting abnormal vascularity. Superficial lesions require the use of a high-frequency linear transducer (9–11 MHz) and a sufficient amount of coupling gel to achieve optimal acoustic transmission, particularly for small, superficial structures (Figs. 2.2 and 2.3). Waterbath or standoff technique may be helpful for superficial lesions as well. Standoff technique involves placing a gel pad or a water-filled glove between the transducer and the patient's skin, thereby increasing the distance between the probe and the surface being examined. In contrast, deeper lesions—such as those located within the abdomen or

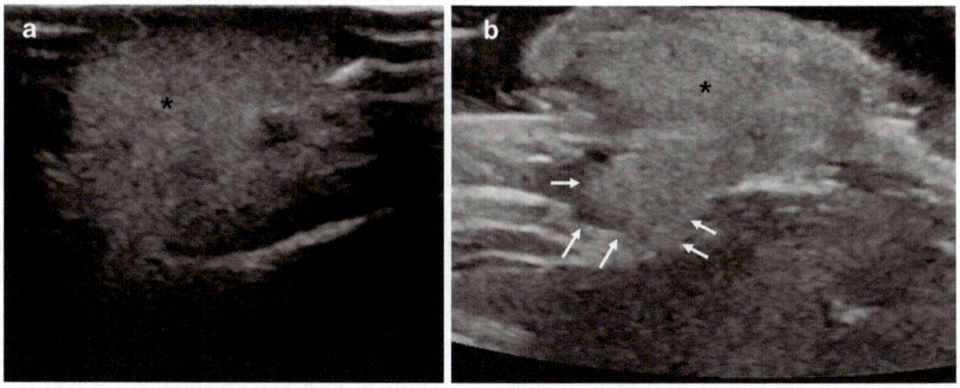

Fig. 2.2 Ultrasound of a 26-month-old boy with cutaneous infantile hemangioma (asterisk) using a superficial high-frequency probe without (**a**) and with (**b**) adequate coupling gel. Adequate gel improves visualization of lesion margins and deep extensions. The lesion appears as well-defined hyperechoic mass (asterisk) involves the skin and extends to the subcutaneous tissue (arrows)

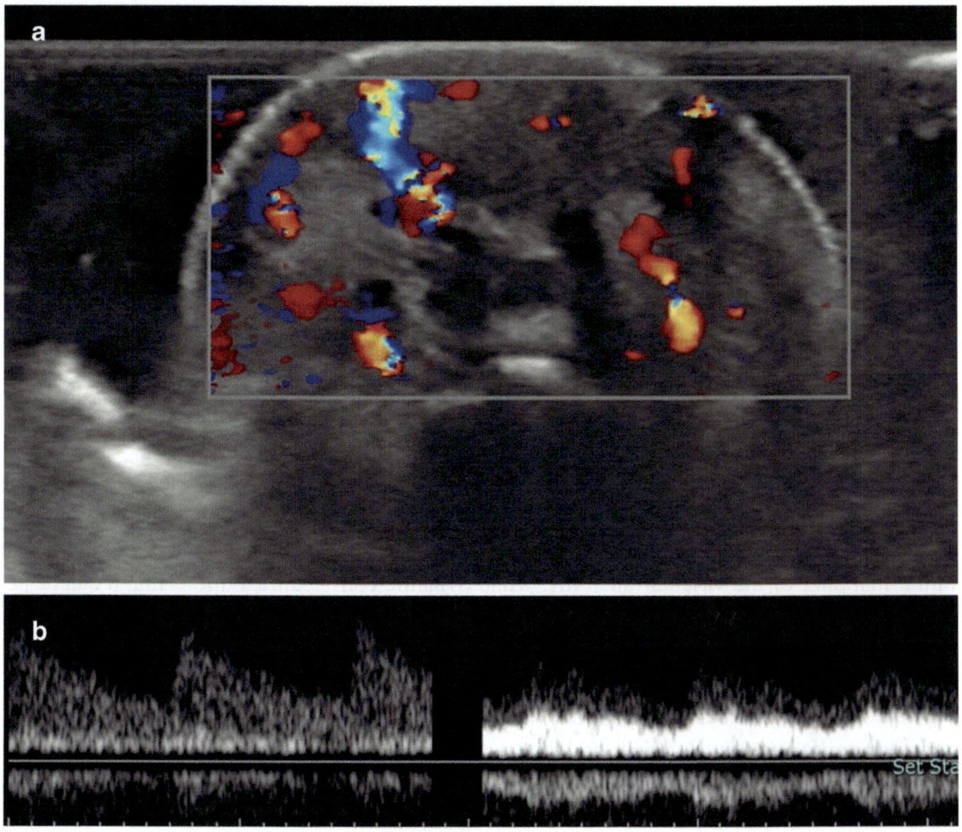

Fig. 2.3 Arteriovenous malformation of the ring finger. (**a**) Color Doppler ultrasound performed with ample gel and minimal compression, demonstrating skin and subcutaneous thickening with increased vascularity. (**b**) Spectral Doppler showing a low-resistance arterial waveform together with a pulsatile venous waveform denoting arteriovenous shunting

liver—are typically evaluated using a low-frequency sector transducer (5–7 MHz). However, in neonates and young infants, a linear probe may still provide high-resolution imaging of deep lesions due to their smaller body size (Fig. 2.4) [3].

Imaging Technique

Imaging begins with gray-scale ultrasound evaluation, acquiring images in both transverse and longitudinal planes. Initial scans are performed without annotations to preserve image clarity, followed by annotated images for documentation. Key lesion characteristics—such as location (cutaneous, subcutaneous, or involving deeper structures), echogenicity, and the presence of cysts, calcification, necrosis, or hemorrhage—can be clearly assessed (Fig. 2.5). For well-defined localized lesions, dimensions including length, width, and thickness are measured and archived. Ultrasound has the capability of doing dynamic maneuvers. Applying compression, tourniquet for lesions in the extremities, Trendelenburg position for lesions in the head and neck are helpful maneuvers in lesion differentiation (Fig. 2.6, Supplementary Video 2.1).

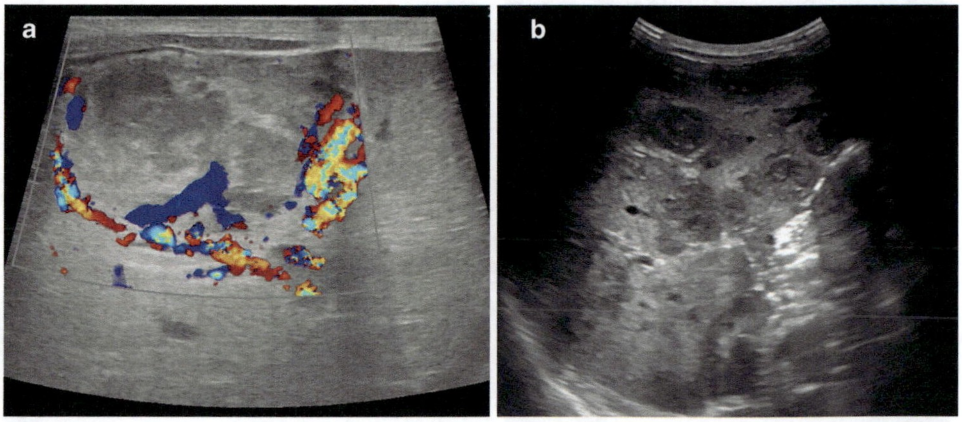

Fig. 2.4 Use of ultrasound probes in hepatic hemangiomas. (**a**) High-frequency superficial probe in a 7-day-old neonate with congenital hepatic hemangioma, demonstrating the lesion with peripheral vascularity. (**b**) Deep probe in a 20-month-old boy with multifocal hepatic hemangioma appear as multiple hypoechoic focal lesions

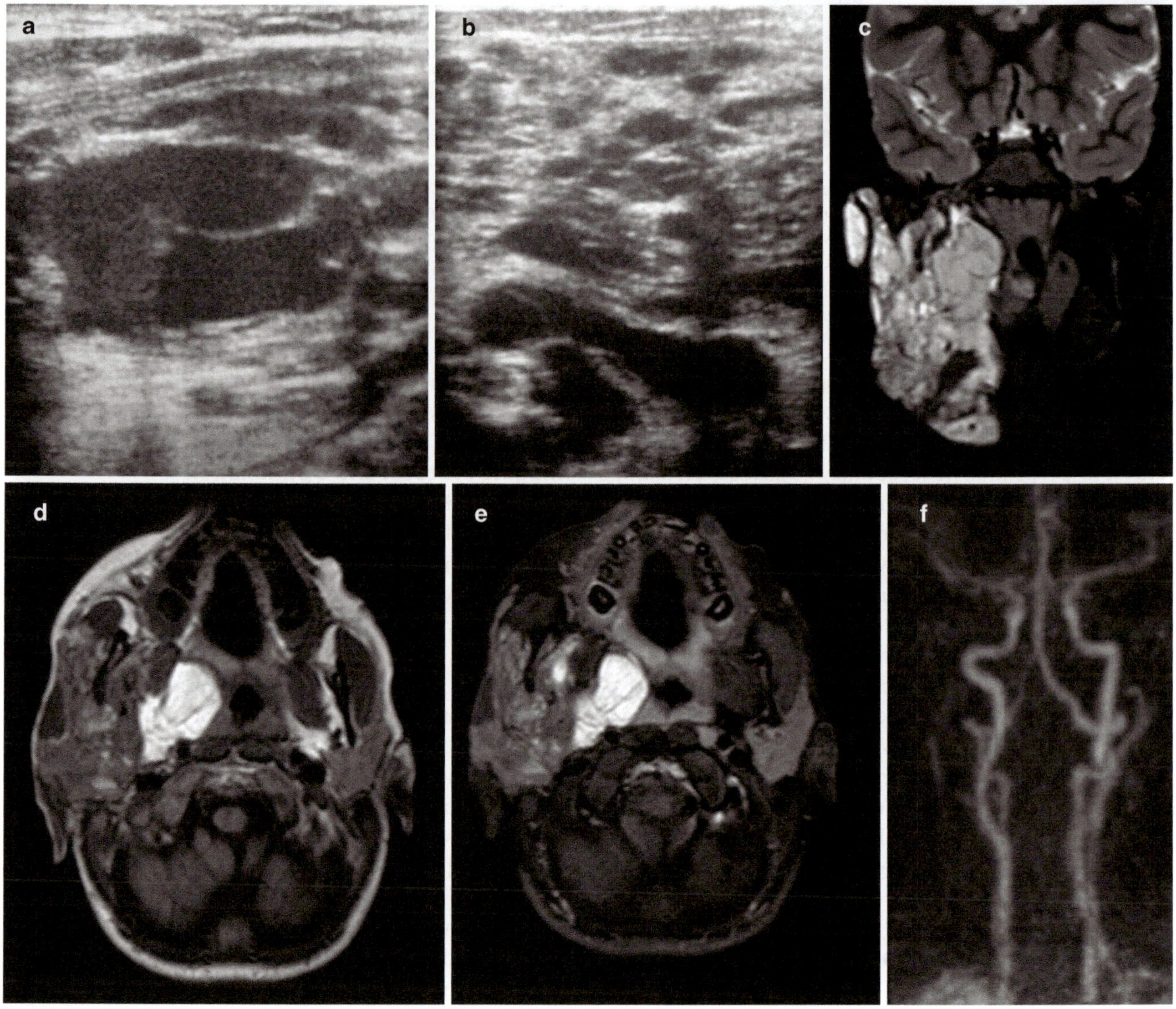

Fig. 2.5 Mixed macrocystic and microcystic lymphatic malformation in an 8-year-old boy. (**a** and **b**) Ultrasound shows multiple variable-sized anechoic cystic spaces with smooth walls and thin septa. (**c**) Coronal MRI (STIR) demonstrates bright signal cystic spaces with trans-spatial extension. (**d**) Axial T1-weighted image shows predominantly hypointense signal, with some cysts hyperintense due to high-protein/hemorrhagic content; lesion extends into the parapharyngeal spaces. (**e**) Fat-suppressed contrast-enhanced axial T1-weighted image shows no significant enhancement; apparent brightness relative to non–fat-suppressed T1 may mimic enhancement. This is clarified on precontrast fat-suppressed T1 (not shown). (**f**) Coronal maximum intensity projection of arterial phase dynamic contrast-enhanced T1 shows no abnormal arterial enhancement, confirming the low-flow nature of the lesion

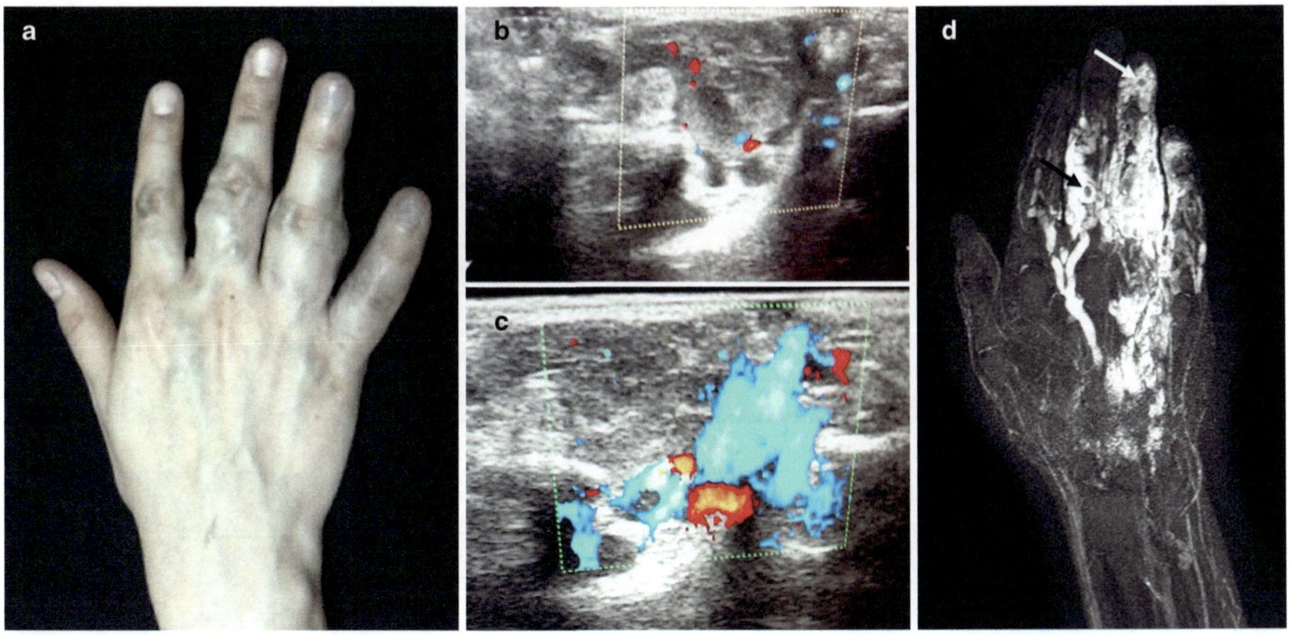

Fig. 2.6 Venous malformation in a 20-year-old woman. (**a**) Clinical photograph shows congested veins with bluish discoloration. (**b** and **c**) Color Doppler ultrasound without (**b**) and with augmentation (**c**) showing hypoechoic venous spaces with hyperechoic areas that denotes very slow venous flow with reduced color density, augmentation (**c**) increases color flow. (**d**) Coronal maximum intensity projection of STIR image depicts the full trans-spatial extent of the malformation with bright signal, dilated veins and phleboliths (arrows)

Color Doppler can determine the vascularity of the lesion and pulsed Doppler permits quantification of the arterial and venous flow velocities. Color Doppler examination starts with low flow color Doppler setting with low pulse repetition frequency to increase sensitivity for detection of weak vascularity. Pulse repetition frequency may be increased if aliasing occurs. Power Doppler imaging is a valuable adjunct due to its enhanced sensitivity to blood flow, particularly in low-flow states. In some cases, low flow can also be appreciated as moving internal echoes on real-time grayscale ultrasound (Supplementary Video 2.2). The degree of vascularity can be assessed by counting the number of color Doppler pixels (visible vessels) per square centimeter within a region of interest that corresponds to the area of greatest intralesional vascularity (Supplementary Videos 2.2 and 2.3). Doppler gate is then placed for pulsed Doppler analysis. Doppler ultrasound is essential for differentiating between high-flow and low-flow vascular anomalies, a crucial aspect of sonographic interpretation [15] (Figs. 2.7, 2.8, and 2.9).

Magnetic Resonance Imaging

Magnetic resonance imaging is known for its high soft tissue resolution capabilities, lacking ionizing radiation making it an ideal imaging modality for imaging children with vascular anomalies. However, due to relatively prolonged scan time compared to CT, sedation may be required, especially in young children and infants. MRI can differentiate between high-flow and low-flow lesions. It determines extensions through tissue planes and the relations to surrounding anatomical structures. Dynamic contrast-enhanced MRI and MR angiography can demonstrate flow dynamics [16].

Imaging Protocol and Optimization

Optimizing the imaging protocol and selecting the appropriate coil should begin with reviewing clinical photographs or directly examining the patient to assess the extent of the lesion. Physical examination also reinforces the radiologist's role as a key consultant in the patient's management plan. The smallest coil that adequately covers the lesion should be selected. Given the complexity and variability of vascular anomalies, unexpected findings may arise during scanning the patients, who are commonly young, sedated children, making repeated scans and sedation undesirable. Therefore, real-time image evaluation during scanning is crucial to adapt the protocol as needed, especially in infants under sedation [17].

Body phased-array surface coil is used for imaging the chest, abdomen, and pelvis, while other dedicated coils can be used for the imaging extremities and the head and neck regions. Imaging sequences should be prioritized based on their significance in diagnosing and characterizing lesions to ensure that the most important sequences are obtained early in the examination. This is especially important because some patients may not tolerate prolonged scan durations, potentially leading to premature termination of the study [16, 17].

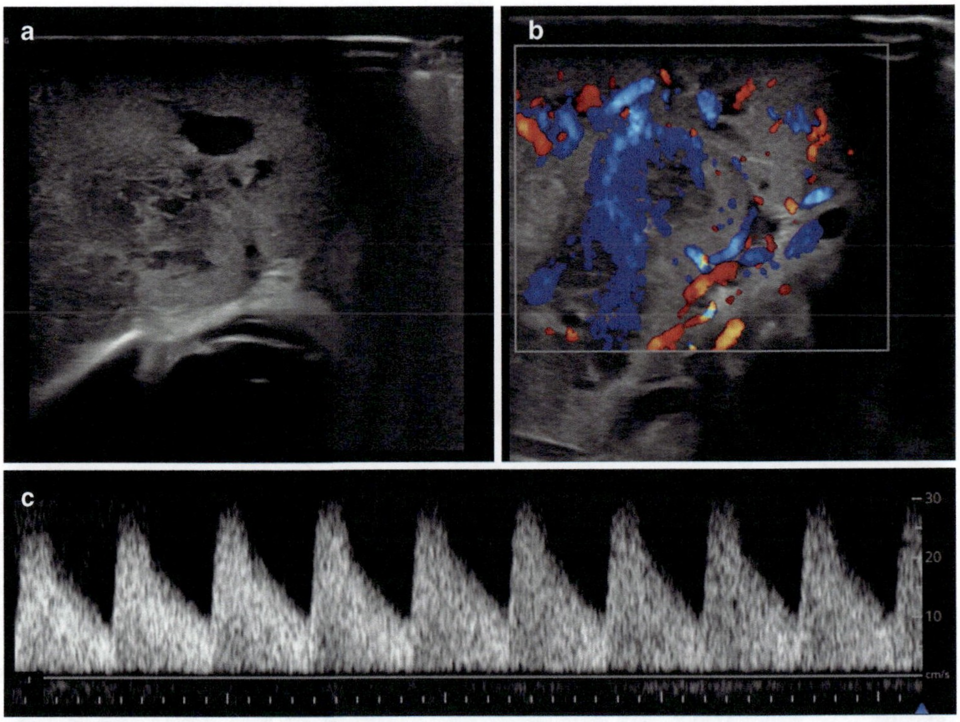

Fig. 2.7 Rapidly involuting congenital hemangioma (RICH) in a 17-day-old boy. (**a** and **b**) Ultrasound reveals soft tissue mass with mixed echogenicity and prominent vascular spaces (this finding is more commonly described in congenital hemangioma and rarely seen in infantile hemangioma). (**b**) Color Doppler reveals increased vascular density in the lesion (**c**) Spectral Doppler reveals low resistance arterial flow within the lesion. The diagnosis of RICH is determined on the basis of lesion involution during follow up visits

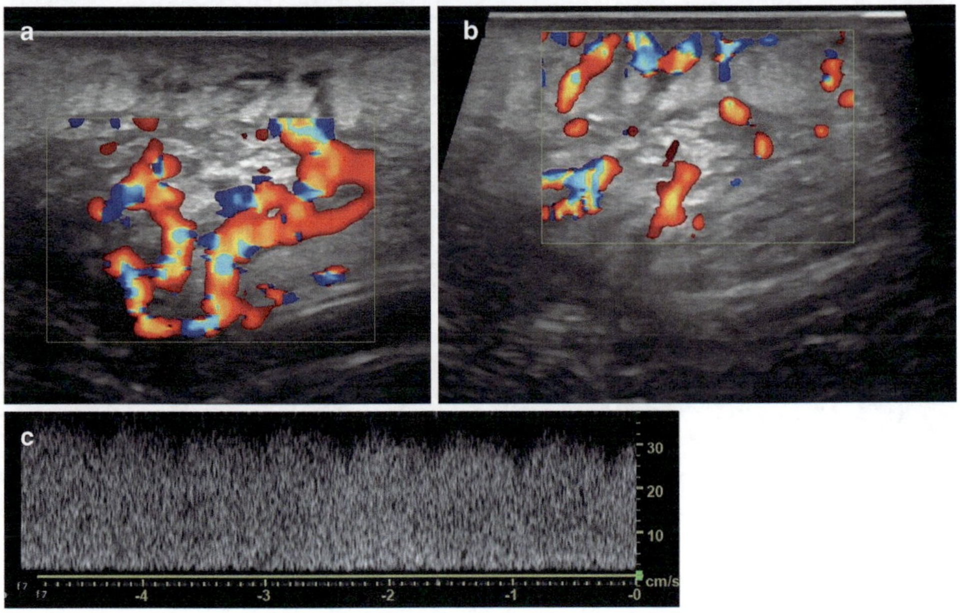

Fig. 2.8 Arteriovenous malformation in the back in a 7-year-old boy. (**a** and **b**) Color Doppler shows diffuse soft tissue thickening with multiple vascular channels. (**c**) Spectral Doppler shows high velocity arterial blood flow with low resistance pattern, denoting arteriovenous shunting

Among these sequences, T2-weighted imaging (T2-WI) plays a crucial role within the imaging protocol. It effectively identifies soft tissue components, vascular flow voids, phleboliths, and fluid levels, all of which are essential for accurately characterizing vascular anomalies. Therefore, T2-WI should be the initial step in any imaging protocol for vascular anomalies. Since the majority of vascular anomalies exhibit high signal intensity on T2-weighted sequences, incorporating fat suppression enhances lesion detectability and improves assessment of their extent. The imaging study should begin with longitudinal scans—either in the coronal or sagittal planes. Coronal scans are preferred for lesions with mediolateral extension (Figs. 2.10, 2.11, 2.12, 2.13, and 2.14), while sagittal scans are suitable for those with antero-posterior extension. These longitudinal images are essential for delineating the full extent of the lesion, which aids in planning subsequent sequences and helps identify deeper components that may not be clinically apparent. When the lymphatic malformation is diagnosed based on T2-WI, dynamic contrast-enhanced sequences may not be required (Fig. 2.14) [1, 16].

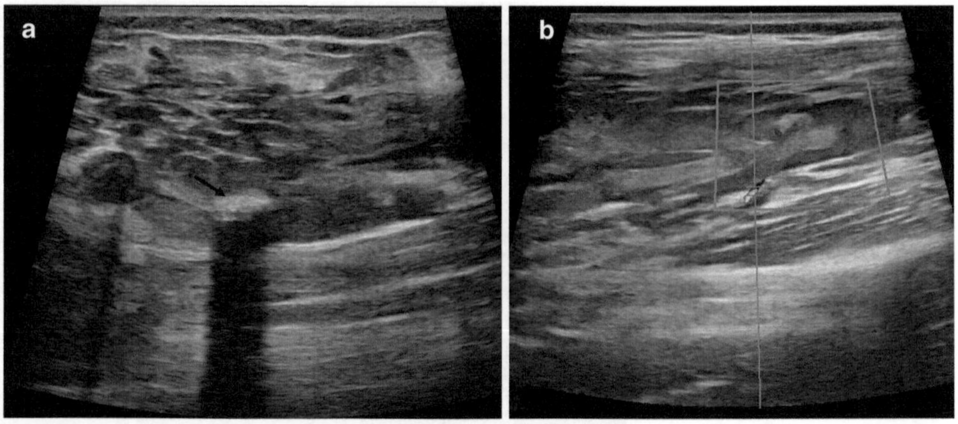

Fig. 2.9 Intramuscular venous malformation in a 12-year-old girl. (**a**) Longitudinal ultrasound shows hypoechoic venous spaces separated by hyperechoic septa. Hyperechoic areas indicate slow flow. Note the associated calcific focus (arrow) with posterior acoustic shadow indicating phlebolith. (**b**) Color Doppler ultrasound reveals no significant vascularity in the lesion

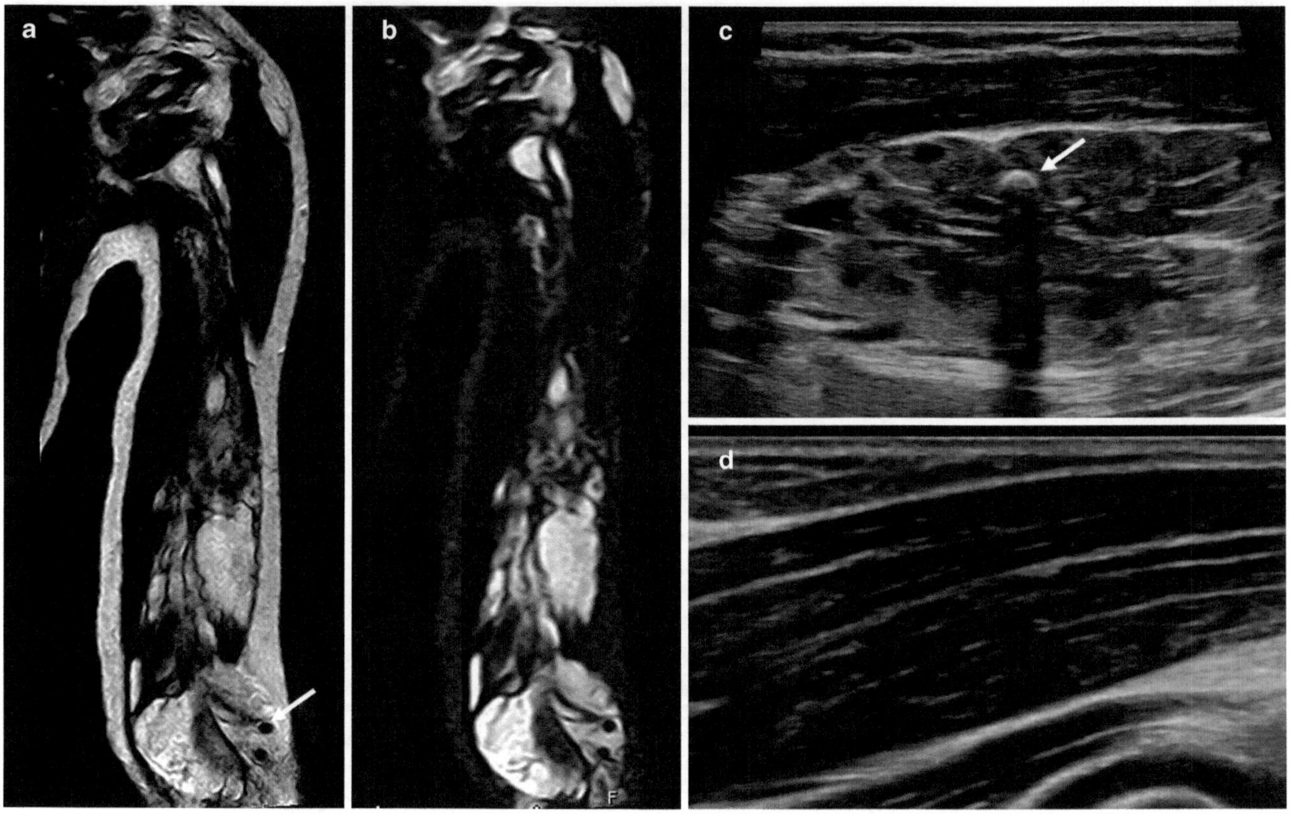

Fig. 2.10 Left upper limb venous malformation in 1 2-year-old girl. (**a**) Coronal T2-WI, (**b**) Coronal STIR demonstrate the full extension of the lesion with its trans-spatial nature. The lesion exhibits bright signal with low signal phleboliths (arrow). (**c**) Longitudinal ultrasound shows the lesion as mixed hypoechoic and hyperechoic vascular spaces with internal septa and phlebolith (arrow) that appears as echogenic focus with posterior acoustic shadow. (**d**) Longitudinal ultrasound of the normal muscle for comparison reveals normal arrangement of the muscle fibers

Fat suppression can be performed by three different techniques: Short tau inversion recovery (STIR) has the advantage of being insensitive to magnetic field inhomogeneities, rendering it suitable for lesions in anatomical areas having multiple tissue interfaces, large lesions requiring large field of view, and lesions with off-center imaging (those beside the body in the arm, elbow, and hand) (Figs. 2.10 and 2.15). STIR sequence has longer scan times with lower resolution. On the other hand, chemical shift fat suppression has better imaging resolution, but it is sensitive to magnetic field inhomogeneity. DIXON is a relatively newly adopted technique of chemical shift imaging that has better resolution and a higher signal-to-noise ratio, although it requires longer scan times. Hybrid method of fat suppression incorporates inversion recovery and chemical shift imaging. It has higher imaging resolution than STIR with less sensitivity to magnetic field inhomogeneity, but with longer scan time [18].

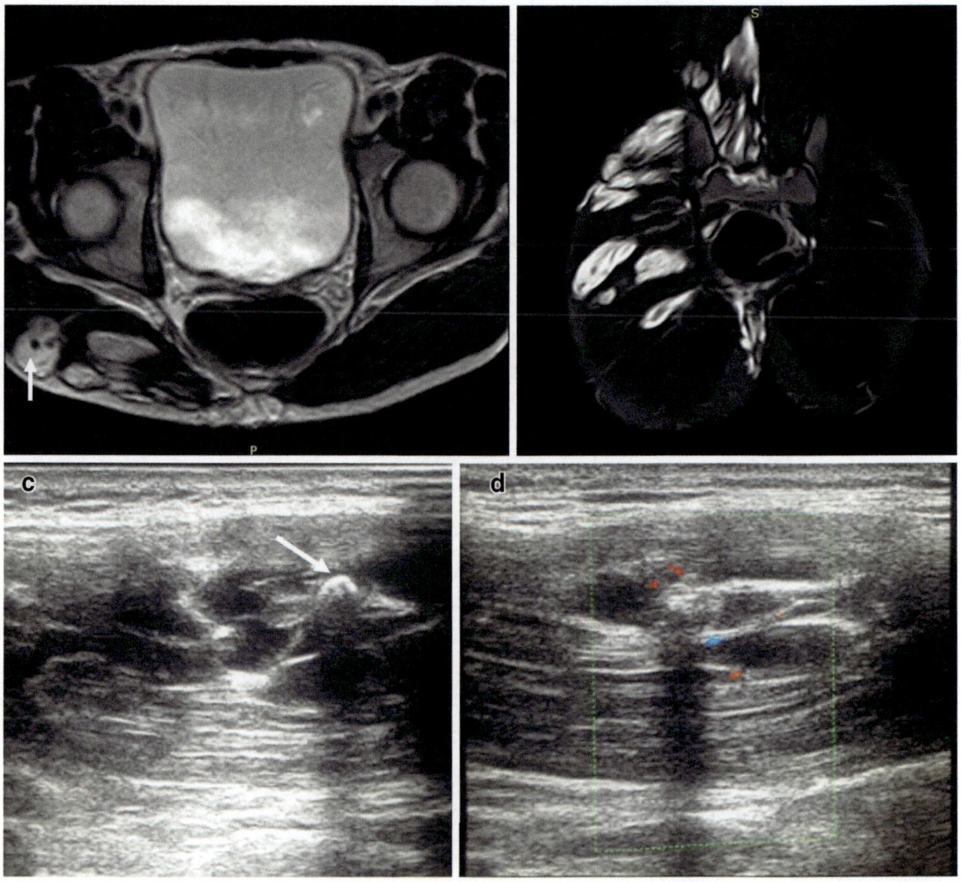

Fig. 2.11 Venous malformation in the gluteal region. (**a**) Axial T2-weighted image shows an intramuscular lesion with bright signal and a hypointense phlebolith (arrow). (**b**) Coronal STIR image demonstrates the lesion's extent. (**c**) B-mode ultrasound reveals intramuscular hypoechoic venous spaces with echogenic phlebolith (arrow). (**d**) Color Doppler shows decreased color density, characteristic of a low-flow lesion

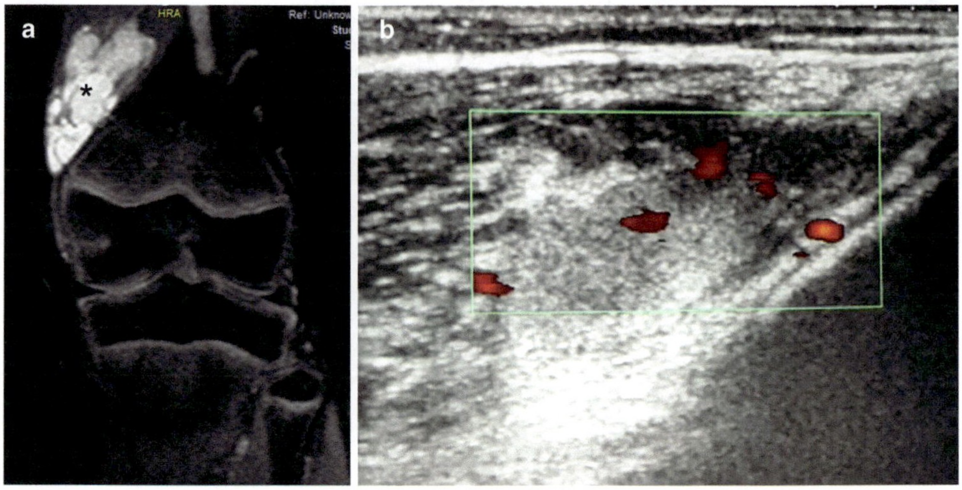

Fig. 2.12 Venous malformation adjacent to the knee joint without intra-articular extension. (**a**) Coronal STIR shows venous malformation (asterisk) at the medial aspect of the thigh exhibiting characteristic bright signal. (**b**) Color Doppler shows decreased color density within the venous spaces

T1-weighted imaging is important to define the fat planes surrounding the lesions (Fig. 2.16). Non-contrast T1 fat suppression may be acquired as well to precisely detect enhancement in contrast enhanced sequences. This is crucial to differentiate venous malformation which typical shows patchy enhancement from lymphatic malformation which shows little if any enhancement (Fig. 2.17) [16].

Non-contrast MR angiography can be performed as an initial anatomical survey prior to contrast-enhanced studies. It aids in defining the field of view and optimizing the timing of contrast administration for dynamic sequences. Three-dimensional Time-of-Flight (3D-TOF) is the preferred non-contrast MR angiography technique for evaluating cerebral vessels, whereas two-dimensional Time-of-Flight (2D-TOF) is more suitable for imaging the extremities (Fig. 2.18) [9].

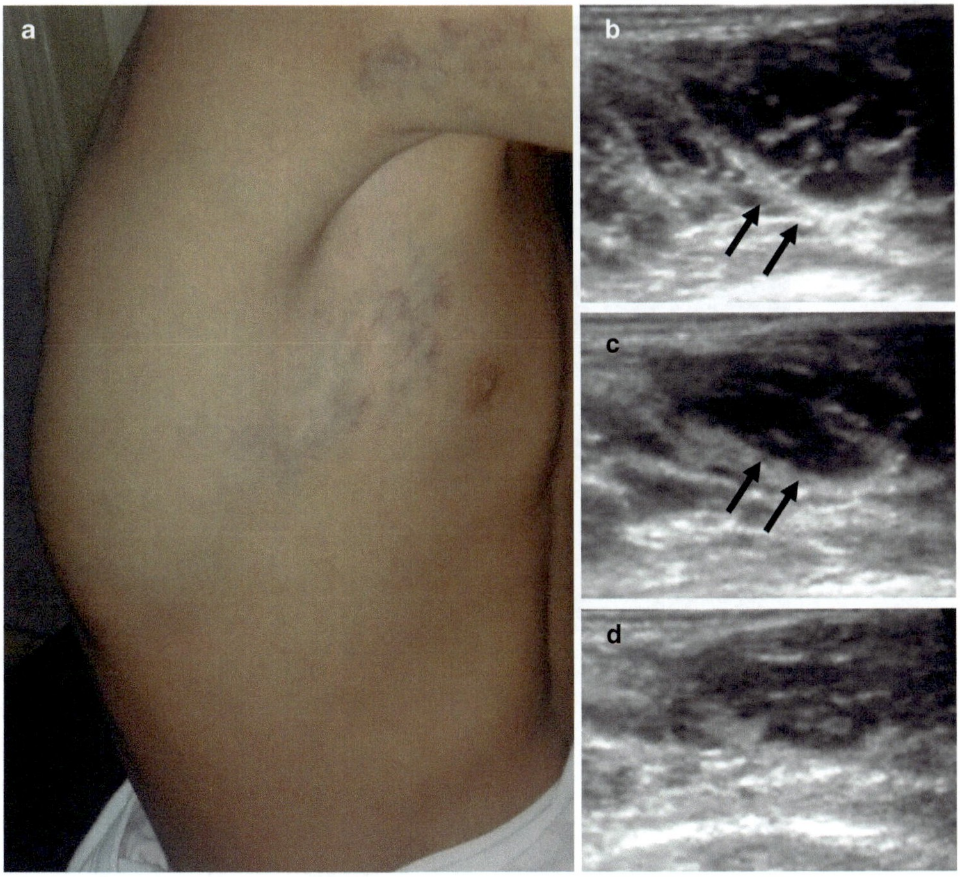

Fig. 2.13 Venous malformation in 10-year-old child. (**a**) Clinical photogram shows a swelling with bluish discoloration in the arm and posterolateral aspect of the chest wall. (**b–d**) B-mode ultrasound without compression (**b**) with progressive compression (**b** and **c**) demonstrates compressible nature of the lesion (arrows). (**e** anb **f**) Coronal STIR (**e**) and axial T2 (**f**) depicts the lesion extension. It shows bright signal intensity associated with low signal intensity phleboliths (arrow). (**g** and **h**) Coronal (**g**), axial (**h**) fat-suppressed contrast-enhanced T1-WI show patchy enhancement

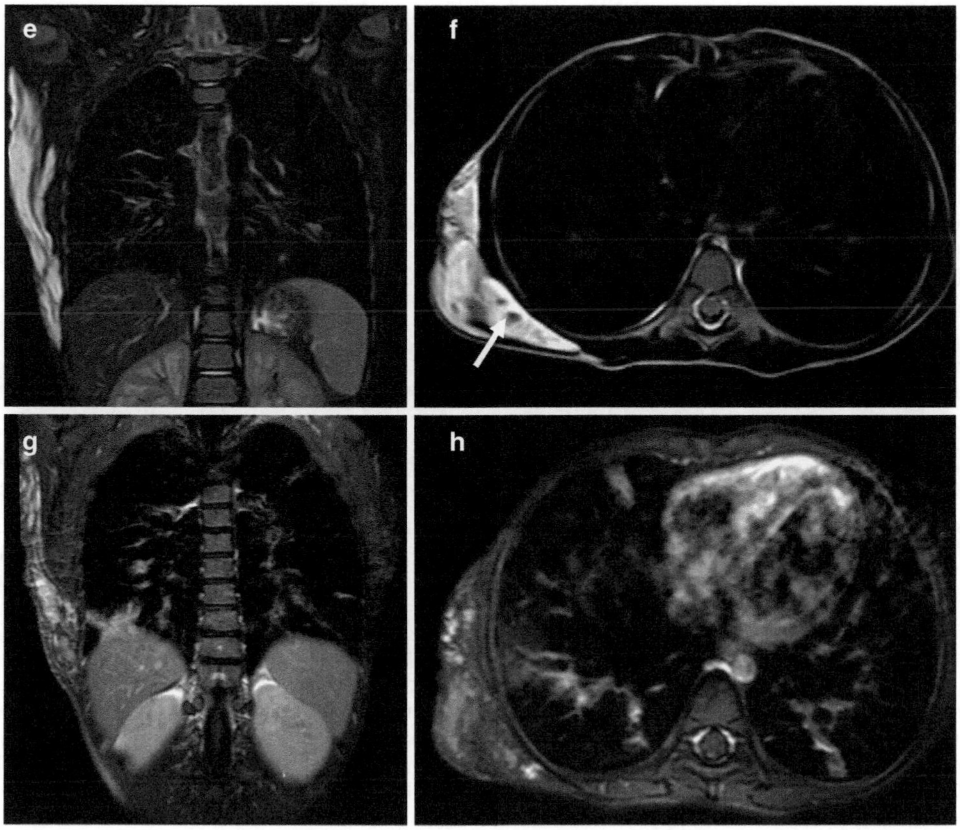

Fig. 2.13 (continued)

Fig. 2.14 Macrocystic lymphatic malformation in a 7-day-old girl. (**a** and **b**) Coronal and axial STIR shows multilocular cystic lesion displaying bright signal with internal septations

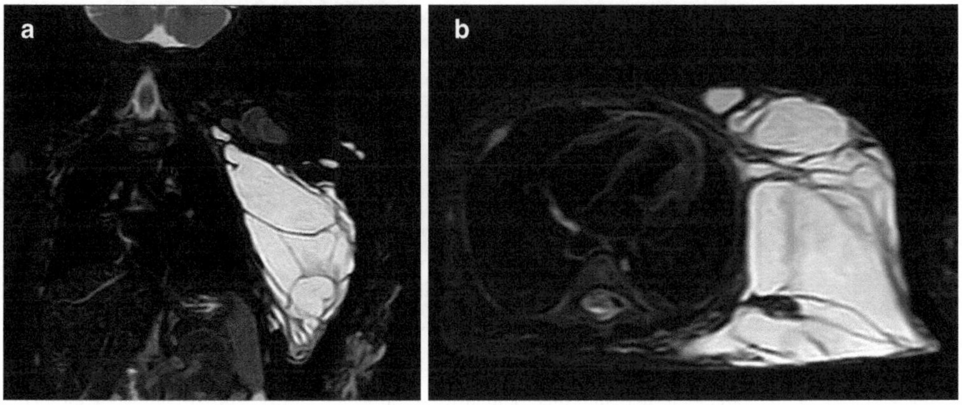

Dynamic contrast-enhanced imaging, when combined with subtraction techniques—where contrast-enhanced images are subtracted from pre-contrast ones—eliminates non-enhancing soft tissue signal, thereby enhancing the visualization of vascular structures. These dynamic sequences are essential for differentiating high flow lesions from low flow malformations and for evaluating contrast flow dynamics and detecting arteriovenous shunting in high flow lesions Coronal dynamic MRA is usually acquired in the coronal plane (Figs. 2.19, 2.20, and 2.21) [4, 19–21] Thirty phases are typically acquired following injection of 0.1 mmol/Kg of gadolinium-based MRI contrast agent (0.2 ml/kg of gadoterate meglumine; Dotarem), with flow rate of 1.5–3 ml/s followed by 10–20 ml saline flush. Dynamic scans have temporal resolution of one dynamic per second, with 1–2 mm slice thickness. The scanning starts simultaneously with automatic power injection of the contrast medium. Due to faster circulation time in infants and children, arterial and venous enhancements are identified based on visual assessment rather than determination of cut-off values of 5–6 s, as previously postulated. Thirty phases are usually acquired. Visualization of the contrast medium exclusively within the nearby non-involved systemic arteries is identified as the arterial phase, while visualization of the enhanced systemic veins marks the venous phase [20, 22] (Supplementary Videos 2.4,

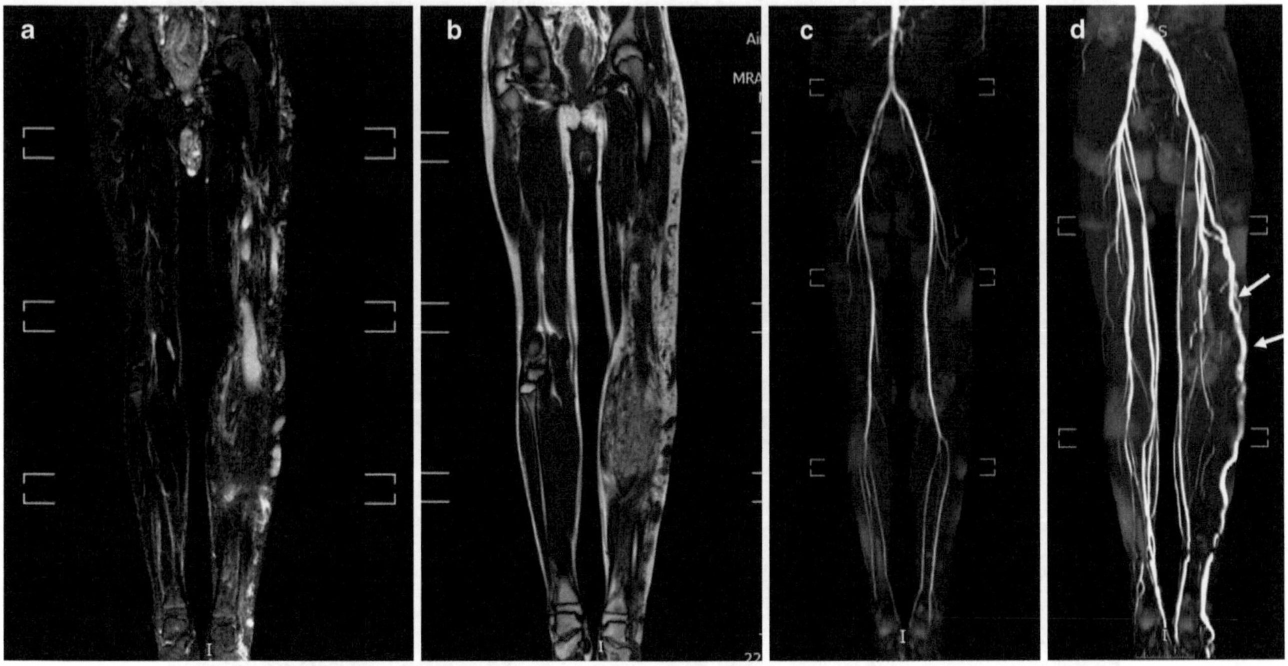

Fig. 2.15 Capillary venous lymphatic malformation (Klippel-Trenaunay syndrome) in a 15-year-old boy. The patient has cutaneous port-wine stain (not shown), venous varicosities and soft tissue hypertrophy. (**a** and **b**) Coronal STIR (**a**) and Coronal T1-WI shows dilated venous channels. (**c**) Coronal maximum intensity projection (MIP) non-contract MR angiography (two-dimensional time of flight; 2D-TOF) shows normal arterial tree. (**d**) Coronal MIP of non-contrast MR venography (2D-TOF) shows persistent embryonic lateral marginal vein of Servelle (arrow) with hypoplastic deep venous system

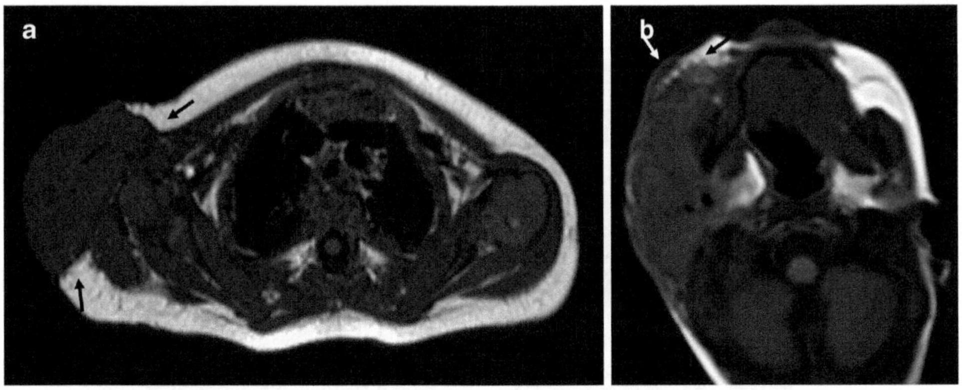

Fig. 2.16 The value of T1-weighted image. (**a**) axial T1-WI of a 1-year-old boy with congenital hemangioma demonstrates a well-defined hypointense lesion. The surrounding fat planes are clear (arrows). (**b**) A 2-month-old boy with kaposiform hemangioenfothelioma with stranding of the surrounding fat planes (black arrow) and overlying cutaneous thickening (white arrow)

2.5, and 2.6). After acquiring dynamic scan, delayed post-contrast fat-saturated T1-weighted image is then acquired.

Diffusion weighted imaging can be added to the study protocol in cases with suspected vascular tumors other than hemangioma. The presence of diffusion restriction is an alarming sign and may suggest malignant neoplastic lesion (such as rhabdomyosarcoma). Diffusion-weighted imaging should be interpreted in the view of other sequences, as presence of hemorrhage within the lesion may be related to intralesional hemorrhage (Figs. 2.22, 2.23, and 2.24), susceptibility-weighted imaging may help in this context [17].

Concerns for Special Locations

Vascular Anomalies of the Head and Neck

When examining vascular anomalies of the head and neck region, special concerns may be required. 3D-TOF is required for searching for associated cerebrovascular anomalies as part of PHACE syndrome. Diffusion-weighted imaging is important to detect acute strokes in these patients as well. Adding susceptibility-weighted imaging in cases with Sturge-Weber syndrome and facial venous malformation may be required to detect associated cerebral calcification

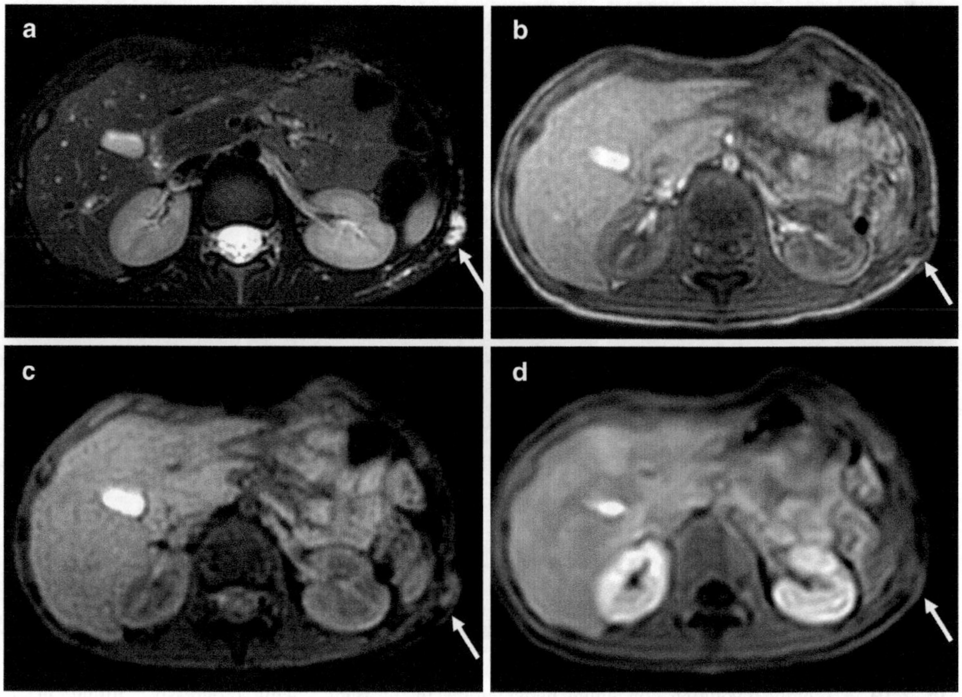

Fig. 2.17 MRI of a 6-year-old girl with microcystic lymphatic malformation demonstrating the value of non-contrast fat suppressed T1-WI. (**a** and **b**) Axial STIR (**a**), and T1-WI (**b**) showing small cystic lesions (arrow) in the subcutaneous tissue exhibiting bright signal on STIR and hypointense signal on T1-WI. (**c**) Axial non-contrast fat-suppressed T1-WI showing that the lesion (arrow) exhibits apparent hyperintense signal when compared to T1-WI without fat suppression (**b**). (**d**) Axial contrast-enhanced fat-suppressed T1-WI showing non-enhancing lesions (arrow) when compared to fat-suppressed precontrast T1-WI (**c**)

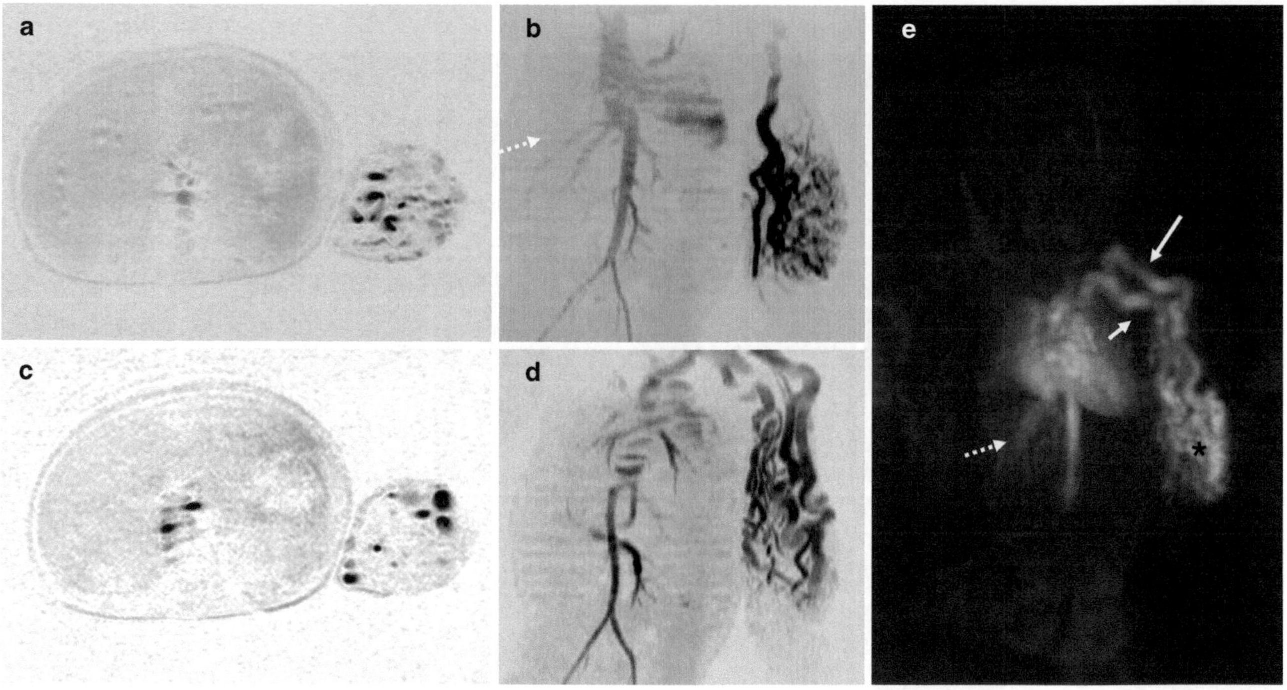

Fig. 2.18 A 9-day-old girl with arteriovenous malformation. Non-contrast MR angiography by using two-dimensional time of flight (2D-TOF) technique. (**a** and **b**) axial TOF arteriography (**a**) and coronal maximum intensity projection (MIP) showing dilated brachial artery multiple branches supplying the nidus. (**c** and **d**) axial TOF venography (**a**) and coronal MIP showing multiple dilated draining veins. (**e**) Coronal MIP of dynamic contrast enhanced MR angiography (4D TRAK, Philips Healthcare) showing the nidus (asterisk), dilated feeding artery (short arrow) and an early appearing draining vein (long arrow) denoting arteriovenous shunting. Note is made to cardiomegaly and retrograde filling of the hepatic veins (dashed arrow) due to high output cardiac failure

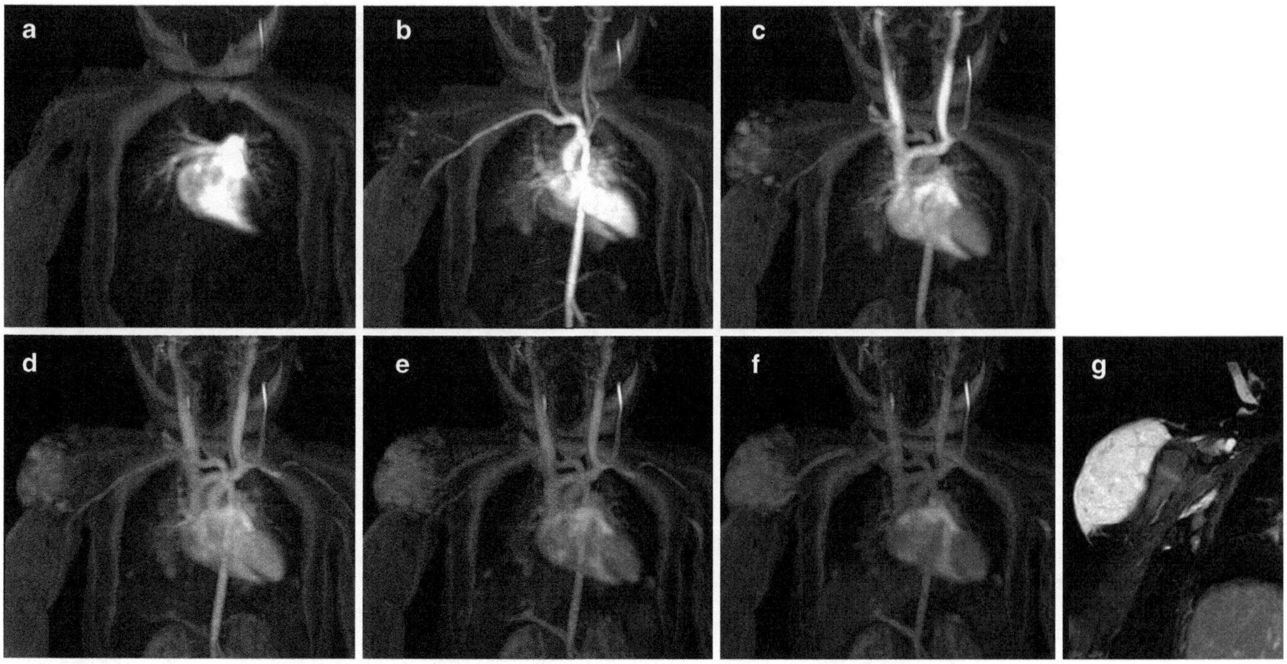

Fig. 2.19 A rapidly involuting congenital hemangioma in the right shoulder. (**a–f**) Sequential phases of dynamic contrast-enhanced MR angiography (4DTRAK, Philips Healthcare) show early enhancement with progressive filling in. (**g**) Delayed contrast-enhanced fat-suppressed coronal T1-WI shows intense enhancement of the lesion

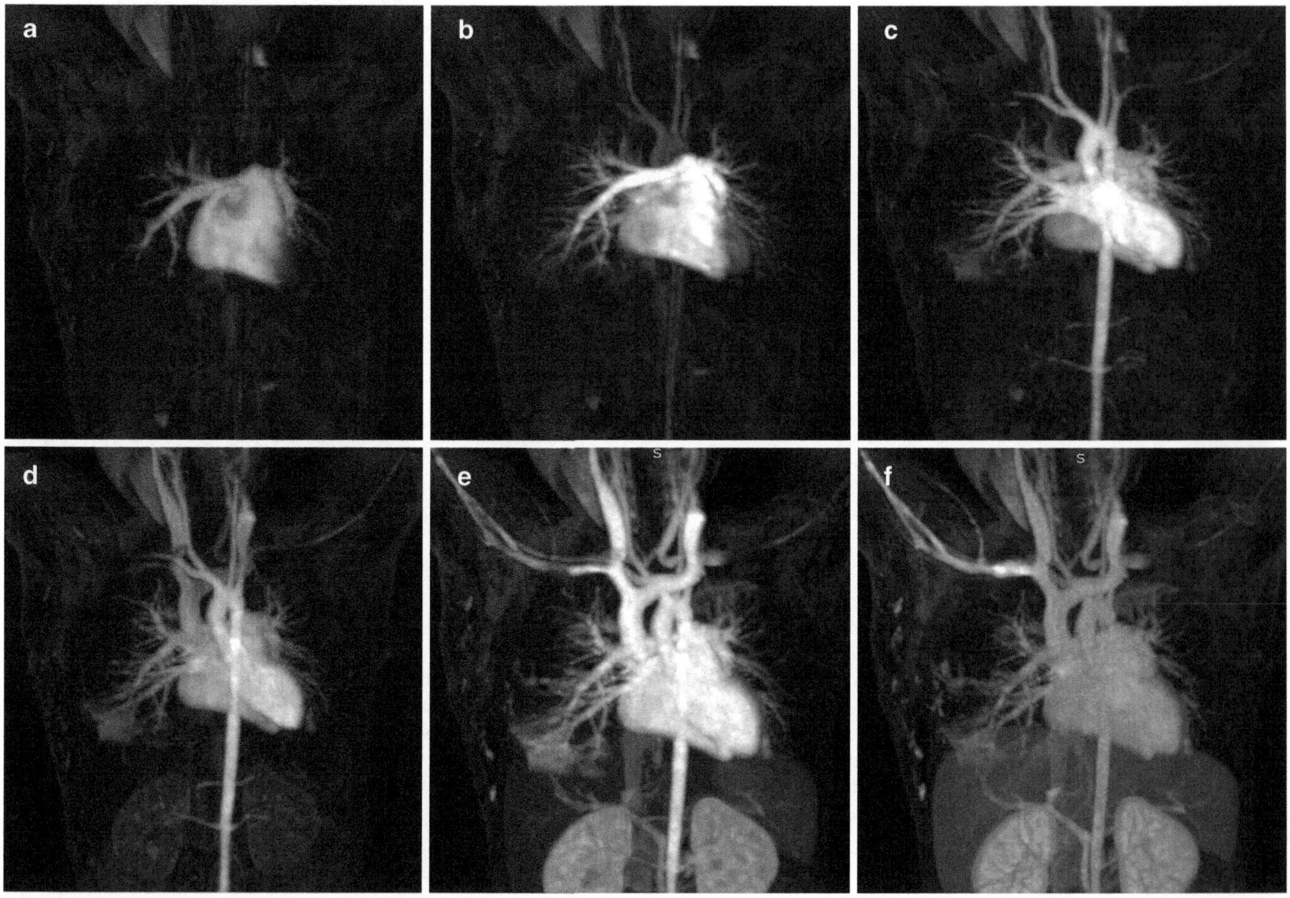

Fig. 2.20 Venous malformation in chest wall. (**a–f**) Sequential phases of dynamic contrast-enhanced MR angiography (4DTRAK, Philips Healthcare) show delayed patchy enhancement (arrows)

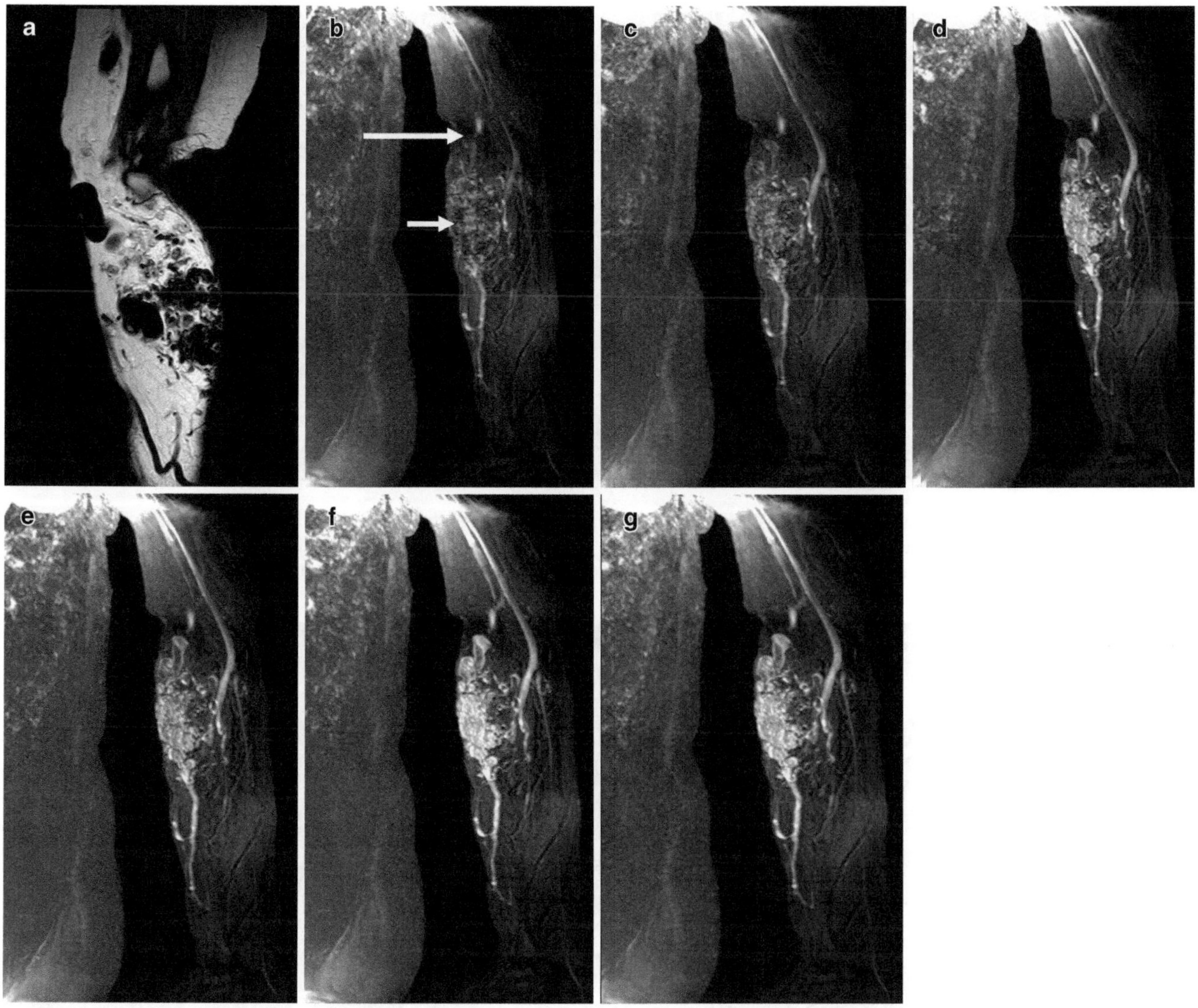

Fig. 2.21 Arterioveous malformation in the left upper limb. (**a**) Sagittal T2-WI shows a subcutaneous lesion with multiple flow voids without associated soft tissue mass. (**b–f**) Sequential phases of dynamic contrast-enhanced MR angiography (4DTRAK, Philips Healthcare) show early arterial enhancement (short arrow) with early venous drainage (long arrow) denoting arteriovenous shunting

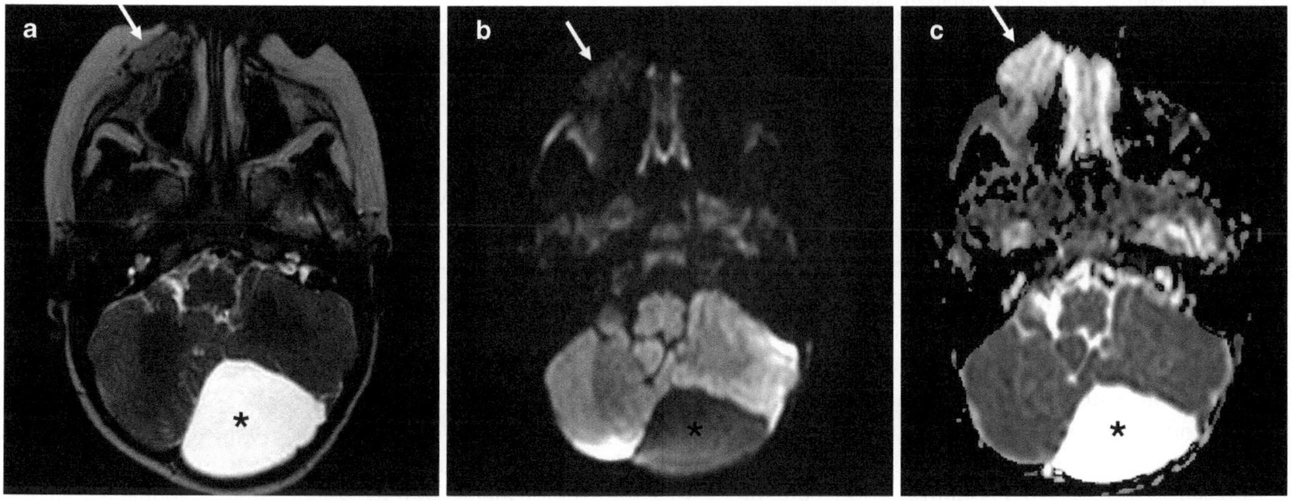

Fig. 2.22 Facial hemangioma and PHACE syndrome in a one-year-old girl. (**a**) Axial T2-WI shows the hemangioma (arrow) exhibiting hyperintense signal with multiple flow voids. (**b** and **c**) Axial diffusion weighted image (DWI) (**b**) and apparent diffusion coefficient (ADC) show that the hemangioma exhibits low signal intensity on DWI (arrow in **b**) and bright signal on ADC denoting facilitated diffusion (arrow on **c**). Note the associated cerebellar hypoplasia and posterior fossa arachnoid cyst (asterisk)

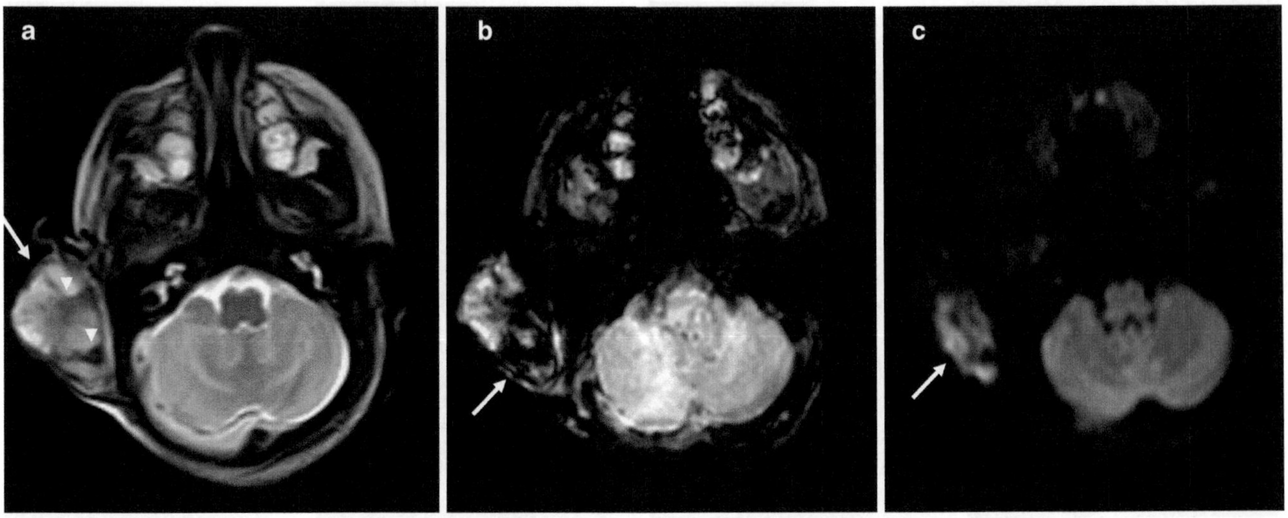

Fig. 2.23 Congenital hemangioma in a neonate. (**a**) Axial T2WI shows that the lesion (arrow) exhibits predominantly hyperintense signal on T2-WI with areas of low signal (arrowheads). (**b**) Axial susceptibility weighted image reveals low signal intensity blooming (arrow) consistent with hemorrhage. (**c**) Axial diffusion weighted image shows diffusion restriction in the areas of hemorrahge (arrow)

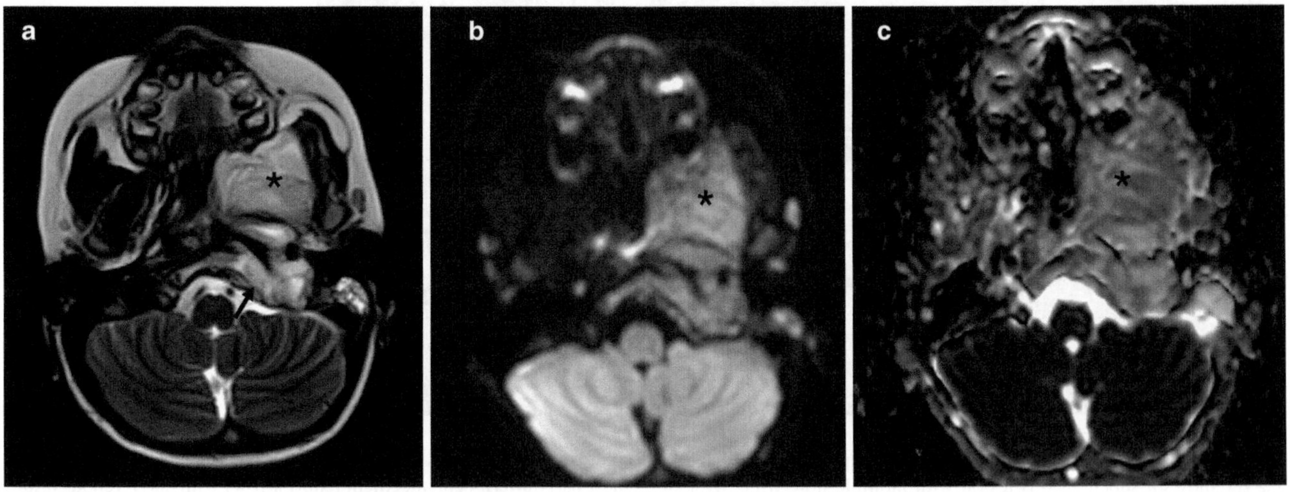

Fig. 2.24 Rhabdomyosarcoma in a 5-year-old boy. Axial T2-WI (**a**) shows soft tissue lesion (asterisk) in the left masticator space extending to the left parapharyngeal space and skull base (arrow). The lesion (asterisk) shows bright signal on DWI (**b**) and low signal on apparent diffusion coefficient (ADC = 0.88 mm2/s) (**c**)

and developmental venous anomalies as in cases with cerebrofacial venous metameric syndrome (Fig. 2.25) [17].

Cerebral Vascular Malformation

In addition to routine sequences of brain imaging, patients with cerebral vascular malformation require 3D-TOF and phase-contrast at a low velocity encoding, which are required for demonstrating arterial and venous anatomy, respectively. Dynamic time-resolved MR angiography is also required to study the flow dynamics and to detect the arteriovenous shunting [23, 24]. Perfusion imaging sequences can be employed to assess cerebral perfusion in conditions such as PHACE syndrome and Moyamoya disease. Arterial Spin Labeling (ASL), a non-contrast perfusion technique, helps differentiate vascular anomalies based on perfusion characteristics. Hemangiomas typically show increased perfusion, while venous and lymphatic malformations exhibit minimal or no perfusion. ASL can also reveal arteriovenous shunting in high-flow lesions. Additionally, contrast-enhanced MRI perfusion techniques can be used to evaluate cerebral perfusion. In addition, contrast-enhanced FLAIR sequence perfectly shows enhancing leptomeningeal angiomatosis, especially in children with Sturge-Weber syndrome (Fig. 2.26) [25, 26].

Extensive Vascular Malformation

Imaging patients with extensive vascular anomalies involving large body regions poses significant challenges. In syndromic conditions—such as Klippel–Trénaunay syndrome

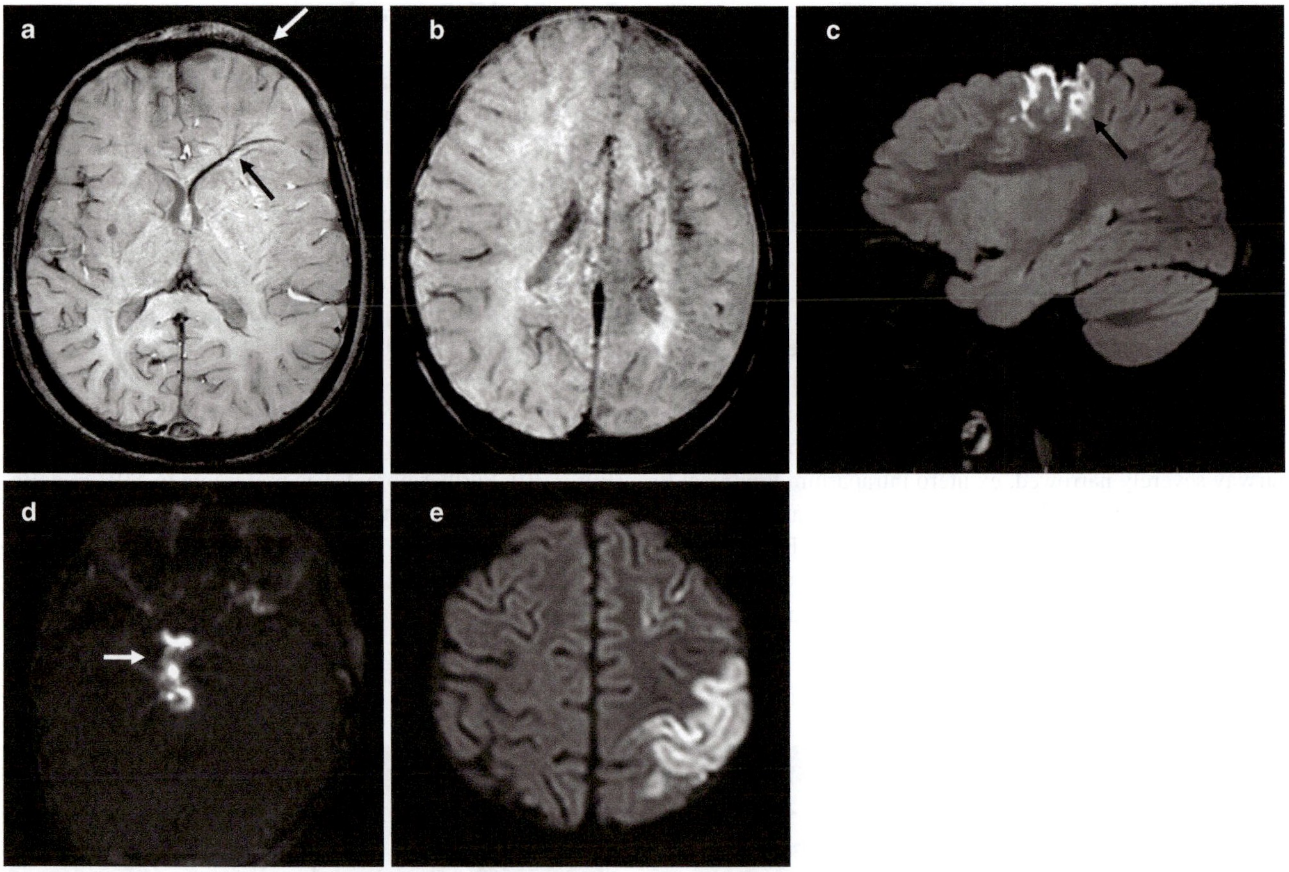

Fig. 2.25 The utility of different pulse sequences in diagnosing intracranial vascular malformation (**a**) Axial SWI in a 9-year-old boy with capillary malformation (white arrow) in the forehead associated with developmental venous anomaly (black arrow). (**b**) Axial T2* in a one-year-old boy with Sturge-Weber syndrome shows calcifications and dilated medullary veins in the left cerebral hemisphere. (**c**) Sagittal contrast-enhanced FLAIR in a 5-year-old boy nicely shows leptomeningeal angiomatosis (arrow). (**d**) Axial non-contrast Time-of-flight angiography shows tortuous anomalous cerebral vessels in a child with PHACE syndrome. (**e**) Axial diffusion weight image shows acute infarction in a child with Moya-Moya disease

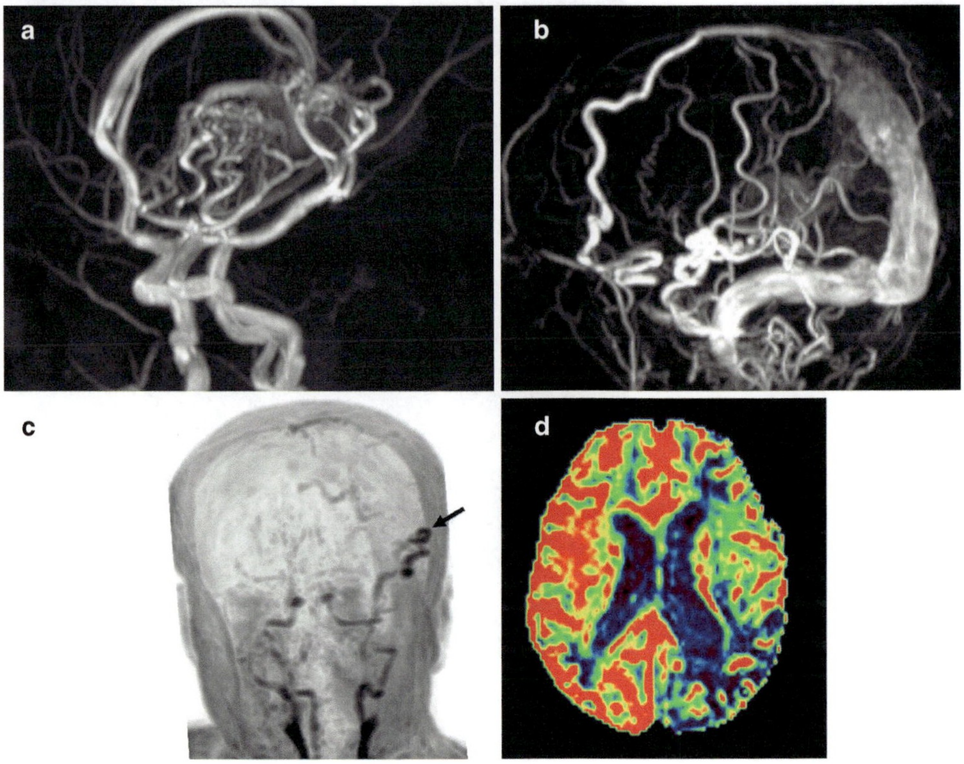

Fig. 2.26 The utility of different pulse sequences in diagnosing intracranial vascular malformation. (**a** and **b**) Mixumum intensity projection (MIP) of MR arteriography (**a**) and venography (**b**) in a 7-year-old boy with vein of Galen aneurysmal malformation. (**c**) Coronal MIP of the arterial phase of dynamic contrast-enhanced angiography shows arteriovenous shunting (arrow) in child with dural arteriovenous fistula. (**d**) Axial cerebral blood volume (CBV) color map in a child with Moyamoya disease showing greater reduction of CBV in the left hemisphere compared to the right

or PIK3CA-related overgrowth spectrum—or in non-syndromic extensive malformations, lesions may affect entire limbs and extend into the trunk, necessitating a wide field of view or whole-body imaging. In such cases, using a multichannel coil system is often required to image multiple anatomical regions with adequate spatial resolution. Images are usually acquired in the coronal plane (Figs. 2.27 and 2.28) [17, 27].

Fetal Imaging

Vascular anomalies can be detected during antenatal screening ultrasounds. MRI may be required for further characterization and management planning. Examination of the airway is crucial for large vascular anomalies of the neck. If airway severely narrowed, ex utero intrapartum treatment to airway procedure (EXIT) can be adopted. Fetal MRI is performed by acquiring T2-weighted single-shot FSE. 2-D fast steady-state acquisition and T1-weighted fast spoiled gradient recalled echo are additional sequences that can be utilized (Fig. 2.29) [28].

Computed Tomography

Due to its associated radiation risk—particularly in pediatric patients—CT is not the first-line imaging modality for vascular anomalies but is reserved for specific clinical indications. However, compared with MRI, CT provides higher spatial resolution, enabling accurate visualization of vascular structures, including feeding arteries and draining veins. This capability is further enhanced by post-processing methods such as multiplanar reformatting, maximum intensity projection, and three-dimensional surface rendering. As such, CT is especially valuable in pre-interventional planning for arteriovenous malformations, significantly reducing both procedure time and radiation exposure (Fig. 2.30). Furthermore, CT is preferable to MRI in delineation of vascular anomalies of the intestine and lung (Figs. 2.31 and 2.32). Additionally, CT is effective in detecting phleboliths, osseous abnormalities associating vascular anomalies, especially of the craniofacial region and extremities (Fig. 2.33). Being faster than MRI, CT may be indicated in uncooperative patients with unstable cardio-

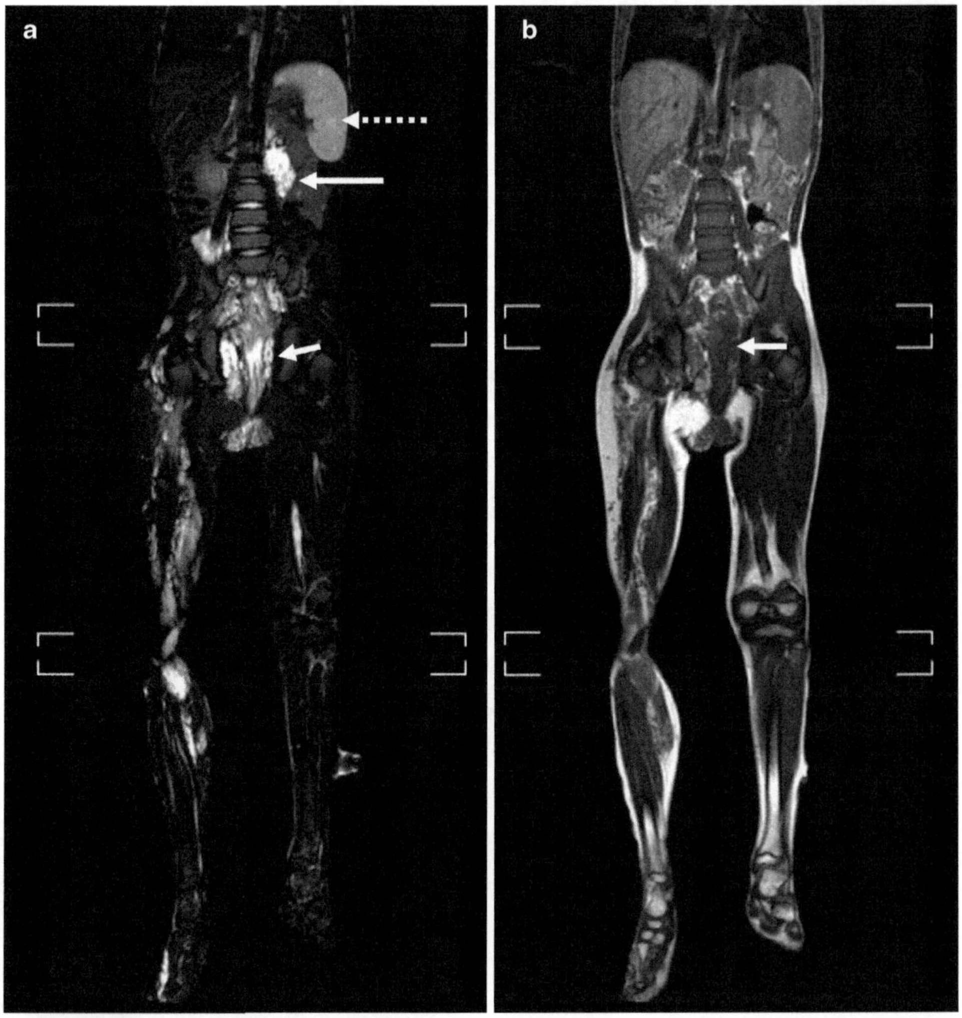

Fig. 2.27 Capillary-lymphatic-venous malformation (Klippel-Trenaunay-Syndrome) in a 6-year-old boy. (**a** and **b**) Coronal STIR (**a**) and Coronal T1-WI (**b**) shows venous malformation of the lower limb, perineum, gluteal region (not shown), with intrapelvic extension and rectal involvement (short arrow). There is associated lymphatic malformation (dashed arrow) in the spleen and left paraspinal region (long arrow)

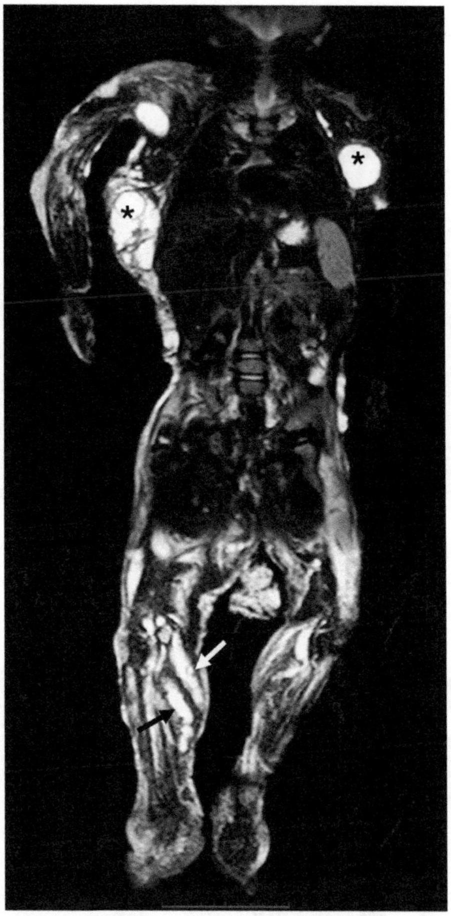

Fig. 2.28 A 3-year-old boy with soft tissue overgrowth syndrome (CLOVES syndrome: Congenital Lipomatous Overgrowth, Vascular malformations, Epidermal naevi, Skeletal/Scoliosis/Spinal anomalies). Whole body MRI (STIR) shows soft tissue-overgrowth dilated anomalous veins (arrows), multiple cysts (asterisks) representing lymphatic malformation involving the right upper limb, trunk and both lower limbs

vascular or respiratory condition or patients with any MRI contraindication [28, 29].

Arteriography

Digital Subtraction Angiography (DSA) offers high-resolution imaging that clearly delineates the vascular anatomy of arteriovenous malformations, including precise identification of feeding arteries and draining veins. However, its role is generally reserved for therapeutic intervention following initial diagnosis and characterization using CT or MR angiography [30].

Diagnostic Algorithm

When a vascular anomaly is suspected on imaging, the initial step is to classify the lesion as either high-flow or low-flow (Fig. 2.34). A high-flow lesion is identified by the presence of low-resistance arterial flow on Doppler or dynamic imaging. If the lesion consists of multiple high-flow vessels without an associated soft tissue mass, this is characteristic of an AVM (Figs. 2.3 and 2.8, Supplementary Video 2.5).

On imaging, AVM appears as multiple serpentine vessels with high vascular density on Doppler ultrasound and appears as flow voids across all pulse sequences on MRI. Dynamic time-resolved MR angiography demonstrates the malformation and the arteriovenous shunting (Fig. 2.21, Supplementary Video 2.5). If a soft tissue mass is present alongside high-flow vessels, the lesion represents a vascular tumour—with hemangioma being the prototypical example. On ultrasound, hemangioma appears as soft tissue mass of variable echogenicity with increased vascular density (Figs. 2.4 and 2.7; Supplementary Video 2.4). On MRI, hemangioma appears as well-defined soft tissue mass, hyperintense on T2-weighted images, with multiple flow voids and early, persistent contrast enhancement (Fig. 2.19, Supplementary Video 2.4).

On the contrary, lymphatic and venous malformations are low-flow lesions lacking the high-flow vessels. Lymphatic malformation appears as a cystic lesion composed of macrocysts, microcysts, or a mix (Fig. 2.5). On MRI, lymphatic malformation appears as a T2 hyperintense multiloculated cystic spaces with septal enhancement (Fig. 2.14). Venous malformation is characterized by slow venous flow, often augmented by dependency, compression, or Valsalva (Figs. 2.6, 2.11, and 2.12, Supplementary Video 2.6). On MRI venous malformation appears as a T2 hyperintense lesion with phleboliths and patchy delayed enhancement (Figs. 2.10, 2.11, 2.12, and 2.13, Supplementary Video 2.6). Further details will be discussed in the following chapters.

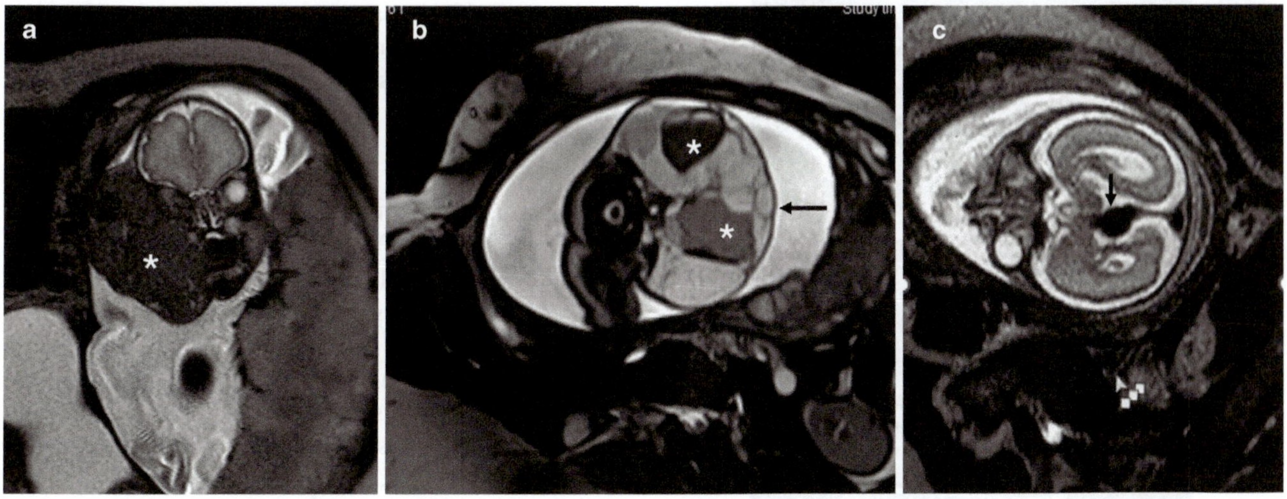

Fig. 2.29 Fetal MRI showing vascular anomalies (**a**) Coronal SSFP shows a right facial venous malformation (asterisk) with intralesional hemorrhage. (**b**) Axial SSFP shows lymphatic malformation (arrow) with intralesional hemorrhage (asterisk). (**c**) axial T2-WI shows vein of Galen aneurysmal malformation (arrow)

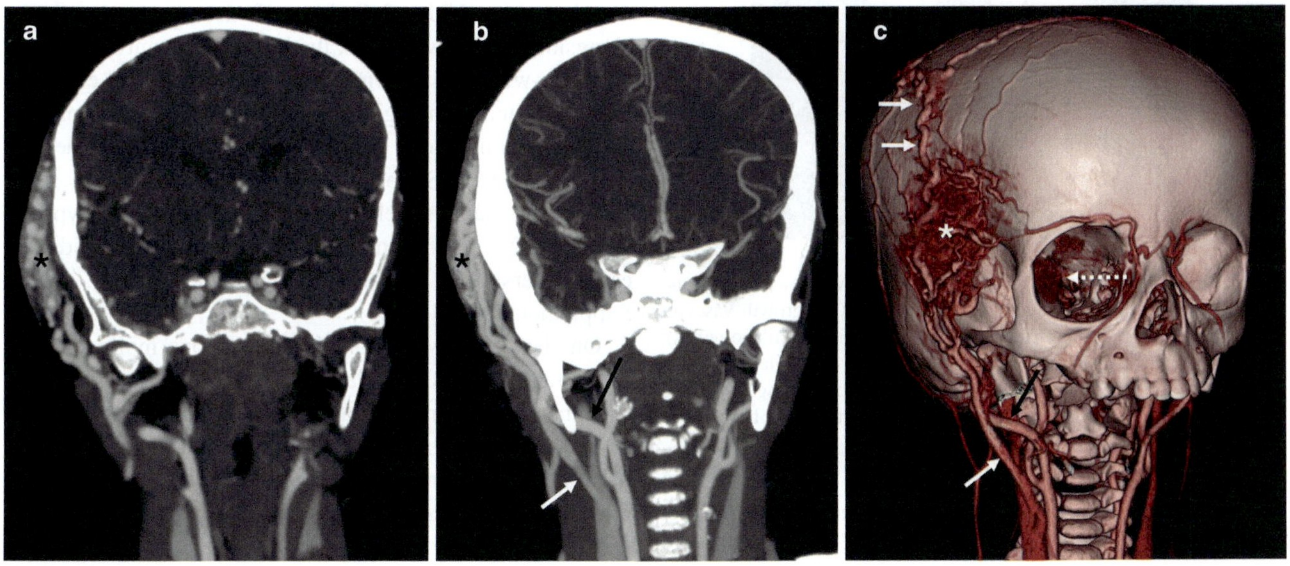

Fig. 2.30 Multiple arteriovenous malformations in the right temporal region and orbit in one-year-old boy. (**a** and **b**) Coronal contrast-enhanced CT (**a**), coronal maximum intensity projection (**b**) of contrast enhanced CT angiography shows arteriovenous malformation with feeding vessel arising from the external carotid artery (black arrow) and draining vein (white arrow) into the internal jugular artery. (**c**) three-dimensional reconstruction shows the right temporal nidus, feeding vessel and multiple draining veins (arrows). Note associated orbital arteriovenous malformation (dashed arrow)

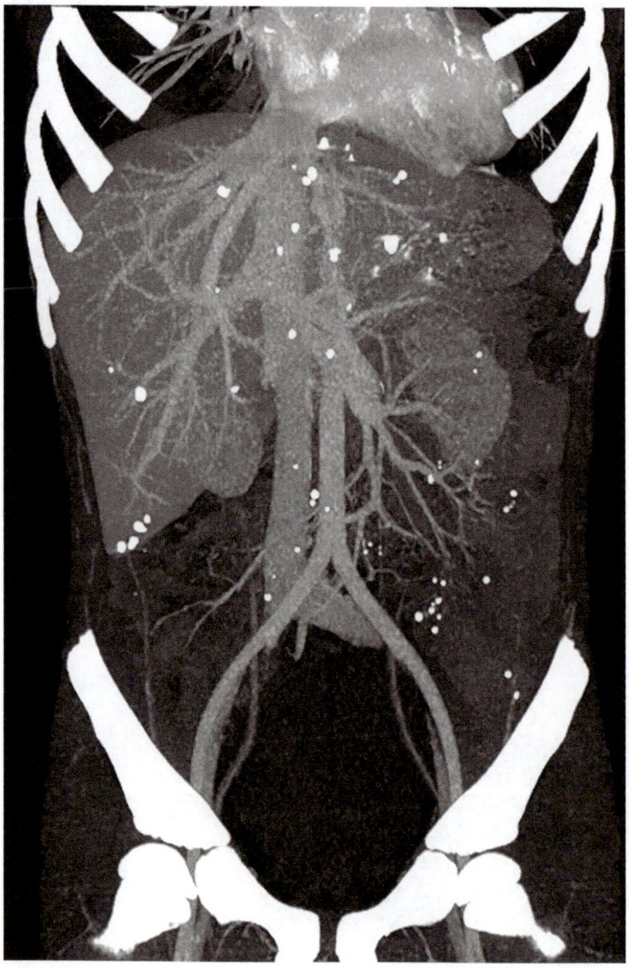

Fig. 2.31 A 9-year-old boy with blue rubber bleb nevus syndrome. Coronal maximum intensity projection shows scattered rounded calcification involving the liver and small bowel signifying phleboliths in multiple venous malformation

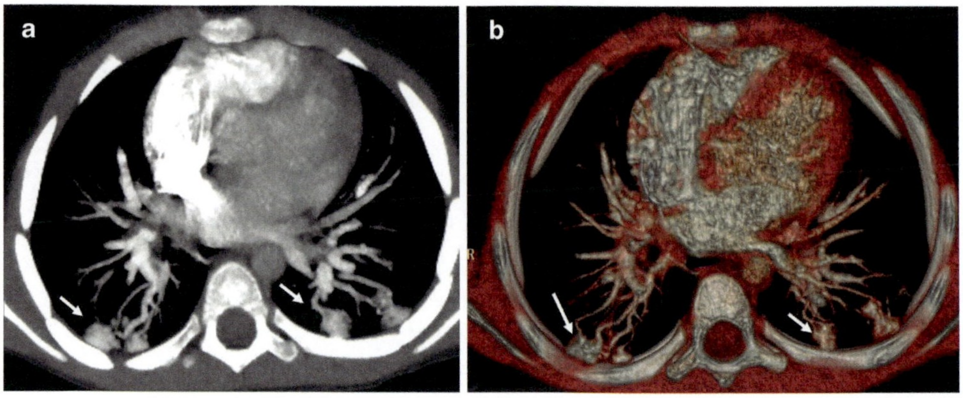

Fig. 2.32 A 5-year-old boy with hereditary hemorrhagic telangiectasia. (**a** and **b**) Axial maximum intensity projection (**a**) and three-dimensional reconstruction (**b**) of contras-enhanced CT show multiple pulmonary arteriovenous malformations (arrows)

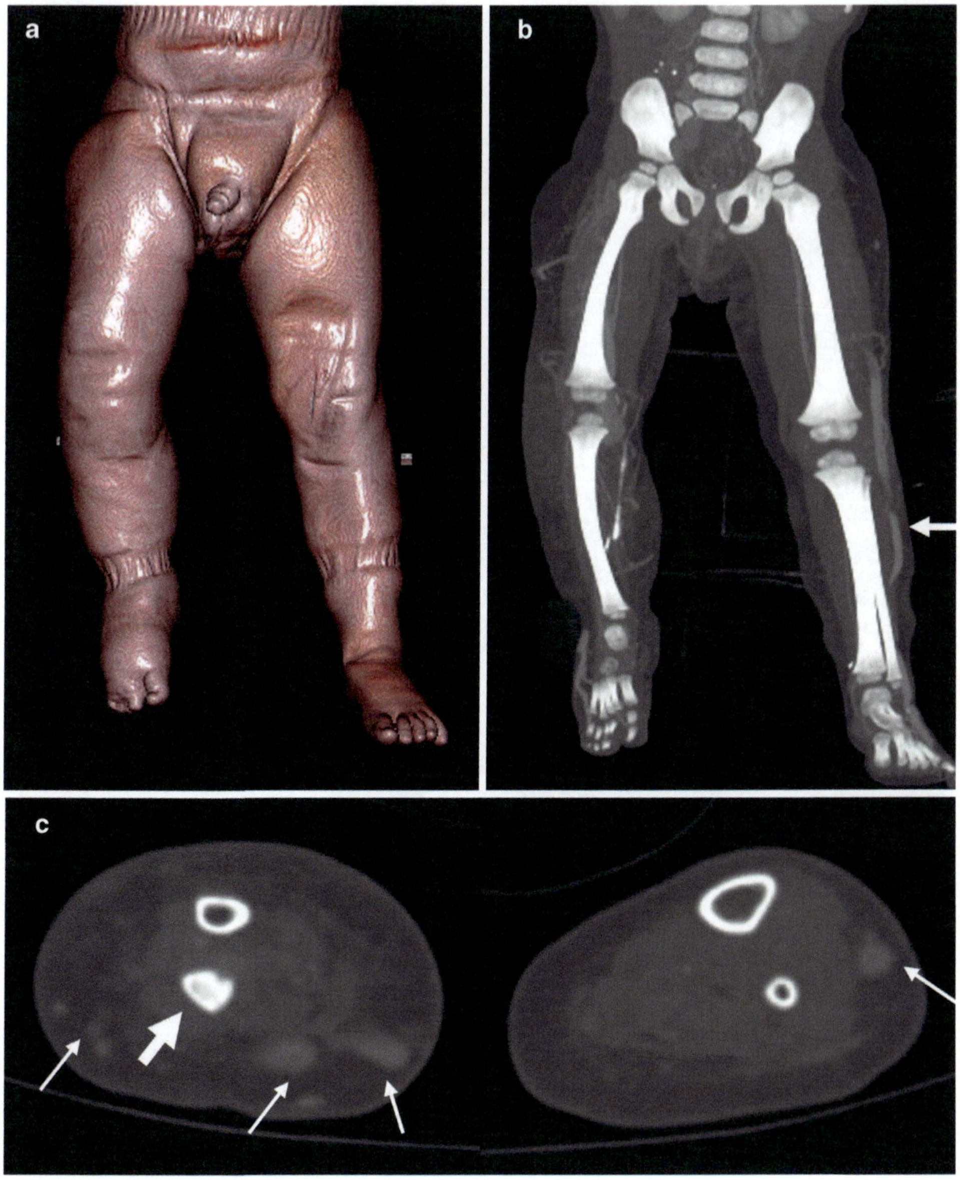

Fig. 2.33 Capillary-lymphatic-venous malformation (Klippel-Trenuanay syndrome) in 1-year-old boy. (**a**) three-dimensional surface reformat of CT of both lower limbs, (**b**) Coronal maximum intensity projection of contrast enhanced CT shows soft tissue over growth and limb-length discrepancy. Note the dilated lateral marginal vein (arrow). (**c**) Axial contrast-enhanced CT of both legs shows soft tissue overgrowth, subcutaneous stranding and dilated anomalous veins (thin arrows). Note the abnormal increase of bone density of the right fibula (thick arrow)

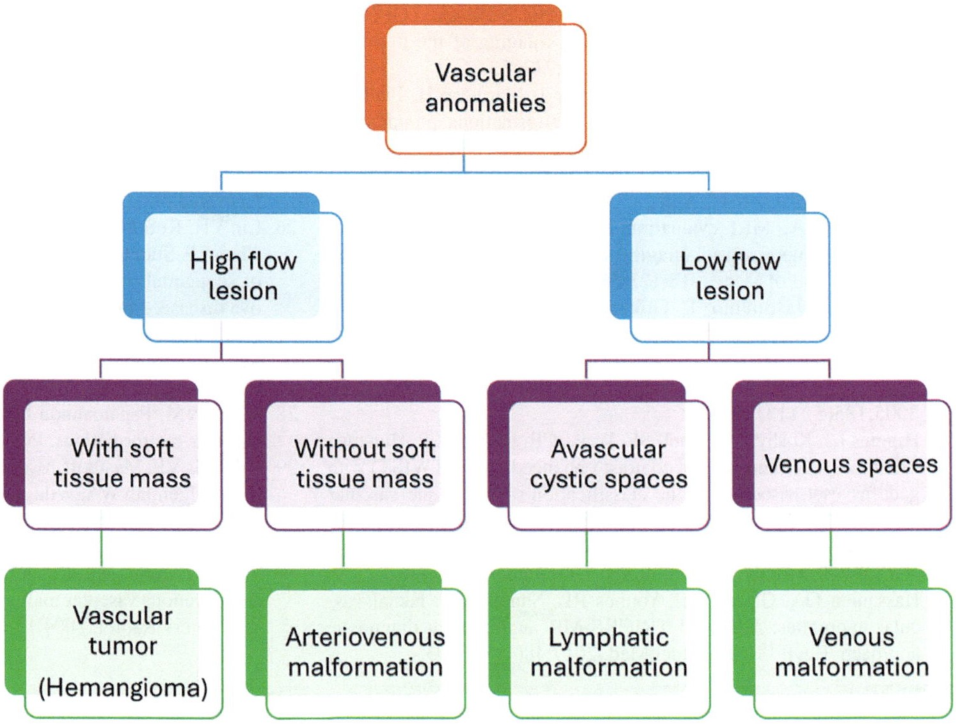

Fig. 2.34 Simplified approach for the diagnosis of vascular anomalies. High flow lesions are demarcated from low flow lesions by the presence of high vascular density on ultrasound color Doppler, and multiple flow voids and early contrast enhancement on MRI

References

1. Fishman SJ, Burrows BE. Treatment of visceral vascular tumors. In: Mulliken JB, Burrows PE, Fishman SJ, editors. Mulliken & Young vascular anomalies: hemangioms and malformations. Oxford University Press; 2013. p. 239–58.
2. Mamlouk MD, Anavim A, Goodwin SC. Radiology residents rounding with the clinical teams: a pilot study to improve the radiologist's visibility as a consultant. J Am Coll Radiol. 2014;11:326–8.
3. Johnson CM, Navarro OM. Clinical and sonographic features of pediatric soft-tissue vascular anomalies part 1: classification, sonographic approach and vascular tumors. Pediatr Radiol. 2017;47(9):1184–95.
4. Bardo DM, Gill AE, Iyer RS, Chan SS, Cooper ML, Dasgupta RA, Guimaraes CV, Hammer MR, Krowchuk DP, Levin TL, Liang MG. ACR appropriateness criteria® soft tissue vascular anomalies: vascular malformations and infantile vascular tumors (non-CNS)-child. J Am Coll Radiol. 2024;21(6):S310–25.
5. Léauté-Labrèze C, Baselga Torres E, Weibel L, Boon LM, El Hachem M, van der Vleuten C, Roessler J, Troilius Rubin A. The infantile hemangioma referral score: a validated tool for physicians. Pediatrics. 2020;145(4)
6. Koplewitz BZ, Springer C, Slasky BS, Avital A, Uwyyed K, Piccard E, Bar-Ziv J. CT of hemangiomas of the upper airways in children. Am J Roentgenol. 2005;184(2):663–70.
7. Iacobas I, Phung TL, Adams DM, Trenor CC III, Blei F, Fishman DS, Hammill A, Masand PM, Fishman SJ. Guidance document for hepatic hemangioma (infantile and congenital) evaluation and monitoring. J Pediatr. 2018;203:294–300.
8. Kollipara R, Dinneen L, Rentas KE, et al. Current classification and terminology of pediatric vascular anomalies. AJR Am J Roentgenol. 2013;201:1124–35.
9. Vilanova JC, Barceló J, Villalón M. MR and MR angiography characterization of soft tissue vascular malformations. Curr Probl Diagn Radiol. 2004;33(4):161–70.
10. Johnson JB, Cogswell PM, McKusick MA, Binkovitz LA, Riederer SJ, Young PM. Pretreatment imaging of peripheral vascular malformations. J Vasc Diagn. 2014;2014:121–6.
11. Merrow AC, Gupta A, Patel MN, Adams DM. 2014 Revised classification of vascular lesions from the international society for the study of vascular anomalies: radiologic-pathologic update. Radiographics. 2016;36:1494–516.
12. Lidsky ME, Spritzer CE, Shortell CK. The role of dynamic contrast enhanced magnetic resonance imaging in the diagnosis and management of patients with vascular malformations. J Vasc Surg. 2012;56:757–764 e1.
13. van Rijswijk CS, van der Linden E, van der Woude HJ, van Baalen JM, Bloem JL. Value of dynamic contrast-enhanced MR imaging in diagnosing and classifying peripheral vascular malformations. AJR Am J Roentgenol. 2002;178:1181–7.
14. Wiesinger I, Schreml S, Wohlgemuth WA, Stroszczynski C, Jung EM. Perfusion quantification of vascular malformations using contrastenhanced ultrasound (CEUS) with time intensity curve analysis before and after treatment: first results. Clin Hemorheol Microcirc. 2015;62:283–90.
15. Dubois JE, Patriquin HB, Garel L, Powell J, Filiatrault D, David M, Grignon A. Soft-tissue hemangiomas in infants and children: diagnosis using Doppler sonography. AJR Am J Roentgenol. 1998;171(1):247–52.
16. Flors L, Leiva-Salinas C, Maged IM, Norton PT, Matsumoto AH, Angle JF, Hugo Bonatti MD, Park AW, Ahmad EA, Bozlar U, Housseini AM. MR imaging of soft-tissue vascular malformations: diagnosis, classification, and therapy follow-up. Radiographics. 2011;31(5):1321–40. BibTeX
17. Mamlouk MD, Nicholson AD, Cooke DL, Hess CP. Tips and tricks to optimize MRI protocols for cutaneous vascular anomalies. Clin Imaging. 2017;45:71–80.

18. Del Grande F, Santini F, Herzka DA, AroMR DCW, Gold GE, et al. Fat-suppression techniques for 3-T MR imaging of the musculoskeletal system. Radiographics. 2014;34:217–33.
19. Madani H, Farrant J, Chhaya N, Anwar I, Marmery H, Platts A, Holloway B. Peripheral limb vascular malformations: an update of appropriate imaging and treatment options of a challenging condition. Br J Radiol. 2015;88(1047):20140406.
20. Schicchi N, Tagliati C, Agliata G, Esposto Pirani P, Spadari R, Giovagnoni A. MRI evaluation of peripheral vascular anomalies using time-resolved imaging of contrast kinetics (TRICKS) sequence. Radiol Med. 2018;123:563–71. BibTeX
21. Ohgiya Y, Hashimoto T, Gokan T, Watanabe S, Kuroda M, Hirose M, Matsui S, Nobusawa H, Kitanosono T, Munechika H. Dynamic MRI for distinguishing high-flow from low-flow peripheral vascular malformations. Am J Roentgenol. 2005;185(5):1131–7.
22. Higgins LJ, Koshy J, Mitchell SE, Weiss CR, Carson KA, Huisman TA, Tekes A. Time-resolved contrast-enhanced MRA (TWIST) with gadofosveset trisodium in the classification of soft-tissue vascular anomalies in the head and neck in children following updated 2014 ISSVA classification: first report on systematic evaluation of MRI and TWIST in a cohort of 47 children. Clin Radiol. 2016;71(1):32–9.
23. Hassanien OA, Ghieda UE, Younes RL, Shaban EA. Facial vascular anomalies; MRI and TRICKS-MR angiography diagnostic approach. Egyp J Radiol Nucl Med. 2017;48(4):885–95.
24. Cellerini M, Mascalchi M, Mangiafico S, Ferrito GP, Scardigli V, Pellicanò G, Quilici N. Phase-contrast MR angiography of intracranial dural arteriovenous fistulae. Neuroradiology. 1999;41:487–92.
25. Boulouis G, Dangouloff-Ros V, Boccara O, Garabedian N, Soupre V, Picard A, et al. Arterial spin-labeling to discriminate pediatric cervicofacial soft-tissue vascular anomalies. AJNR Am J Neuroradiol. 2017;38:633.
26. Lin YH, Kuo MF, Lu CJ, Lee CW, Yang SH, Huang YC, Liu HM, Chen YF. Standardized MR perfusion scoring system for evaluation of sequential perfusion changes and surgical outcome of moyamoya disease. Am J Neuroradiol. 2019;40(2):260–6.
27. Kaddah RO, Lotfi U, Haggag M, Ghani HA. The role of radiology in the planning management of Klippel Trenaunay Syndrome (KTS). Egyp J Radiol Nucl Med. 2011;42(2):201–10.
28. Klein WM, Papaioannou G. Magnetic resonance imaging of fetal vascular malformations. Pediatr Radiol. 2025;55(4):633–43.
29. Schmidt VF, Masthoff M, Czihal M, Cucuruz B, Häberle B, Brill R, Wohlgemuth WA, Wildgruber M. Imaging of peripheral vascular malformations—current concepts and future perspectives. Mol Cell Pediatr. 2021;8:1–8.
30. Tan KT, Simons ME, Rajan DK, Terbrugge K. Peripheral high-flow arteriovenous vascular malformations: a single-center experience. J Vasc Interv Radiol. 2004;15:1071–80.

Part II

Vascular Tumors

Infantile Hemangioma

3

Introduction

Infantile hemangiomas (IH) are benign, self-resolving vascular tumors affecting mostly the skin (either cutaneous and/or subcutaneous) (Fig. 3.1). Less commonly, infantile hemangiomas may be found within internal organs or deeper tissue planes—such as the liver, intestines, mediastinum, or pelvis—which will be covered in the following chapter (Chap. 4). The incidence of infantile hemangiomas ranges from approximately 10% in full-term infants up to 20% in premature infants, with a noted female predominance [1, 2]. Typically, skin lesions are absent or minimal at birth [1, 2]. They are usually noticed within the first few days of life and follow a characteristic natural course comprising three phases: an initial rapid proliferative phase (during the first 5–8 months); a plateau or slow involuting phase; and finally, a phase of spontaneous involution typically completed by 5–9 years of age (Fig. 3.2) [1–3]. This characteristic behavior of IH has been described by Mulliken and Bischoff as "A Play in Three Acts" [4]. Management is typically conservative; however, active treatment is indicated when functional or cosmetic complications arise, such as ulceration (Figs. 3.3 and 3.4), significant distortion (Fig. 3.5), or obstruction of vision (Fig. 3.6) or vital structures [1–3].

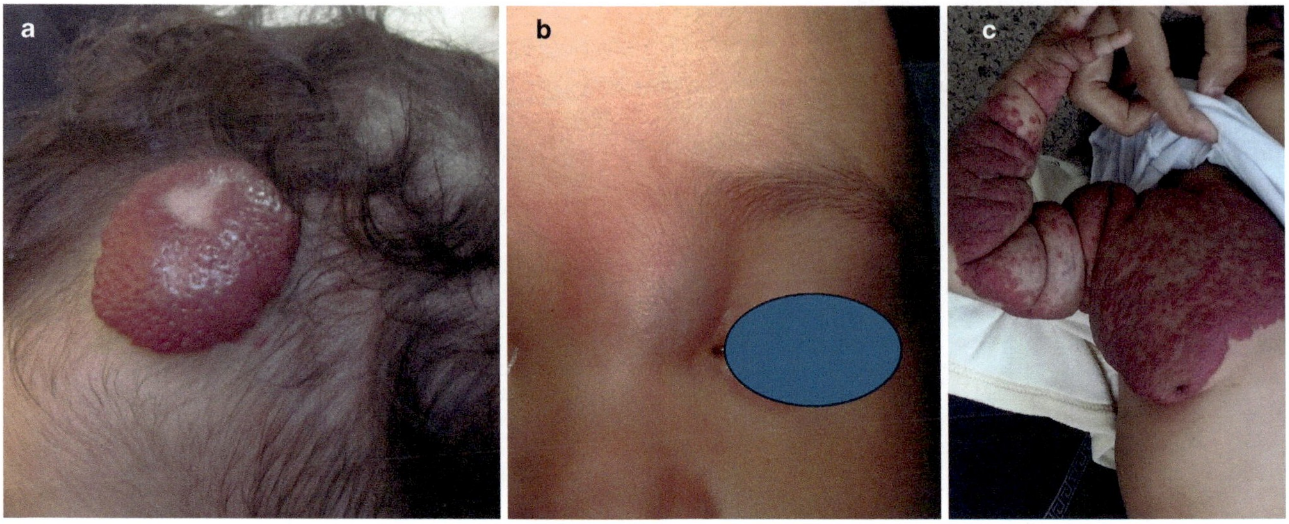

Fig. 3.1 Clinical variations of infantile hemangiomas in three different cases. Panel (**a**) shows a localized cutaneous lesion, (**b**) depicts a localized subcutaneous lesion, and (**c**) demonstrates a segmental diffuse lesion

A. A. AbouZeid et al., *Atlas of Pediatric Vascular Anomalies*, https://doi.org/10.1007/978-3-032-30866-5_3

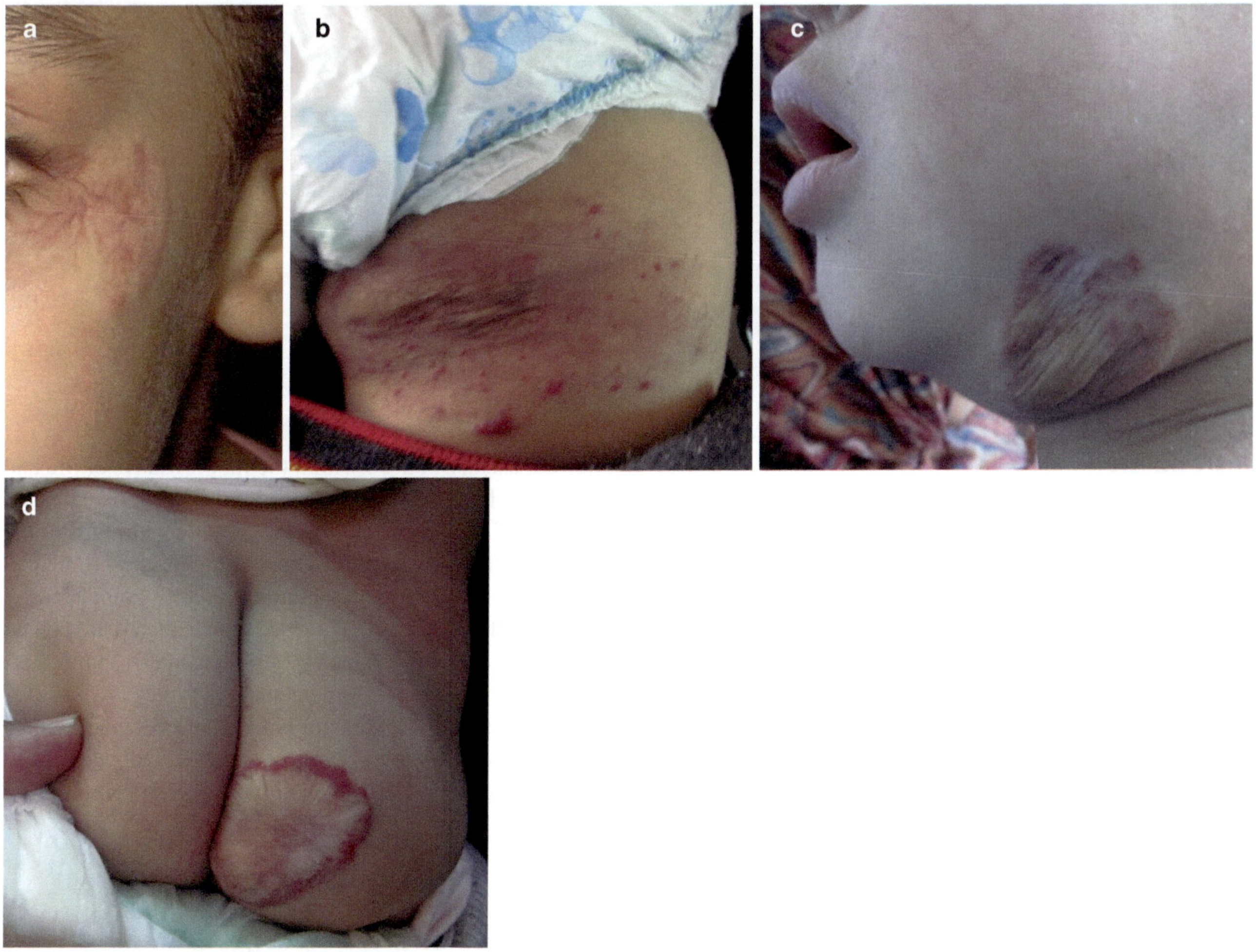

Fig. 3.2 Infantile hemangiomas at various stages of involution in different locations: periorbital (**a**), posterior thigh (**b**), submandibular (**c**), and gluteal (**d**)

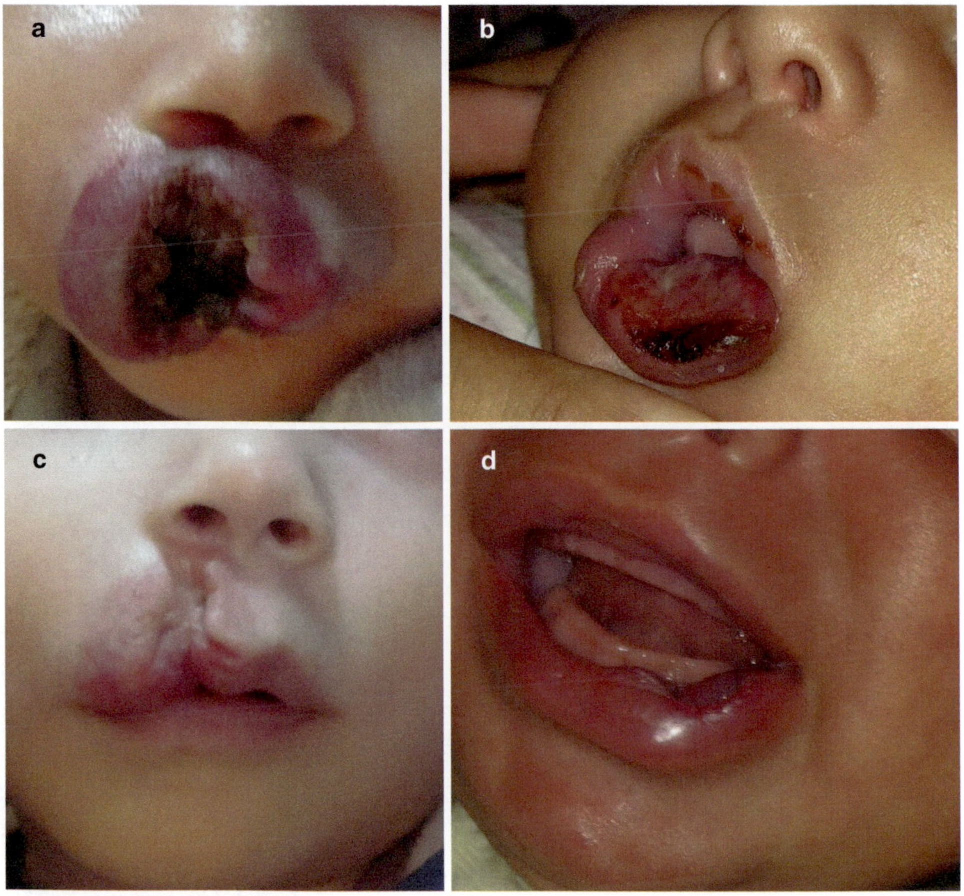

Fig. 3.3 Ulcerated infantile hemangiomas of the upper (**a**) and lower (**b**) lips in two different cases during the proliferative phase, with follow-up images (**c** and **d**, respectively) showing healing after oral propranolol therapy

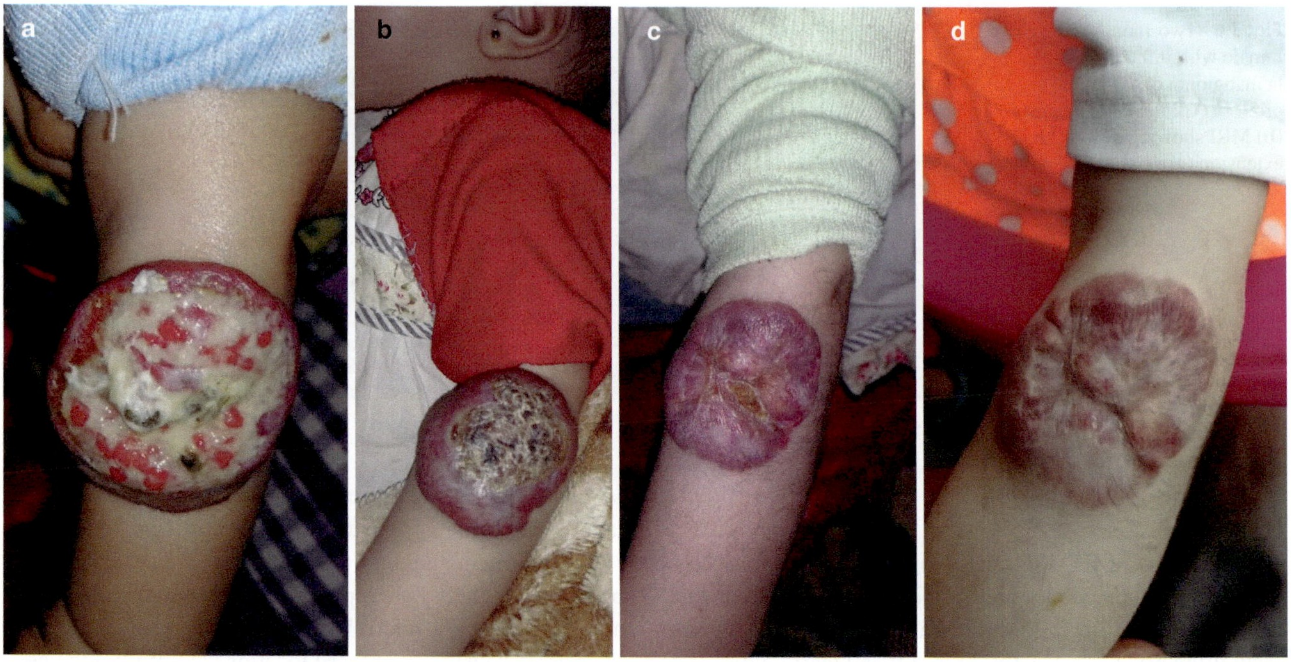

Fig. 3.4 Infantile hemangioma of the upper limb in the same patient. (**a**) At 3 months with ulceration during the proliferative phase; (**b** and **c**) gradual healing with dressings and oral propranolol; (**d**) regression at 18 months. (Reproduced from AbouZeid et al. [2])

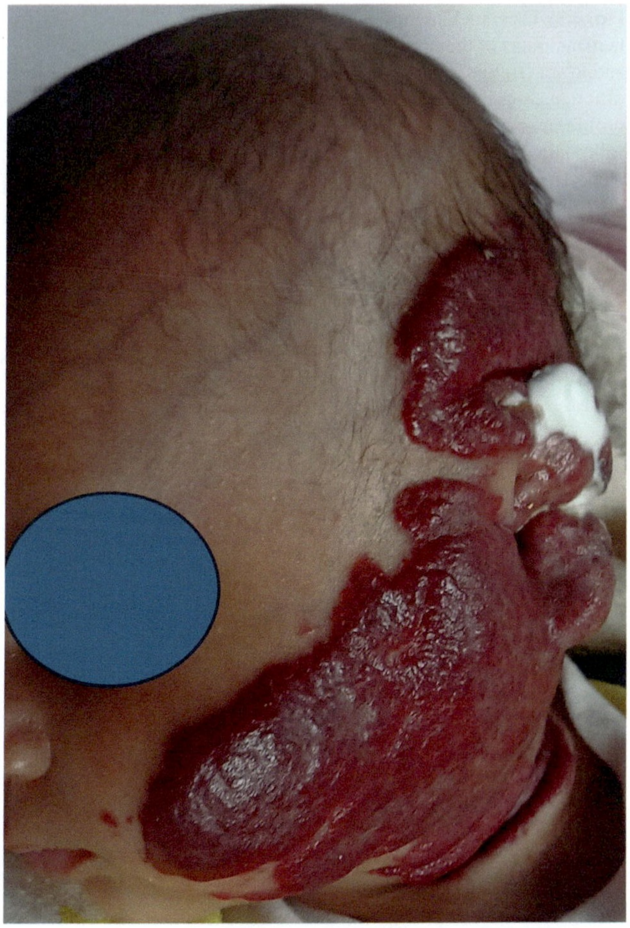

Fig. 3.5 Diffuse segmental infantile hemangioma with ulceration over the ear pinna in a 35-day-old female

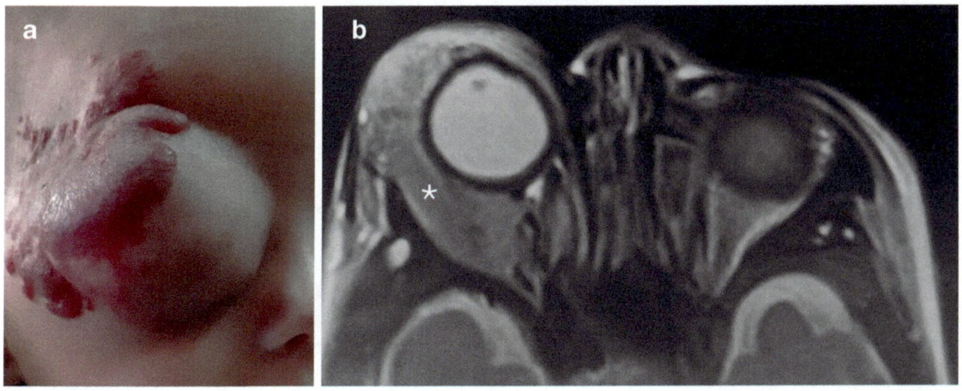

Fig. 3.6 Two-month-old female with infantile hemangioma of the right orbit. (**a**) Clinical appearance; (**b**) MRI showing deep orbital extension (asterisk)

Diagnosis

The diagnosis of IH is usually a clinical diagnosis based on characteristic appearance and typical history (absent or small skin lesions at birth followed by rapid proliferative phase in early infancy) [1–3]. The tumor is soft and warm with a typical bright red color when situated on the skin surface (strawberry nevus) (Fig. 3.1a). Subcutaneous lesions may have blue tinge or no color (Fig. 3.1b) [1]. Infantile hemangiomas may appear as either localized lesions or as diffuse/segmental lesions involving large areas of the skin (Fig. 3.1); the latter form is more prone to complications (Fig. 3.5) [1–3].

Infantile hemangiomas (IH) can occur in any region of the body. Although they are reported more frequently in the head and neck [1, 2], a referral bias cannot be excluded due to their greater visibility in these locations [1]. Within the head and neck region, infantile hemangiomas tend to occur more frequently at specific sites (Table 3.1): periorbital (Figs. 3.6 and 3.7), parotid (Fig. 3.8), scalp (Fig. 3.9), lips (Fig. 3.10), and nose (Fig. 3.11). The trunk (Fig. 3.12), limbs (Figs. 3.4,

3.13, and 3.14), and perineum (Fig. 3.15) are other common locations in the rest of the body. Facial lesions typically raise greater cosmetic concerns, particularly when located near natural orifices such as the eyes, nose, or lips or when they are large or ulcerated (Fig. 3.16). Specific complications related to the location of lesions can be summarized below:

Orbital/periorbital: Lesions involving the upper eyelid may cause visual distortion or obstruction on the affected side. Large lesions, posing a risk of amblyopia, represent one of the rare critical situations in the management of infantile hemangiomas (Fig. 3.6). Retro-ocular lesions present with exomphalos (Fig. 3.17).

Parotid: Especially when bilateral (beard distribution) may be associated with airway involvement and risk of respiratory complications (Fig. 3.18).

Table 3.1 The distribution of infantile hemangioma through different parts of the body among cases attending the vascular anomaly clinic over the last 10 years

Head and neck		Other parts of the body		
Periorbital	38	Trunk	21	
Parotid	33	Upper limb	17	
Scalp	29	Gluteal/lower limb	12	
Lip	29	Breast	5	
Nose	13	Perineal/genitalia	11	
Cheek	11	Sacrum	2	
Periauricular	7			
Neck	5			
Submandibular	2			
Diffuse lesions in the face	19			
Total	186	Total	68	254

Ear and nose: Ulceration of skin lesions may cause underlying cartilage necrosis (Figs. 3.16 and 3.19). Ulceration of the columella can result in collapse of nasal tip (Fig. 3.11c) [5].

Segmental lesions in the face may be associated with PHACE syndrome (Fig. 3.20) [6]. This is a well-known neurocutaneous disorder that will be covered in Chap. 4.

Lower back/Sacrum: It may be associated with underlying vertebral and spinal lesions (Fig. 3.21).

Multiple cutaneous hemangiomas (more than 3, Fig. 3.22) may be associated with visceral hemangiomas (liver).

Investigations are usually not required except for cases with doubtful diagnoses (atypical presentations), or when searching for associated anomalies or deeper extensions [7, 8]. During the proliferative phase, infantile hemangiomas typically appear on ultrasound as a homogeneous solid mass containing numerous high-flow vessels traversing the lesion (Figs. 3.23, 3.24, and 3.25) [9]. Magnetic Resonance Imaging (MRI) and Computed Tomography (CT) can demonstrate more anatomical details, especially for lesions with deeper extensions (e.g., the parotid and back; Figs. 3.26 and 3.27). MRI may be superior for its high soft tissue resolution and lack of ionizing radiation but requires general anesthesia. Typical MRI features of proliferative-phase infantile hemangiomas (Fig. 3.28) include a well-defined mass with characteristic 'flow voids'; the mass appears isointense to muscle on T1-weighted images, hyperintense on T2-weighted images, and shows intense, uniform enhancement following intravenous gadolinium administration [8–10].

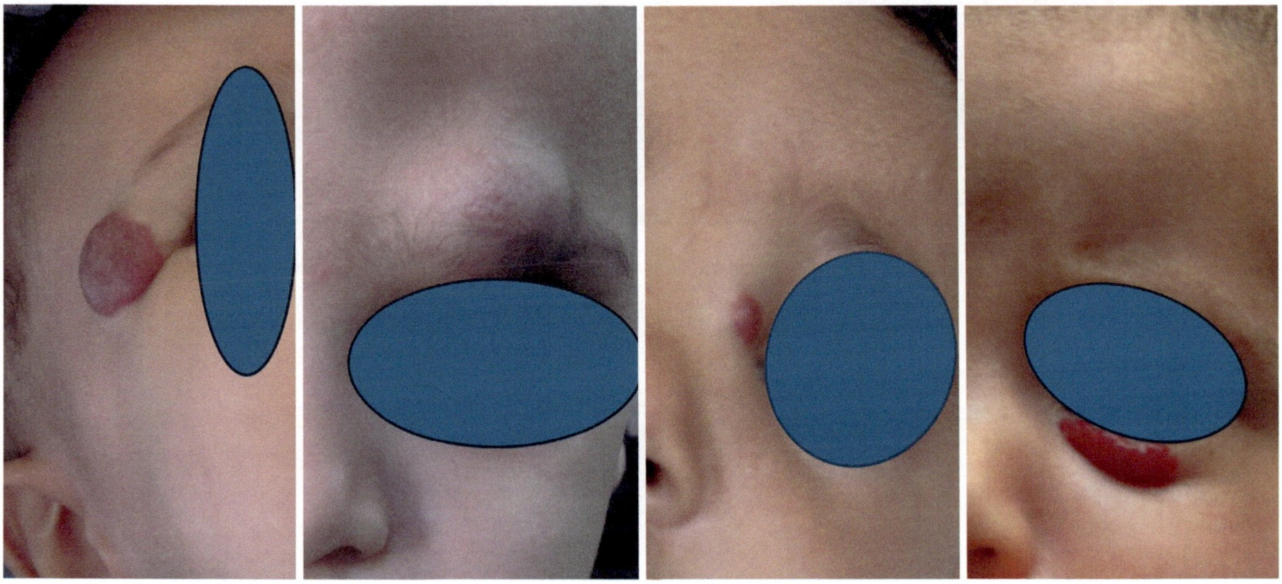

Fig. 3.7 Periorbital infantile hemangiomas in different cases and locations

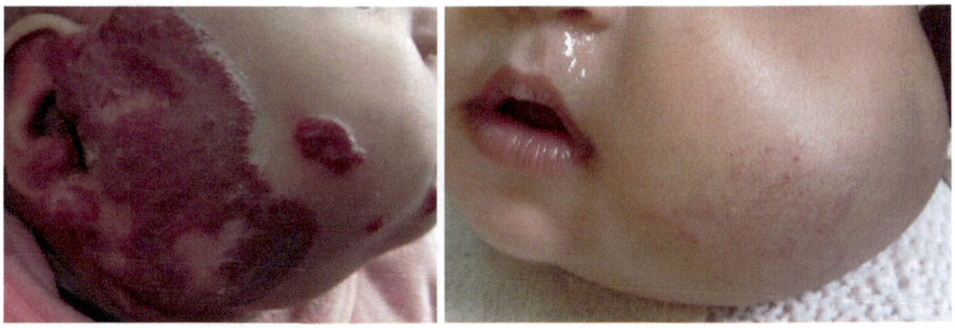

Fig. 3.8 Infantile hemangiomas of the parotid region in two different cases

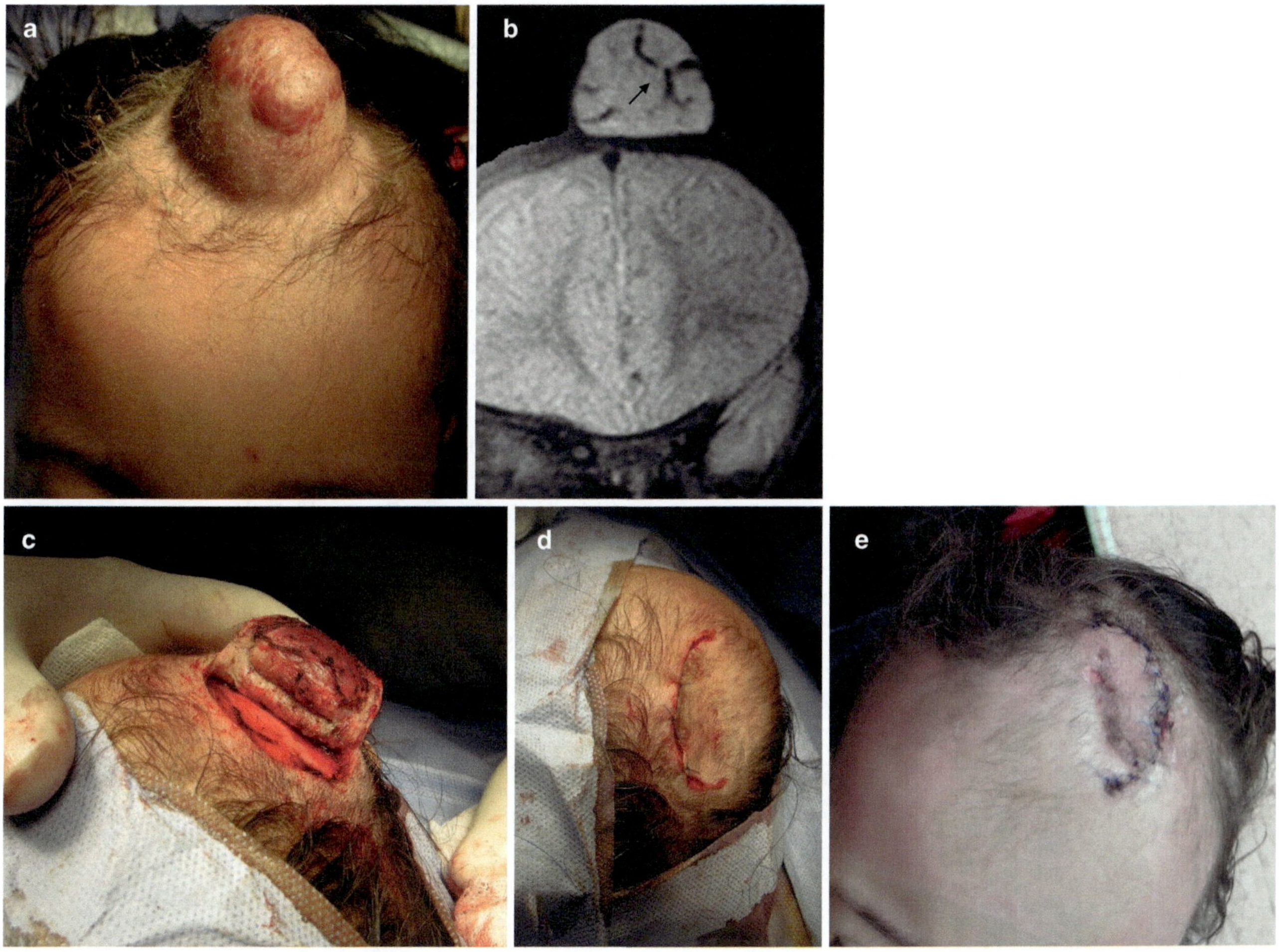

Fig. 3.9 Infantile hemangioma of the scalp. (**a**) Clinical appearance; (**b**) MRI showing a hyperintense mass with flow voids (arrow); (**c**–**e**) lack of response to medical therapy (propranolol, intralesional steroid/bleomycin) leading to surgical excision at 3 years, with skin flap preservation for defect coverage. (Reproduced from AbouZeid et al. [2]

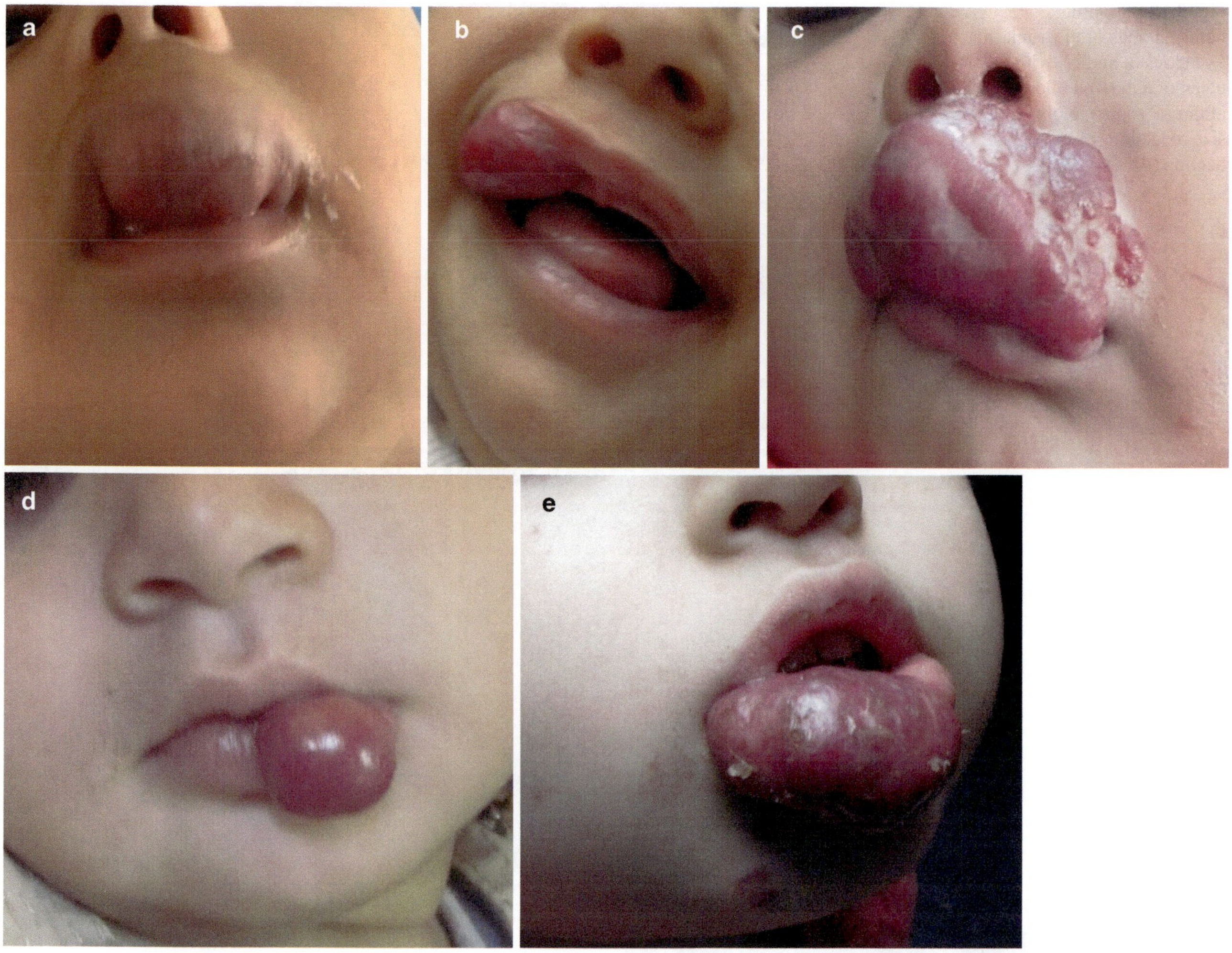

Fig. 3.10 Infantile hemangiomas of the upper lip in three cases (**a**–**c**) and of the lower lip in two cases (**d** and **e**)

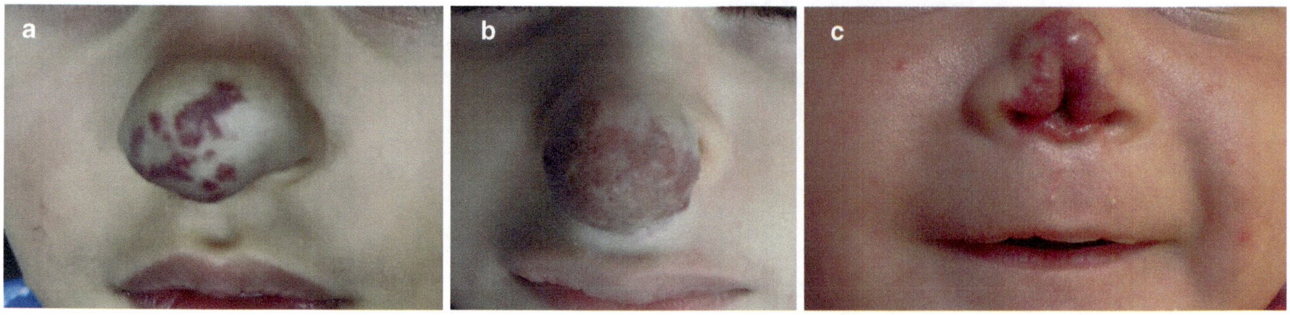

Fig. 3.11 Infantile hemangiomas of the nose in three cases (**a**–**c**), with columellar ulceration in (**c**)

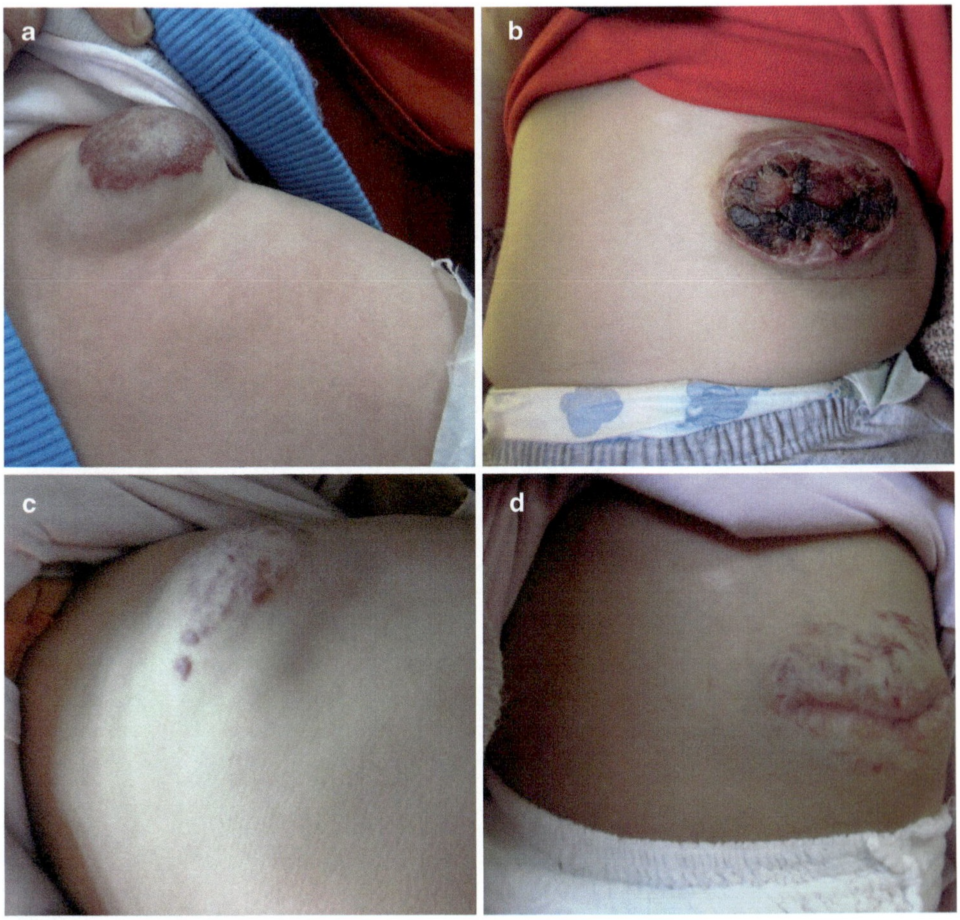

Fig. 3.12 Infantile hemangiomas of the trunk in two cases (**a** and **b**), with ulceration in (**b**). Follow-up after oral propranolol shows size reduction (**c**) and ulcer healing (**d**)

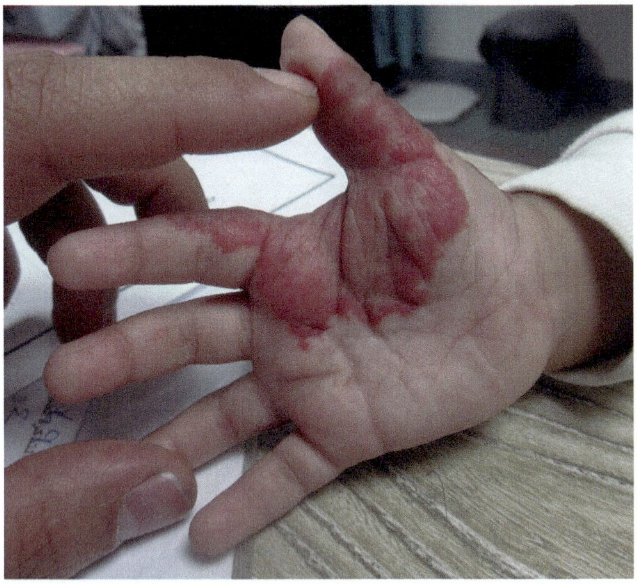

Fig. 3.13 Infantile hemangioma of right hand

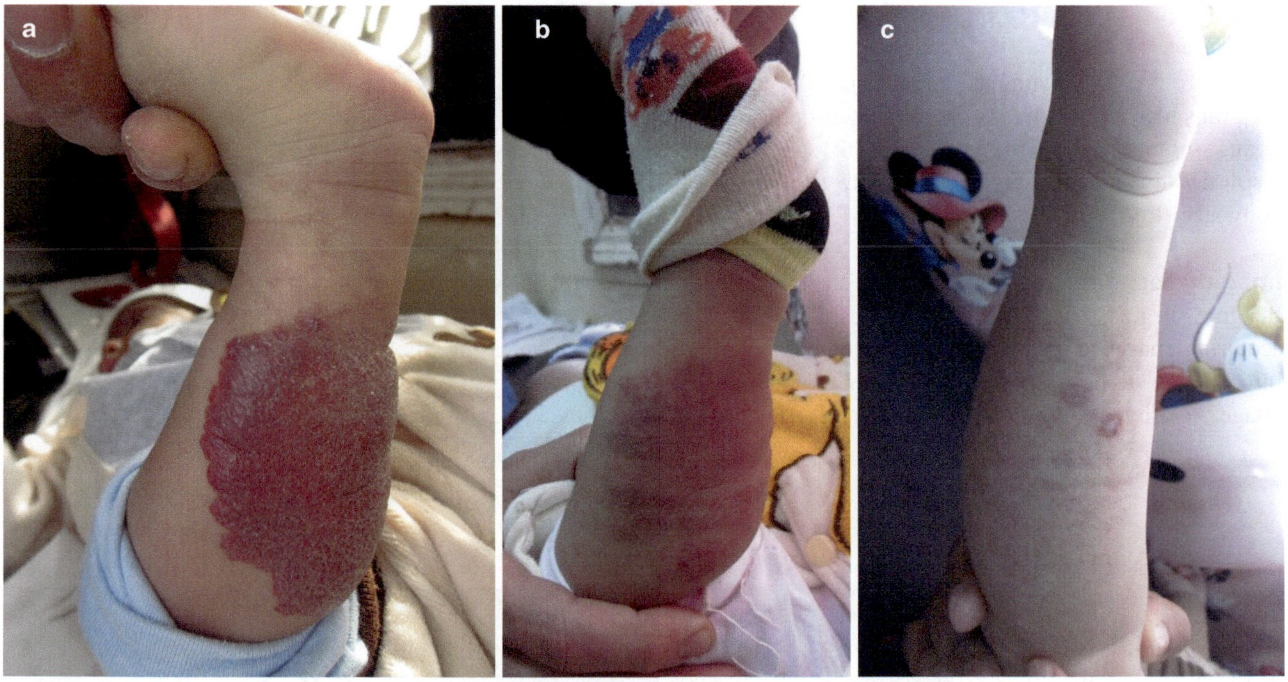

Fig. 3.14 Infantile hemangioma of the lower limb in the same patient showing excellent response to propranolol. (**a**) Proliferative phase at 2.5 months; (**b**) at 7 months; (**c**) regression at 12 months. (Reproduced from AbouZeid et al. [2])

Fig. 3.15 Infantile hemangiomas of the perineum in two cases

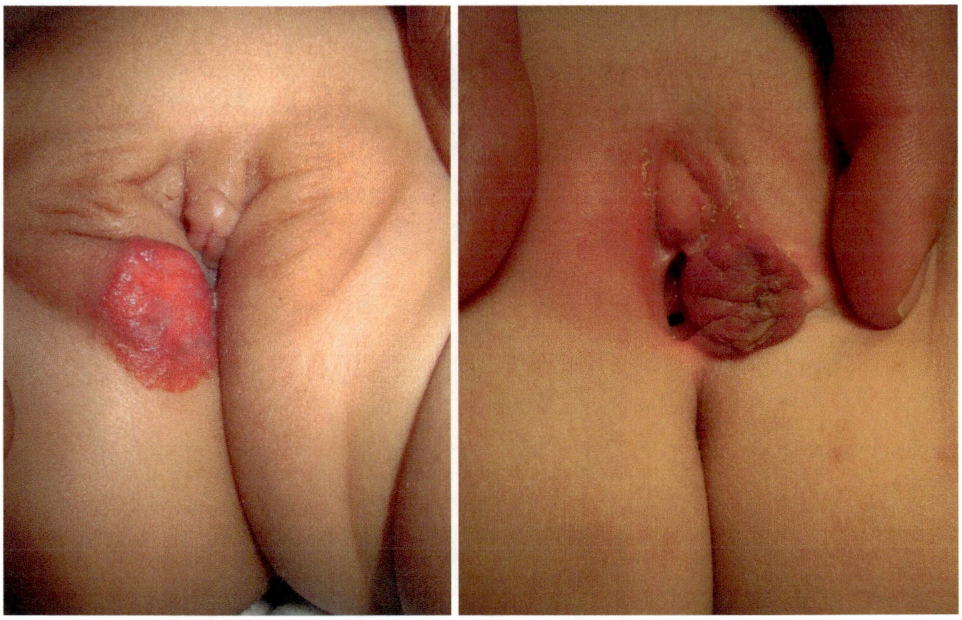

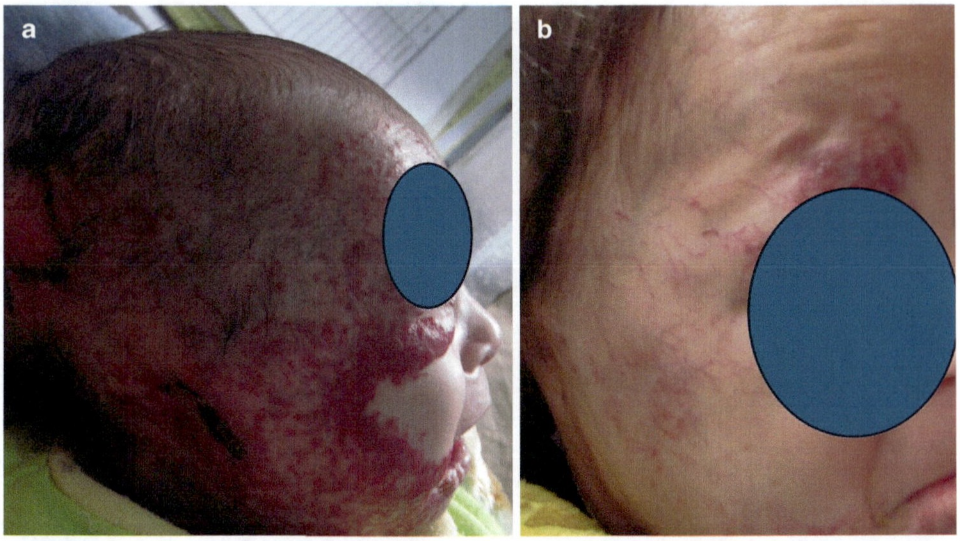

Fig. 3.16 Newborn with diffuse segmental infantile hemangioma complicated by skin ulceration and ear cartilage necrosis (**a**). Follow-up at 2 years after oral propranolol treatment (**b**)

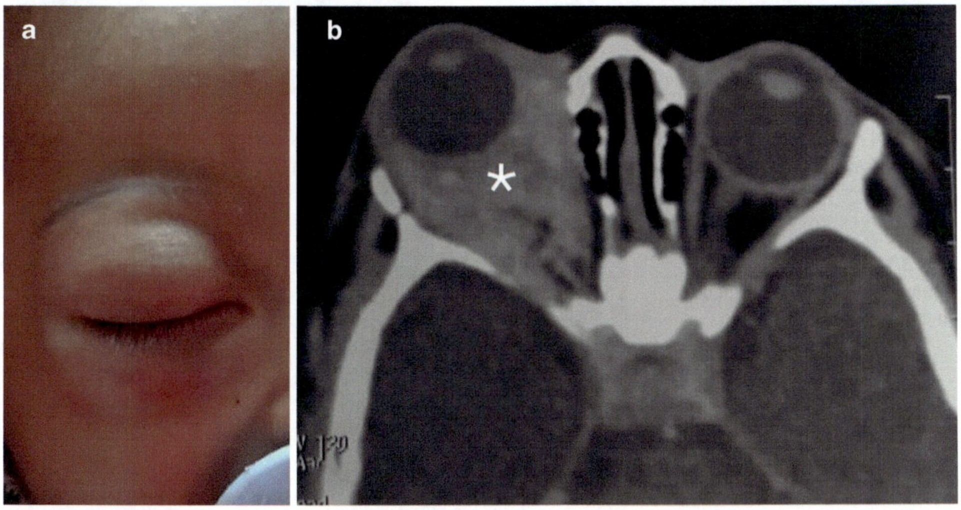

Fig. 3.17 Three-month-old girl with right retro-orbital infantile hemangioma presenting with proptosis (**a**). CT scan shows the retro-orbital lesion (asterisk) (**b**)

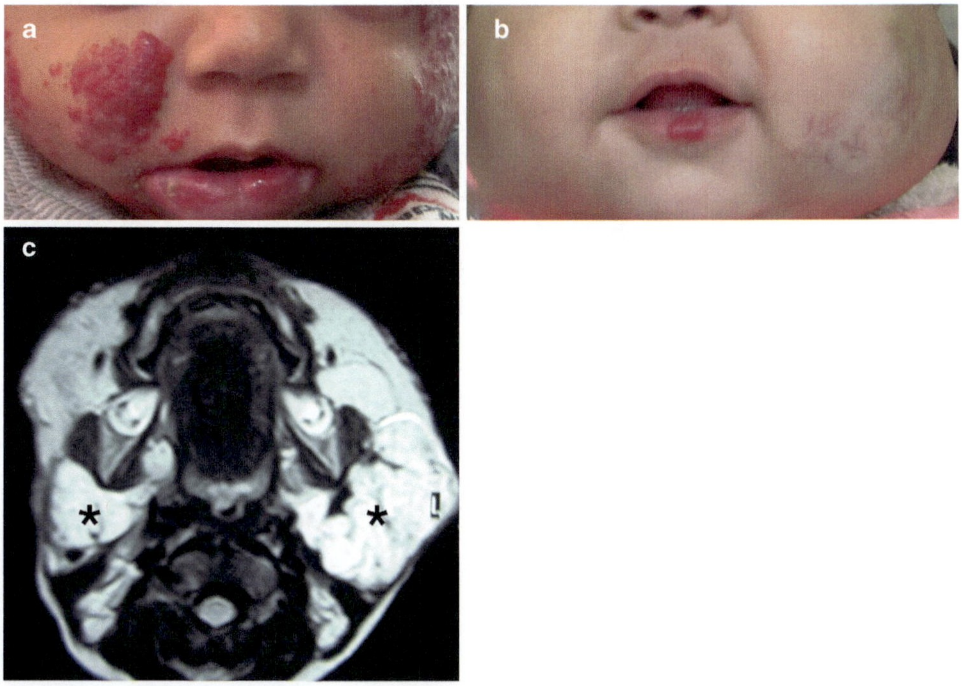

Fig. 3.18 Bilateral parotid infantile hemangiomas in two cases (**a** and **b**). (**c**) MRI of case (**a**) shows deep extension of the lesions (asterisks)

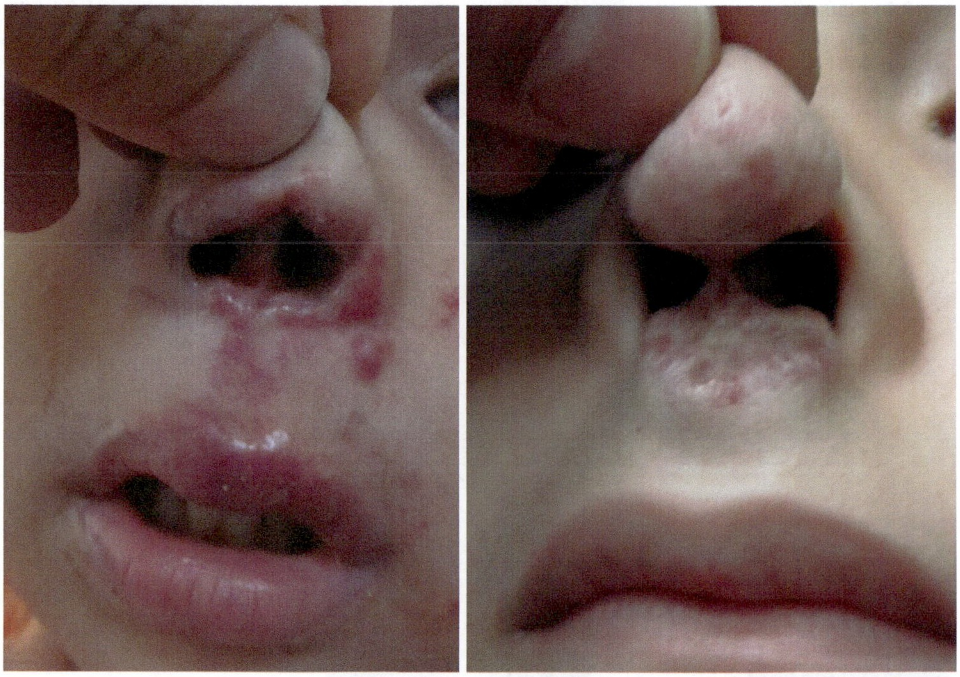

Fig. 3.19 Infantile hemangiomas of the nose in two cases, complicated by ulceration and nasal septal skin loss

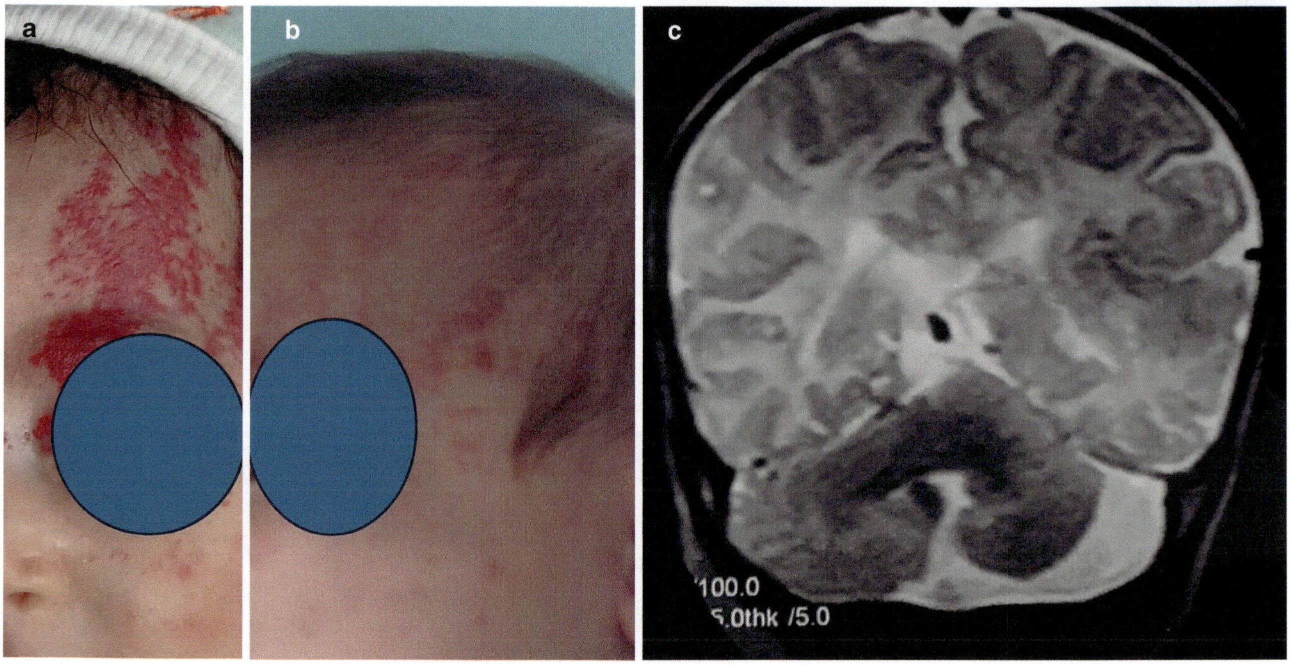

Fig. 3.20 Segmental facial hemangioma associated with posterior fossa anomalies (PHACE syndrome). (**a**) Skin lesion at 40 days; (**b**) good response to propranolol at 2 months; (**c**) MRI showing cerebellar hypoplasia

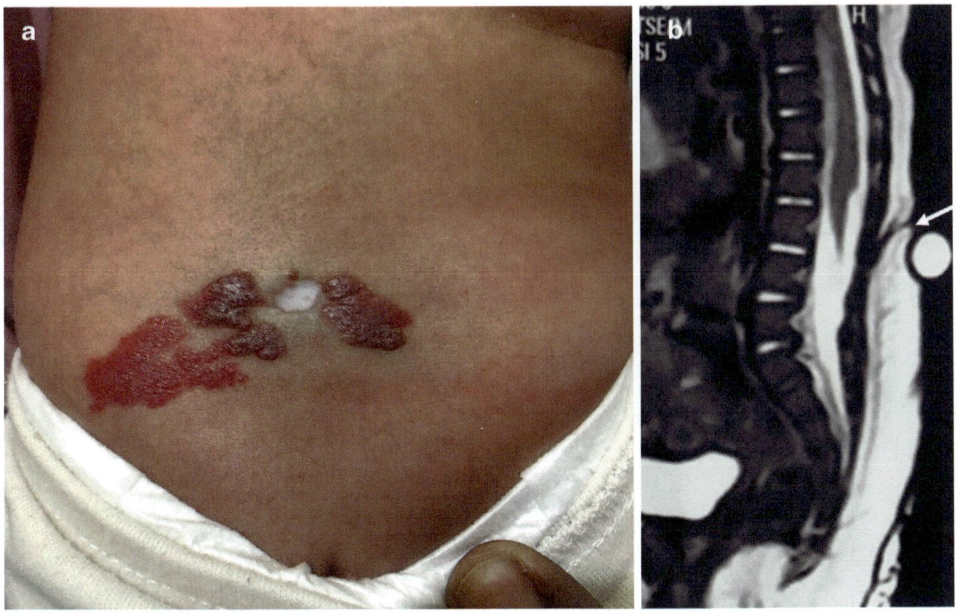

Fig. 3.21 Infantile hemangioma of the lower back (**a**). MRI of the same patient shows an associated dermal sinus (arrow) (**b**)

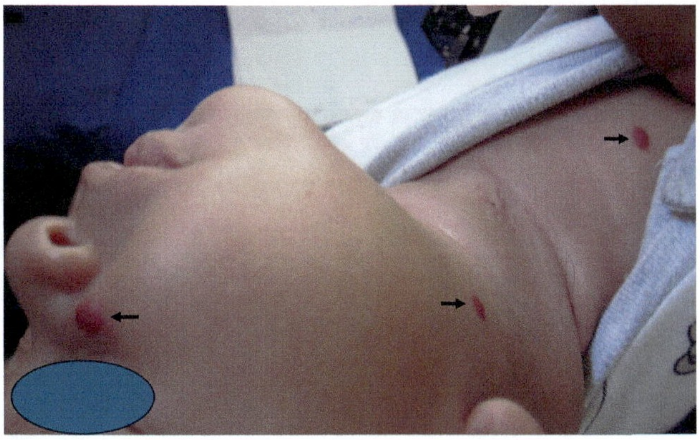

Fig. 3.22 Multiple cutaneous hemangiomas (arrows) may be associated with hepatic hemangioma

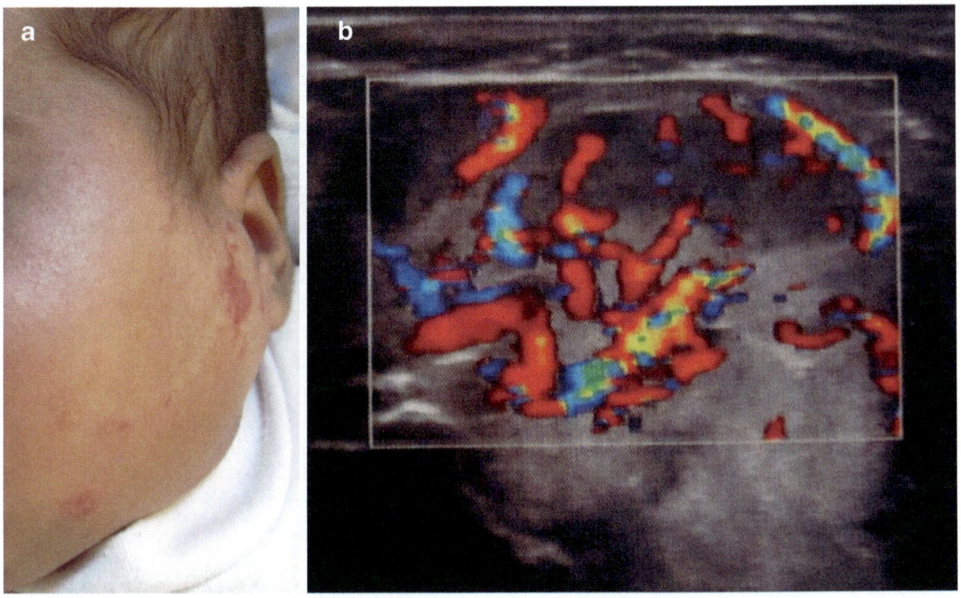

Fig. 3.23 Forty-day-old girl with parotid infantile hemangioma (**a**). Ultrasound shows a homogeneous solid mass with multiple high-flow vessels (**b**)

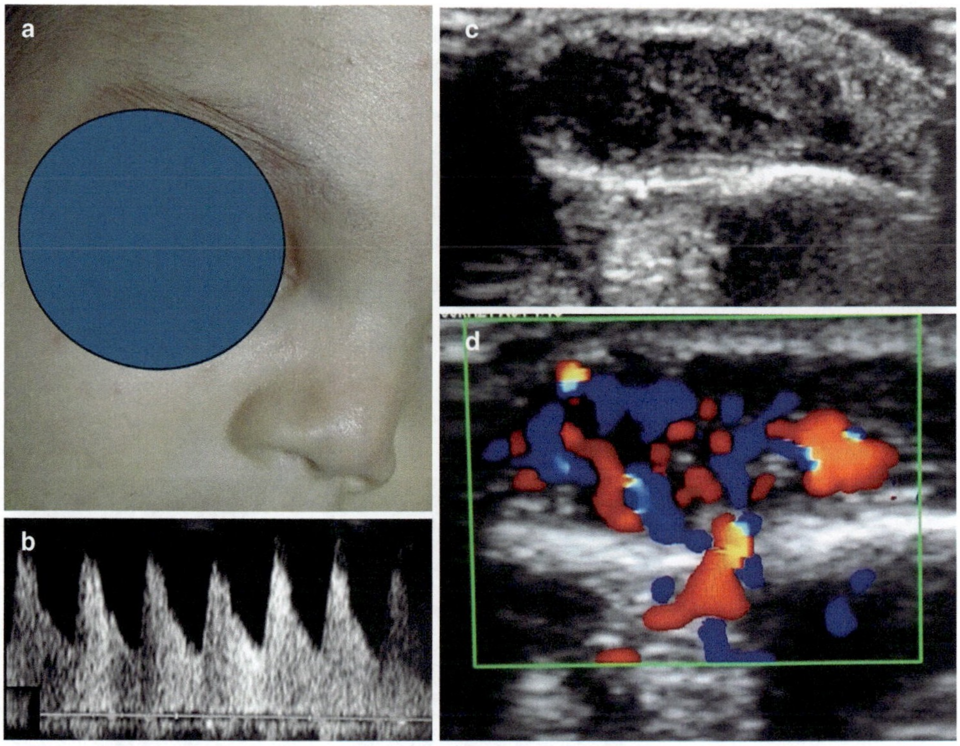

Fig. 3.24 Subcutaneous right internal angular infantile hemangioma. (**a**) Clinical appearance; (**b**) B-mode ultrasound showing a homogeneous hypoechoic soft tissue mass; (**c**) spectral Doppler demonstrating low-resistance arterial flow; (**d**) color Doppler showing increased vascularity

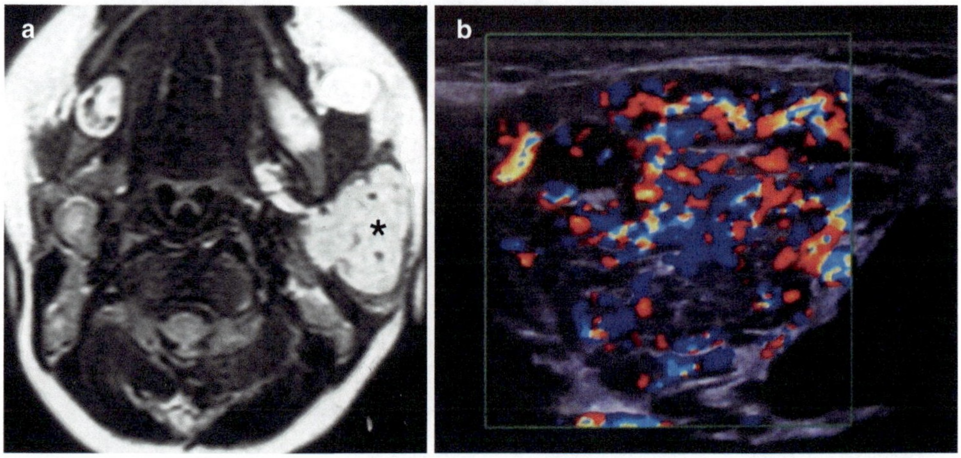

Fig. 3.25 Imaging of left parotid hemangioma. (**a**) Axial T2-weighted MRI shows a well-defined hyperintense mass with flow voids (asterisk); (**b**) ultrasound demonstrating multiple high-flow vessels

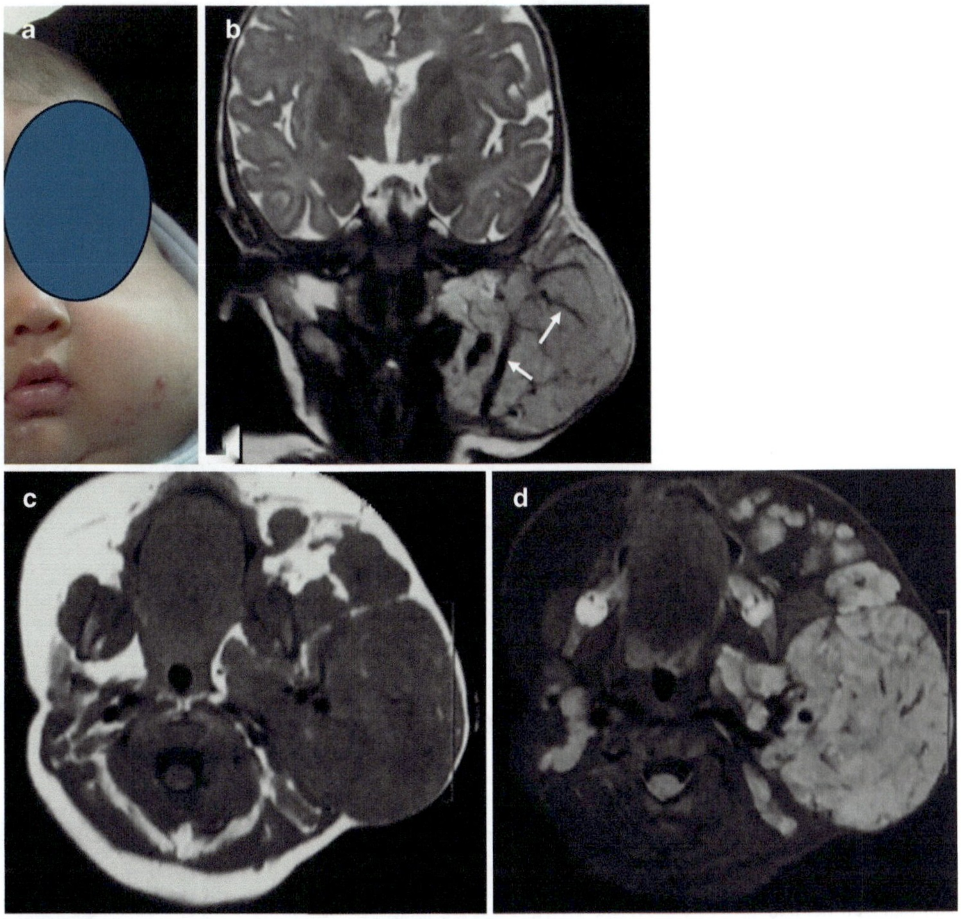

Fig. 3.26 Left parotid hemangioma. MRI shows a well-defined homogeneous mass with flow voids (arrows), hyperintense on T2-weighted images (**b**), isointense to muscle on T1 (**c**), and better localized on axial T2 with fat suppression (**d**)

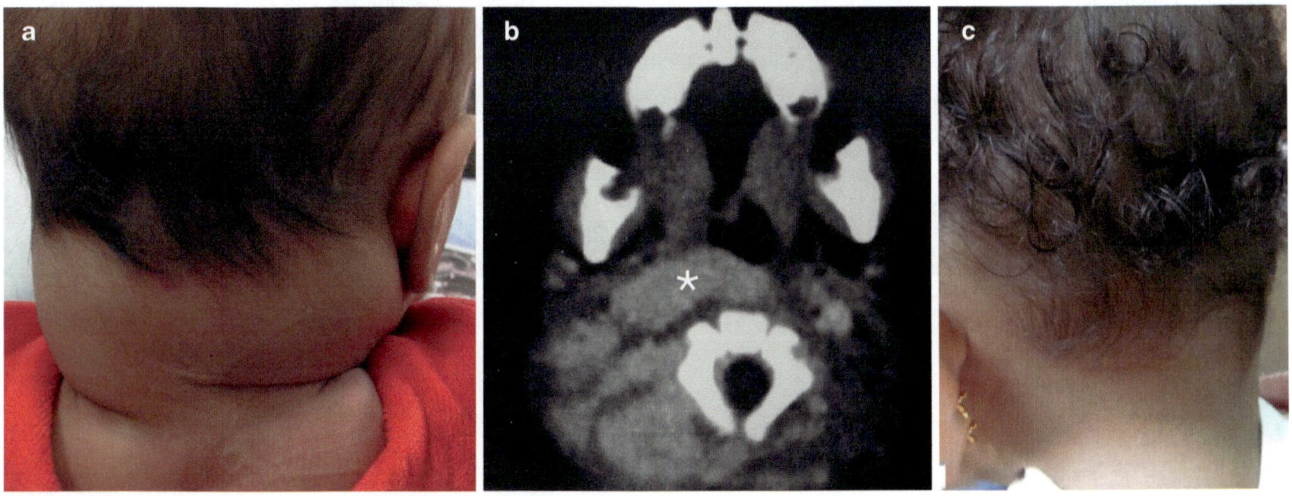

Fig. 3.27 Infantile hemangioma at the nape of a 3-month-old girl (**a**). CT shows deep prevertebral extension (asterisk) (**b**). Follow-up at 2 years after oral propranolol demonstrates regression (**c**)

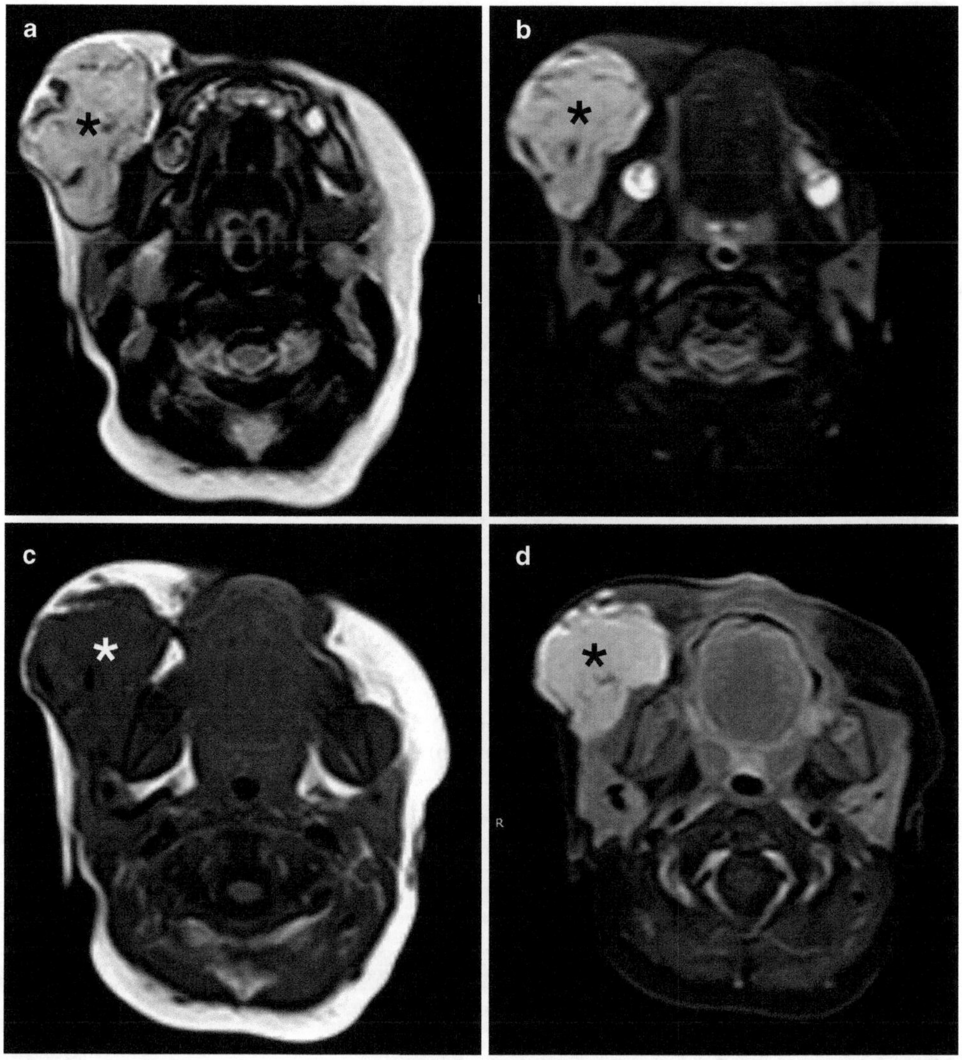

Fig. 3.28 MRI of infantile hemangioma. The lesion (asterisk) is a well-circumscribed soft tissue mass. It demonstrates hyperintense signal on T2-weighted and STIR sequences (**a** and **b**), hypointense signal on T1-weighted image (**c**), and intense, homogeneous contrast enhancement (**d**). Multiple internal flow voids indicate high vascularity, while preserved fat planes confirm absence of invasion

Treatment

Generally, IH requires no treatment (expectant treatment), waiting for spontaneous involution [1–3, 11]. Repeated reassurance for parents is required, as complete regression may be delayed up to the age of 7–9 years [1, 2]. Active intervention is necessary in specific situations: large lesions causing significant distortion, ulceration, airway involvement with risk of stridor, eye occlusion, or, commonly, social stress on the child and his family from lesions, particularly in the face [1–3].

Medical treatment In the early proliferative phase (within the first year of life), propranolol is the first-line treatment when clinically indicated [12]. An oral dose of 1–3 mg/kg/day in three divided doses is generally well tolerated (Figs. 3.29, 3.30, and 3.31) [1, 2]. Based on clinical response (tumor regression) and site-specific complications, oral propranolol can be tapered and discontinued between the ages of 1 and 2 years [2]. Alternatively, small superficial lesions may be treated with a topical timolol maleate solution or gel [13].

Intralesional injection Intralesional steroid injection (triamicinolone 2 mg/kg) can be used as a second line of treatment to accelerate tumor regression (Figs. 3.32 and 3.33) [1–3]. Alternatively, intralesional bleomycin injection 0.2–0.5 mg/kg (per dose) may be used for cases showing poor response to steroid injection [14].

Surgical treatment Surgery remains a valid option for lesions amenable to resection (localized lesions using hidden scars) (Figs. 3.34, 3.35, and 3.36) [1–3]. When indicated, surgical intervention is generally considered a second- or third-line treatment option between the ages of 2 and 4 years (Fig. 3.9).

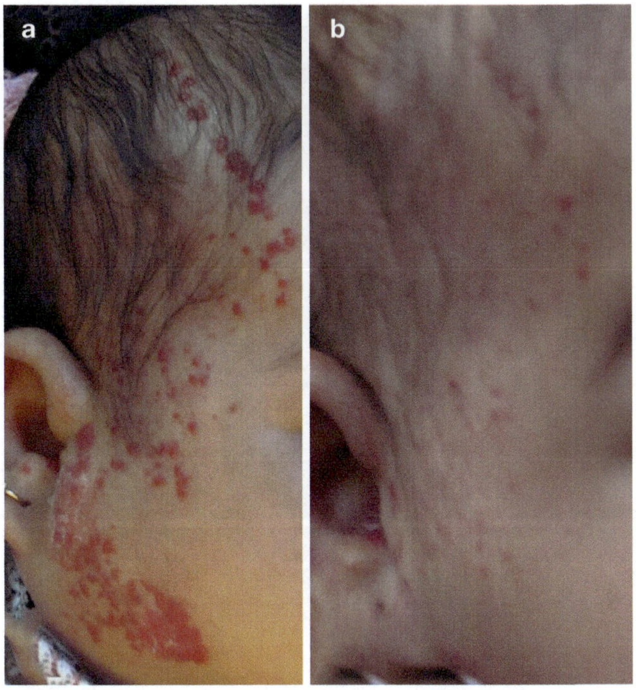

Fig. 3.29 Parotid hemangioma in a 2-month-old girl (**a**). Follow-up after 2 months shows good response to oral propranolol (**b**)

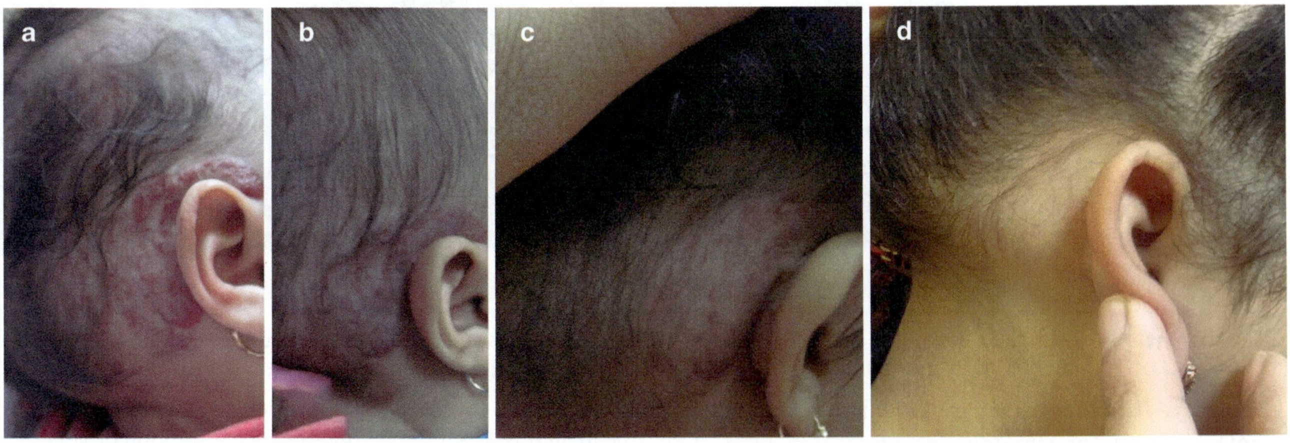

Fig. 3.30 Retro-auricular infantile hemangioma in a 3-month-old girl (**a**). Good response to oral propranolol (**b** and **c**). Follow-up at 4 years (**d**)

Fig. 3.31 Infantile hemangioma of the nasal tip (**a**) with good response to oral propranolol (**b**)

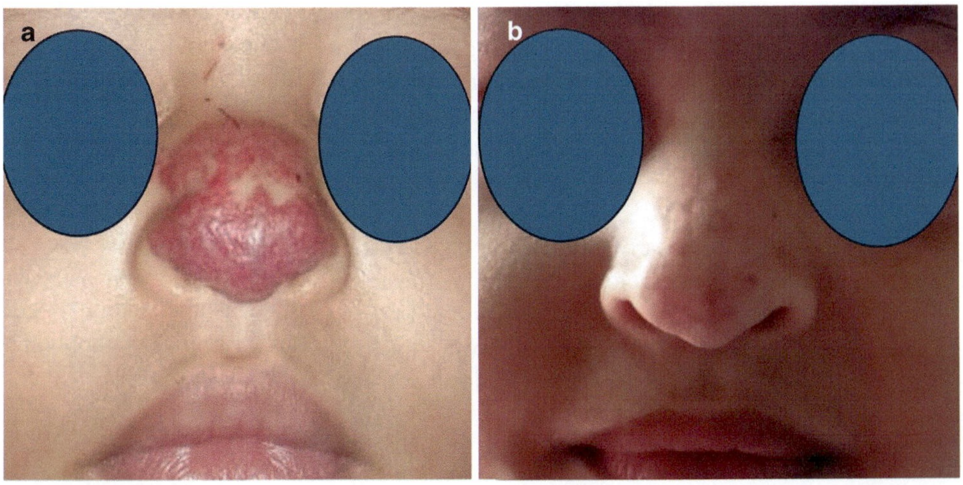

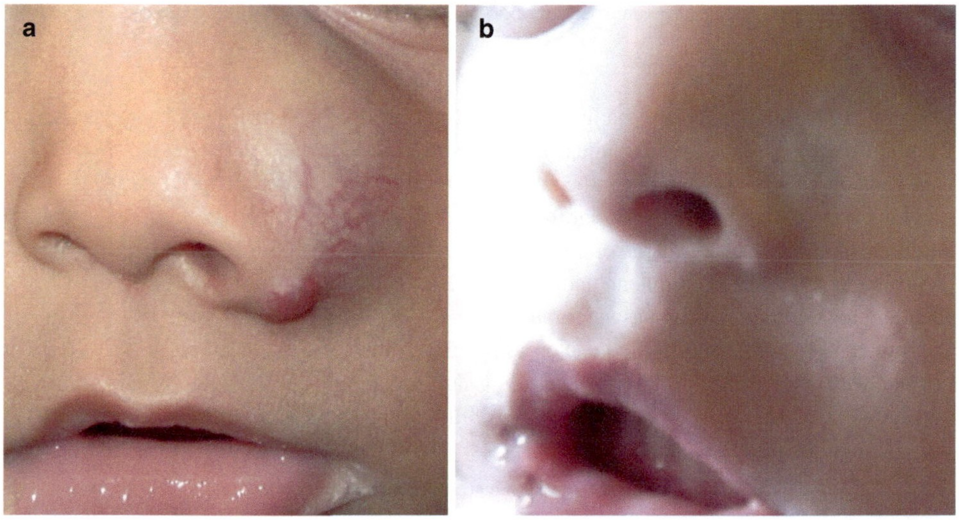

Fig. 3.32 Infantile hemangioma of the left nasolabial fold (**a**) with good response to local steroid injection (**b**)

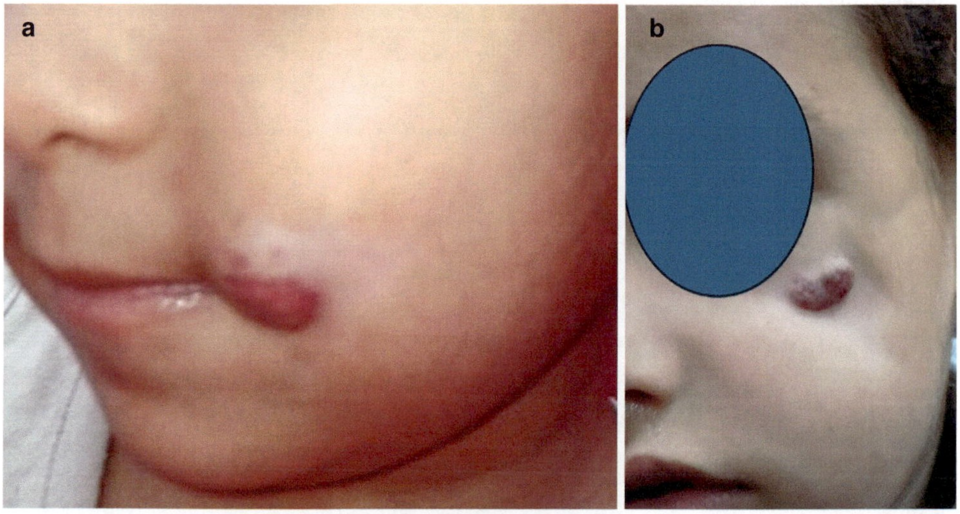

Fig. 3.33 Complications of local steroid injection in two patients: hypopigmentation (**a**) and skin atrophy (**b**)

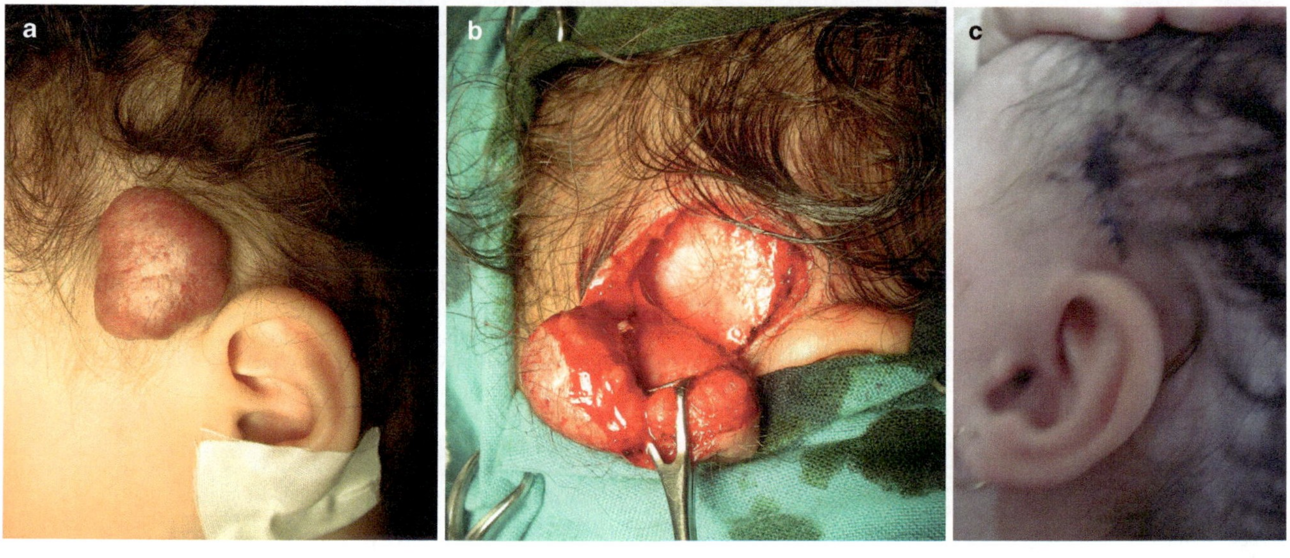

Fig. 3.34 Surgical excision of infantile hemangioma

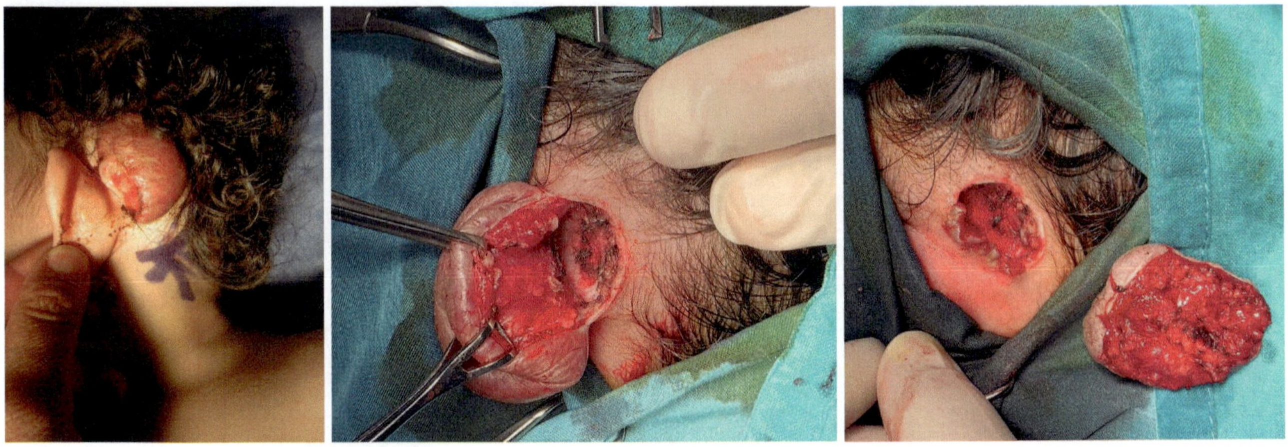

Fig. 3.35 Surgical excision of infantile hemangioma (post-auricular)

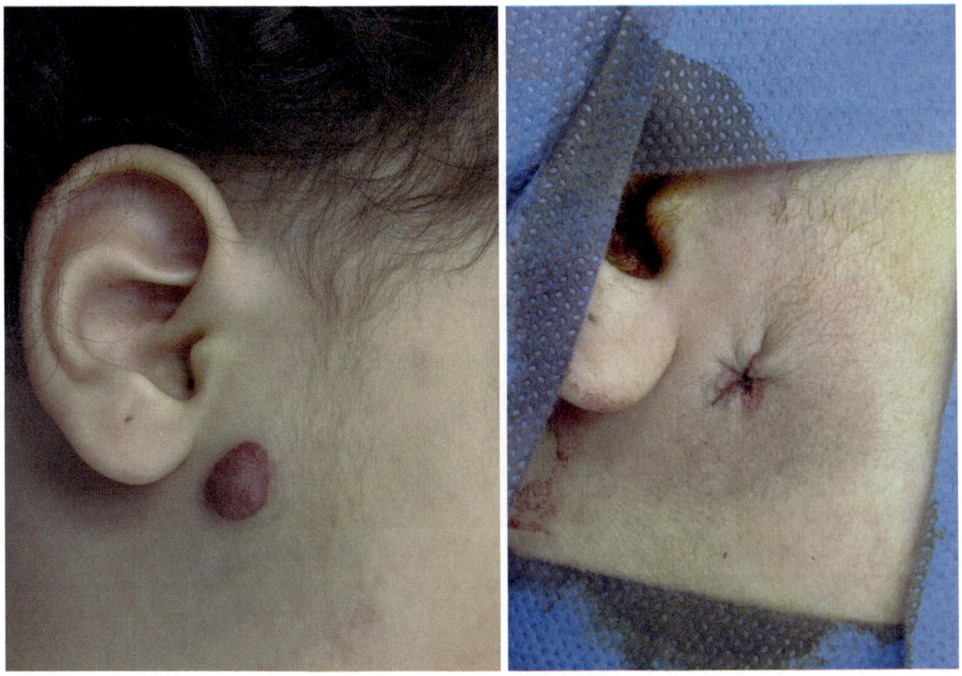

Fig. 3.36 Surgical excision of infantile hemangioma with purse string wound closure

References

1. Gokani VJ, Sivakumar B, Kangesu L. Vascular anomalies. Surgery (Oxford). 2018;36:314–23.
2. AbouZeid AA, Ragab IA, Mohammad SA, et al. Infantile haemangioma: 5-year experience at the vascular anomaly clinic. Egypt Pediatric Association Gaz. 2021;69:16. https://doi.org/10.1186/s43054-021-00062-2.
3. Strub G, Sidbury R, Bauman N. Vascular tumors: infantile hemangioma. In: Perkins JA, Balakrishnan K, editors. Evidence-based management of head and neck vascular anomalies. Springer; 2018. p. 37–46.
4. Mulliken JB, Bischoff J. Pathogenesis of infantile hemangioma. In: Mulliken JB, Burrows PE, Fishman SJ, editors. Mulliken & Young's vascular anomalies: hemangiomas and malformations. Oxford University Press; 2013. p. 43–67.
5. Waner M, Teresa MO. Nasal and lip infantile hemangiomas. In: Perkins JA, Balakrishnan K, editors. Evidence-based management of head and neck vascular anomalies. Springer; 2018. p. 121–30.
6. Gupta D, Rosbe K. PHACE syndrome. In: Perkins JA, Balakrishnan K, editors. Evidence-based management of head and neck vascular anomalies. Springer Nature Switzerland; 2018. p. 245–52.
7. Flors L, Park AW, Norton PT, Hagspiel KD, Leiva-Salinas C. Soft-tissue vascular malformations and tumors Part 1: classification, role of imaging and high-flow lesions. Radiologia (English edition). 2019;61:4–15.
8. Mohammad SA, AA AZ, Fawzi AM, et al. Magnetic resonance imaging of head and neck vascular anomalies: pearls and pitfalls. Ann Pediatr Surg. 2017;13:116–24.
9. Burrows PE, Paltiel HJ. Radiological imaging of hemangiomas and related vascular tumors. In: Mulliken JB, Burrows PE, Fishman SJ, editors. Mulliken & Young's vascular anomalies: hemangiomas and malformations. Oxford University Press; 2013. p. 111–60.

10. Mamlouk MD, Nicholson AD, Cooke DL, Hess CP. Tips and tricks to optimize MRI protocols for cutaneous vascular anomalies. Clin Imaging. 2017;45:71–80.
11. Sadick M, Wohlgemuth WA, Huelse R, et al. Interdisciplinary management of head and neck vascular anomalies: clinical presentation, diagnostic findings and minimal invasive therapies. Euro J Radiol Open. 2017;4:63–8.
12. Leaute-Labreze C, et al. Propranolol for severe hemangiomas of infancy. N Engl J Med. 2008;358:2649–51.
13. Herlihy E, Hochman M. Periocular vascular tumors: infantile hemangioma. In: Perkins JA, Balakrishnan K, editors. Evidence-based management of head and neck vascular anomalies. Springer; 2018. p. 105–11.
14. Pienaar C, Graham R, Geldenhuys S, Hudson DA. Intralesional bleomycin for the treatment of hemangiomas. Plast Reconstr Surg. 2006;117(1):221–6. https://doi.org/10.1097/01.prs.0000194906.61805.b0.

Segmental Hemangiomas and Common Associations

4

Introduction

Infantile hemangiomas (IHs) are the most prevalent tumors in infancy, characterized by a distinct biological behavior of initial rapid proliferation, followed by spontaneous regression, and non-recurrence [1]. They typically appear as cutaneous lesions, which may be either localized or segmentally distributed. In most cases, we can expect a benign course with a favorable and predictable outcome. Segmental hemangiomas may be more liable for complications. A famous example is segmental hemangiomas on the face (Fig. 4.1), which may be associated with brain and cardiac anomalies, a condition known as PHACE syndrome [2]. Another example is segmental hemangiomas located in the mandibular region "beard distribution" that have been linked to airway involvement [3]. Additionally, the presence of multiple cutaneous hemangiomas may indicate the existence of visceral hemangiomas, most commonly in the liver [4]. In this chapter, we are going to highlight these specific associations with cutaneous infantile hemangiomas.

Segmental Face Hemangiomas and "PHACE" Syndrome

PHACE is an acronym representing a constellation of anomalies: **P**osterior fossa brain malformations (Fig. 4.2), **H**emangiomas, **A**rterial anomalies, **C**ardiac defects including **C**oarctation of the aorta, and **E**ye abnormalities [5]. When **S**ternal defects are present, the condition is sometimes referred to as PHACES [2]. Typical presentations involve large facial infantile hemangiomas (exceeding 5 cm in diameter) that follow a segmental distribution, commonly affecting the frontotemporal, maxillary, or mandibular regions

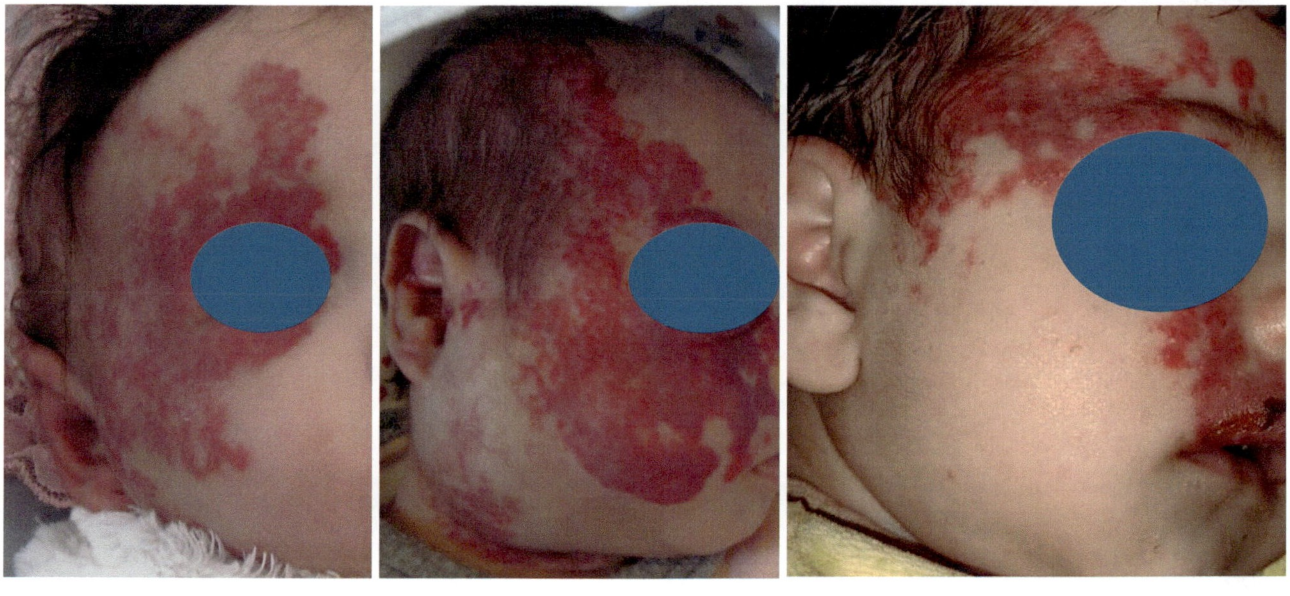

Fig. 4.1 Segmental facial hemangiomas in three different cases

A. A. AbouZeid et al., *Atlas of Pediatric Vascular Anomalies*, https://doi.org/10.1007/978-3-032-30866-5_4

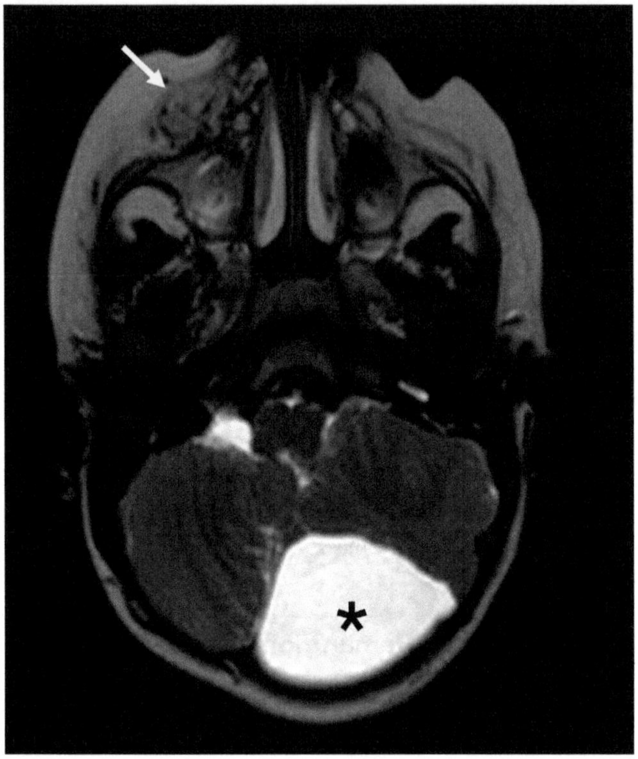

Fig. 4.2 Facial hemangioma with PHACE syndrome in a one-year-old girl. Axial T2-weighted MRI shows the hemangioma (arrow) with internal flow voids, associated with left cerebellar hypoplasia and a posterior fossa cyst (asterisk)

(Fig. 4.3) [2]. In some cases, hemangiomas associated with PHACE syndrome may be smaller in size or appear in atypical locations such as the scalp, neck, or chest wall [6, 7].

One of the key diagnostic criteria for PHACE syndrome involves anomalies in the major cerebral arteries, such as their absence, moderate to severe underdevelopment (hypoplasia), or an abnormal origin or course (Figs. 4.3 and 4.4) [2]. The presence of such cerebral vascular anomalies poses a potential risk for vascular events, such as stroke (Fig. 4.5) [8, 9]. In such cases, initiating propranolol treatment for facial hemangiomas at lower doses with a slower titration schedule is recommended [2].

Evaluation for PHACE syndrome:

- Brain imaging to diagnose structural anomalies: posterior fossa brain anomalies (Fig. 4.2), Dandy-Walker complex (Fig. 4.6).
- Magnetic Resonance Angiography (MRA) of cerebral, head, and neck vessels (Fig. 4.4).
- Echocardiography/CT angiography (aortic arch anomalies, coarctation of aorta) (Fig. 4.7).
- Ocular examination (retinal vascular anomalies, optic nerve hypoplasia).
- Appropriate airway evaluation (direct laryngoscopy) especially with segmental facial hemangiomas in the mandibular region (also known as beard distribution, Fig. 4.8).

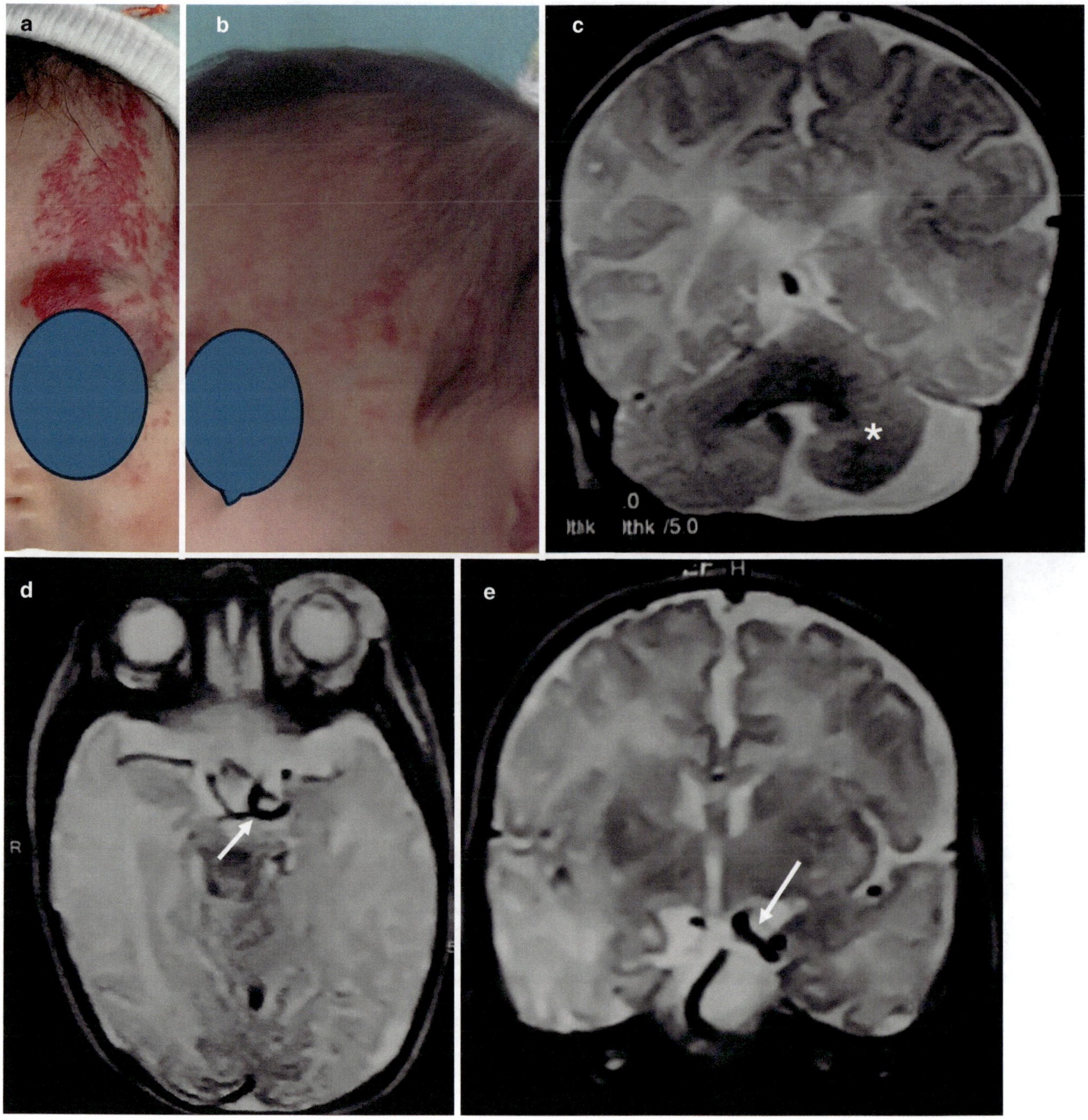

Fig. 4.3 Forty-day-old girl with infantile hemangioma and PHACE syndrome. Clinical photos at presentation (**a**) and after 2 months of oral propranolol (**b**). (**c**–**e**) Coronal T2-WI (trans-cerebellar plane) shows the "tilted telephone receiver" sign with upward displacement and hypoplasia of the left cerebellar hemisphere (asterisk). Axial and coronal T2-WI demonstrate tortuous major cerebral vessels (arrows)

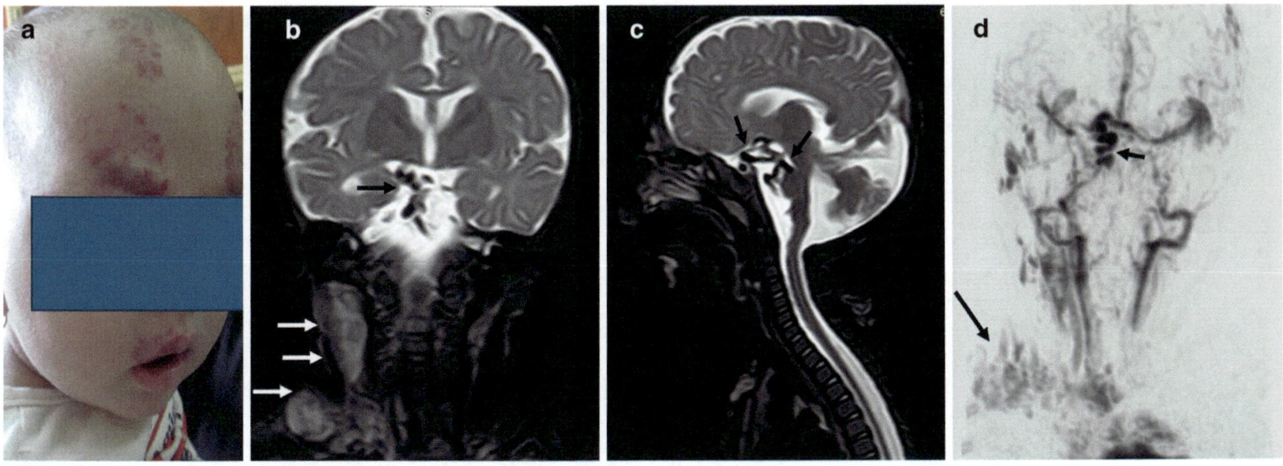

Fig. 4.4 Infantile hemangioma with PHACE syndrome. (**a**) Clinical photo showing cutaneous hemangioma. (**b**, **c**) Coronal and sagittal T2-WI demonstrate a hyperintense hemangioma (white arrows) with tortuous basilar and posterior cerebral vessels (black arrow). (**d**) Coronal (maximum intensity projection) from arterial-phase contrast-enhanced MRA shows early arterial enhancement of the hemangioma (long arrow) and basilar artery tortuosity (short arrow)

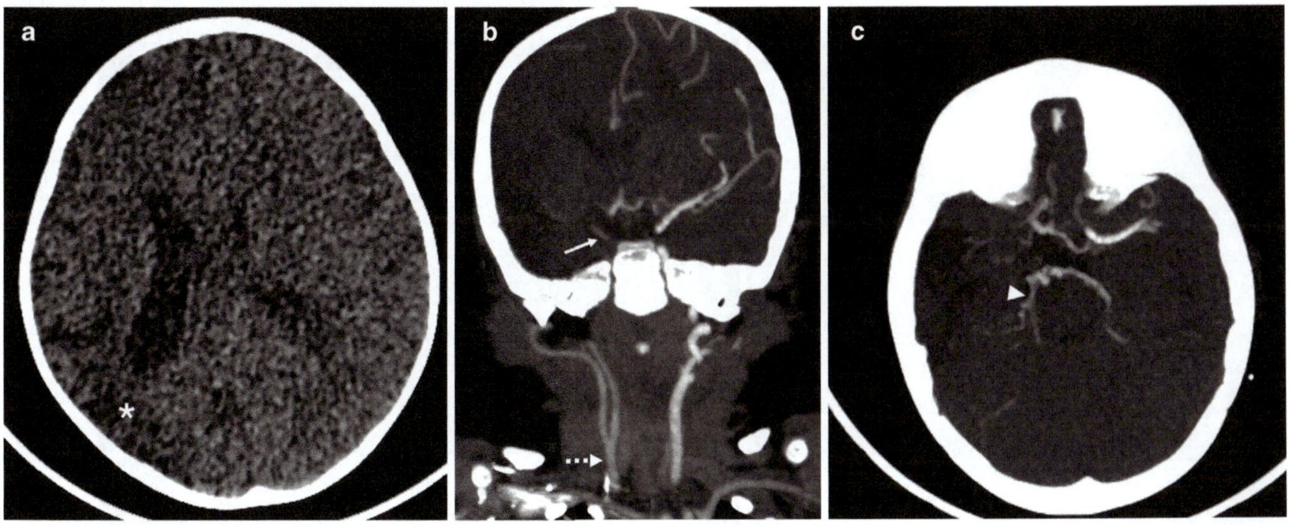

Fig. 4.5 Infantile hemangioma with PHACE syndrome in a 2-month-old girl. (**a**) Axial CT shows atrophy of the right cerebral hemisphere with area of encephalomalacia (asterisk) denoting old infarction. (**b**, **c**) Coronal and axial CT angiography demonstrate hypoplastic right carotid artery (dashed arrow), markedly attenuated right internal carotid artery (solid arrow), absent opacification of the right middle cerebral artery, and tortuous right posterior cerebral artery (arrowhead)

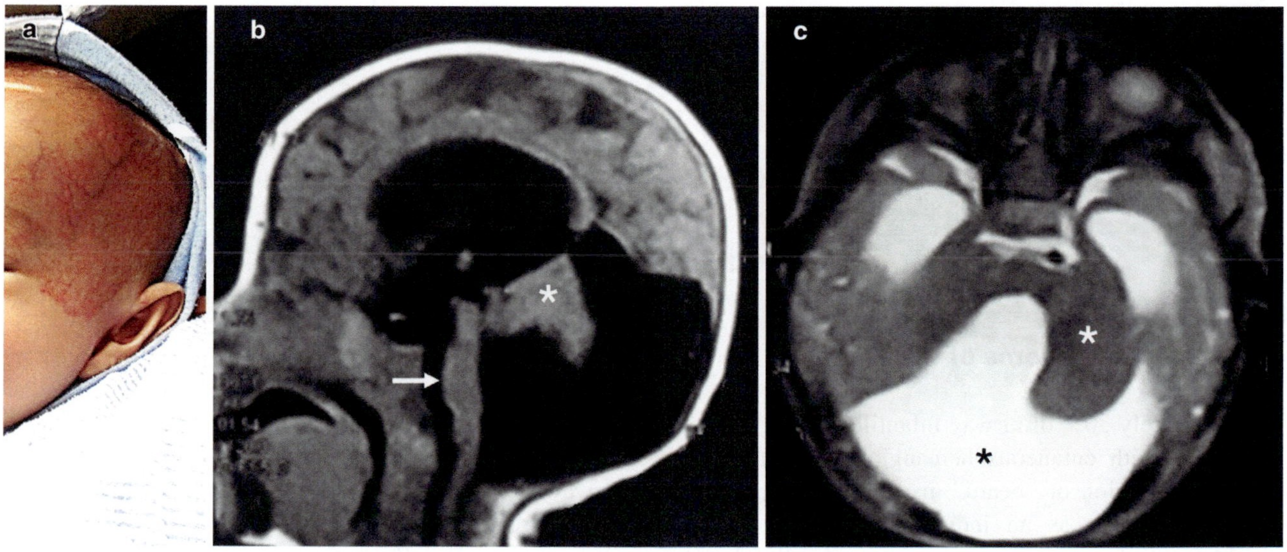

Fig. 4.6 Infantile hemangioma associated with Dandy–Walker malformation and PHACE syndrome. (**a**) Clinical photograph showing a cutaneous hemangioma. (**b**, **c**) Sagittal T1-weighted and axial T2-weighted images demonstrate cerebellar hypoplasia (white asterisk), brainstem hypoplasia (arrow), a large posterior fossa cyst (black asterisk), and dilatation of the ventricular system

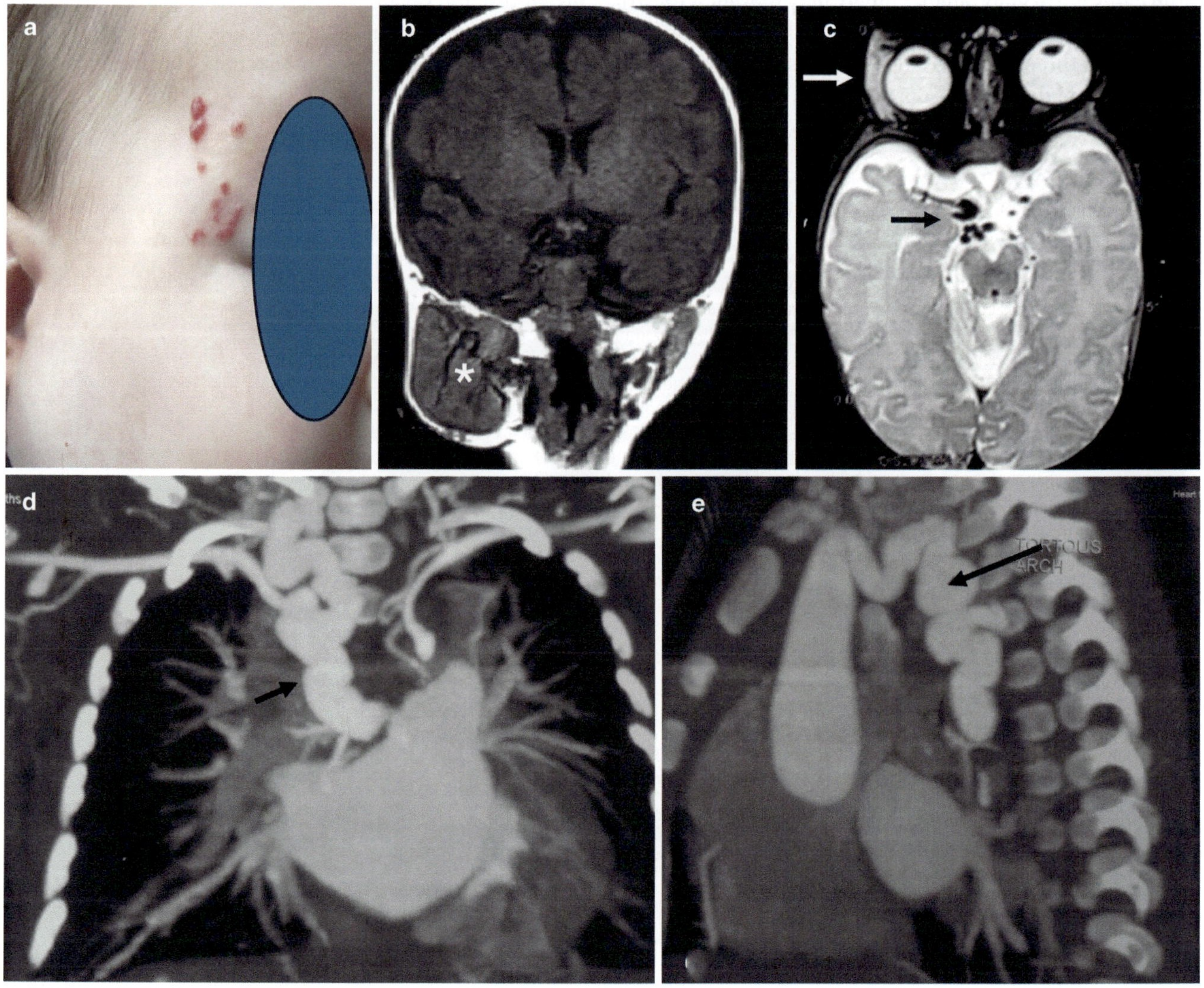

Fig. 4.7 Two-month-old girl with PHACE syndrome. (**a**) Clinical photograph shows parotid enlargement with a small cutaneous hemangioma. (**b**) Coronal T1-weighted image demonstrates a hypointense lesion in the parotid gland with multiple flow voids (hemangioma, asterisk). (**c**) Axial T2-weighted image reveals a hyperintense hemangioma in the right orbit (white arrow) with associated tortuosity of the arteries of the circle of Willis (black arrow). (**d**, **e**) Coronal and sagittal CT angiography demonstrate tortuosity and dilatation of the thoracic aorta (arrow)

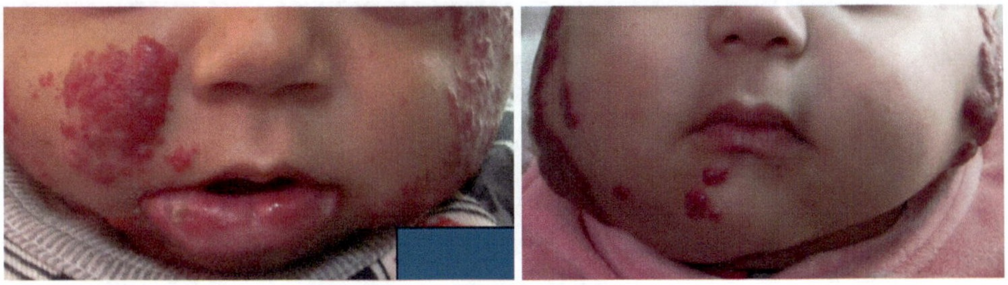

Fig. 4.8 Segmental facial hemangiomas in the mandibular region (beard distribution)

Infantile Hemangioma of the Airway

Approximately 50% of airway infantile hemangiomas are associated with cutaneous hemangiomas located in the mandibular region or "beard" distribution (Fig. 4.8) [3]. The latter serves as an indicator suggesting potential involvement of the airway. Lesions are usually absent or barely noticeable at birth, but they tend to grow rapidly during the first few months of life, potentially leading to airway obstruction and resulting in respiratory distress [3]. Mild cases are asymptomatic; others may present with stridor, cough, wheezing, or croup. Definitive diagnosis depends on direct laryngoscopy demonstrating characteristic lesions in the glottis, supra- or infra-glottic regions [2, 3], while cross-sectional imaging (CT/MRI) is occasionally needed to assess extra-tracheal and mediastinal involvement (Figs. 4.9 and 4.10) [2, 3]. The primary aim of treatment is to decrease the size of the lesions to preserve airway patency until they naturally regress. Oral propranolol is currently the first-line treatment [10], which has been shown to be more effective and have less side effects than steroids (Fig. 4.11). More recently, the newly introduced m-TOR inhibitors (sirolimus) have been used successfully to treat resistant cases [11, 12]. Surgery may represent a last resort for severe symptomatic cases after failure of various drug therapies [2, 3]. Surgical options include excision, laryngeal reconstruction, or tracheostomy (Fig. 4.9).

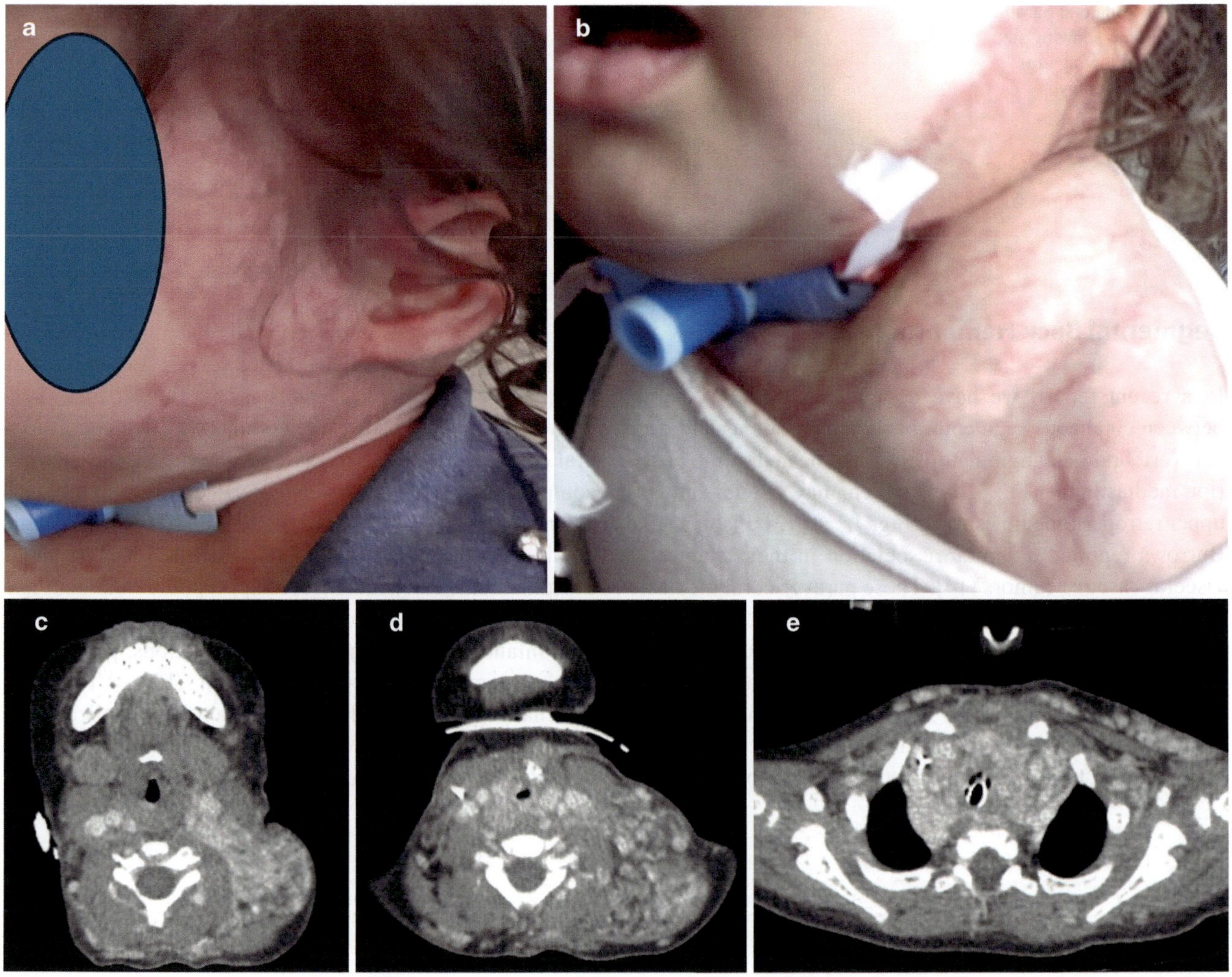

Fig. 4.9 (**a**, **b**) Three-month-old girl with facial hemangioma (beard distribution, extending to upper chest) presenting with severe stridor requiring tracheostomy. (**c**–**e**) CT shows deep extension of hemangiomas in the neck and mediastinum encasing the airway as an enhancing soft tissue mass

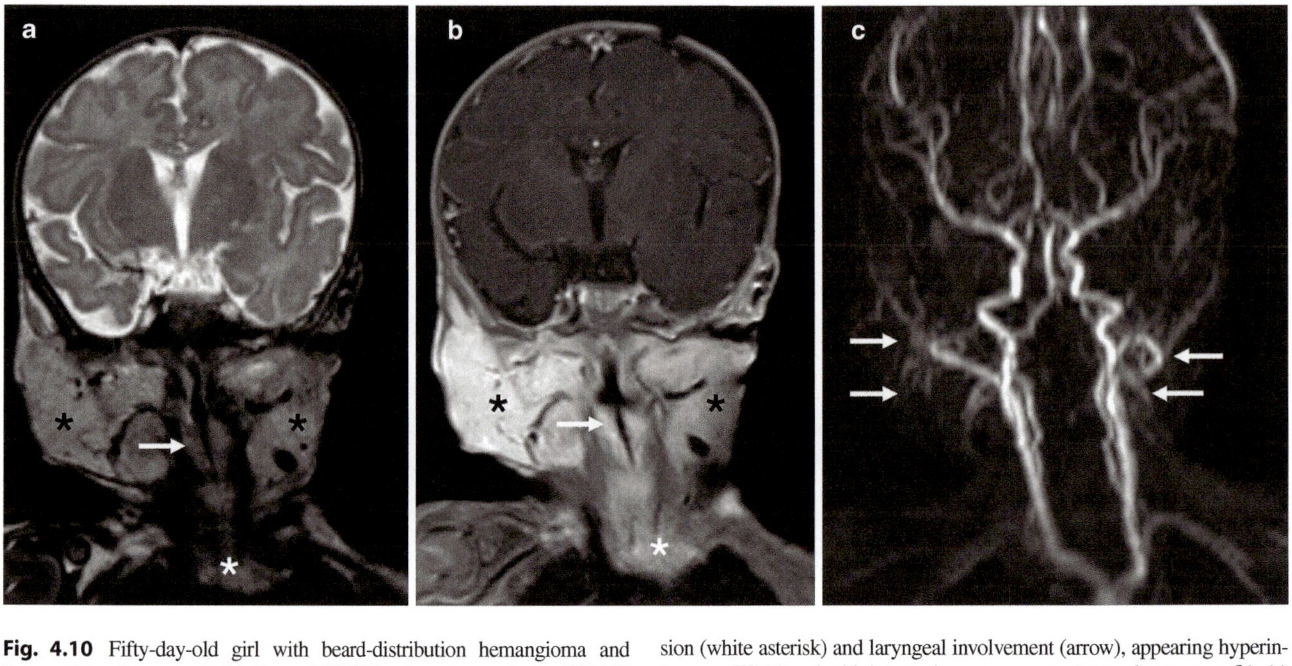

Fig. 4.10 Fifty-day-old girl with beard-distribution hemangioma and laryngeal involvement. (**a**, **b**) Coronal T2-WI and contrast-enhanced T1-WI show bilateral parotid hemangiomas (black asterisk) with mediastinal extension (white asterisk) and laryngeal involvement (arrow), appearing hyperintense on T2 (**a**) and with intense homogenous contrast enhancement (**b**). (**c**) MR angiography shows increased vascularity (arrows)

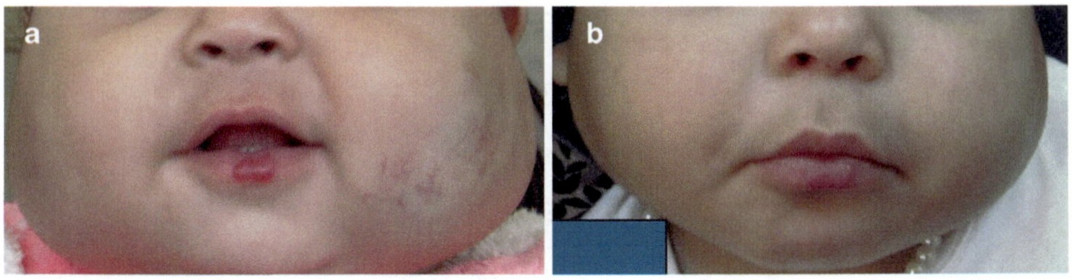

Fig. 4.11 Bilateral parotid hemangiomas showing size reduction following oral propranolol therapy

Segmental Back Hemangiomas

In a recent report, we have demonstrated an association between cutaneous segmental back hemangiomas and deep paravertebral hemangiomatous lesions located in the posterior mediastinum (Fig. 4.12), which may extend into the upper retroperitoneum as well (Fig. 4.13) [13]. Fishman and Burrows reported a similar association in their chapter on visceral vascular tumors [14]. These paravertebral mediastinal masses can raise suspicion for malignancy, particularly neuroblastoma [13]. However, awareness of this association, in addition to the typical imaging characteristics of hemangioma [15], can help resolve this diagnostic confusion. In doubtful situations, invasive diagnostic biopsy may turn out to be necessary [13]. Moreover, the rapid proliferation of hemangiomas in this critically deep location encasing the airway (Fig. 4.14) and major vessels (Fig. 4.15), can result in compression manifestations (mediastinal syndrome). Segmental back hemangiomas with deep paravertebral components have been associated with various serious complications, including respiratory distress, intraspinal extension (Figs. 4.14 and 4.16), scoliosis (Fig. 4.17), and renal atrophy (Fig. 4.13) [13]. Given the risk of such serious complications, early initiation of appropriate treatment and careful ongoing follow-up are essential after diagnosis. As with infantile hemangiomas in other locations, propranolol is considered the first-line treatment (Fig. 4.18) [10]. Alternatively, in cases that are resistant or complicated by propranolol-related side effects, steroids and, more recently, mTOR inhibitors may be employed [11–13].

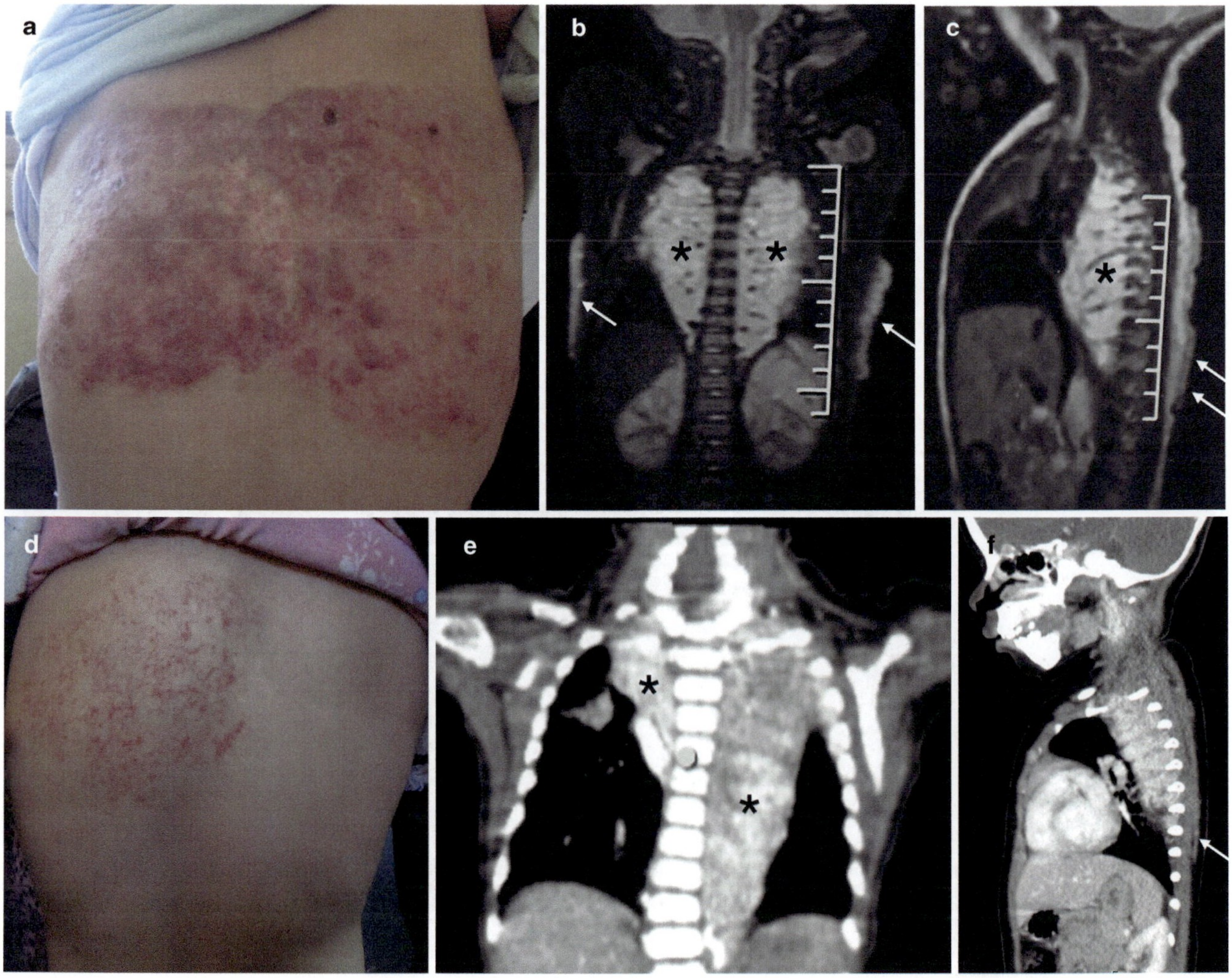

Fig. 4.12 Infantile hemangioma of the back with mediastinal extension in two patients. (**a–c**) Case 1: Clinical photo, MRI (coronal STIR), and MRI sagittal contrast-enhanced T1. Note the paraspinal extension (asterisk) in (**b**, **c**), and intense contrast enhancement in (**c**); white arrows are pointing to cutaneous lesions. (**d–f**) Case 2: Clinical photo and coronal and sagittal contrast-enhanced CT show enhancing paraspinal lesion (asterisk) with associated cutaneous component (arrow)

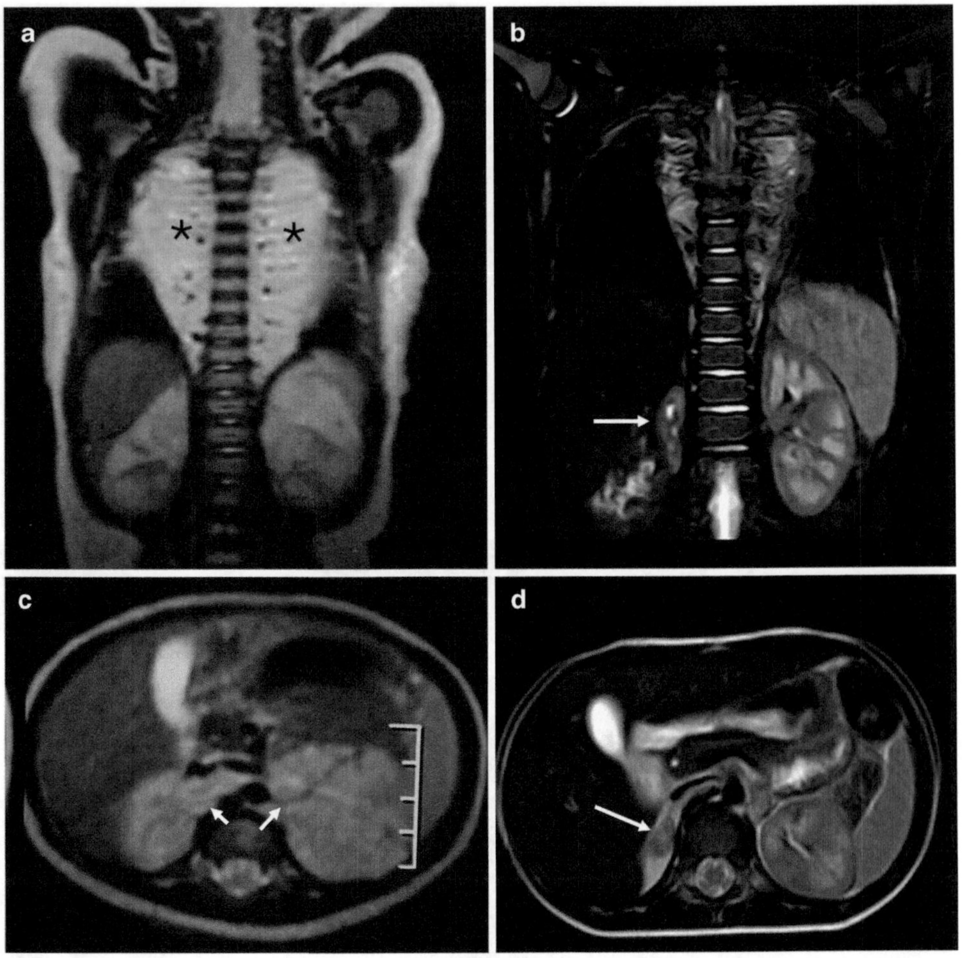

Fig. 4.13 Posterior mediastinal hemangioma with retroperitoneal extension. (**a**, **c**) Initial MRI (coronal and axial T2-WI) shows bilateral paraspinal hemangiomas (asterisk) with hyperintense signal, internal flow voids, and retroperitoneal extension (short arrows in c). (**b**, **d**) Follow-up MRI (coronal STIR and axial T2-WI) demonstrates marked size reduction after treatment but associated right renal atrophy (long white arrow)

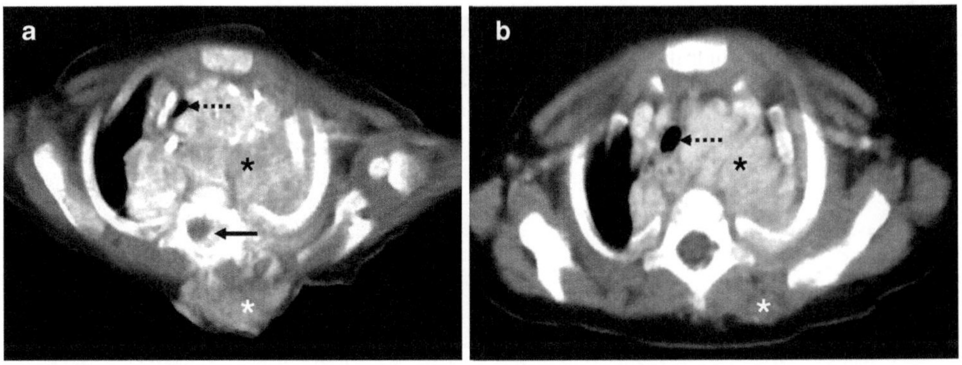

Fig. 4.14 Contrast-enhanced CT of infantile hemangioma of the back with mediastinal extension. (**a**) At presentation, an avidly enhancing mediastinal mass (black asterisk) causes tracheal compression and deviation (dashed arrow), with epidural extension (solid arrow) and dorsal component (white asterisk). (**b**) On follow-up, the lesion (black asterisk) shows interval reduction with relief of tracheal compression, resolution of epidural extension, and decreased dorsal component with fatty replacement

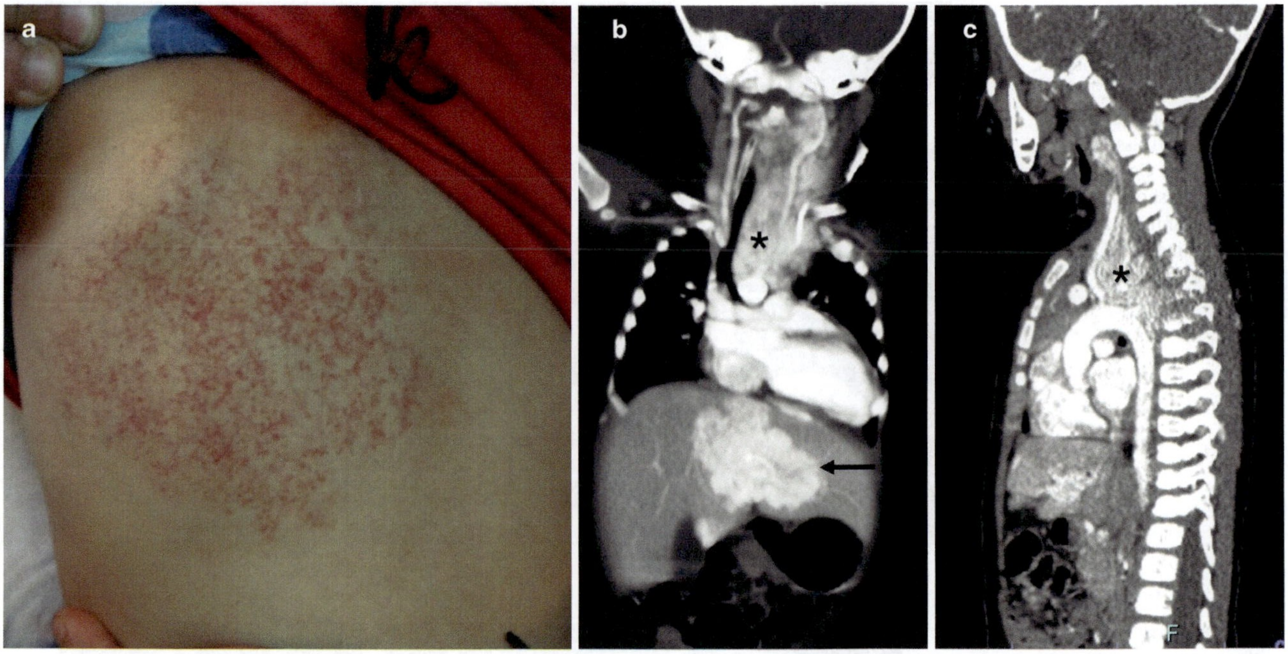

Fig. 4.15 Dorsal hemangioma (**a**) Clinical photograph (**b**, **c**) Coronal and sagittal contrast-enhanced CT show avidly enhanced mediastinal hemangioma (asterisk) causing tracheal deviation and vascular encasement. There is an associated liver hemangioma (arrow)

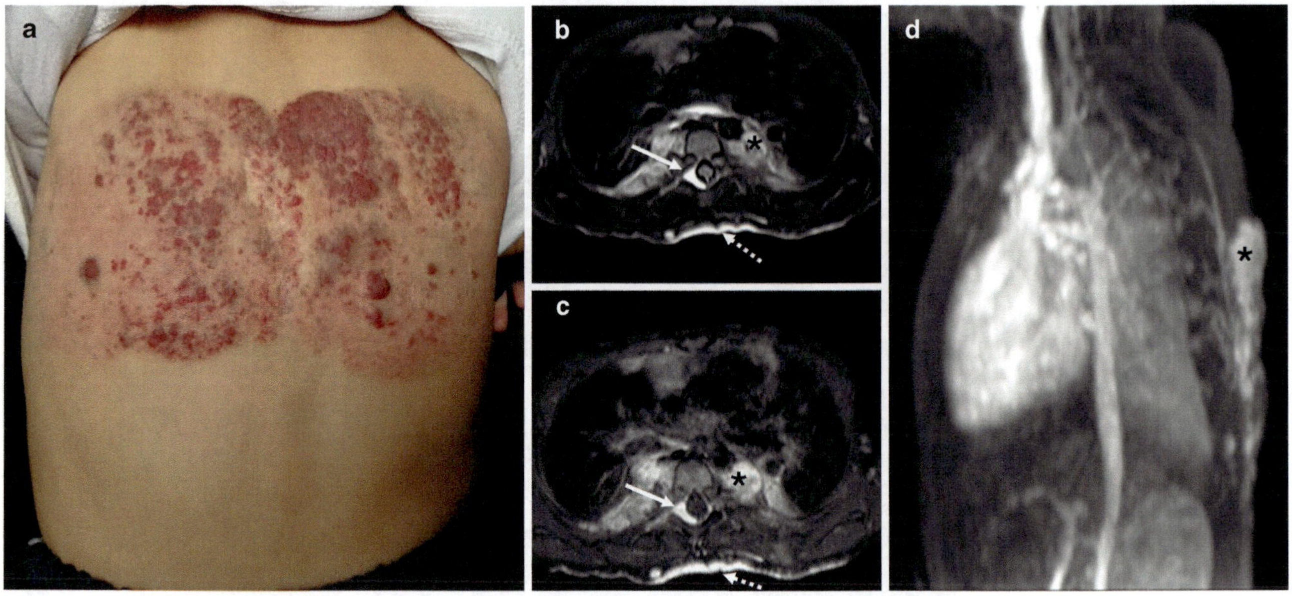

Fig. 4.16 Dorsal hemangioma with associated paraspinal component (**a**) Clinical photograph (**b**, **c**) Axial STIR and axial contrast-enhanced fat-suppressed T1-WI show hyperintense cutaneous lesion (dashed arrow) with paraspinal (asterisk) and epidural (solid arrow) components and appreciable contrast enhancement. (**d**) Sagittal maximum intensity projection of the arterial phase of the dynamic contrast-enhanced MRI shows early arterial enhancement (asterisk)

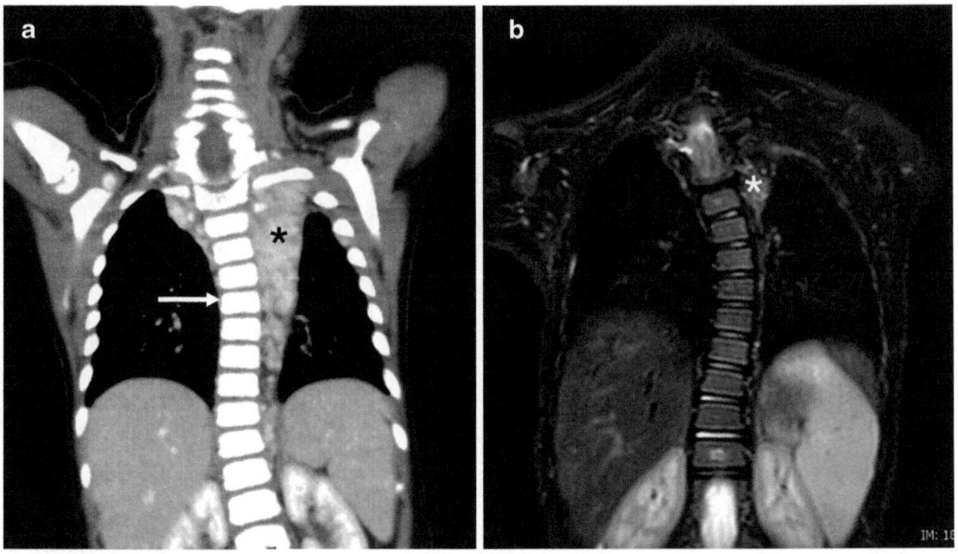

Fig. 4.17 Paraspinal hemangioma associated with dorsal scoliosis (**a**) Coronal contrast-enhanced CT at presentation shows avidly enhancing soft tissue mass (asterisk). (**b**) Coronal STIR at follow-up shows decrease in the size of the mass and more prominence of the scoliotic curve

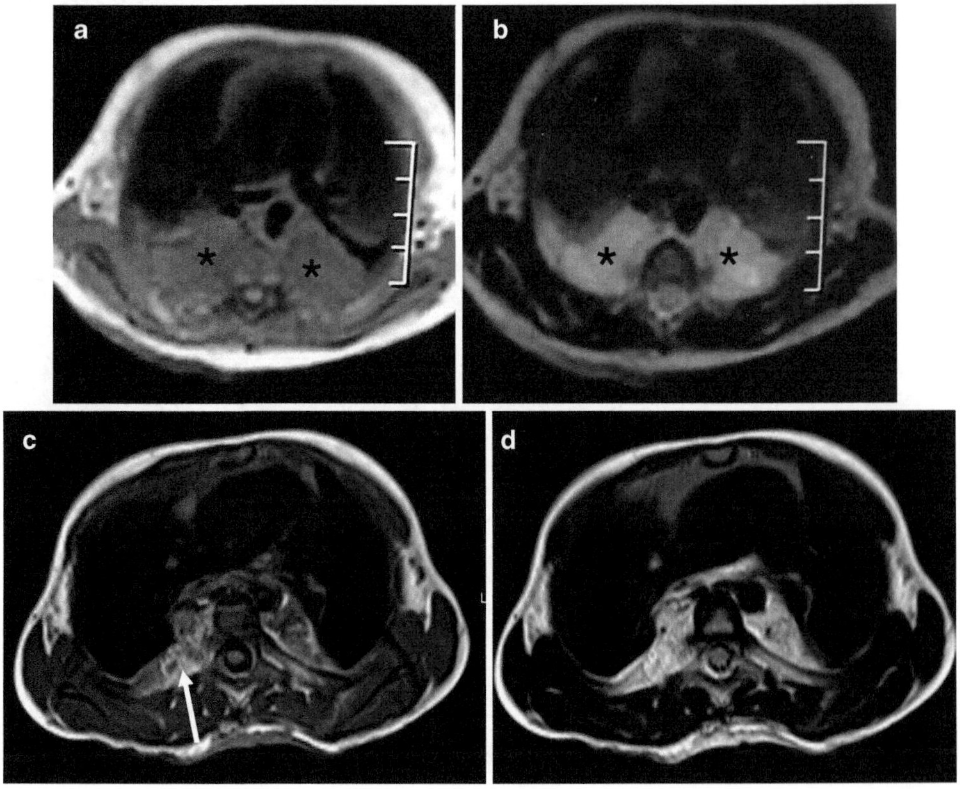

Fig. 4.18 Back hemangioma with paraspinal component. (**a**, **b**) MRI axial T1- and T2-weighted images at presentation show a paraspinal hemangioma (asterisk) appearing hypointense on T1WI and hyperintense on T2WI. (**c**, **d**) Follow-up MRI axial T1- and T2-weighted images demonstrate reduction in size with fatty infiltration (arrow), which appears hyperintense on both T1- and T2-weighted sequences

Segmental Lumbosacral Hemangioma

LUMBAR syndrome is an acronym referring to a constellation of clinical findings: **L**ower-body hemangioma (Fig. 4.19), **U**rogenital abnormalities/**U**lceration, **M**yelopathy of the spinal cord, **B**ony deformities, **A**norectal malformations (Fig. 4.20) and **A**rterial anomalies, **R**enal anomalies. The diagnosis of the syndrome relies on the presence of a characteristic segmental cutaneous infantile hemangioma (IH). Partial manifestations of LUMBAR syndrome have also been described using different acronyms: PELVIS and SACRAL [15, 16]. LUMBAR syndrome represents one of the rare neurocutaneous disorders, which may be considered the lower body counterpart of the other, upper-body PHACE syndrome [15].

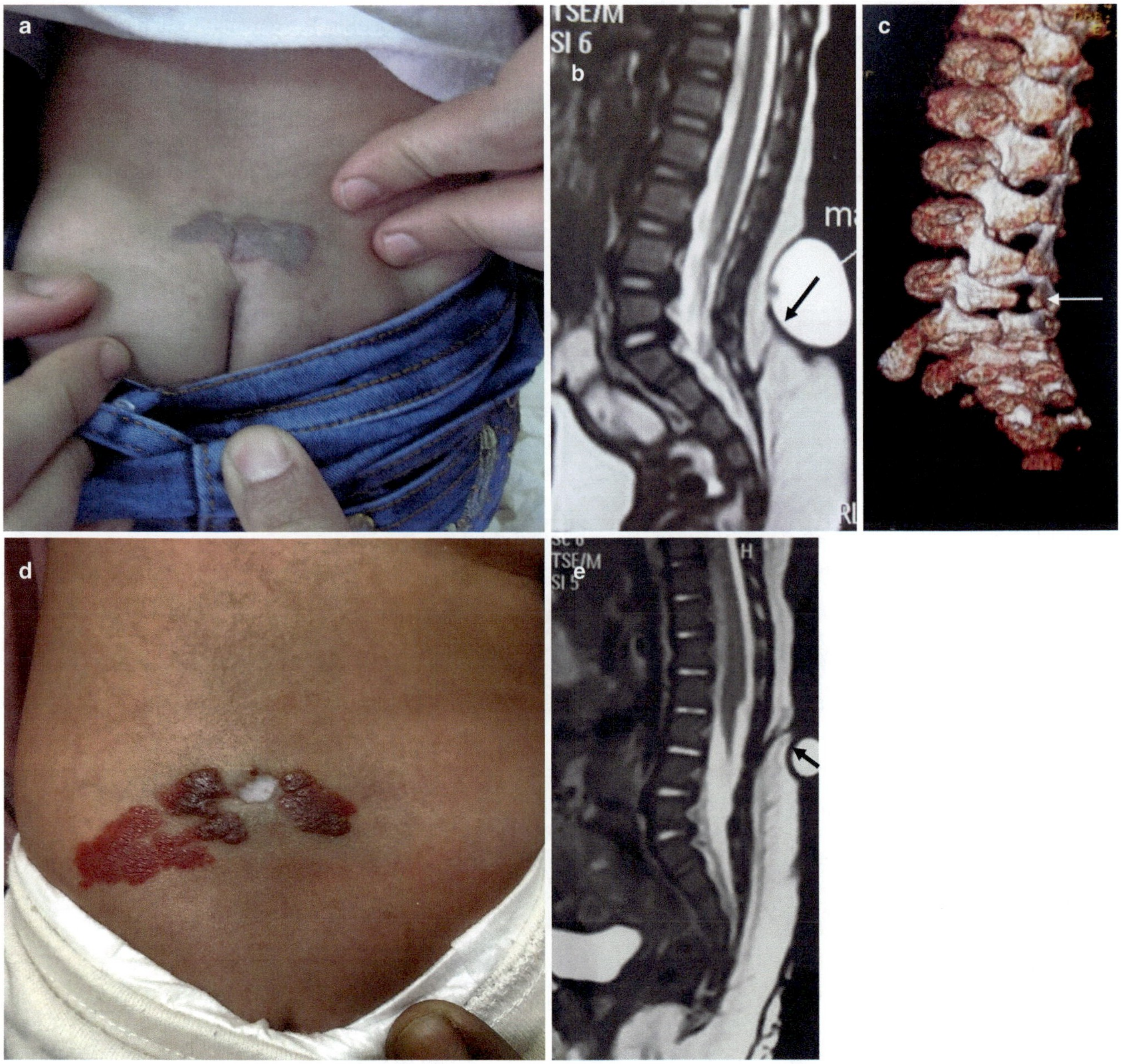

Fig. 4.19 Lower back hemangiomas in two cases. (**a**, **d**) Cutaneous lesions. (**b**, **e**) MRI shows underlying dorsal dermal sinus with external marker at the lesion site (black arrow). (**c**) 3D lumbar sine reconstruction demonstrates spina bifida occulta in the first case (white arrow)

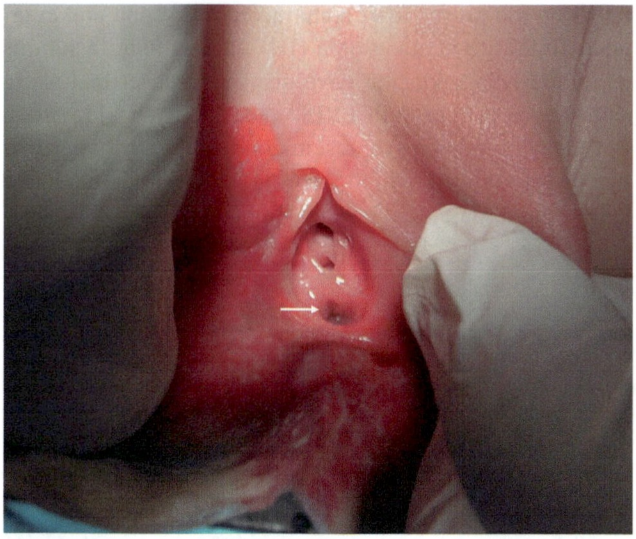

Fig. 4.20 Eight-month-old girl with vestibular anus (arrow) and perineal hemangioma

Liver and Gastrointestinal Hemangiomas

Infants who present with multiple cutaneous hemangiomas (more than three) should undergo screening for potential associated visceral hemangiomas. Liver hemangiomas are the most prevalent type and are easily identifiable using various imaging techniques such as ultrasound, MRI, or CT (Fig. 4.21) [14]. Liver hemangiomas may present as focal, multifocal, or diffuse lesions that will be discussed in detail in Chap. 6. On the other hand, intestinal hemangiomas are much less common. Small, even multifocal mucosal hemangiomas are difficult to detect by imaging. Endoscopy is inherently restricted to the evaluation of the proximal and distal segments of the gastrointestinal tract. CT (with intravenous but not oral contrast) can reveal large hemangiomas affecting the mesentery and large portions of the bowel (Figs. 4.22 and 4.23). The treatment of intestinal hemangiomas is usually medical, like other infantile hemangiomas

Fig. 4.21 Infant with multiple cutaneous hemangiomas. (**a**) Clinical photo. (**b**) Axial T2-WI MRI shows hyperintense hepatic hemangioma (arrow)

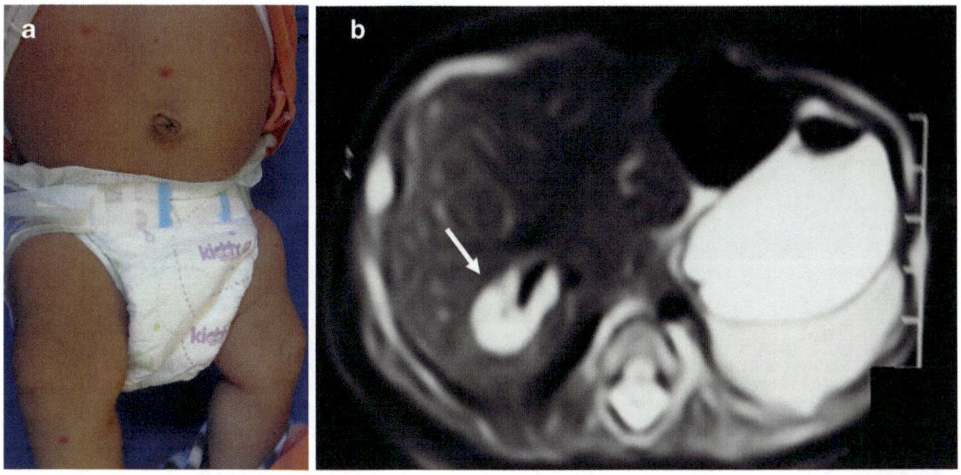

Fig. 4.22 Infant with visceral hemangioma. (**a**, **b**) Contrast-enhanced abdominal CT shows pancreatic enlargement with intense enhancement (asterisk) and associated involvement of the mesentery and bowel loops (arrows)

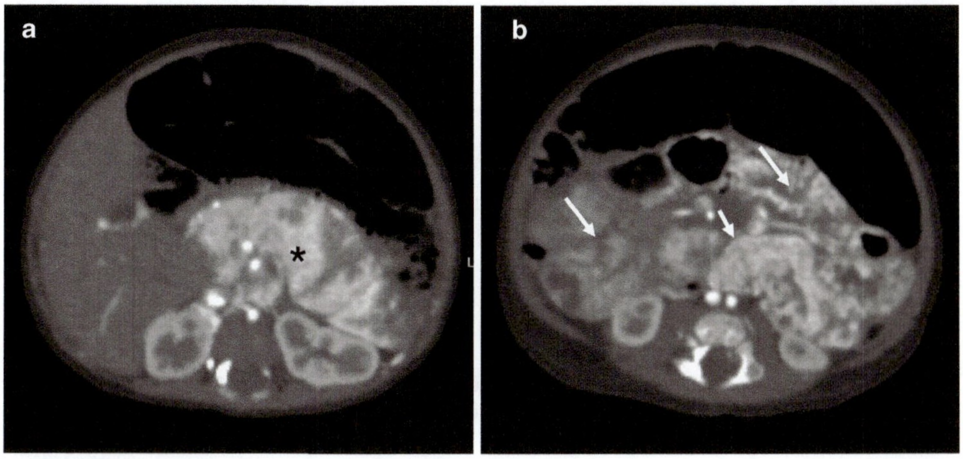

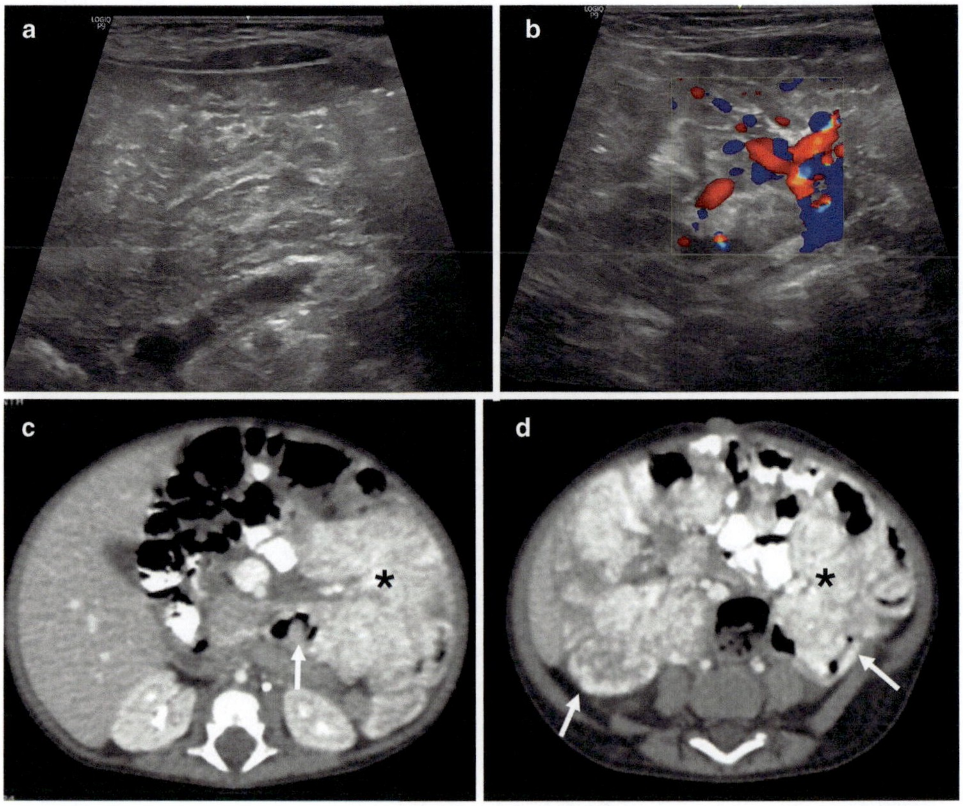

Fig. 4.23 Six-month-old girl with mesenteric hemangioma. (**a**) B-mode ultrasound shows a mixed echogenic mesenteric mass. (**b**) Color Doppler demonstrates increased vascularity. (**c**, **d**) Contrast-enhanced CT reveals an avidly enhancing mesenteric mass (asterisk) with bowel involvement (arrows)

elsewhere (propranolol, corticosteroids). Focal lesions can be removed surgically; however, resection of long bowel segments can result in short bowel syndrome [14].

References

1. Enjolras O, Mulliken JB, Kozakewich HPW. Vascular tumors and tumor-like lesions. In: Mulliken JB, Burrows PE, Fishman SJ, editors. Mulliken & Young's vascular anomalies: Hemangiomas and malformations. Oxford University Press; 2013. p. 259–324.
2. Gupta D, Rosbe K. PHACE syndrome. In: Perkins JA, Balakrishnan K, editors. Evidence-based management of head and neck vascular anomalies. Springer Nature Switzerland; 2018. p. 245–52.
3. Elluru RG. Vascular tumors of the airway. In: Perkins JA, Balakrishnan K, editors. Evidence-based management of head and neck vascular anomalies. Springer Nature Switzerland; 2018. p. 131–7.
4. Strub G, Sidbury R, Bauman N. Vascular tumors: infantile hemangioma. In: Perkins JA, Balakrishnan K, editors. Evidence-based management of head and neck vascular anomalies. Springer Nature Switzerland; 2018. p. 37–46.
5. Frieden IJ, Reese V, Cohen D. PHACE syndrome: the association of posterior fossa brain malformations, hemangiomas, arterial anomalies, coarctation of the aorta and cardiac defects, and eye abnormalities. Arch Dermatol. 1996;132:307–11.
6. Chan YC, Eichenfield LF, Malchiodi J, Friedlander SF. Small facial hemangioma and supraumbilical raphe—a forme fruste of PHACES syndrome? Br J Dermatol. 2005;153:1053–7.
7. Nabatian AS, Milgraum SS, Hess CP, Mancini AJ, Krol A, Frieden IJ. PHACE without face? Infantile hemangiomas of the upper body region with minimal or absent facial hemangiomas and associated structural malformations. Pediatr Dermatol. 2011;28:235–41.
8. Garzon MC, Epstein LG, Heyer GL, et al. PHACE syndrome: consensus-derived diagnosis and care recommendations. J Pediatr. 2016;178:24–33.
9. Siegel DH, Tefft KA, Kelly T, et al. Stroke in children with posterior fossa brain malformations, hemangiomas, arterial anomalies, coarctation of the aorta and cardiac defects, and eye abnormalities (PHACE) syndrome: a systematic review of the literature. Stroke. 2012;43:1672–4.
10. Leaute-Labreze C, et al. Propranolol for severe hemangiomas of infancy. N Engl J Med. 2008;358:2649–51.
11. Adams DM. Practical genetic and biologic therapeutic considerations in vascular anomalies. Tech Vasc Interventional Rad. 2019;22:Article 100629.
12. Ragab IA, Abdel-Kader SM, AbouZeid AA, Mohammad SA, Abdel Raheem HG, Aly NH. A successful tale of sirolimus treatment in refractory vascular tumors. J Pediatr Surg Case Rep. 2022;78:102180.
13. AbouZeid AA, Mohammad SA, Aly HG, Ragab IA. Posterior mediastinal and cutaneous back hemangiomas in infants: a new association. Eur J Pediatr Surg Rep. 2021;9(01):e37–40.
14. Fishman SJ, Burrows BE. Treatment of visceral vascular Tumors. In: Mulliken JB, Burrows PE, Fishman SJ, editors. Mulliken & Young's vascular anomalies: hemangiomas and malformations. Oxford University Press; 2013. p. 239–58.
15. Mohammad SA, AbouZeid AA, Fawzi AM, et al. Magnetic resonance imaging of head and neck vascular anomalies: pearls and pitfalls. Ann Pediatr Surg. 2017;13:116–24.
16. Metry D, Copp HL, Rialon KL, Iacobas I, Baselga E, Dobyns WB, Drolet B, Frieden IJ, Garzon M, Haggstrom A, Hanson D. Delphi consensus on diagnostic criteria for LUMBAR syndrome. J Pediatr. 2024;272:114101.

Congenital Hemangioma

5

Introduction

Congenital hemangiomas are uncommon vascular tumors. In contrast to infantile hemangiomas (see Chap. 3), congenital hemangiomas are usually present at birth and do not exhibit postnatal growth (Fig. 5.1) [1, 2]. Congenital hemangiomas can present anywhere on the skin with a predilection for the head (Fig. 5.1), neck (Fig. 5.2), and limbs (Fig. 5.3) [1, 2].

Congenital hemangioma is usually diagnosed based on clinical evaluation. At birth, the lesion is fully developed and can range in size from a few centimeters to over 20 centimeters (Fig. 5.4) [1]. Congenital hemangioma typically appears as a solitary, raised, red-purple vascular mass (Figs. 5.1, 5.2 and 5.3), often surrounded by a peripheral rim of pallor (Fig. 5.5) and may be accompanied by overlying dilated vessels (Fig. 5.6) [1–3]. Ulceration is rare but can occur in lesions with higher blood flow (Fig. 5.7) [4].

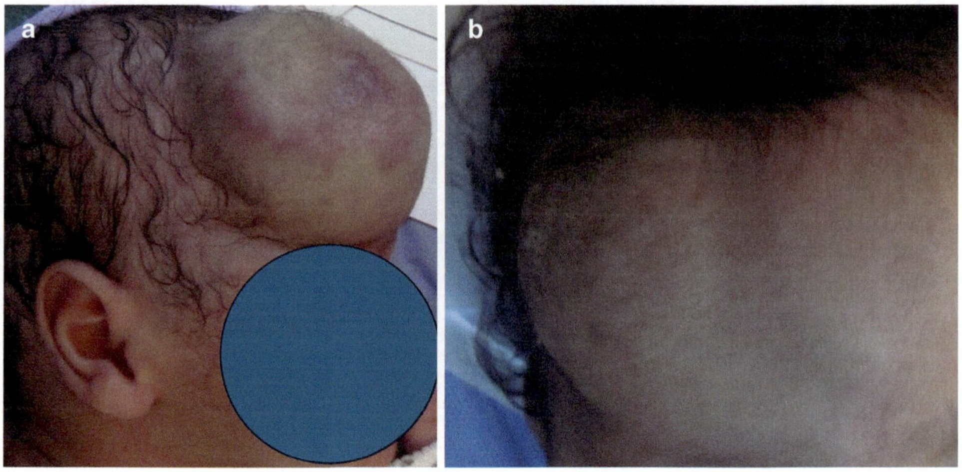

Fig. 5.1 Congenital hemangioma in a neonate. (**a**) Scalp swelling at birth. (**b**) Follow-up at 7 months shows spontaneous regression

A. A. AbouZeid et al., *Atlas of Pediatric Vascular Anomalies*, https://doi.org/10.1007/978-3-032-30866-5_5

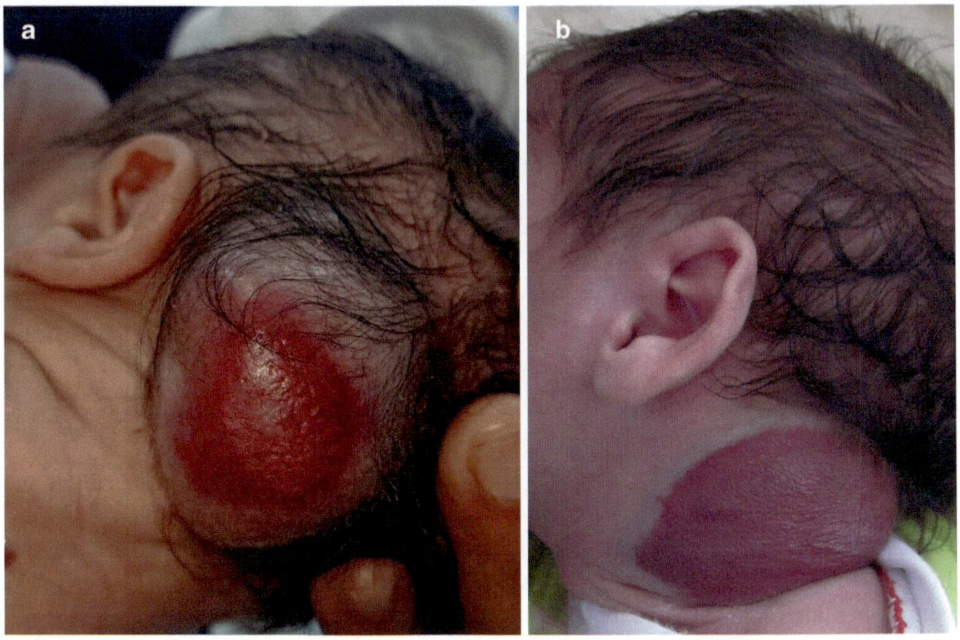

Fig. 5.2 Congenital hemangiomas in two neonates, located at the back of the neck (**a**, **b**)

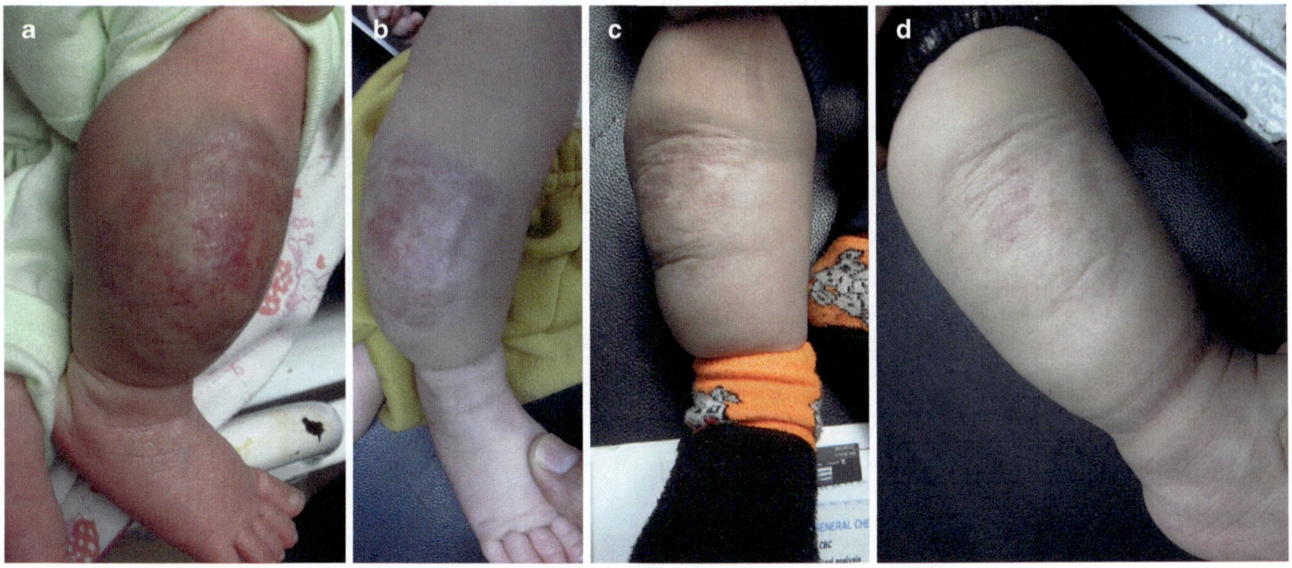

Fig. 5.3 Congenital hemangioma (RICH) of the leg showing spontaneous regression. Clinical images at birth (**a**), 2 months (**b**), 7 months (**c**), and 9 months (**d**)

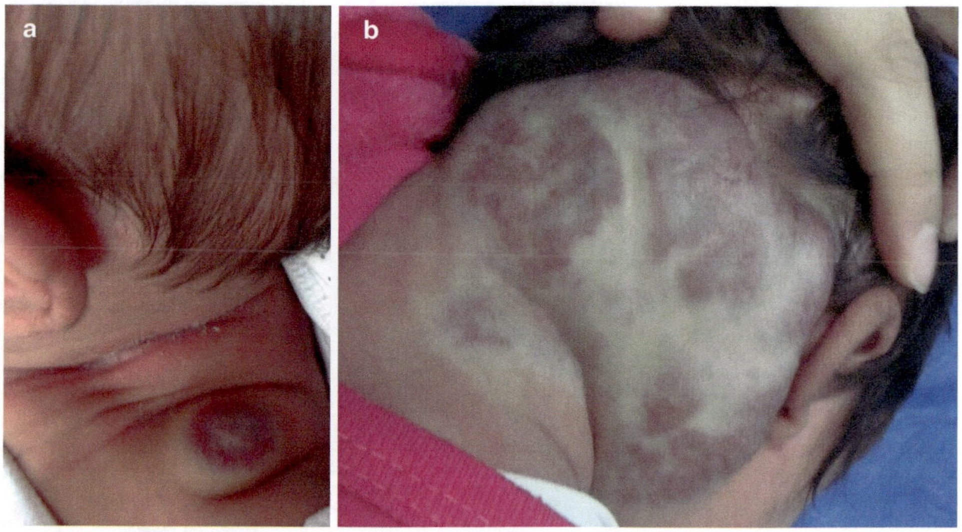

Fig. 5.4 Congenital hemangiomas in two neonates (**a**, **b**), showing size variation and central pallor

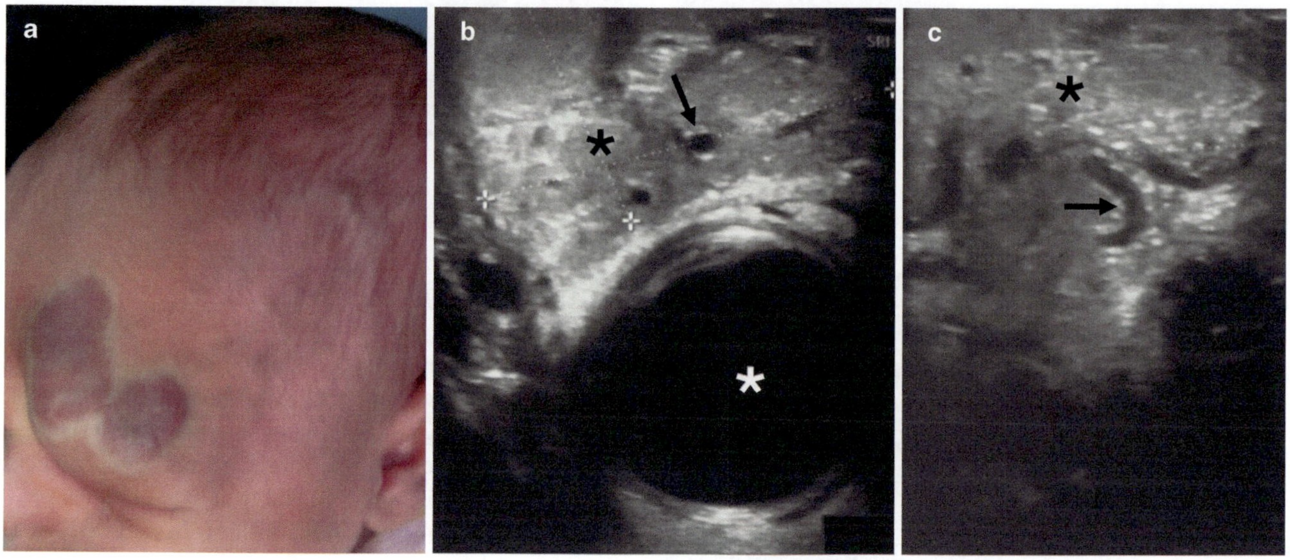

Fig. 5.5 Congenital hemangioma. (**a**) Clinical photo shows characteristic peripheral rim of pallor. (**b**, **c**) B-mode ultrasound demonstrates an echogenic soft tissue mass (black asterisk) with internal vascularity (arrows) extending over the eye globe (white asterisk)

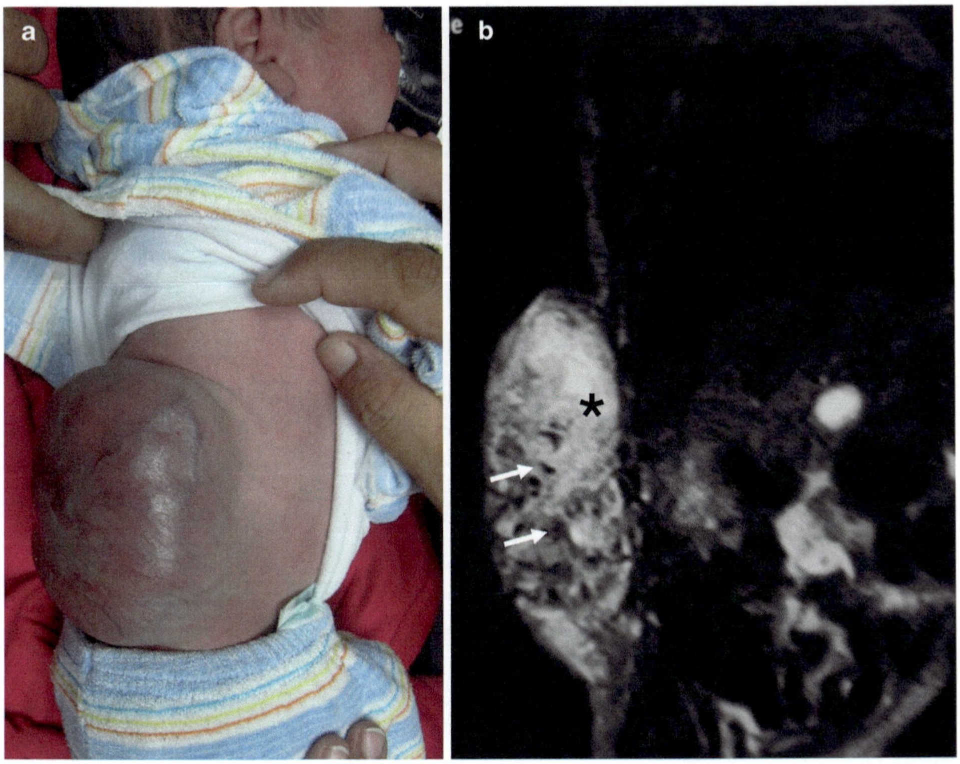

Fig. 5.6 Congenital hemangioma. (**a**) Clinical photo of the mass. (**b**) Sagittal T2-WI MRI of the thoraco-abdominal region shows a hyperintense mass (asterisk) with internal flow voids indicating high vascularity (arrows)

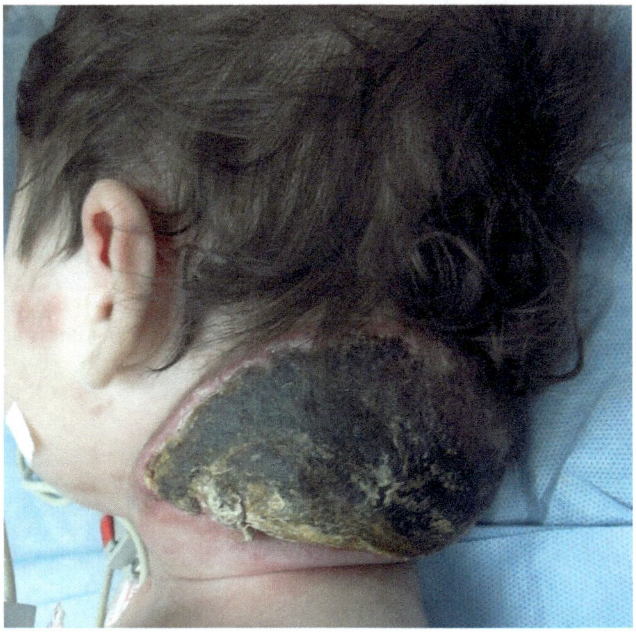

Fig. 5.7 Congenital hemangioma with overlying skin ulceration

Natural History

Congenital hemangiomas are classified into two main types: rapidly involuting congenital hemangioma (RICH) and non-involuting congenital hemangioma (NICH) [1–3]. RICH typically begins to involute within days to weeks after birth (Figs. 5.8 and 5.9) and usually completes involution by the age of 1 year (Fig. 5.3) [5]. In contrast, NICH persists and grows proportionately with the child (Fig. 5.10) [1]. Thrombocytopenia is occasionally observed in cases of large RICH, but it is typically transient and self-limiting [6, 7].

Investigations are indicated when the diagnosis is uncertain. The differential diagnosis of congenital hemangioma includes other vascular tumors or malformations, as well as non-vascular tumors (benign or malignant) [1, 8]. Ultrasound and MRI are the investigations of choice. The former is cheaper and readily available (Figs. 5.8, 5.9, 5.10 and 5.11), while the latter is superior in demonstrating the anatomy in

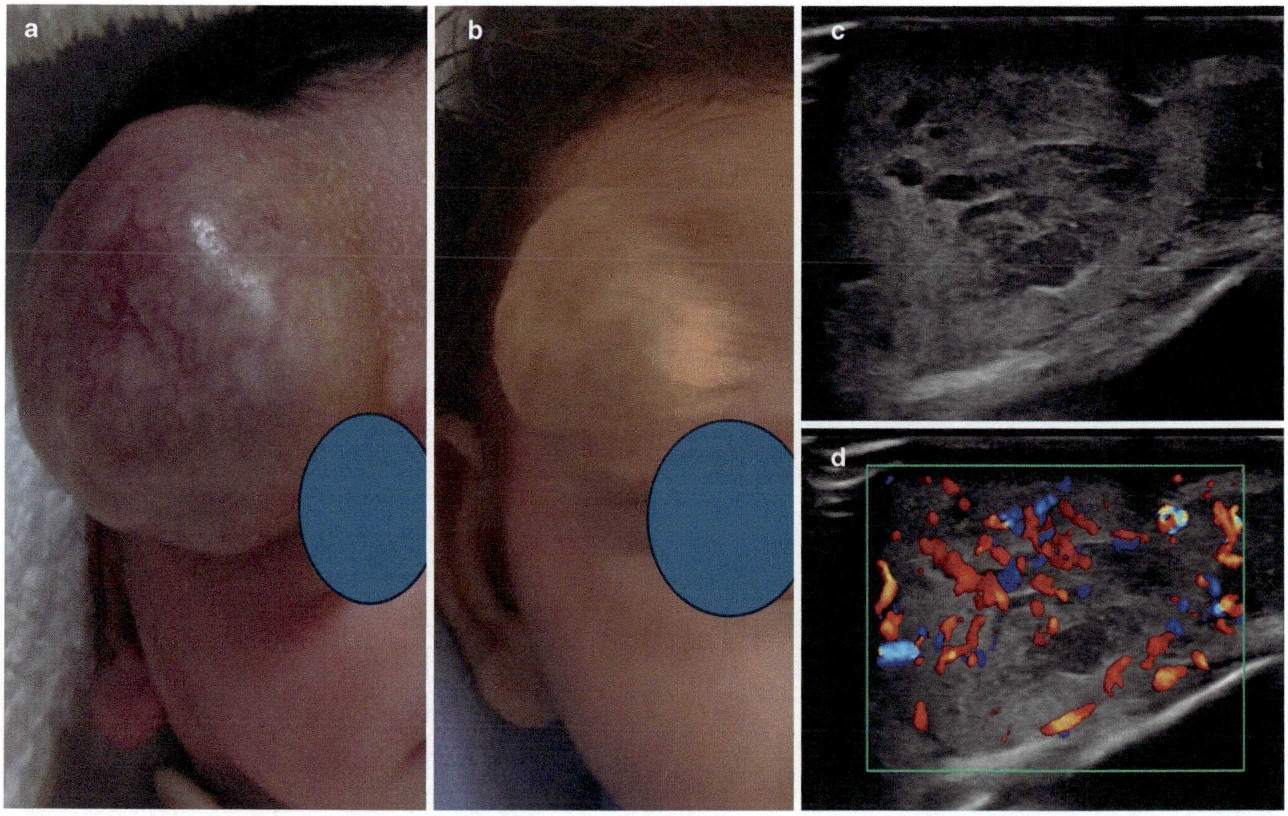

Fig. 5.8 Congenital hemangioma (RICH). (**a**) Clinical photo at presentation and (**b**) follow-up at 5 months. (**c**, **d**) B-mode ultrasound and color Doppler show an echogenic mass with vascular lakes and increased vascularity

multiple planes with high soft tissue resolution and dynamic post-contrast details (Figs. 5.12 and 5.13). Typical imaging features of congenital hemangiomas include a well-circumscribed heterogeneous mass with visible blood vessels demonstrating high flow in ultrasound and flow voids in MRI with homogeneous postcontrast enhancement (Fig. 5.13) [1, 9]. Biopsy reveals the histopathological features of congenital hemangiomas, including benign neoplastic proliferation with numerous thin-walled, ectatic vascular spaces lined by endothelial cells [1]. Congenital hemangioma stains negative for glucose transporter (GLUT-1) protein, which represents a differentiating point from infantile hemangioma [1–3].

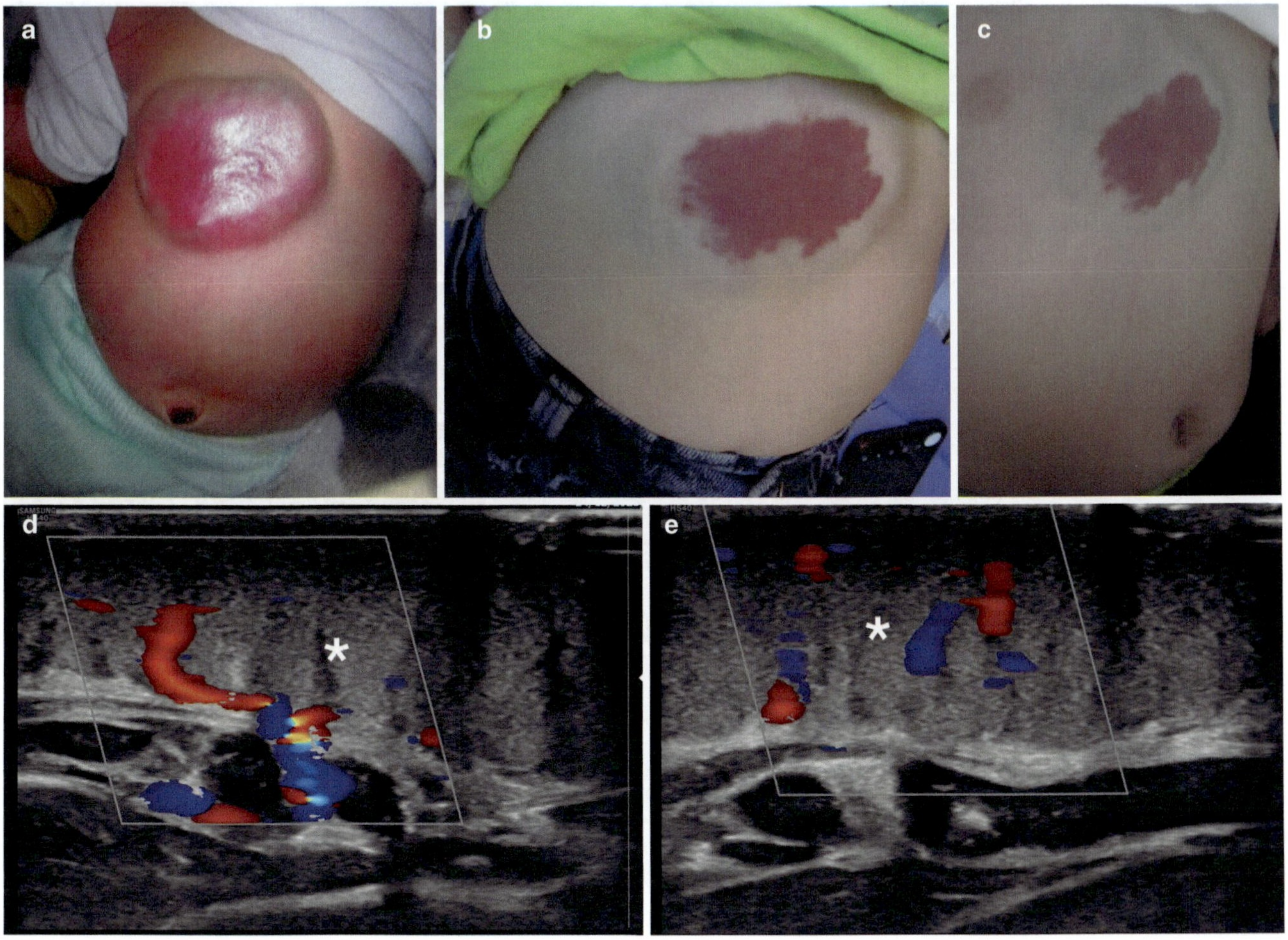

Fig. 5.9 Congenital hemangioma (RICH). (**a**–**c**) Clinical photos at presentation, 4 months, and 5 months. (**d**, **e**) Color Doppler ultrasound shows an echogenic mass with internal vascularity

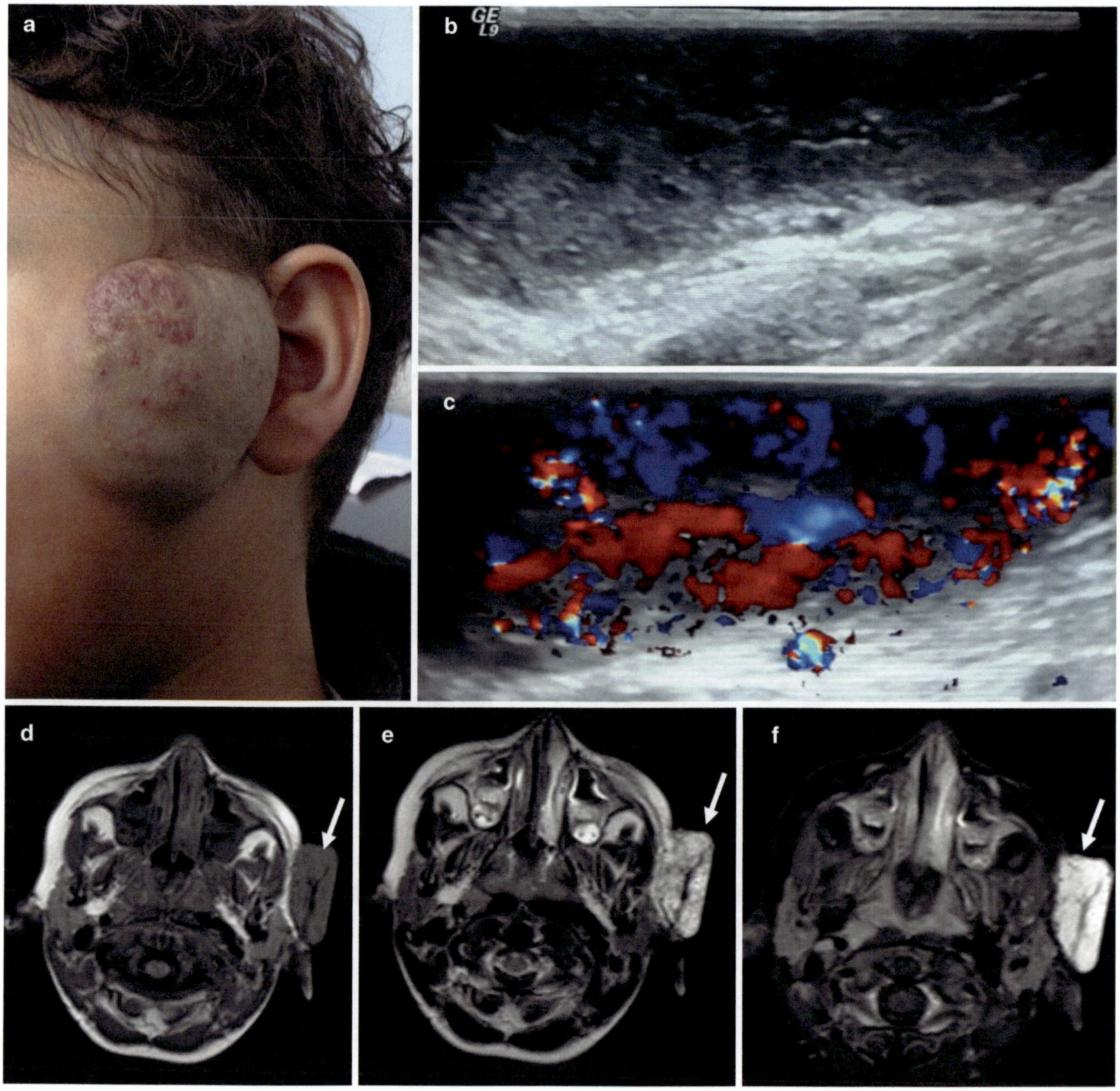

Fig. 5.10 Non-involuting congenital hemangioma in an 8-year-old boy. (**a**) Clinical photo. (**b**, **c**) B-mode ultrasound and color Doppler show an echogenic mass with increased vascularity. (**d–f**) Axial MRI (T1, T2, contrast-enhanced T1) demonstrates a soft tissue mass (arrow) with T1 hypointensity, T2 hyperintensity, and intense homogeneous contrast enhancement

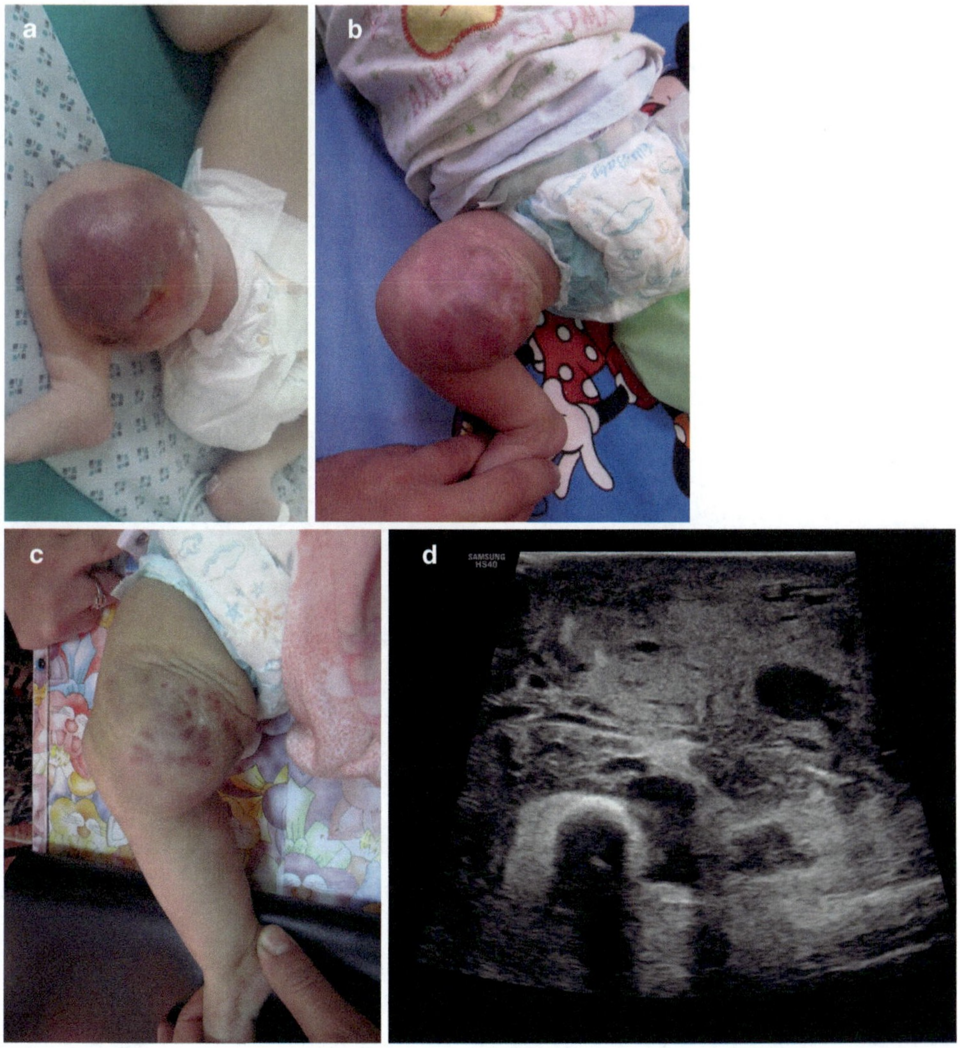

Fig. 5.11 Congenital hemangioma. (**a**–**c**) Clinical photos at presentation, 2 months, and 4 months. (**d**) Transverse B-mode ultrasound shows an echogenic mass with internal vascular lakes

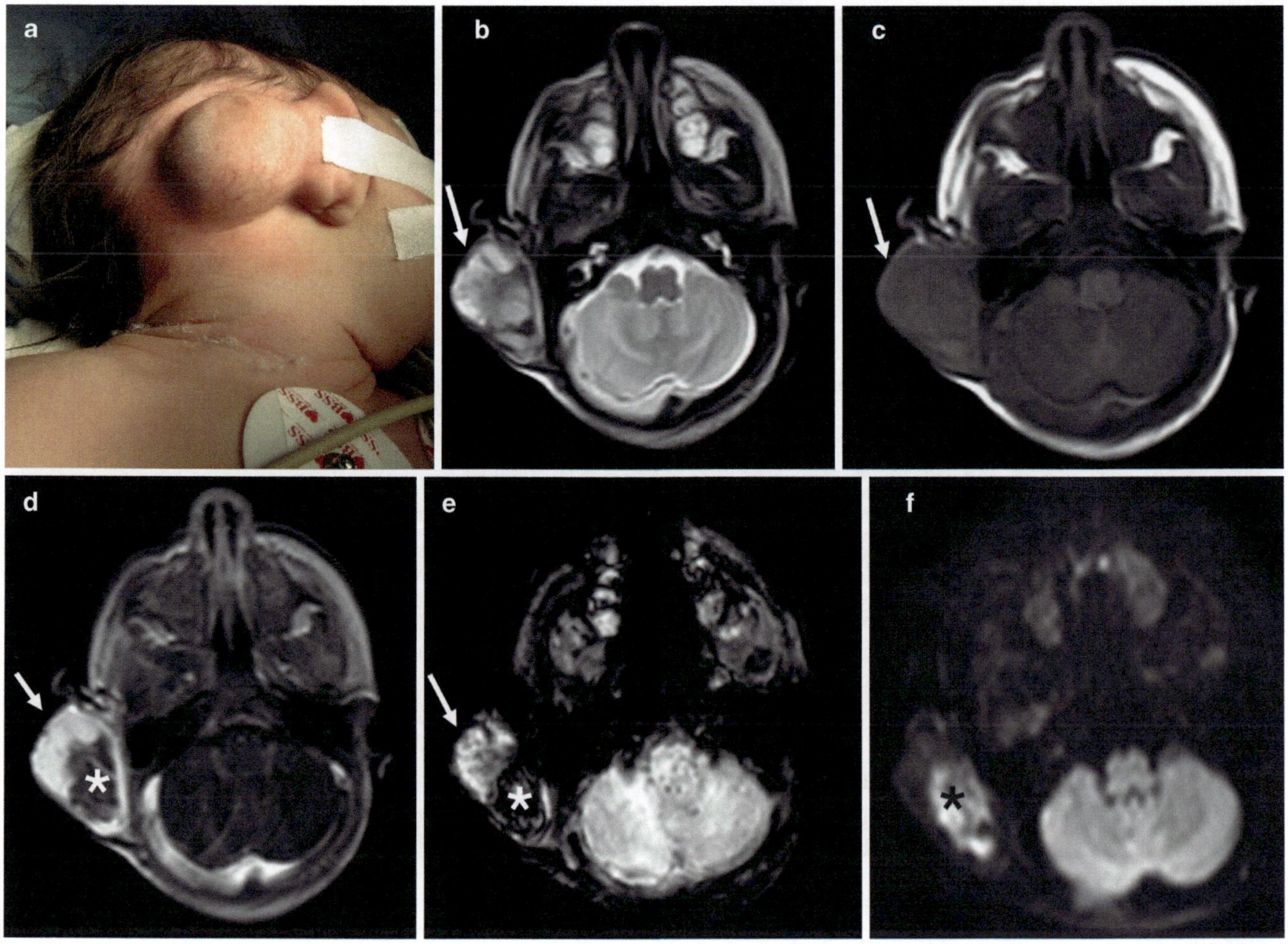

Fig. 5.12 Congenital hemangioma. (**a**) Clinical photo shows post-auricular swelling. (b–d) MRI demonstrates a well-defined soft tissue mass (arrow) with T2 hyperintensity (**b**), T1 intermediate signal (**c**), and intense contrast enhancement (**d**). A non-enhancing central area (asterisk) represents internal hemorrhage, showing intermediate-to-low T2 signal (**b**), blooming on susceptibility weighted image (**e**), and diffusion restriction (**f**)

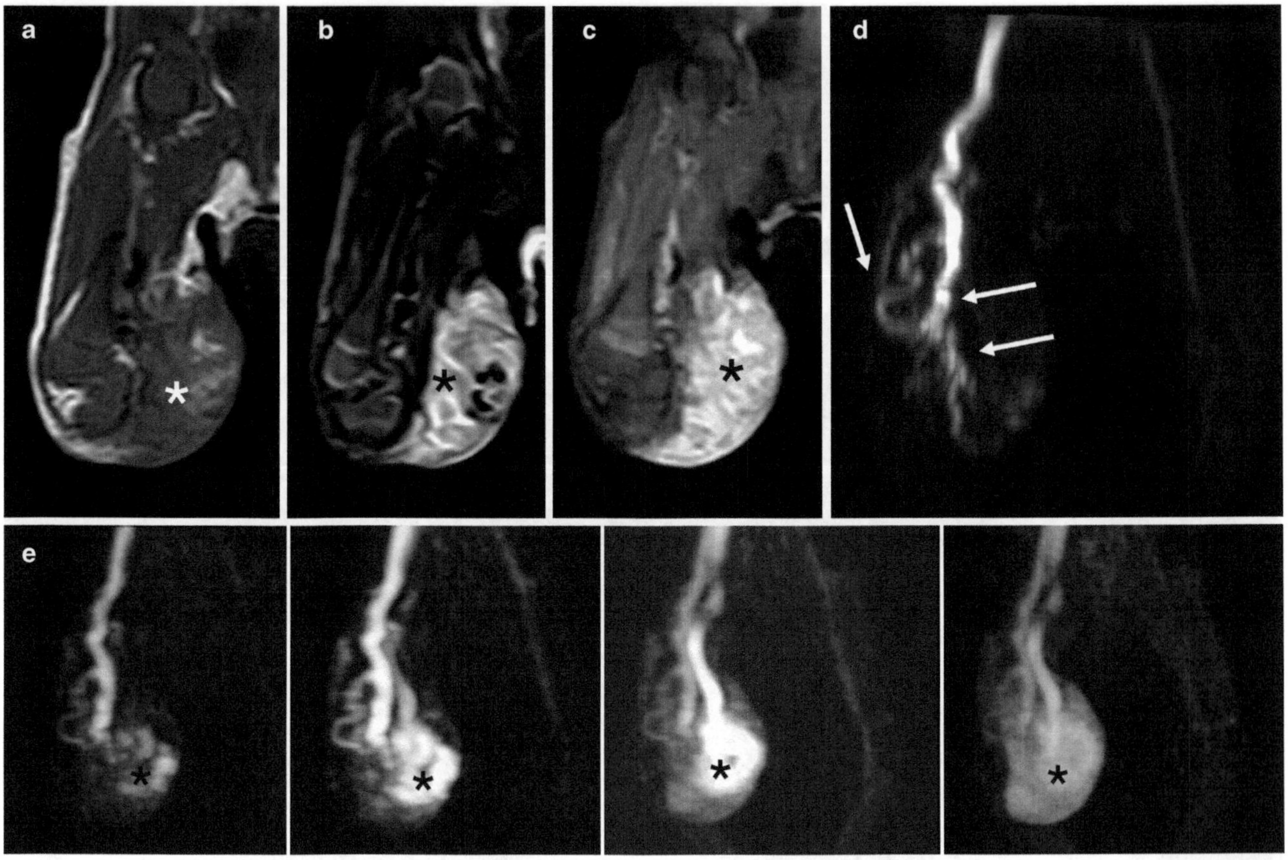

Fig. 5.13 MRI of congenital hemangioma (same case as Fig. 5.11). (**a**) T1-WI shows a soft tissue mass (asterisk) with intermediate signal. (**b**) STIR image shows hyperintensity. (**c**) Contrast-enhanced MRI demonstrates intense homogeneous enhancement. (**d**) Non-contrast MR angiography shows increased vascularity (arrow). (**e**) Dynamic MR angiography reveals early arterial enhancement with progressive filling (asterisk)

Treatment

In general, uncomplicated RICH requires no treatment (Fig. 5.3) [1]. Systemic corticosteroids and propranolol are generally thought to be ineffective in treating congenital hemangiomas; however, they may be used in critical life-threatening complications (thrombocytopenia, associated arrhythmia). Surgery may be indicated for large non-involuting congenital hemangiomas (Fig. 5.10). Embolization may be used alone in complicated cases or adjunctively with surgical removal [6, 7, 10, 11].

References

1. Tollefson MM. Congenitle hemangioma. In: Perkins JA, Balakrishnan K, editors. Evidence-based management of head and neck vascular anomalies. Springer Nature Switzerland; 2018. p. 46.
2. Gokani VJ, Sivakumar B, Kangesu L. Vascular anomalies. Surgery (Oxford). 2018;36:314–23.
3. Flors L, Park AW, Norton PT, Hagspiel KD, Leiva-Salinas C. Soft-tissue vascular malformations and tumors Part 1: Classification, role of imaging and high-flow lesions. Radiologia (English edition). 2019;61:4–15.
4. Vildy S, et al. Life-threatening hemorrhaging in neonatal ulcerated congenital hemangioma: two case reports. JAMA Dermatol. 2015;151(4):422–5.
5. Krol A, MacArthur CJ. Congenital hemangiomas: rapidly involuting and noninvoluting congenital hemangiomas. Arch Facial Plast Surg. 2005;7(5):307–11.
6. Baselga E, et al. Rapidly involuting congenital haemangioma associated with transient thrombocytopenia and coagulopathy: a case series. Br J Dermatol. 2008;158(6):1363–70.
7. Rangwala S, et al. Rapidly involuting congenital hemangioma associated with profound, transient thrombocytopenia. Pediatr Dermatol. 2014;31(3):402–4.
8. AbouZeid AA, Mohammad SA, Aly NH, et al. Differential diagnostic features between congenital haemangioma, KHE, and congenital fibrosarcoma: a single-Centre experience. Eur J Pediatr. 2021;180:2581–9. https://doi.org/10.1007/s00431-021-04119-7.
9. Mohammad SA, AbouZeid AA, Fawzi AM, et al. Magnetic resonance imaging of head and neck vascular anomalies: pearls and pitfalls. Ann Pediatr Surg. 2017;13:116–24.
10. Sur A, et al. Multiple successful angioembolizations for refractory cardiac failure in a preterm with rapidly involuting congenital hemangioma. AJP Rep. 2016;6(1):e99–e103.
11. Browning JC, Metry DW. Rapidly involuting congenital hemangioma: case report and review of the literature. Dermatol Online J. 2008;14(4):11.

6 Hemangioma of the Liver and Differential Diagnosis

Introduction

Hepatic hemangioma represents the most prevalent primary hepatic neoplasm in neonates and infants. According to the classification system established by the International Society for the Study of Vascular Anomalies (ISSVA), hepatic hemangiomas are stratified into congenital and infantile subtypes based on the timing of clinical presentation. Congenital hepatic hemangiomas (CHH) are fully developed in utero, often identifiable on prenatal imaging, and are present at birth. In contrast, infantile hepatic hemangiomas (IHH) manifest within the early postnatal period. Two distinct phenotypes of CHH were initially delineated: rapidly involuting congenital hemangioma (RICH) and non-involuting congenital hemangioma (NICH). A third subtype—partially involuting congenital hemangioma—was formally recognized by ISSVA in 2018. IHH exhibits a characteristic pattern of postnatal proliferation followed by a spontaneous involution phase, typically commencing between two and 5 years of age [1–3].

Different types of hemangioma have different molecular characteristics. Immunohistochemical staining showing positivity for glucose transporter 1 (GLUT-1) consistently differentiates infantile hemangioma at all stages from congenital hemangioma. The insulin-like growth factor 2 gene (IGF2) is weakly expressed in congenital hemangioma. IGF2 promotes expression of hypoxia-induced factor 1α, which in turn increases levels of GLUT1 mRNA. That's why congenital hemangioma is negatively stained for GLUT-1. On the contrary, mRNA levels for membrane-associated FLT-1 gene (which encodes vascular endothelial growth factor receptor 1) was found to be uniformly higher in congenital hemangiomas than in the proliferating or involuting phase of infantile hemangioma [4].

The use of the term "infantile hemangioendothelioma" of the liver should be discouraged for the following reasons: Infantile liver hemangioma and cutaneous hemangioma have the same natural history and pathological features; hence, they should have the same term, also when the term "Hemangioendothelioma" is used, it might be mistaken for two distinct conditions: epithelioid hemangioendothelioma and kaposiform hemangioendothelioma [2, 5].

Ultrasound with color Doppler is the first-line imaging technique used to diagnose hepatic hemangiomas. If imaging findings are inconclusive, the clinical history is not suggestive of hemangioma, or if the lesion is identified beyond infancy, dynamic contrast-enhanced MRI or CT may be utilized, with MRI being the preferred option due to the radiation risks associated with CT [6]. By imaging, hepatic hemangioma can be classified into focal, multifocal, or diffuse [7]. Congenital hepatic hemangioma is typically focal, whereas infantile hepatic hemangiomas tend to present in multifocal or diffuse forms. Knowing different types of hepatic hemangiomas, their age of presentation and clinical behavior, as well as their characteristic imaging features and the possible differential diagnoses, is crucial for setting the accurate diagnosis, aiming for proper patients' managements [2–8].

This chapter will explore various types of hepatic hemangiomas in infants (Table 6.1), as well as differentiate them from other hepatic masses and vascular abnormalities. Hepatic vascular anomalies are summarized in Figs. 6.1 and 6.2.

A. A. AbouZeid et al., *Atlas of Pediatric Vascular Anomalies*, https://doi.org/10.1007/978-3-032-30866-5_6

Table 6.1 Differences between different types of hepatic hemangioma in neonates and infants

	Focal	Multifocal	Diffuse
Time of presentation	Present antenatally or during neonatal period	Postnatal (early infancy)	Postnatal (early infancy)
Clinical presentation	Often asymptomatic; palpable abdominal mass or incidental imaging finding. May involute spontaneously (congenital types have variable involution).	May be asymptomatic or cause hepatomegaly; skin cutaneous IH often present (multiple cutaneous hemangiomas).	Marked hepatomegaly, abdominal distension; high risk of systemic effects (cardiac, metabolic)
Possible complications	High-output cardiac failure Intratumoral bleeding Thrombocytopenia Hypofibrinogenemia	High-output cardiac failure	Abdominal compartment syndrome *Consumptive hypothyroidism* (due to type 3 deiodinase activity in tumor) High-output cardiac failure, significant anemia, consumptive coagulopathy, cholestasis, respiratory compromise, and liver failure
Investigations	*At diagnosis*: CBC Fibrinogen AFP Liver function tests If there are imaging features of shunts or the patient is symptomatic (echocardiography)	*At diagnosis*: CBC AFP Liver function tests TSH and free T4 Echocardiography if there are imaging features of shunts or the patient is symptomatic	
	Follow up tests Serial liver ultrasound If hemangioma increases in size (CBC) To rule out hepatoblastoma (AFP) Liver function tests as needed	*Follow up tests* Serial liver ultrasound TSH and free T4 are repeated monthly in diffuse disease at least until 6 months of age, while in multifocal disease, monitoring is needed if there is progression or development of new symptoms AFP repeated monthly until normalized CBC as needed Liver function tests as needed	
Length of monitoring	Monitor for at least 1 year until two consecutive ultrasounds show stable size and vascularity	Continue follow-up until complete hemangioma involution is reached	

AFP alpha feto-protein, *CBC* complete blood count, *TSH* thyroid stimulating hormone

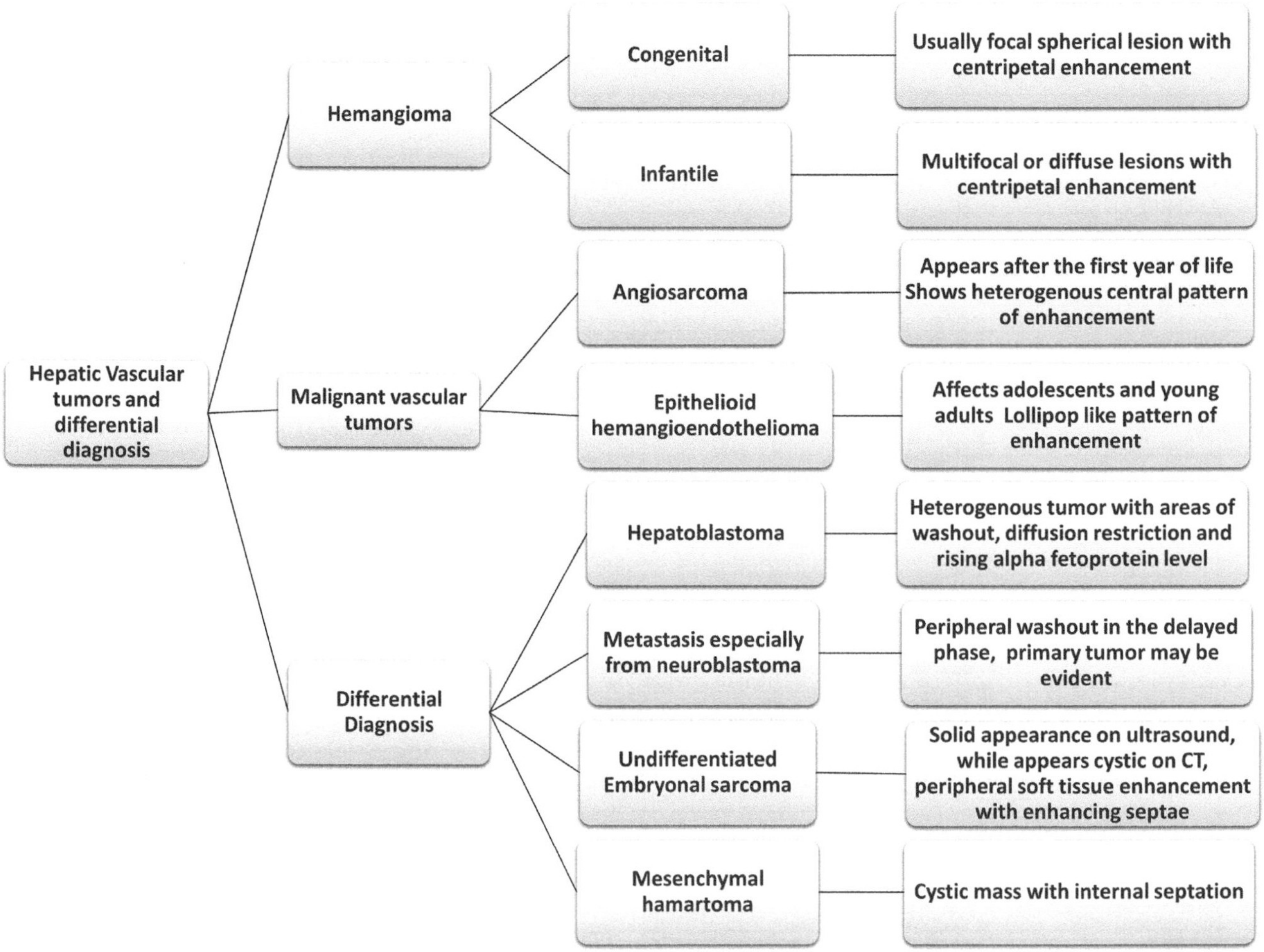

Fig. 6.1 Schematic representation of hepatic Vascular tumors and their differential diagnosis

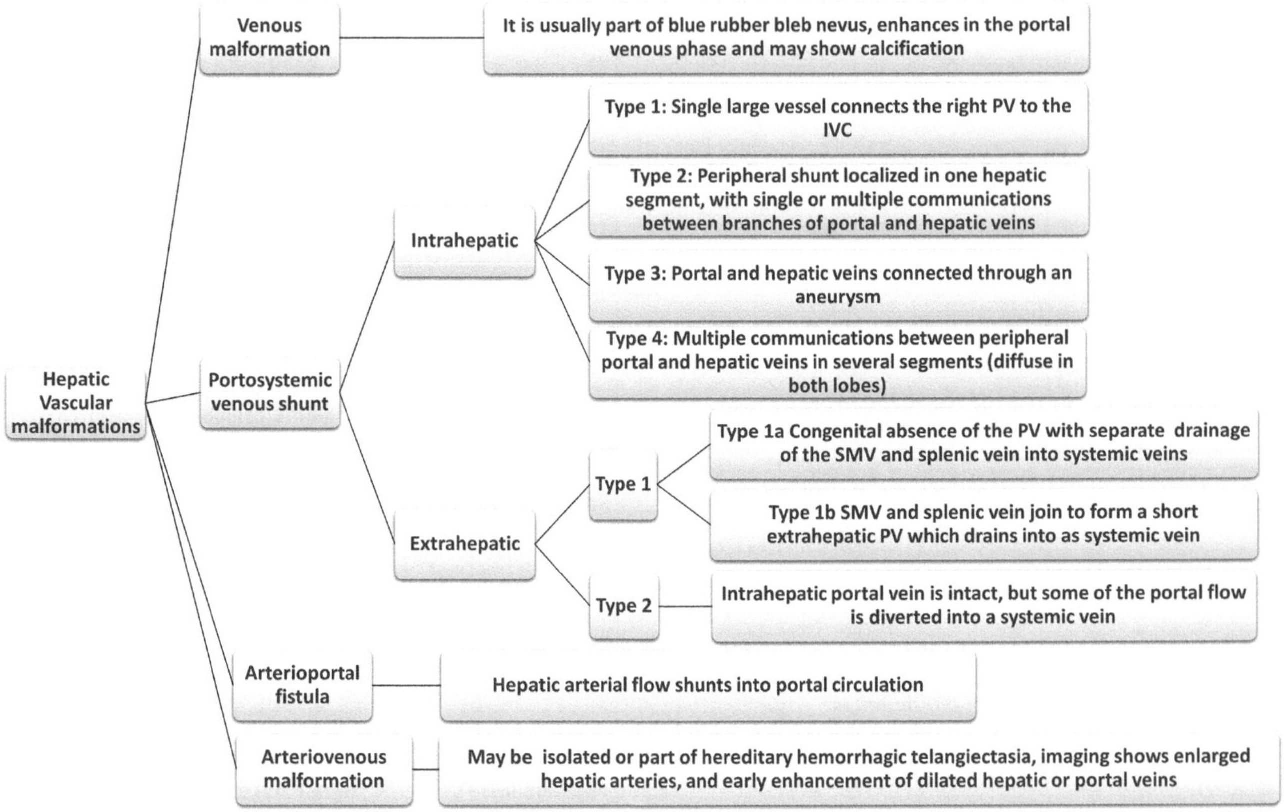

Fig. 6.2 Schematic representation of hepatic vascular malformations

Hepatic Hemangioma

Focal Hepatic Hemangioma

Focal hepatic hemangioma is usually congenital benign high-flow vascular tumor that proliferates in utero and may be identified through antenatal screening or diagnosed at birth. It usually involutes rapidly during the first year of life, similar to its cutaneous counterpart, "rapidly involuting congenital hemangioma (RICH)" [10].

In the neonatal period, patients usually present with abdominal enlargement and less commonly high-output cardiac failure due to arteriovenous shunting. The arteriovenous shunts may occur between branches of the hepatic artery and portal or hepatic veins. Patients may also have anemia and thrombocytopenia, which are not as severe as in Kasabach-Merritt phenomenon of Kaposiform hemangioendothelioma, and disseminated intravascular coagulopathy is uncommon. Thrombocytopenia is related to platelet consumption in the formation of central thrombosis rather than trapping by the tumor itself. Spontaneous rise of platelets typically occurs within a week [11].

Diagnosis of congenital hepatic hemangioma is established when the imaging features are typical for hemangioma, with successive decline of the lesion size and alpha-fetoprotein (AFP) level obviating the need for biopsy. As AFP is normally high in neonates (often well over 100,000 ng/ml), it declines with time in cases of hemangioma opposed to hepatoblastoma with half-life of about 1 week [9].

At ultrasound, CHH appears usually as focal liver lesion of large size. It displays mixed echogenicity with possible calcification. Color Doppler analysis reveals increased peripheral vascularity with less vascularized central portion. It also demonstrates congested hepatic veins with arteriovenous shunting (Figs. 6.3 and 6.4). Contrast-enhanced ultrasound is adequately justified in neonatal period and may obviate the need for other imaging modalities [12, 13].

MRI is the recommended cross-sectional imaging modality for further evaluation of hepatic lesions in neonates and young infants. CHH appears as heterogeneous mass lesion on T2WI with flow voids. Heterogeneous signal is related to the presence of hemorrhage, fibrosis, and calcification (Fig. 6.5). When MRI is not available, CT may be appropriate. By CT, CHH appears as hypoattenuating mass lesion. Dynamic contrast-enhanced sequence reveals early intense peripheral nodular contrast enhancement (Peripheral discontinuous nodular type of arterial phase hyperenhancement) of variable thickness with little if any central enhancement in delayed scans

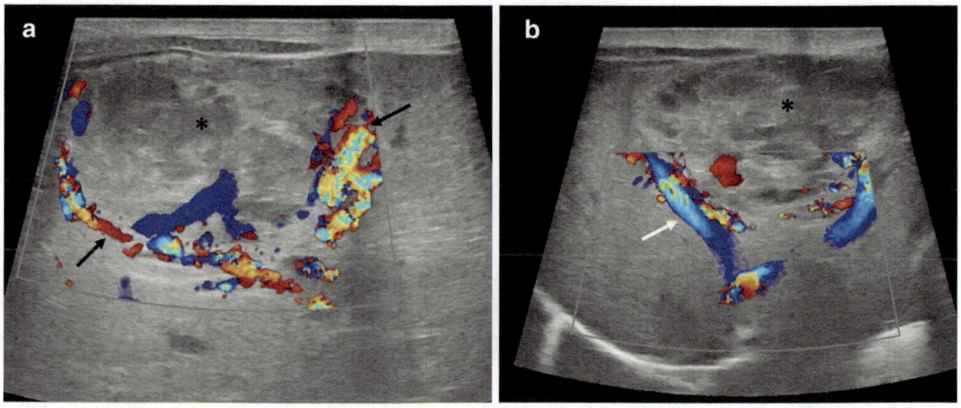

Fig. 6.3 A 14-day-old boy with rapidly involuting congenital hepatic hemangioma (**a**) Axial ultrasound of the liver shows a solid mass with peripheral vascularity (arrows) and absence of central color flow reflecting thrombosis/necrosis (asterisk). (**b**) Axial ultrasound at a higher level shows increased venous outflow (arrow) indicating increased arteriovenous shunting

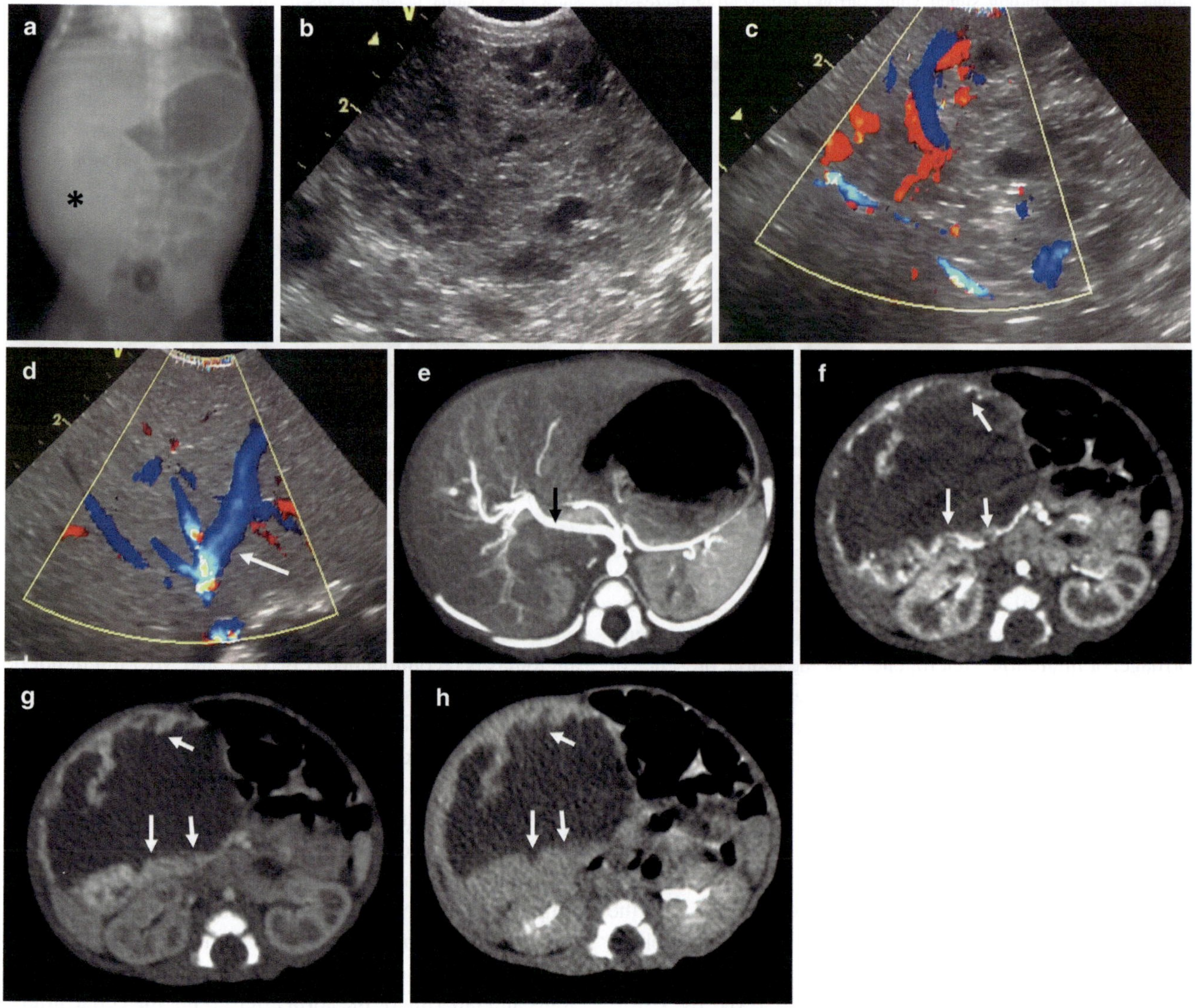

Fig. 6.4 A 7-day-old neonate with rapidly involuting congenital hemangioma. (**a**) Coronal average intensity projection shows opacity (asterisk) occupying the right side of the abdomen and displacing the bowel loops. (**b**) Ultrasound image shows a large mass of heterogenous echopattern. (**c**) Color doppler interrogation shows peripheral vascularity. (**d**) Colour Doppler at the level of hepatic veins shows congested hepatic veins (arrow). (**e**) Axial maximum intensity projection at the arterial phase of contrast-enhanced CT shows dilated hepatic artery (arrow). (**f, g, h**) Dynamic contrast enhanced CT at the arterial, portal venous and delayed phases respectively shows peripheral nodular hyperenhancement in the arterial phase with progressive filling (arrows). Note the persistent large non enhancing central portion of the tumor reflecting thrombosis and hemorrhage

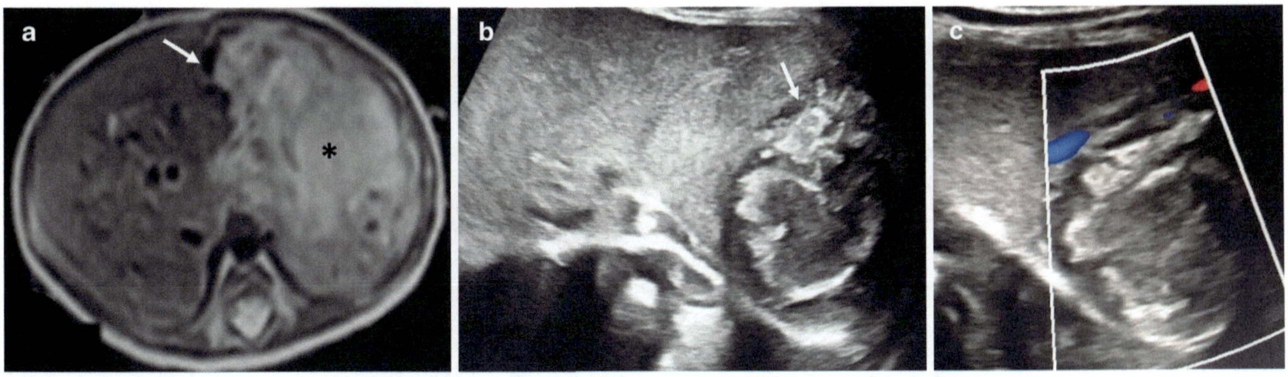

Fig. 6.5 Congenital hepatic hemangioma. (**a**) axial T2-WI MRI at the age of 30 days shows a large lesion (asterisk) exhibiting hyperintense signal with surrounding signal voids (arrow) representing increased peripheral vascularity. (**b**) follow-up sonogram at the age of three months show decrease the size of the mass (arrow). (**c**) Color Doppler shows few residual peripheral vascularity

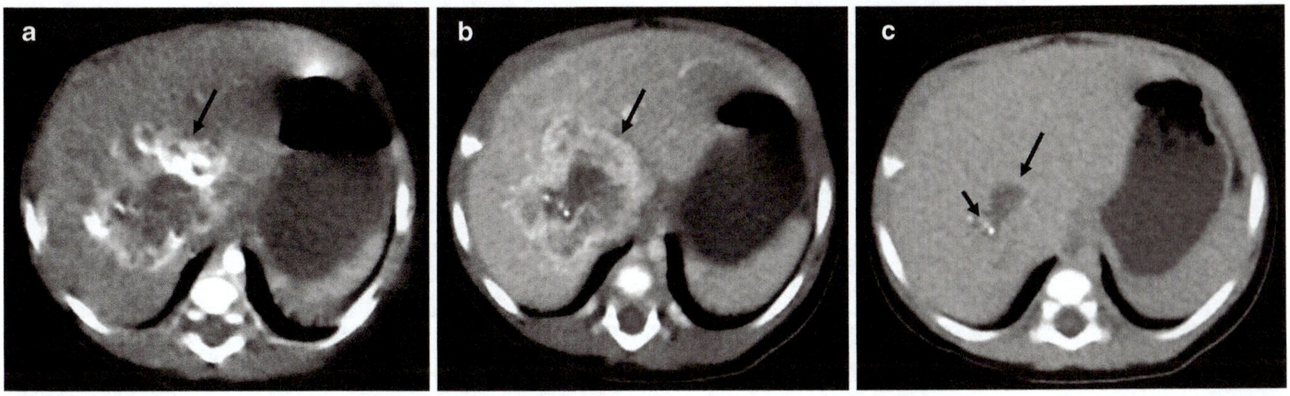

Fig. 6.6 A 1-month-old boy with rapidly involuting congenital hemangioma of the liver. (**a–c**) Dyanmic contrast enhanced CT shows a large mass (long arrow) with peripheral hyperenhancement at the arterial phase (**a**) with progressive centripetal filling throughout venous (**b**) and delayed phase (**c**). Note the presence of foci of calcification (short arrow)

(Figs. 6.4 and 6.6). The central non-enhancing regions correspond pathologically to the presence of central fibrosis, hemorrhage, or infarction. Heterogeneity of the lesion, presence of calcification, and the little central enhancement in the delayed phases of post-contrast dynamic study may differentiate congenital from infantile hemangioma [14].

Multifocal Hepatic Hemangioma

Multifocal hepatic hemangioma is clinically similar to the cutaneous infantile hemangioma. It has proliferative phase that starts shortly after birth (approximately 4–8 weeks) and extends for 9–12 months. This phase is followed by a slow involution over years. Multifocal hemangioma may enlarge with time, progressing into diffuse hemangioma. Multifocal hepatic hemangioma can cause cardiomegaly and high cardiac output failure due to the associated arteriovenous shunting. Multifocal infantile hemangioma usually is associated with multiple cutaneous hemangiomas. Hence, ultrasound screening of children having more than five cutaneous hemangiomas is recommended (Fig. 6.7), and MRI might not be necessary in this instance [15].

The lesions are usually imaged during the progressive phase. Ultrasound reveals multiple hypoechoic or echolucent masses that are associated with high vascularity (Fig. 6.7). IHH are usually hypodense to the liver parenchyma at CT and display homogenous hypointense and hyperintense signals on T1 and T2W MRI, respectively (Figs. 6.8 and 6.9). Signal voids may be seen within or nearby the lesions, reflecting high-flow arteriovenous shunts. This is associated with enlarged hepatic arteries and veins and tapering of the aorta after giving the celiac artery. IHH shows rapid filling with centripetal pattern of enhancement during dynamic scans (Fig. 6.8). Calcification and hemorrhage are not common in IH compared to CHH. Involuting hemangiomas show fatty replacement with minimal enhancement [8, 9].

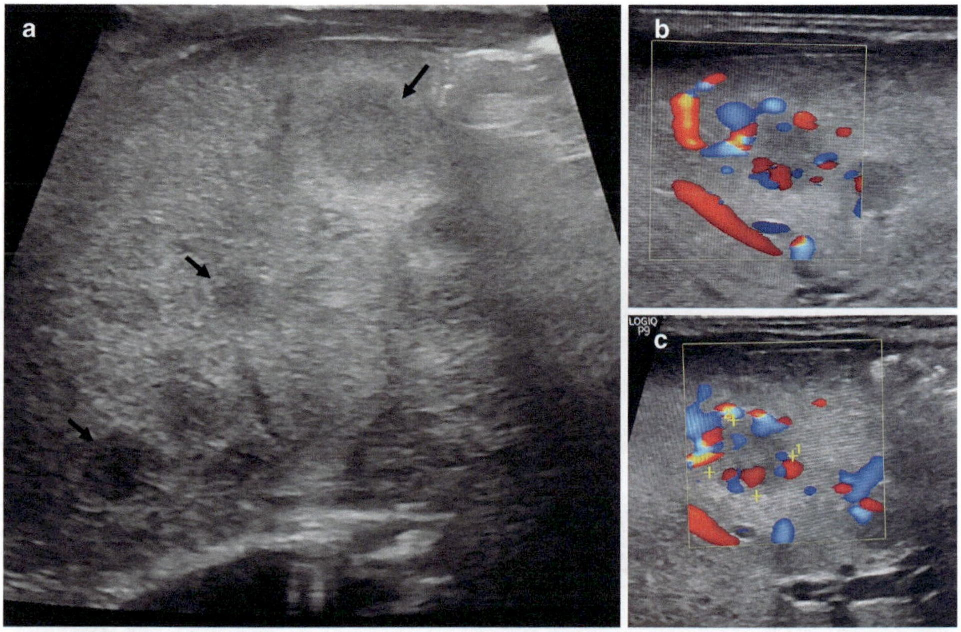

Fig. 6.7 A 6-month-old girl with multiple cutaneous hemangiomas, ultrasound is requested for screening. (**a**) Axial B-mode ultrasound reveals multiple hypoechoic focal lesions (arrows) scattered throughout the liver, with intervening normal parenchyma. (**b**, **c**) Axial color Doppler images demonstrate increased vascularity

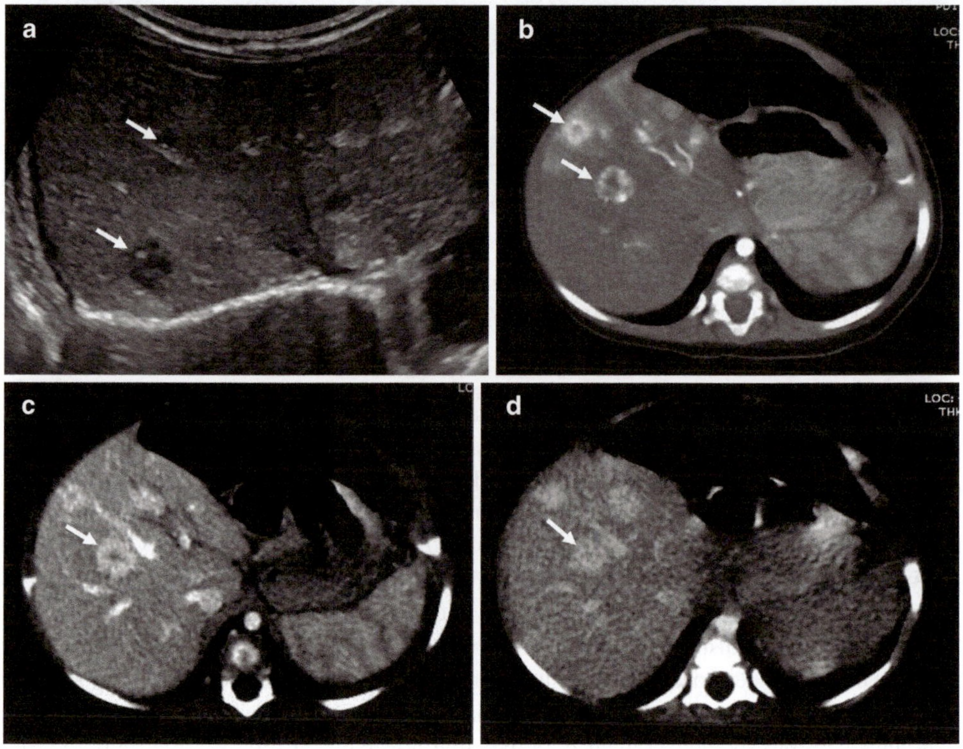

Fig. 6.8 A 4-month-old girl with multifocal hepatic hemangioma (**a**) axial ultrasound shows multiple hypoechoic focal lesions (arrows). (**b**–**d**) axial contrast-enhanced CT in the arterial, venous, and delayed phases respectively demonstrate early arterial enhancement with progressive centripetal filling (arrows)

Diffuse Hepatic Hemangioma

Diffuse hepatic hemangiomas show extensive liver involvement with almost total replacement of hepatic parenchyma, differentiating them from multifocal hemangiomas. Unlike multifocal hemangioma, high-flow shunts are not typically seen with diffuse hemangioma, and morbidity is related not to high cardiac output failure but to massive liver enlargement leading to abdominal compartment syndrome, which may hinder ventilation even with mechanical ventilatory support. Replacement of the hepatic parenchyma also leads to acute liver decompensation [6].

Diffuse hepatic hemangioma shares the imaging characteristics of multifocal hepatic hemangioma with centripetal enhancement and gradual centripetal filling (Fig. 6.10). When the lesions are confluent and their margins are ill-defined, the term hemangiomatosis may be applied [2, 15]. Ultrasound imaging of hemangiomatosis reveals a heteroge-

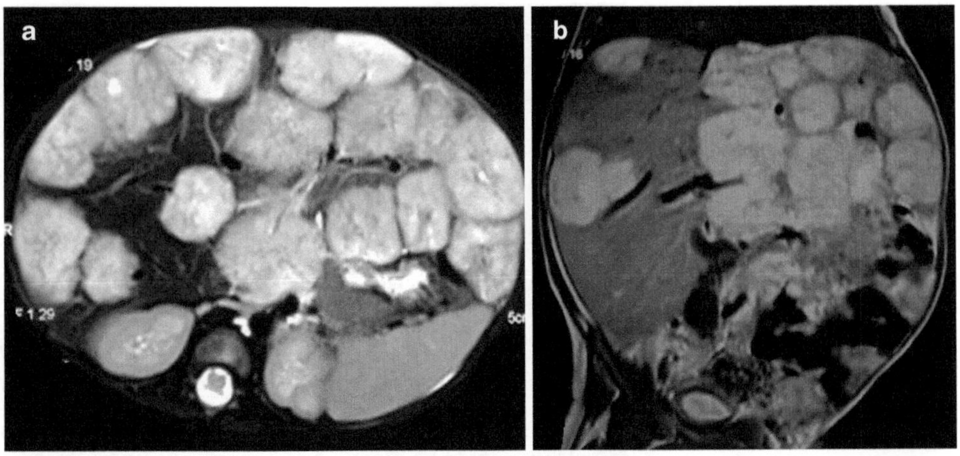

Fig. 6.9 A 7-month-old boy with multiple innumerable hepatic hemangioma. (**a**) axial T2-fat saturated MRI shows multiple spherical focal lesions exhibiting bright signal. (**b**) Coronal contrast-enhanced T1-WI at the delayed phase shows diffuse enhancement of the lesions

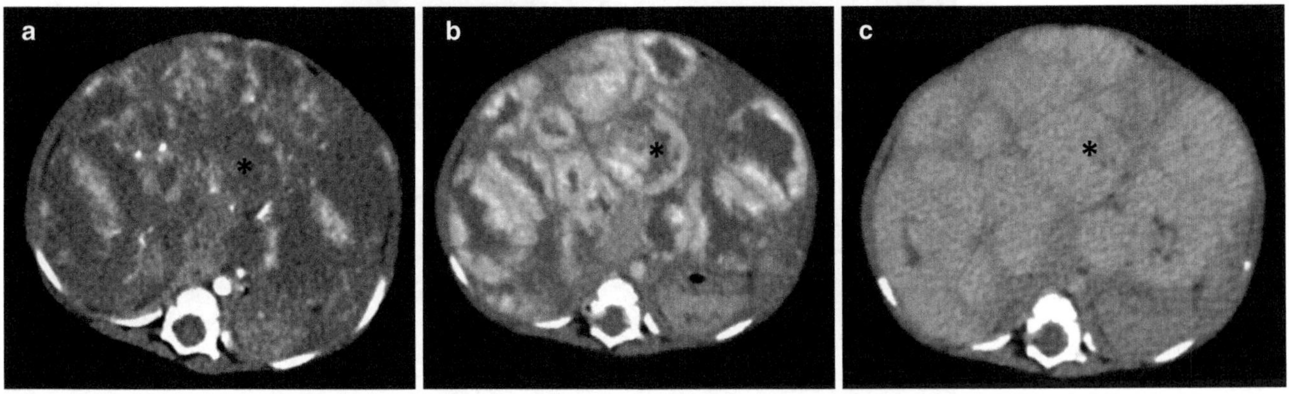

Fig. 6.10 Dynamic contrast-enhanced CT images of a 5-month-old boy with diffuse hepatic hemangioma. (**a**, **b**, **c**) Arterial, venous, and delayed phase images, respectively, show multiple hepatic focal lesions (asterisk) demonstrating early peripheral enhancement with progressive centripetal filling. Note the near-complete replacement of normal liver parenchyma by these lesions

neous liver parenchyma without distinct mass lesions, while dynamic contrast-enhanced studies demonstrate early arterial phase heterogeneous enhancement with diffuse hepatic enhancement in the delayed phase (Fig. 6.11). Pathological confirmation may be necessary in doubtful cases [2, 15, 16].

Additionally, the IHH expresses type 3- iodothyronine deiodinase that converts thyroid hormone to its inactive form, leading to hypothyroidism. Hypothyroidism may lead to fatal hypothermia and decreased cardiac function. Hence, all patients with diffuse hepatic hemangioma and large non-hepatic lesions should be screened for hypothyroidism by measuring the serum level of thyroid-stimulating hormone [6].

Management of Infantile and Congenital Hepatic Hemangioma

Observation is the mainstay of treatment of asymptomatic hepatic hemangioma. Follow-up ultrasound scan should be scheduled at 4–6 weeks intervals over the first months of life to evaluate hepatic size and presence of shunting (Figs. 6.12 and 6.13). Imaging is requested at less frequent intervals and may be indicated later to document involution. Medical treatment is initiated if there are imaging signs of high flow shunting even if the patient is asymptomatic. Patients with significant hepatomegaly and cardiac overload do require pharmacotherapy. Historically, corticosteroid was the standard treatment for infants with infantile hemangioma; however, propranolol has become the treatment of choice. Embolization may be required to interrupt high-flow arteriovenous shunts in infants with high cardiac output failure who don't improve with pharmacotherapy. Thyroid replacement is indicated in infants with hepatic hemangioma and hypothyroidism. Mechanical ventilation may be required in infants with large hepatomegaly and compartment syndrome. Surgical resection is rarely required and limited to extremely large tumors with rupture. Urgent surgical resection is indicated in this instance [6, 17].

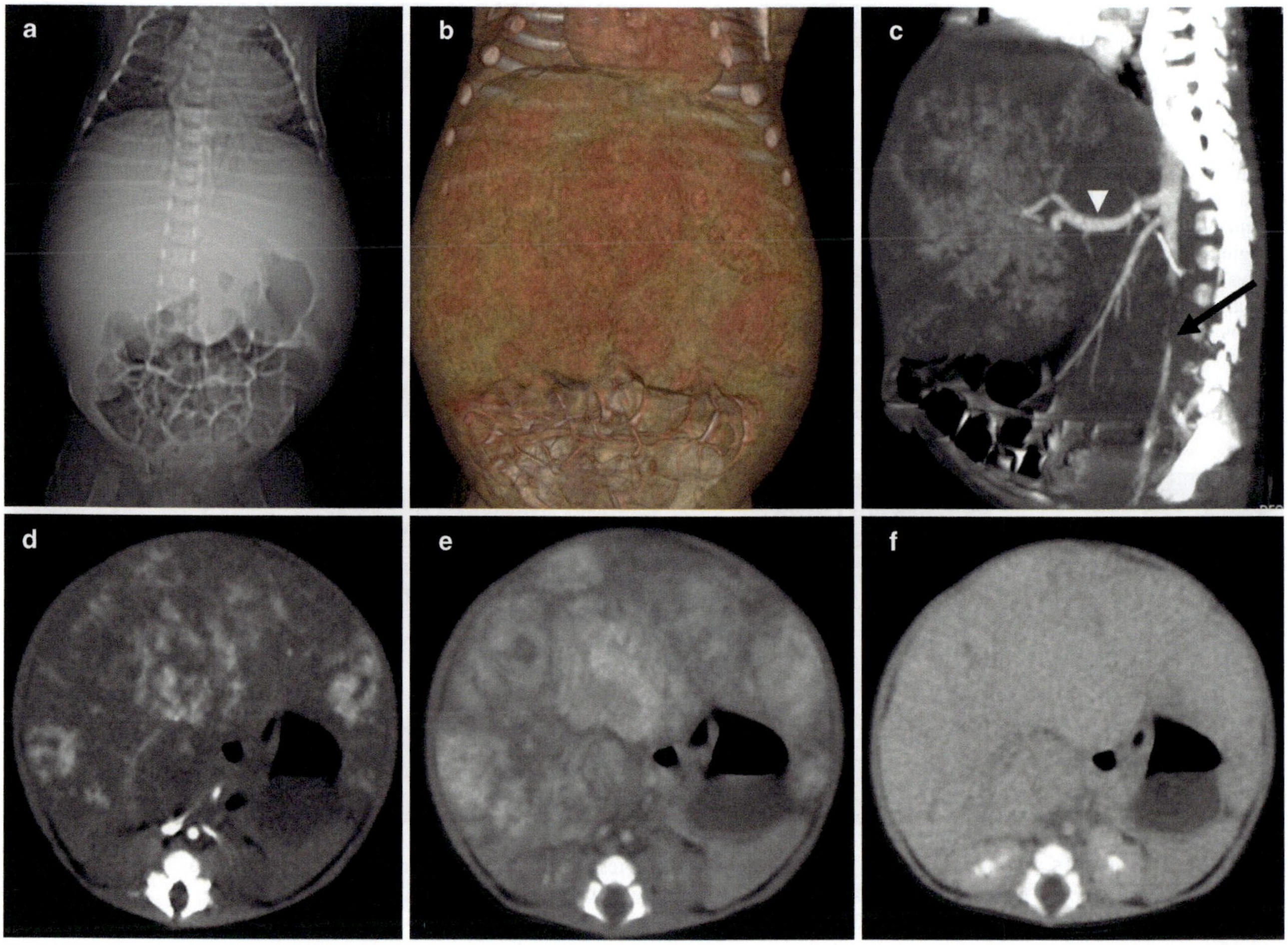

Fig. 6.11 A 34-day-old boy with diffuse hepatic hemangioma (**a**) Scout view of the CT shows enlarged liver. (**b**) Surface rendered three-dimensional reconstruction shows enlarged abdominal circumference by virtue of enlarged liver. (**c**) Sagittal maximum intensity projection of the arterial phase of contrast-enhanced CT reveals enlarged hepatic artery (arrowhead) with decreased caliber of the abdominal aorta after giving the celiac branch (long arrow). (**d, e, f**) Axial sections of the arterial, venous, and delayed phases of contrast-enhanced CT show early intense enhancement in the arterial phase (**d**) with progressive enhancement in the venous phase (**e**) and diffuse liver enhancement in the delayed phase (**f**). Note that the focal lesions are ill-defined with diffuse liver involvement which may be called as hemangiomatosis

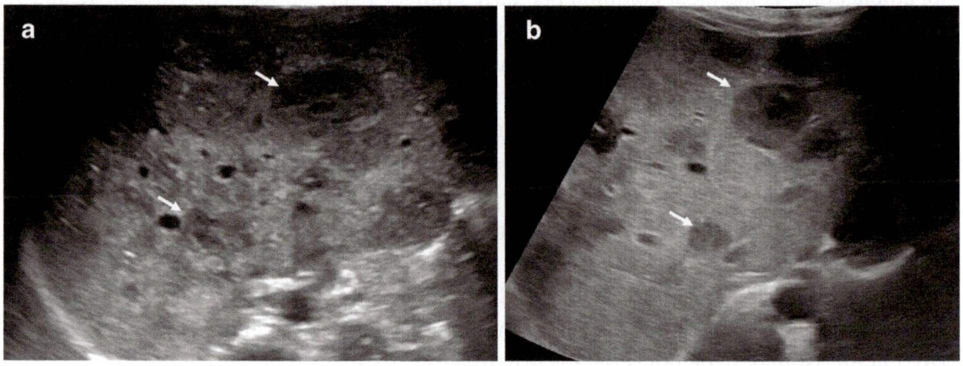

Fig. 6.12 Transverse ultrasound images of an infant with multifocal hepatic hemangiomas (arrows) at 20 months (**a**) and 24 months (**b**) of age. The images demonstrate multiple hypoechoic focal lesions with a noticeable reduction in both size and number on the follow-up scan

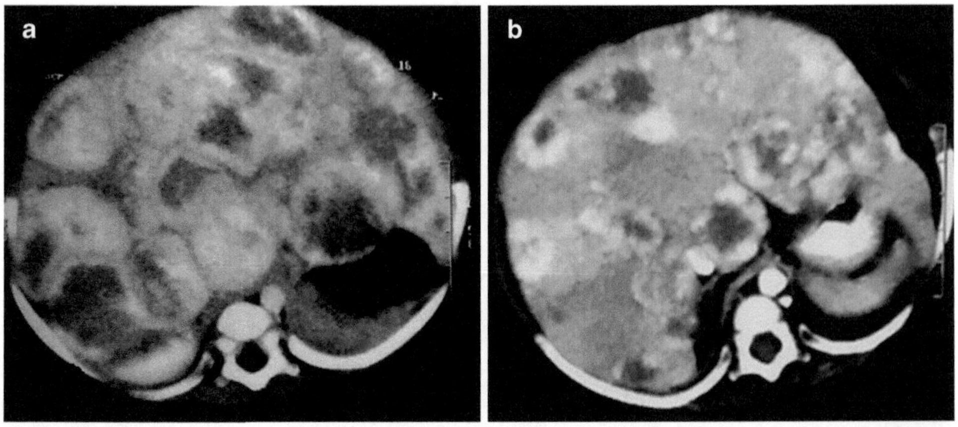

Fig. 6.13 Contrast-enhanced CT images of an infant with diffuse hepatic hemangioma. At 5 months of age (**a**), numerous spherical hepatic lesions exhibit intense enhancement, nearly replacing the normal liver parenchyma. Follow-up imaging at 9 months (**b**) shows a reduction in both the size and number of these lesions

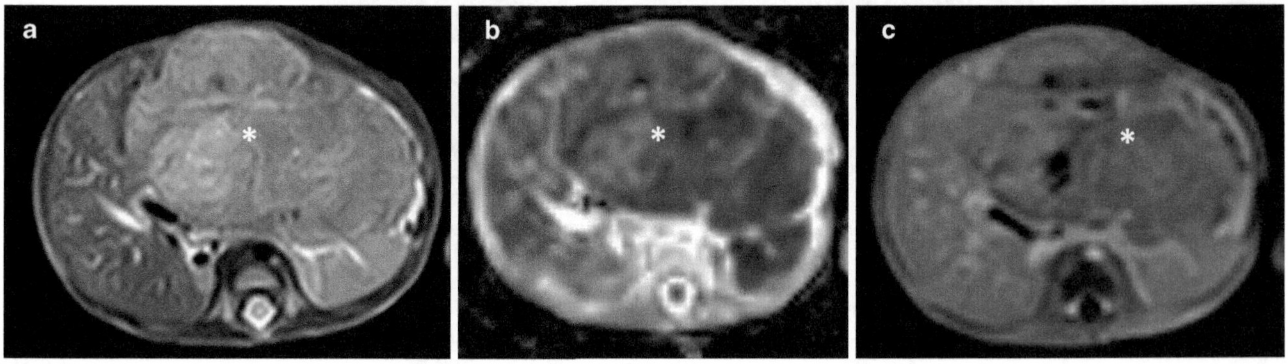

Fig. 6.14 MRI of a 15-day-old male infant with hepatoblastoma (asterisk). The mass appears hyperintense on T2-weighted imaging (**a**), hypointense on the apparent diffusion coefficient map indicating restricted diffusion (**b**), and shows heterogeneous, faint enhancement on post-contrast T1-weighted imaging (**c**)

Differential Diagnosis of Hepatic Hemangioma in Children

Hepatoblastoma

Hepatoblastoma is the most common pediatric primary liver malignancy, usually occurs in the first 2 years of age, and 95% occurs in children younger than 5 years of age. Alpha fetoprotein is an important tumor marker that is elevated in 90% of children at the time of diagnosis. Tumors that don't express AFP are more aggressive with a poorer prognosis. Hepatoblastoma may metastasize to the lungs, or, less commonly, to mediastinal lymph nodes. Metastasis to abdominal lymph nodes is not typical [18].

Imaging is crucial for pretreatment evaluation of tumor extension (PRETEXT) as well as other annotation factors [18]. On ultrasound, hepatoblastoma is usually large, exhibiting variable echo pattern. It usually appears heterogeneous due to the presence of hemorrhage, necrosis, or calcification. However, it may be isoechoic, hypoechoic, or hyperechoic relative to the liver [12, 19]. The MRI signal characteristics of hepatoblastoma vary according to the histological subtype. Epithelial tumors are homogenously hypointense and hyperintense on T1-WI and T2-WI respectively, while mixed epithelial-mesenchymal tumors display heterogeneous signal intensity on both pulse sequences. Heterogeneous signal is attributed to the presence of hemorrhage, necrosis, calcification, and fibrosis. Solid tumor component displays diffusion restriction on diffusion-weighted images (Fig. 6.14). The tumor usually has heterogeneous post-contrast enhancement with areas of early wash due to the presence of arteriovenous shunting. Some large tumors enhance peripherally. But unlike hemangioma, peripheral enhancement is not intense (Figs. 6.15 and 6.16). The arterial and venous phases following contrast administration are helpful for demonstration of vascular anatomy and determination of possible vascular invasion. Compared to bland thrombus, tumor thrombus usually enhances and causes vessel enlargement [12, 14].

Metastasis

Hepatic metastasis in neonates and young infants is typically from neuroblastoma. Hepatic metastasis from neuroblastoma usually occurs in association with stage 4S, and the

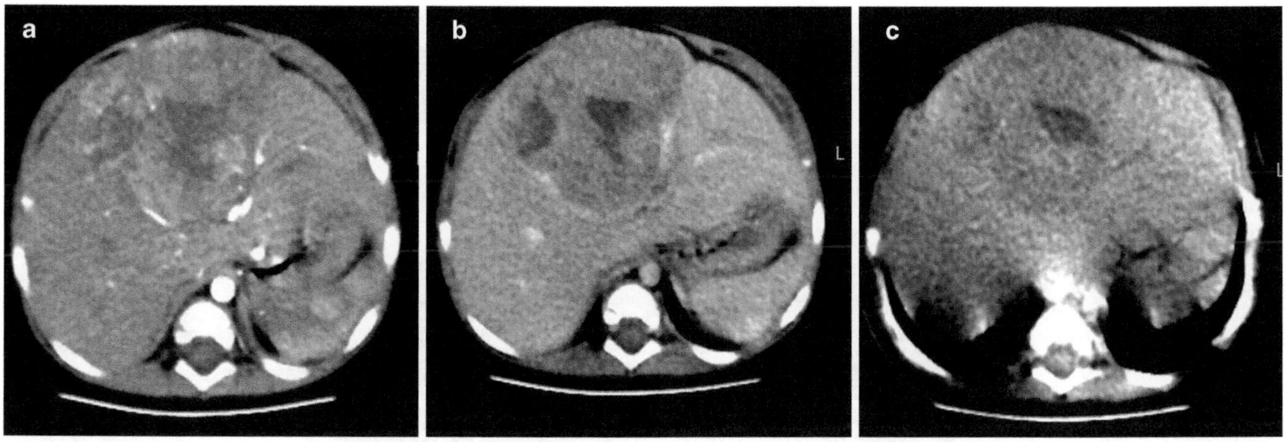

Fig. 6.15 Dynamic contrast-enhanced CT images of an infant with hepatoblastoma. The lesion demonstrates early arterial-phase heterogeneous enhancement (**a**), which is less intense than typically seen in hemangiomas, followed by contrast washout in the venous (**b**) and delayed (**c**) phases

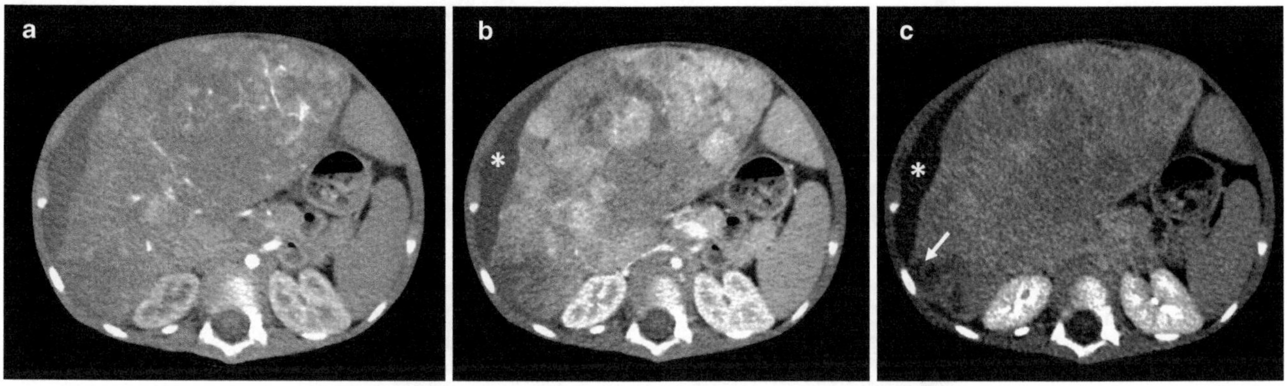

Fig. 6.16 Contrast-enhanced CT images of a 3-year-old boy with hepatoblastoma. Hypervascular masses involving both hepatic lobes demonstrate enhancement in the arterial (**a**) and venous (**b**) phases, followed by washout in the delayed phase (**c**). A subcapsular fluid collection (asterisk) is evident, consistent with tumor rupture (arrow)

primary tumor may not be apparent on imaging. Nevertheless, stage 4S neuroblastoma has relatively a good prognosis.

Neuroblastoma metastases may be solitary or multiple and diffuse, replacing most of the liver's normal parenchyma (Figs. 6.17 and 6.18). They demonstrate peripheral arterial enhancement with progression of enhancement in the portal venous phase; however, unlike hemangioma, they show peripheral washout in the delayed phase. Neuroblastoma metastases may appear isointense to liver parenchyma or may be calcified [20–22]. The detection of diffuse liver metastases may be challenging; they may appear as diffuse liver enlargement with heterogenous parenchyma with patchy contrast enhancement. I-123-MIBG scan shows avid hepatic uptake of the tracer [23]. MRI with hepatobiliary agents is strongly recommended in patients with suspected liver metastasis unless liver function is significantly compromised. Metastasis appears as hypointense in the hepatobiliary phase, augmenting lesion detection and characterization [12, 19].

Mesenchymal Hamartoma

Mesenchymal hamartoma is the second most common benign pediatric hepatic neoplasm, with 80% of cases detected in the first 2 years of age [23]. It is predominantly cystic mass with internal septae; however, predominantly solid tumors do exist; hence, imaging appearance depends on its pathological features. The predominantly cystic type appears as hypodense or hypoechoic on CT and ultrasound respectively. Contrast CT shows enhancing septae (Fig. 6.19). The solid tumors exhibit hypointense signal on T2WI due to its fibrous stroma, while the cystic types exhibit hyperintense signal on T2WI [14, 24]. The existence of proliferating hepatocytes within the tumor may cause the blood level of alpha-fetoprotein to rise; however, this is not the case in the majority of patients. Similarly, Mesenchymal hamartoma seldom exhibits calcification [25].

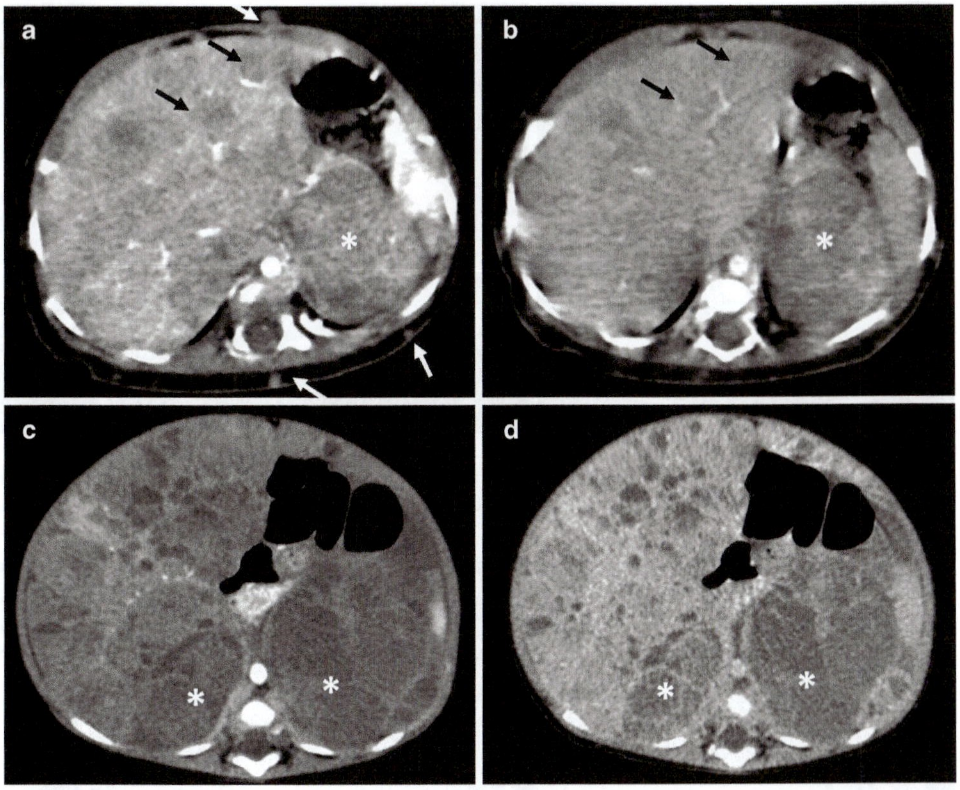

Fig. 6.17 Axial contrast-enhanced CT images of two infants with metastatic neuroblastoma (asterisk). (**a**, **b**) A 5-month-old boy shows multiple faintly enhancing hepatic lesions (black arrows) during the arterial phase (**a**), becoming isodense to the liver in the venous phase (**b**). Cutaneous metastases are also noted (white arrows). (**c**, **d**) Another 5-month-old boy demonstrates diffuse cystic hepatic metastases in the arterial (**c**) and venous (**d**) phases, originating from bilateral cystic neuroblastoma (asterisk)

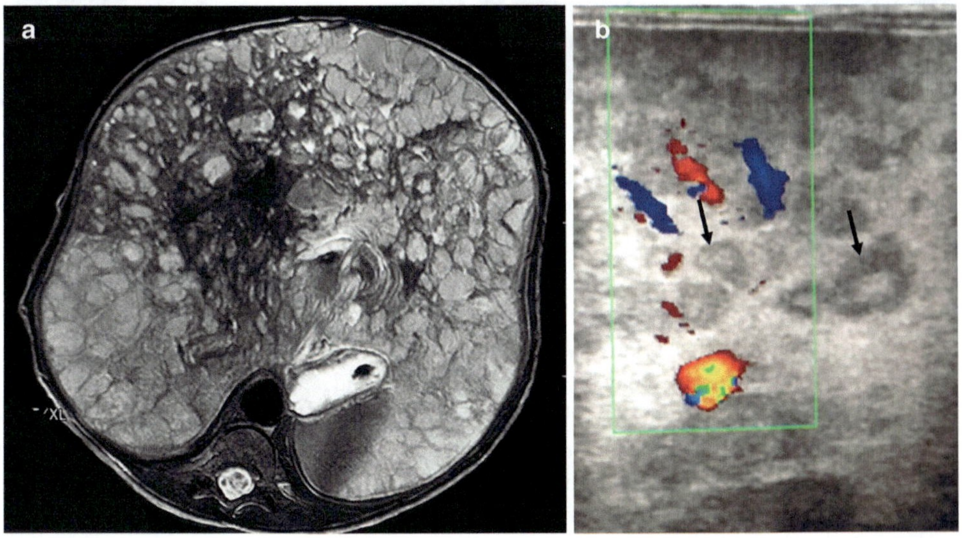

Fig. 6.18 A 3-month-old boy with hepatic metastases from neuroblastoma. (**a**) Axial T2-weighted MRI reveals diffuse liver infiltration with numerous hyperintense focal lesions. (**b**) Axial ultrasound with color Doppler demonstrates multiple hypoechoic lesions, some with a targetoid appearance (arrows)

Biliary Rhabdomyosarcoma

Embryonal rhabdomyosarcoma is the most common sarcoma in children. Biliary rhabdomyosarcoma is usually diagnosed below the age of 5 years. By imaging, it usually appears as a large polypoidal mass projecting into the lumen of the biliary tree (commonly the extrahepatic ducts). At ultrasound, it displays heterogenous hypoechoic pattern with cystic areas. Similarly, it appears as a heterogeneous mass at CT and MRI with prominent fluid density/signal intensity component. It shows variable enhancement patterns ranging from intense to non-enhancement [26].

Hepatic Epithelioid Hemangioendothelioma

Epithelioid hemangioendothelioma is a vascular sarcoma that arises from the endothelium of medium-to-large-sized blood vessels, which affects adolescents and young adults but may occur in children. It has variable clinical behavior. It

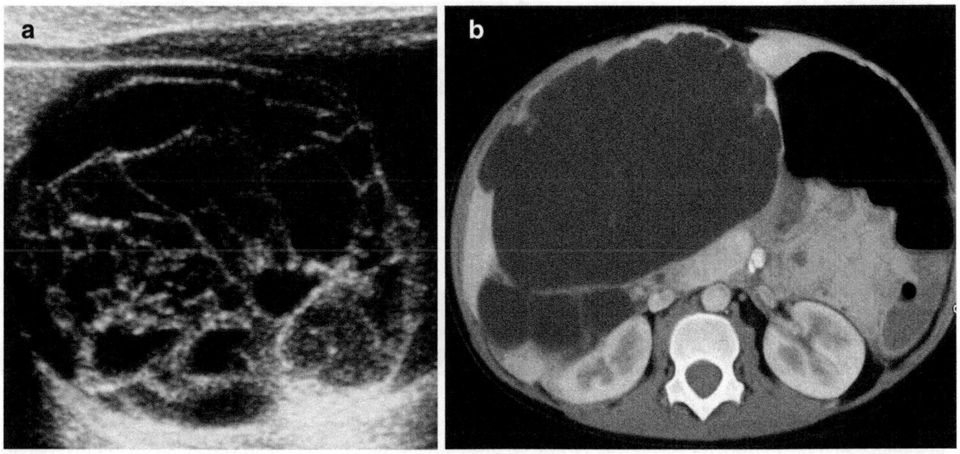

Fig. 6.19 Mesenchymal hamartoma in two infants. (**a**) Ultrasound image demonstrates complex cystic hepatic lesion. (**b**) Axial contrast-enhanced CT reveals a large cystic lesion containing fine internal septations

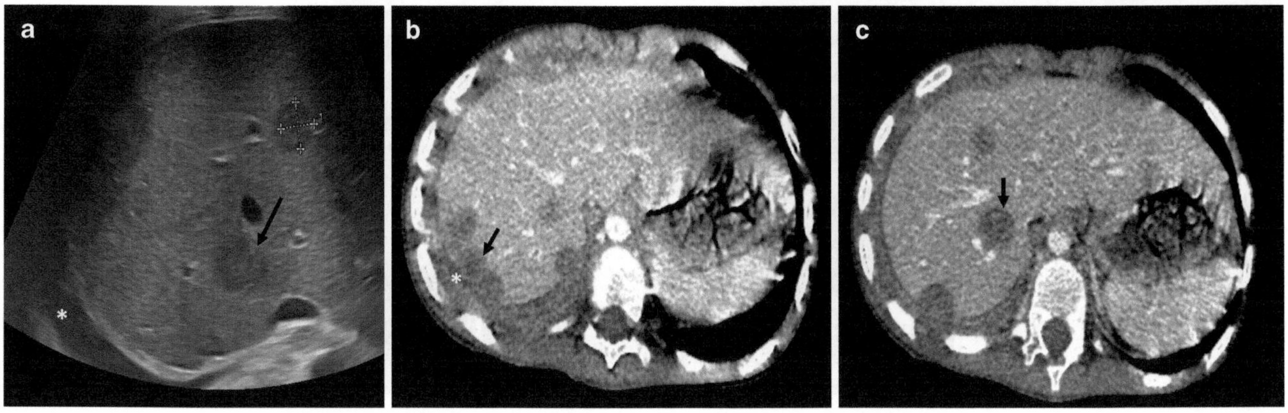

Fig. 6.20 A 9-year-old girl with epithelioid hemangioendothelioma. (**a**) Axial ultrasound reveals multiple hypoechoic hepatic lesions with a targetoid appearance (arrow) and associated pleural effusion (asterisk). (**b**, **c**) Axial contrast-enhanced CT images show mild enhancement of the lesions in a layered or target-like pattern (arrows), with associated pleural metastases (asterisk)

may present as a low-grade malignant tumor or a high-grade sarcoma that has the tendency for recurrence and metastasis to other organs.

On imaging, the tumor is multifocal, scattered in both hepatic lobes. This multifocal nodular pattern is usually observed in the early stages of the disease (Fig. 6.20). However, these multiple lesions progressively enlarge and become confluent masses, forming the diffuse pattern. Peripheral lesions cause capsular retraction because of compensatory hypertrophy of the nearby unaffected liver segments or due to associated fibrosis. Calcifications may be found as well. For solitary lesions, surgery is considered the treatment of choice. However, the response to chemotherapy is usually poor once metastasized [2, 26].

On ultrasound scans, the lesions are most frequently hypoechoic, or have a targetoid appearance, but may have heterogenous echogenicity. On CT, the lesions are hypodense with parenchymal calcifications, and the lesions may show progressive peripheral enhancement (Fig. 6.20). On MRI, the lesions display hypointense signal on T1-WI, with heterogenous bright signal on T2-WI. The lesions may exhibit central hypointense signal due to hemorrhage or calcification, with peripheral bright signal due to tumor viability of edematous changes giving the tumor a targetoid appearance. Dynamic post-contrast study reveals progressive peripheral enhancement with a central nodular enhancement pattern, giving the lesion a lollipop-like pattern [14, 26].

Angiosarcoma

Angiosarcoma is aggressive neoplasm with poor prognosis, presenting after the first year of life. It has variable imaging features. It is mostly multifocal, lacking the typical centripetal enhancement pattern of hemangioma. The enhancement is mostly heterogenous and may be central [27].

Undifferentiated Embryonal Sarcoma

It is considered the third common malignant liver tumor after hepatoblastoma and hepatocellular carcinoma. The majority of undifferentiated embryonal sarcoma (UES) cases are identified in children between the ages of 6 and 10 years.

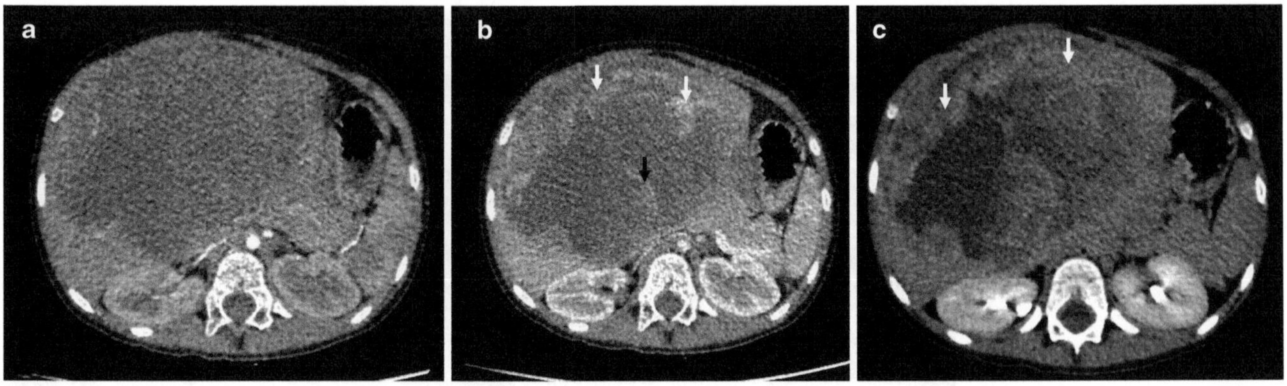

Fig. 6.21 A 9-year-old girl with undifferentiated embryonal sarcoma (**a, b, c**) Dynamic contrast enhanced CT shows despite the early cystic appearance there is peripheral soft tissue (white arrows) and septal enhancement (black arrow) in the venous and delayed phases

Fig. 6.22 A 9-year-old boy with undifferentiated embryonal sarcoma. (**a**) Axial contrast-enhanced CT shows a large hypodense hepatic mass with multiple enhancing internal septations (arrows). (**b**) Axial T2-weighted MRI demonstrates a hyperintense, multiloculated lesion

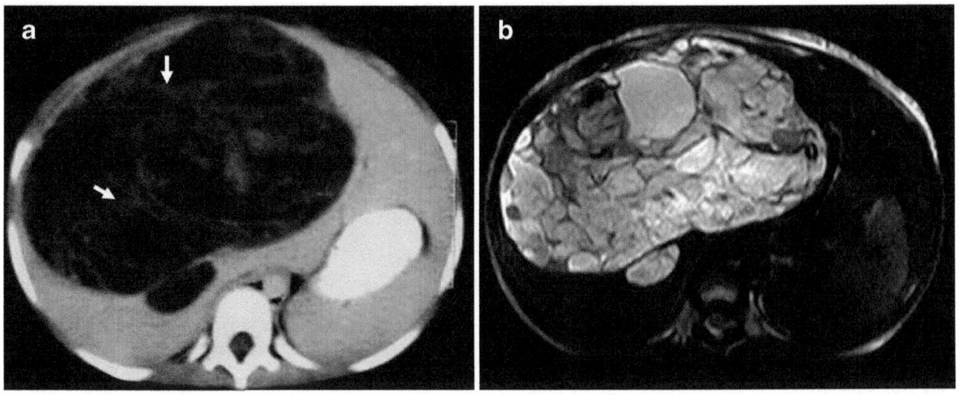

UES characteristically appears solid at ultrasound but cystic at CT due to the high water content of its myxoid stroma. Anechoic areas are also seen at ultrasound due to necrosis. In addition to a predominantly cystic appearance, CT also shows enhanced soft tissue foci at the periphery with septae of variable thickness (Fig. 6.21). Enhanced fibrous pseudocapsule is also noted at the delayed phase following contrast injection. At MRI, UES appears as predominantly hyperintense on T2WI with hypointense fibrous pseudocapsule on T1 and T2WI (Fig. 6.22). UES has imaging characteristics that may be very similar to mesenchymal hamartoma due to its similar pathological origin. Age is the main differentiating point. Mesenchymal hamartoma usually presents in early infancy [14, 26].

Vascular Malformations of the Liver

Venous and Venolymphatic Malformation

Venous malformation of the liver is rare, usually part of blue rubber bleb nevus syndrome. Imaging reveals focal hepatic lesions that show enhancement in the portal venous phase and may contain calcification (phleboliths) (Fig. 6.23). Moreover, patients with abdominal lymphatic malformation may have associated portal vein anomalies (occlusion and varices) [27].

Portosystemic Venous Shunt

Portosystemic venous shunts may be classified based on anatomical location as either intrahepatic or extrahepatic and etiologically as congenital or acquired. Congenital extrahepatic portosystemic shunts, initially reported by Abernethy and Banks, are classified into two types based on whether the portal vein is present. In type I, there is a complete absence of intrahepatic portal blood flow due to an end-to-side connection between the main portal vein and the inferior vena cava (IVC). In this instance, the portal vein shows triphasic pulsatile waveform, reflecting systemic venous flow pattern [28, 29] (Figs. 6.24 and 6.25). In contrast, type II involves only partial diversion of portomesenteric blood into the systemic circulation through congenital shunts, which may include portocaval, gastrorenal, mesenterorenal, splenorenal, or mesenteroiliac pathways. Patients are susceptible to the development of liver tumors (focal nodular hyperplasia, adenoma, and hepatocellular carcinoma) [28, 29] (Fig. 6.24). On the other hand, Park et al. classified congenital intrahepatic portosystemic shunts into four types [30] (Figs. 6.2 and 6.26).

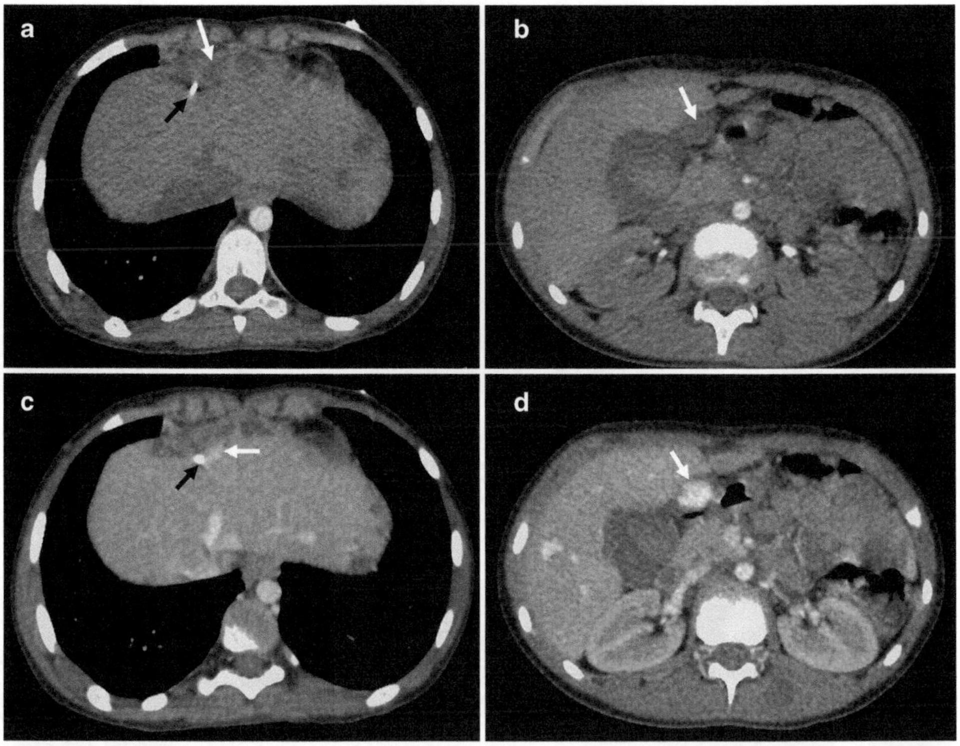

Fig. 6.23 An 11-year-old girl with blue rubber bleb nevus and multiple venous malformations. Axial contrast-enhanced CT at the arterial (**a**, **b**) and venous phases (**c**, **d**) shows multiple focal lesions (white arrows) that show enhancement in the venous phase. Note the associated phlebolith (black arrow)

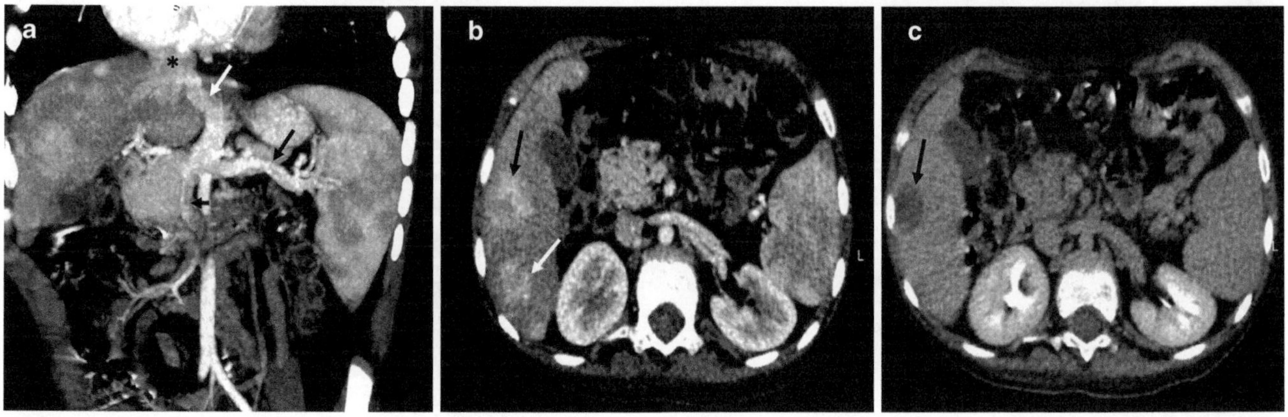

Fig. 6.24 A 5-year-old boy with congenital portosystemic shunt (Abernethy malformation type I) with multiple hepatic focal lesions. a. Oblique coronal CT shows that the splenic vein (long black arrow) joined the superior mesenteric vein (short black arrow) to form the portal vein (white arrow) the latter ends with end to side connection to the inferior vena cava (asterisk). b, c Axial Contrast enhanced CT shows early hyper-enhancing lesion (black arrow) with delayed washout (**c**) suggesting hepatocellular carcinoma. Another focal lesion (white arrow) shows the characteristic central scar (not shown) of focal nodular hyperplasia that shows early hyperenhancement (**b**) and becomes isodense to the liver parenchyma on the delayed phase (**c**)

Acquired portosystemic shunts—such as gastroesophageal, paraesophageal, splenorenal, and mesenterocaval shunts—commonly develop in the setting of portal hypertension or trauma. Imaging reveals dilated and tortuous veins in relation to both the portal venous system and the systemic venous circulation [31, 32]. Cavernous transformation may be observed as a sequel of portal vein thrombosis (Figs. 6.27, 6.28 and 6.29).

Arterioportal Shunt and Arteriovenous Malformation

Congenital arterioportal fistulas represent direct communication of the hepatic artery branch and portal vein branch that may lead to portal hypertension. There may be multiple arterial feeders leading to portal vein varix. Arterioportal shunt may be isolated or associated with connective tissue

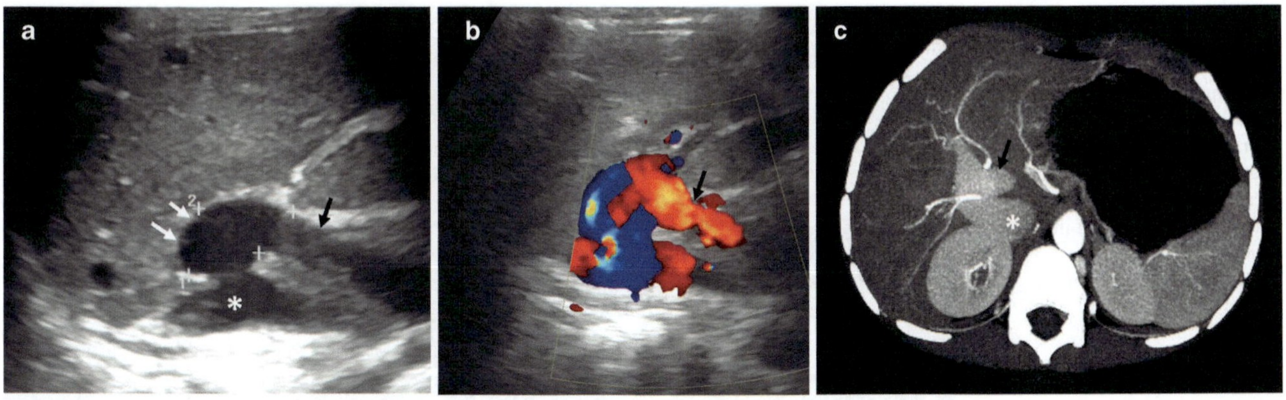

Fig. 6.25 A 10-year-old boy with congenital portosystemic shunt (**a**) Oblique B-mode ultrasound shows anomalous end to side connection (white arrow) between the portal vein (black arrow) and inferior vena cava (asterisk). (**b**) color Doppler interrogation confirms portosystemic connection with turbulent flow. (**c**) Axial contrast enhanced CT confirms the abnormal connection between the portal vein (arrow) and the inferior vena cava (asterisk)

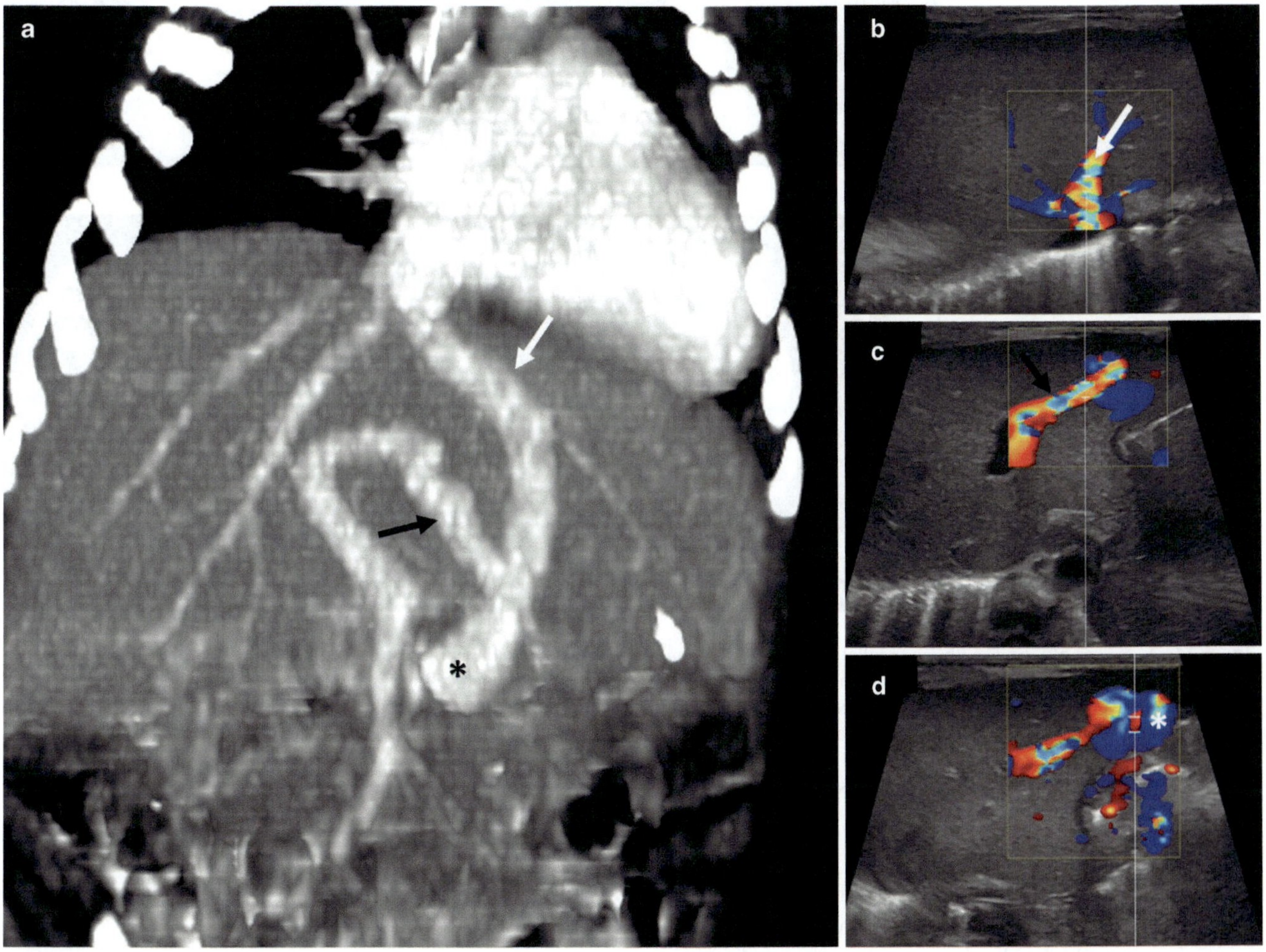

Fig. 6.26 A 27-day-old neonate with intrahepatic portosystemic fistula presenting with jaundice. (**a**) Coronal maximum intensity projection from contrast-enhanced CT demonstrates a connection between the dilated left portal vein (black arrow) and the dilated left hepatic vein (white arrow) via a varix (asterisk). (**b**, **c**, **d**) Consecutive axial ultrasound scans with color Doppler confirm the same vascular communication

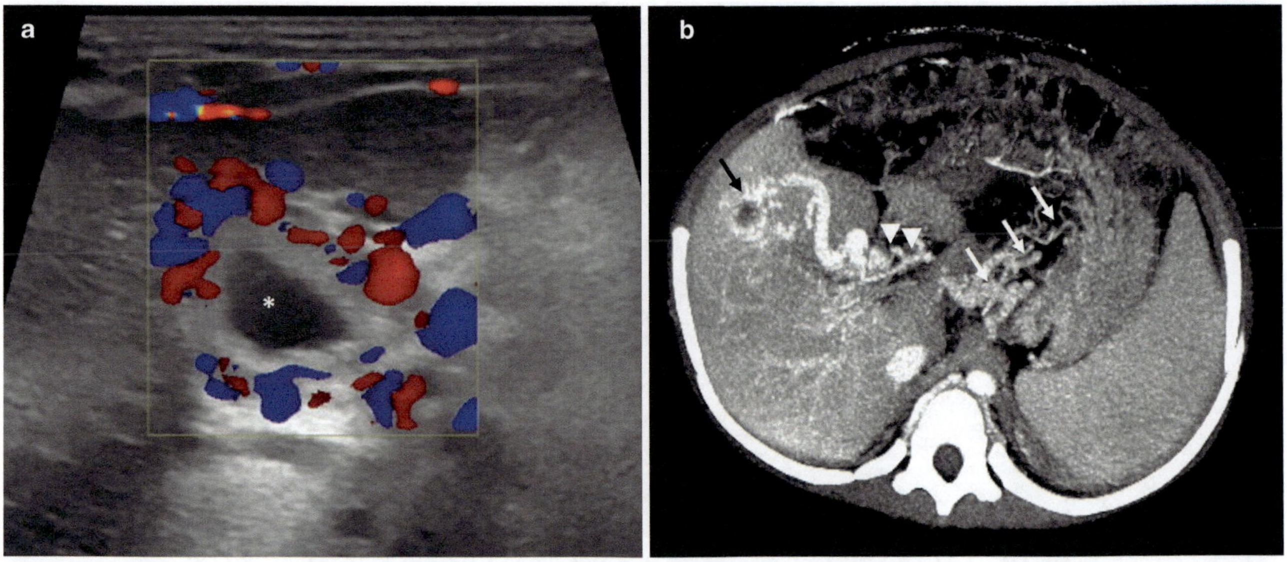

Fig. 6.27 A 3-year-old boy with portal hypertension. (**a**) Axial ultrasound with color Doppler interrogation shows increased vascularity surrounding the gall bladder (asterisk) corresponding to portosystemic collaterals. (**b**) Axial maximum intensity projection of contrast enhanced CT confirms the presence of multiple portosystemic collaterals surrounding the gall bladder (black arow) and along the lesser curvature of the stomach (white arrows). The main portal vein is thrombosed with cavernous transformation (arrow heads)

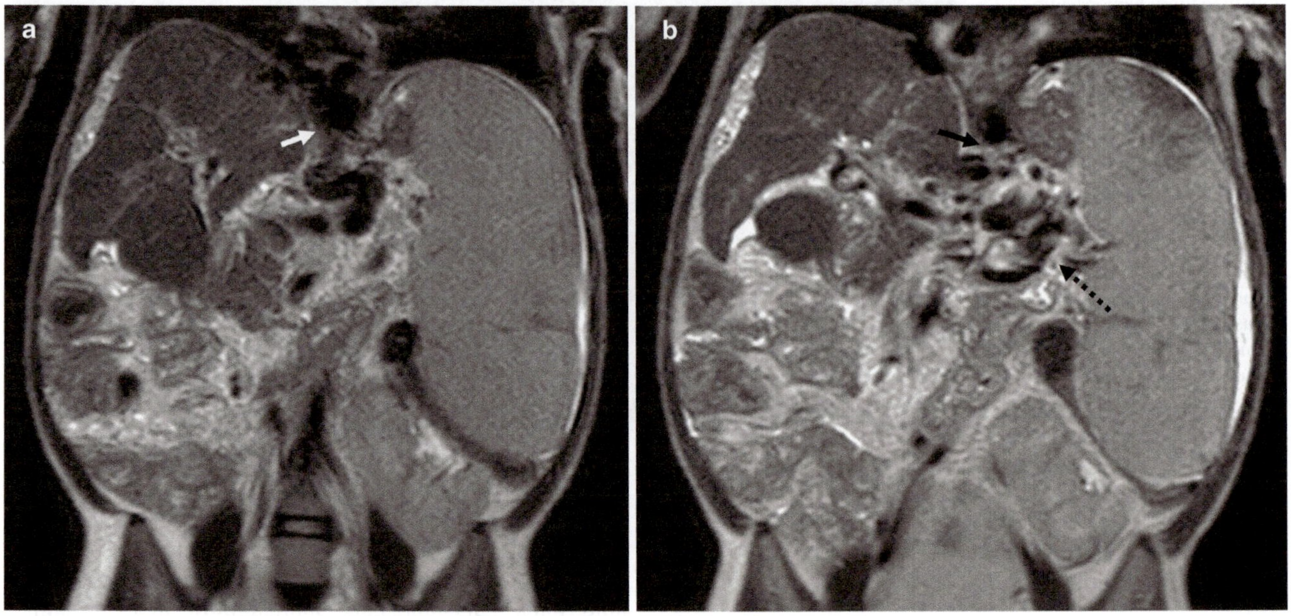

Fig. 6.28 MRI images of an 8-year-old girl with Gaucher disease, portal vein thrombosis, and portal hypertension. (**a, b**) Coronal T2-weighted images demonstrate cirrhotic liver changes, marked splenomegaly, and varices in the paraesophageal (white arrow), perigastric (black arrow), and splenic hilum (dotted arrow) regions

disorders (as Ehlers-Danlos syndrome). It manifests as early visualization of a portal vein branch before the main portal vein with segmental wedge-shaped area of transient hyperenhancement during the arterial phase [29].

The arteriovenous malformation (AVM) of the liver is rare malformation. It may present in the neonatal period with congestive heart failure. Embolization is the treatment of choice of those lesions. In older children, AVM of the liver may present as part of hereditary hemorrhagic telangiectasia. Liver transplantation is recommended in those patients as the AVMs are usually diffuse, and embolization may cause further liver damage. Moreover, the liver of hereditary hemorrhagic telangiectasia patients shows hypervascular lesions (telangiectasias) that demonstrate arterial enhancement, which persists into the portal venous phase (Fig. 6.30). The presence of enlarged arterial branches both inside and outside

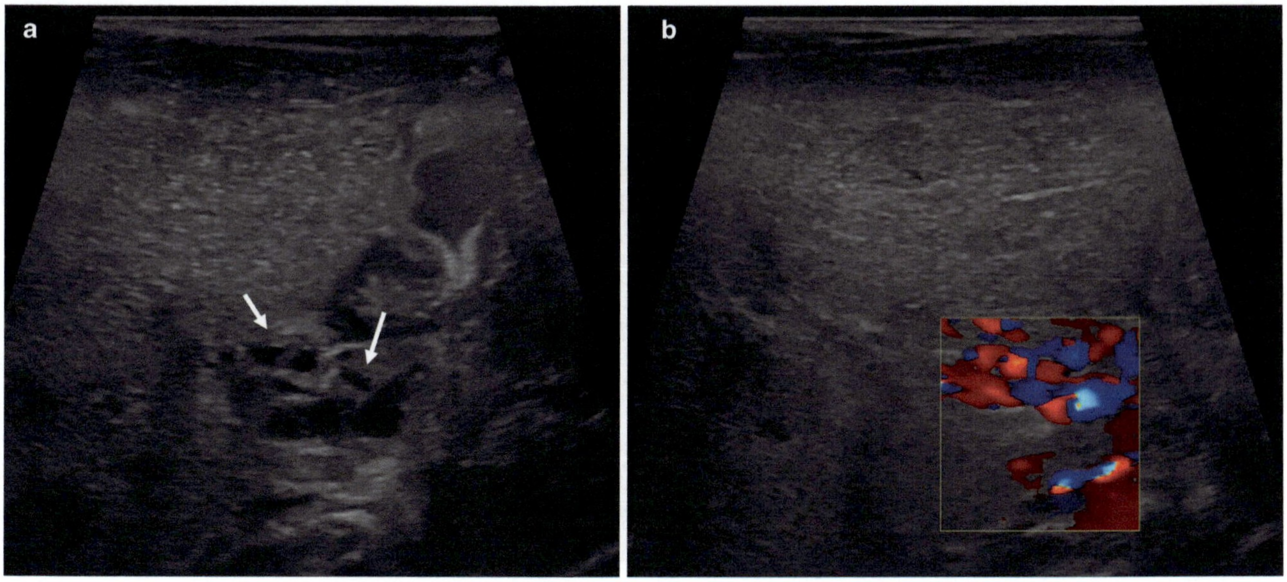

Fig. 6.29 A 50-day-old boy with history of portal vein thrombosis (**a**) axial B-mode and (**b**) color Doppler interrogation reveals multiple tortuous vessels (arrows) at the anatomical location of the portal vein

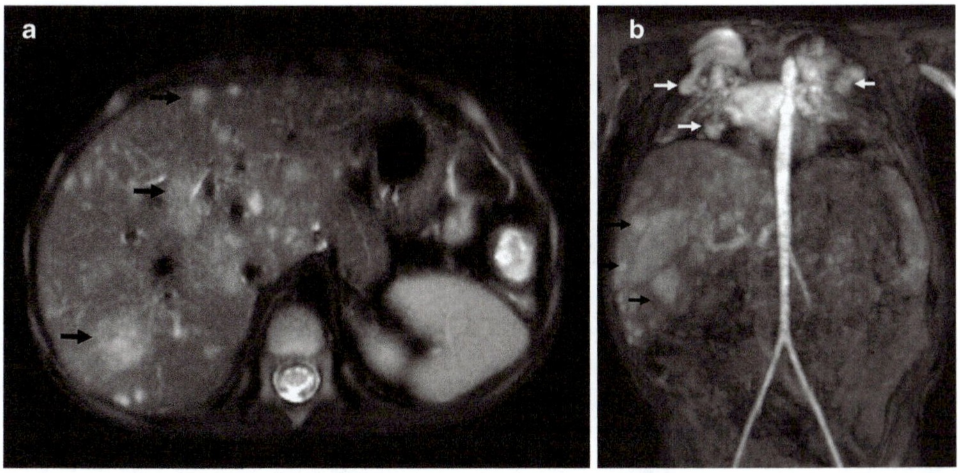

Fig. 6.30 A 5-year-old boy with hereditary hemorrhagic telangiectasia (**a**) axial T2-fat saturated MRI shows multiple variable sized hyperintense hepatic focal lesions (telangiectasia) (arrows). (**b**) Coronal maximum intensity projection of the arterial phase of the dynamic contrast enhanced MRI shows enhancement of those focal lesions (black arrow). Note the associated multiple pulmonary arteriovenous malformations (white arrows)

the liver, along with early opacification of portal or hepatic veins, suggests the presence of associated arterioportal or arteriovenous shunting [27, 32].

Hepatic Hemangioma in Adults

Hepatic hemangioma in adults is the second common liver mass after metastasis. It is essentially venous malformation and doesn't belong to vascular tumors. It is usually small in size and detected incidentally due to unrelated cause. On ultrasound, small lesions appear as a solid, homogeneous, hyperechoic lesion, while large lesions may have heterogeneous echogenicity due to central necrosis and hemorrhage. On CT, it typically shows peripheral nodular hyperenhancement in the arterial phase with progressive centripetal filling [17] (Fig. 6.31).

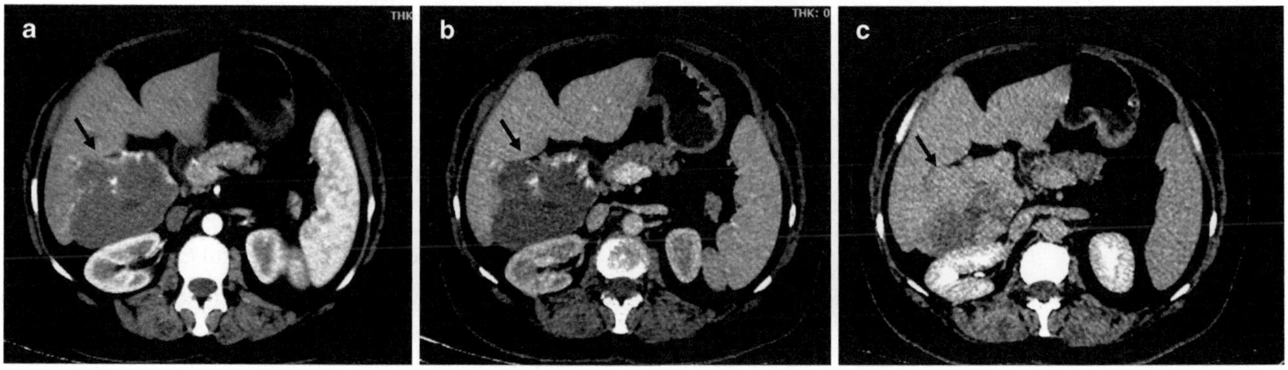

Fig. 6.31 A 57-year-old woman with incidentally discovered hepatic hemangioma during the diagnostic work-up for menorrhagia. Axial contrast-enhanced CT shows early peripheral nodular hyperenhancement (**a**) and progressive filling in the venous (**b**) and delayed phases (**c**)

References

1. ISSVA Classification of Vascular Anomalies ©2018 International Society for the Study of Vascular Anomalies Available at "issva.org/classification". Accessed 6 May 2023.
2. Wildgruber M, Sadick M, Müller-Wille R, Wohlgemuth WA. Vascular tumors in infants and adolescents. Insights Imaging. 2019;10:1–4.
3. Roebuck D, Sebire N, Lehmann E, Barnacle A. Rapidly involuting congenital haemangioma (RICH) of the liver. Pediatr Radiol. 2012;42(3):308–14. https://doi.org/10.1007/s00247-011-2268-z. PMID: 22302317
4. Picard A, Boscolo E, Khan ZA, Bartch TC, Mulliken JB, Vazquez MP, Bischoff J. IGF-2 and FLT-1/VEGF-R1 mRNA levels reveal distinctions and similarities between congenital and common infantile hemangioma. Pediatr Res. 2008;63(3):263–7.
5. ISSVA Classification of Vascular Anomalies ©2025 International Society for the Study of Vascular Anomalies Available at "issva.org/classification". Accessed 9 June 2025.
6. Iacobas I, Phung TL, Adams DM, Trenor IIICC, Blei F, Fishman DS, Hammill A, Masand PM, Fishman SJ. Guidance document for hepatic hemangioma (infantile and congenital) evaluation and monitoring. J Pediatr. 2018;203:294–300.
7. Christison-Lagay ER, Burrows PE, Alomari A, Dubois J, Kozakewich HP, Lane TS, Paltiel HJ, Klement G, Mulliken JB, Fishman SJ. Hepatic hemangiomas: subtype classification and development of a clinical practice algorithm and registry. J Pediatr Surg. 2007;42(1):62–8.
8. Gnarra M, Behr G, Kitajewski A, Wu JK, Anupindi SA, Shawber CJ, Zavras N, Schizas D, Salakos C, Economopoulos KP. History of the infantile hepatic hemangioma: from imaging to generating a differential diagnosis. World J Clin Pediatr. 2016;5(3):273.
9. Pugmire BS, Towbin AJ. Magnetic resonance imaging of primary pediatric liver tumors. Pediatr Radiol. 2016;46(6):764–77.
10. Berenguer B, Mulliken JB, Enjolras O, et al. Rapidly involuting congenital hemangioma: clinical and histopathologic features. Pediatr Dev Pathol. 2003;6:495.
11. Baselga E, Cordisco MR, Garzon M, Lee MT, Alomar A, Blei F. Rapidly involuting congenital haemangioma associated with transient thrombocytopenia and coagulopathy: a case series. Br J Dermatol. 2008;158(6):1363–70.
12. Schooler GR, Squires JH, Alazraki A, Chavhan GB, Chernyak V, Davis JT, Khanna G, Krishnamurthy R, Lungren MP, Masand PM, Podberesky DJ. Pediatric hepatoblastoma, hepatocellular carcinoma, and other hepatic neoplasms: consensus imaging recommendations from American College of Radiology Pediatric Liver Reporting and Data System (LI-RADS) Working Group. Radiology. 2020;296(3):493–7.
13. Squires JH, McCarville MB. Contrast-enhanced ultrasound in children: implementation and key diagnostic applications. AJR Am J Roentgenol. 2021;217(5):1217–31.
14. Vasireddi AK, Leo ME, Squires JH. Magnetic resonance imaging of pediatric liver tumors. Pediatr Radiol. 2022;52(2):177–88.
15. Gong X, Li Y, Yang K, Chen S, Ji Y. Infantile hepatic hemangiomas: looking backwards and forwards. Precision Clin Med. 2022;5(1):pbac006.
16. Kassarjian A, Zurakowski D, Dubois J, Paltiel HJ, Fishman SJ, Burrows PE. Infantile hepatic hemangiomas: clinical and imaging findings and their correlation with therapy. Am J Roentgenol. 2004;182(3):785–95.
17. Fishman SJ, Burrows BE. Treatment of visceral vascular tumors. In: Mulliken JB, Burrows PE, Fishman SJ, editors. Mulliken & Young vascular anomalies: Hemangioms and malformations. Oxford university press; 2013. p. 239–58.
18. Towbin AJ, Meyers RL, Woodley H, Miyazaki O, Weldon CB, Morland B, Hiyama E, Czauderna P, Roebuck DJ, Tiao GM. 2017 PRETEXT: radiologic staging system for primary hepatic malignancies of childhood revised for the Paediatric Hepatic International Tumour Trial (PHITT). Pediatr Radiol. 2018;48(4):536–54.
19. Chavhan GB, Schooler GR, Tang ER, Squires JH, Rees MA, Nguyen HN, Morin CE, Kolbe AB, Khanna G, Infante JC, Alazraki AL. Optimizing imaging of pediatric liver lesions: guidelines from the Pediatric LI-RADS Working Group. Radiographics. 2022;43(1):e220043.
20. Maino C, Vernuccio F, Cannella R, Cortese F, Franco PN, Gaetani C, Giannini V, Inchingolo R, Ippolito D, Defeudis A, Pilato G. Liver metastases: the role of magnetic resonance imaging. World J Gastroenterol. 2023;29(36):5180.
21. Kushner BH. Neuroblastoma: a disease requiring a multitude of imaging studies. J Nucl Med. 2004;45(7):1172–88.
22. Lee SY, Chuang JH, Huang CB, Hsiao CC, Wan YL, Ng SH, Lee TY, Ko SF. Congenital bilateral cystic neuroblastoma with liver metastases and massive intracystic haemorrhage. Br J Radiol. 1998;71(851):1205–7.
23. Brisse HJ, McCarville MB, Granata C, Krug KB, Wootton-Gorges SL, Kanegawa K, Giammarile F, Schmidt M, Shulkin BL, Matthay KK, Lewington VJ. Guidelines for imaging and staging of neuroblastic tumors: consensus report from the International Neuroblastoma Risk Group Project. Radiology. 2011;261(1):243–57.
24. Kim SH, Kim WS, Cheon JE, Yoon HK, Kang GH, Kim IO, Yeon KM. Radiological spectrum of hepatic mesenchymal hamartoma in children. Korean J Radiol. 2007;8(6):498–505.

25. Martins-Filho SN, Putra J. Hepatic mesenchymal hamartoma and undifferentiated embryonal sarcoma of the liver: a pathologic review. Hepat Oncologia. 2020;7:HEP19.
26. Chavhan GB, Siddiqui I, Ingley KM, Gupta AA. Rare malignant liver tumors in children. Pediatr Radiol. 2019;49:1404–21.
27. Burrows PE, Dubois J, Kassarjian A. Pediatric hepatic vascular anomalies. Pediatr Radiol. 2001;31:B533–45.
28. Abernethy J, Banks J. Account of two instances of uncommon formation in the viscera of the human body. Phil Trans R Soc Lond. 1793;83:59–66.
29. Albers BK, Khanna G. Vascular anomalies of the pediatric liver. Radiographics. 2019;39(3):842–56.
30. Park JH, Cha SH, Han JK, Han MC. Intrahepatic portosystemic venous shunt. AJR Am J Roentgenol. 1990;155(3):527–8.
31. Leite AF, Mota JA, Chagas-Neto FA, Teixeira SR, Elias J, Muglia VF. Acquired portosystemic collaterals: anatomy and imaging. Radiol Bras. 2016;49(4):251–6.
32. Elsayes KM, Shaaban AM, Rothan SM, Javadi S, Madrazo BL, Castillo RP, Casillas VJ, Menias CO. A comprehensive approach to hepatic vascular disease. Radiographics. 2017;37(3):813–36.

Kaposiform Hemangioendothelioma and Tufted Angioma

7

Kaposiform Hemangioendothelioma (KHE)

Kaposiform hemangioendothelioma (KHE) represents a distinctive vascular neoplasm classified as benign yet locally aggressive (Fig. 7.1). Although it does not metastasize, KHE frequently demonstrates infiltrative growth across tissue planes, extending into muscle and adjacent soft tissues (Fig. 7.2). Rarely, multifocal presentations have been documented [1]. The histopathological hallmark of KHE is the simultaneous presence of progressive angiogenesis and lymphangiogenesis. Regional lymph node involvement may occur (Fig. 7.3), but distant metastasis has not been reported [2].

KHE typically presents as a progressively enlarging cutaneous or subcutaneous lesion, most commonly involving the face (Fig. 7.1) and extremities (Fig. 7.4). Lesions are often red to violaceous in color (Figs. 7.1a and 7.3a) and may exhibit an erythematous surface resembling an orange peel (Fig. 7.5a). While occasionally congenital, KHE most often arises during infancy, and spontaneous involution is rare.

A critical clinical feature is the association of KHE with Kasabach–Merritt phenomenon (KMP), observed in approximately 70% of cases [3]. KMP is a life-threatening consumptive coagulopathy characterized by profound thrombocytopenia (platelet count <50,000/mm^3), hypofibrinogenemia, elevated D-dimer levels, and prolongation of both prothrombin time and activated partial thromboplastin time [4].

The precise pathophysiology of KMP remains incompletely understood. Current evidence suggests that platelet trapping, activation, and aggregation within the tumor vasculature initiate a cascade of intralesional thrombosis. Subsequent activation of the coagulation system results in factor consumption, hemorrhage, and progressive tumor enlargement. Clinically, these processes are reflected by increasing lesion size, violaceous discoloration, and localized warmth [4].

Cutaneous KHE without KMP shares similar demographic, clinical, radiologic, and pathologic features with KHE associated with KMP [5]. Biopsy is indicated when the diagnosis remains uncertain. Visceral involvement is less common but has been documented in the literature.

Imaging Characteristics

On ultrasound, KHE typically presents as a heterogeneous soft tissue mass with ill-defined margins and trans-spatial extension. Central hypoechoic areas are usually encircled by increased echogenicity and soft tissue thickening. Color Doppler consistently demonstrates increased vascular density (Fig. 7.5) [6, 7].

On MRI, kaposiform hemangioendothelioma (KHE) typically presents as an irregular, infiltrative soft tissue mass (Fig. 7.6). Subcutaneous thickening (Fig. 7.7) and trans-spatial extension into deeper structures such as muscle and fascia are frequently noted (Fig. 7.2). The lesion usually demonstrates an isointense to mildly hyperintense signal relative to muscle on T1-weighted images, occasionally with hyperintense foci suggestive of hemorrhage. On T2-weighted sequences, KHE appears heterogeneously hyperintense (Figs. 7.6, 7.8 and 7.9), reflecting hemosiderin deposition and hyaline stromal reaction. Dynamic contrast-enhanced imaging reveals early progressive enhancement (Fig. 7.10) [8, 9]. Associated findings include subcutaneous reticular stranding, indicative of lymphedema, and overlying skin thickening [8–10].

Treatment and Outcomes

Therapeutic strategies for KHE generally include systemic corticosteroids in combination with vincristine (Figs. 7.1, 7.4 and 7.8) [8]. More recently, sirolimus has been used successfully to induce tumor regression in cases with KHE (Fig. 7.11) [11–13]. Mortality associated with KHE remains low, at approximately 1% [12].

A. A. AbouZeid et al., *Atlas of Pediatric Vascular Anomalies*, https://doi.org/10.1007/978-3-032-30866-5_7

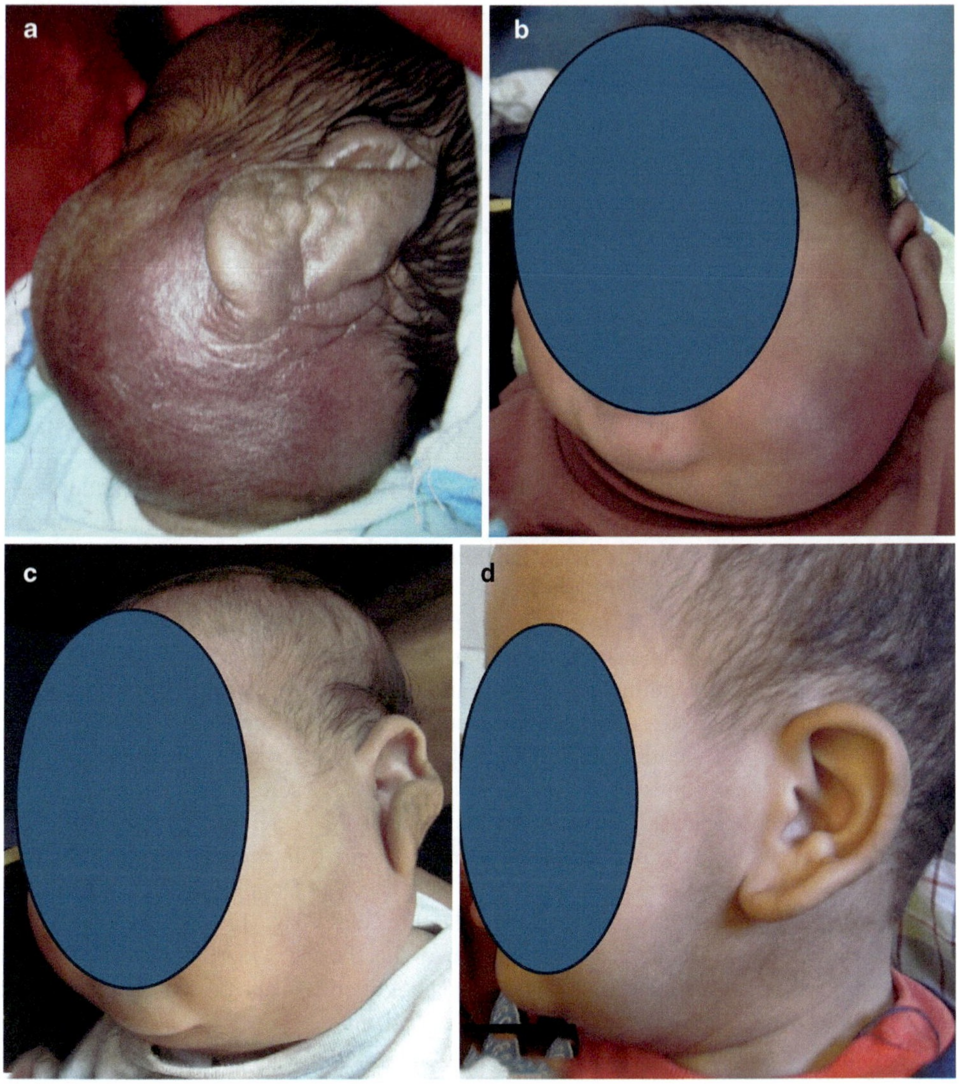

Fig. 7.1 (**a**) Neonate with a facial mass and thrombocytopenia, confirmed as kaposiform hemangioendothelioma (KHE). (**b–d**) Marked regression of the tumor was observed following medical treatment with steroids and vincristine, as shown at 3 months, 8 months, and 1 year of follow-up, respectively

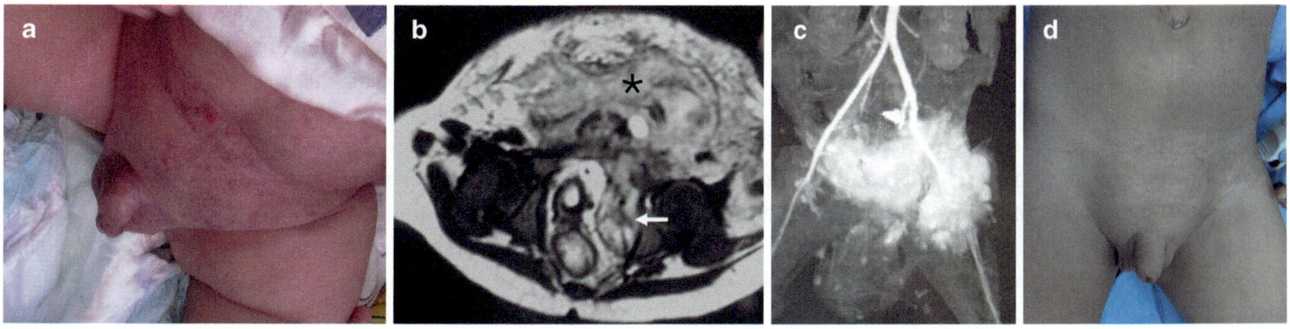

Fig. 7.2 A 1-year-old boy with kaposiform hemangioendothelioma (KHE) presenting as diffuse subcutaneous swelling in the suprapubic region (**a**) and associated thrombocytopenia. (**b**) MRI (T2-weighted image) shows subcutaneous thickening (*) with ill-defined margins and trans-spatial extension into adjacent pelvic structures (arrow). (**c**) Contrast-enhanced magnetic resonance arteriography in the arterial phase demonstrates early, intense, diffuse enhancement of the lesion. (**d**) At 4-year follow-up after successful medical treatment, marked tumor regression is observed with no evidence of recurrence

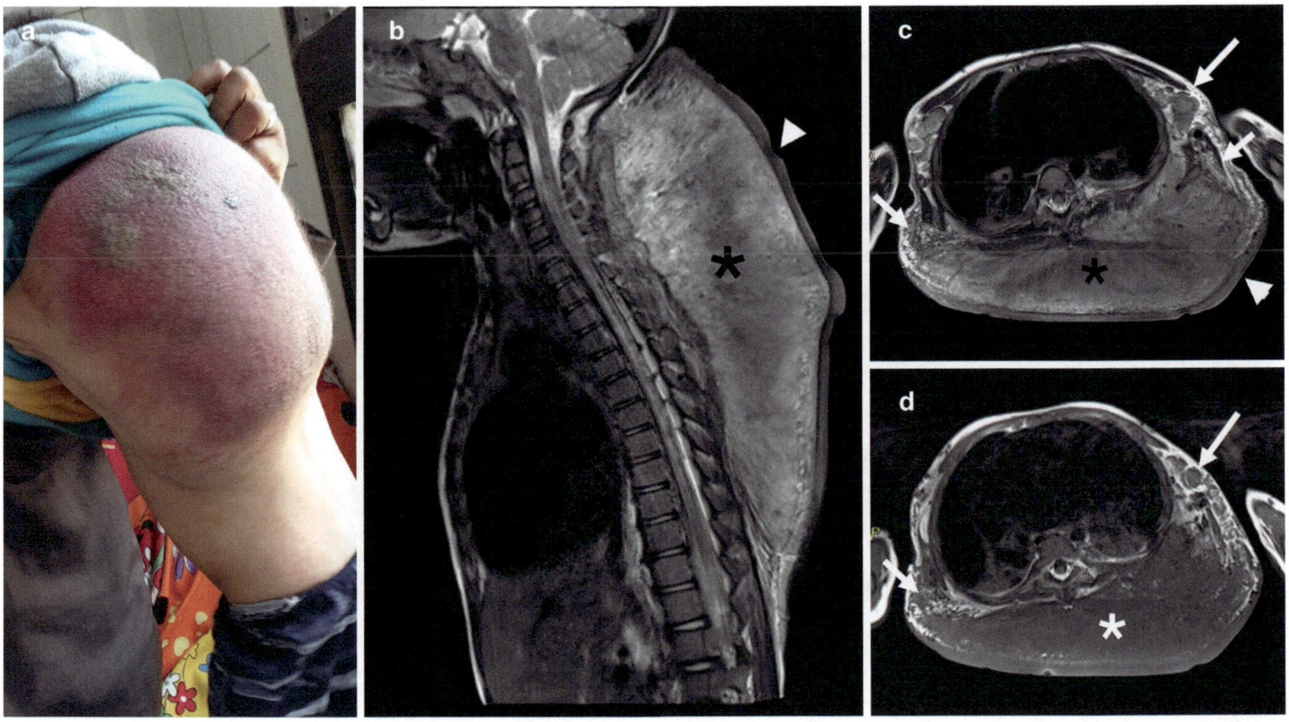

Fig. 7.3 (**a**) A 3-year-old boy with a neglected, large swelling involving the back, confirmed as kaposiform hemangioendothelioma (KHE). (**b–d**) Sagittal T2-weighted image (**b**), axial T2-weighted image (**c**), and axial T1-weighted image (**d**) demonstrate a large soft-tissue mass (asterisk) with infiltrative margins (short arrow) and overlying cutaneous thickening (arrowhead). The lesion shows heterogeneous signal intensity on T2-WI (**b**, **c**) and is isointense to muscle on T1-WI (**d**). Associated enlarged lymph nodes are also noted (long arrow)

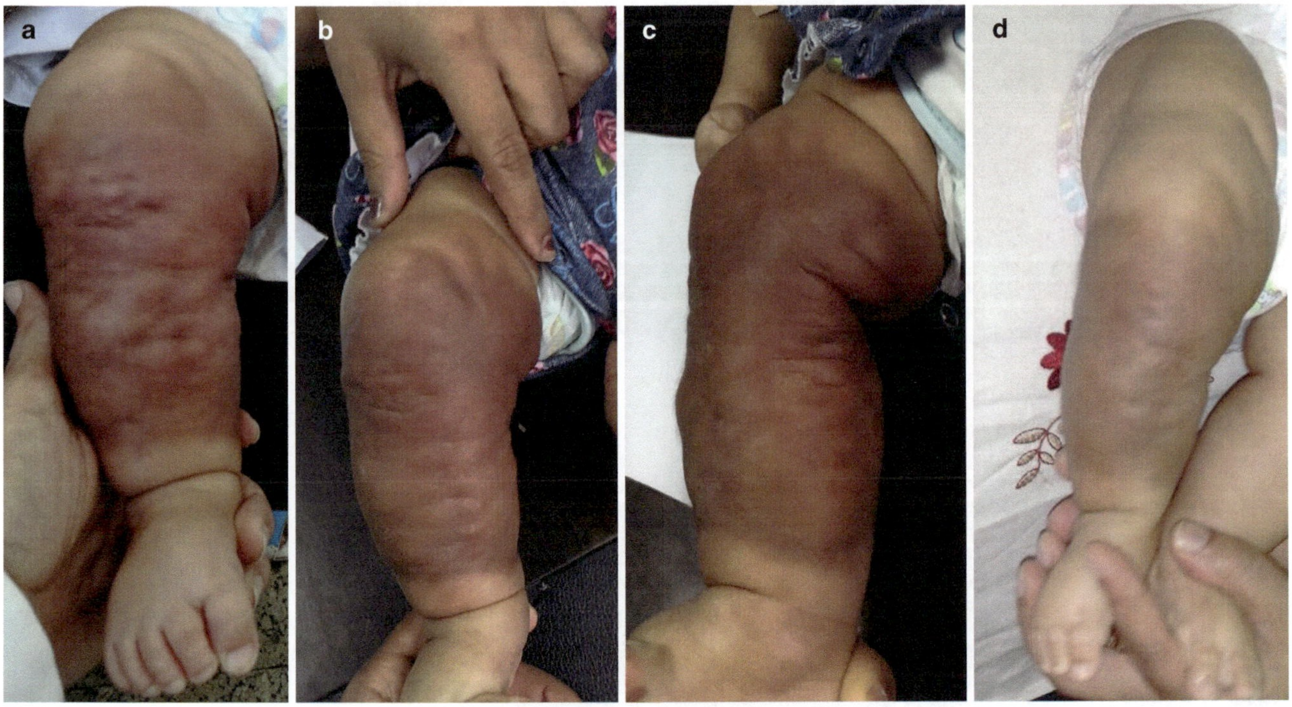

Fig. 7.4 (**a**) 2-month-old girl presenting with dusky-red swelling of the leg and thrombocytopenia, confirmed as kaposiform hemangioendothelioma (KHE). (**b–d**) Follow-up images after initiation of medical treatment with steroids and vincristine at 2 weeks (**b**, **c**) and marked regression after 2 months (**d**)

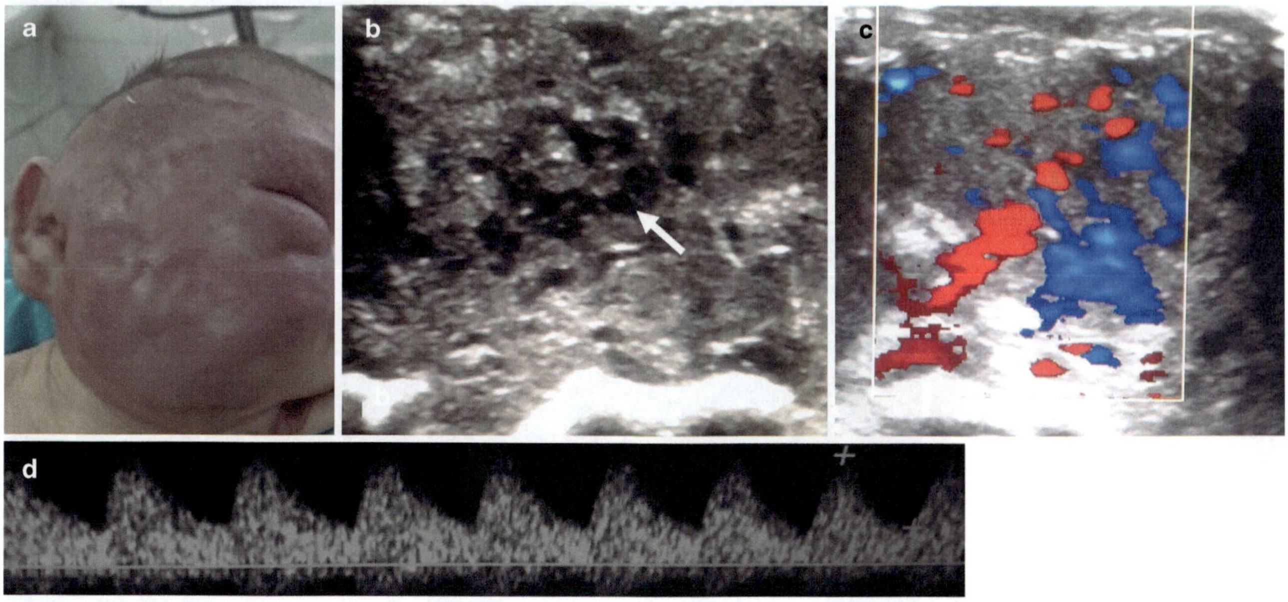

Fig. 7.5 Kaposiform hemangioendothelioma in a 4-week-old girl. (**a**) Clinical image showing a pink facial swelling. (**b**) B-mode ultrasound demonstrating an echogenic mass with internal hypoechoic vascular spaces (arrow). (**c**) Color Doppler revealing increased vascularity. (**d**) Spectral Doppler showing low-resistance arterial flow

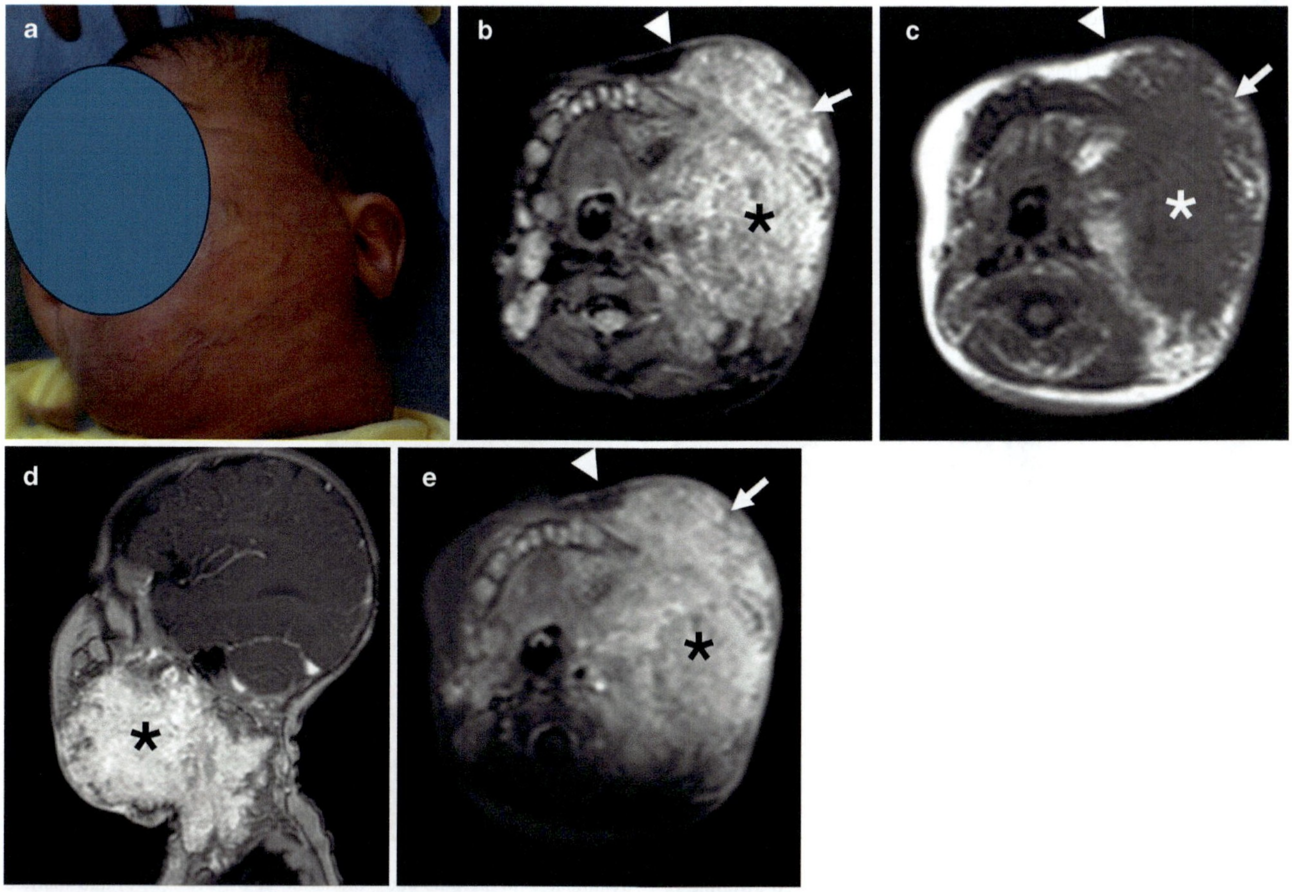

Fig. 7.6 (**a**) Kaposiform hemangioendothelioma in an 8-month-old boy with facial and neck swelling and thrombocytopenia. MRI findings: (**b**) axial STIR, (**c**) axial T1-WI, (**d**) sagittal contrast-enhanced T1-WI, and (**e**) axial contrast-enhanced fat-suppressed T1-WI demonstrating large infiltrative soft tissue mass (asterisk) surrounded by reticular stranding (short arrow) with overlying cutaneous thickening (arrowhead). The lesion and the adjacent reticular stranding exhibit heterogeneous signal on STIR (**b**) and isointense signal to the muscle on T1-WI (**c**) and intense post-contrast enhancement (**d**, **e**)

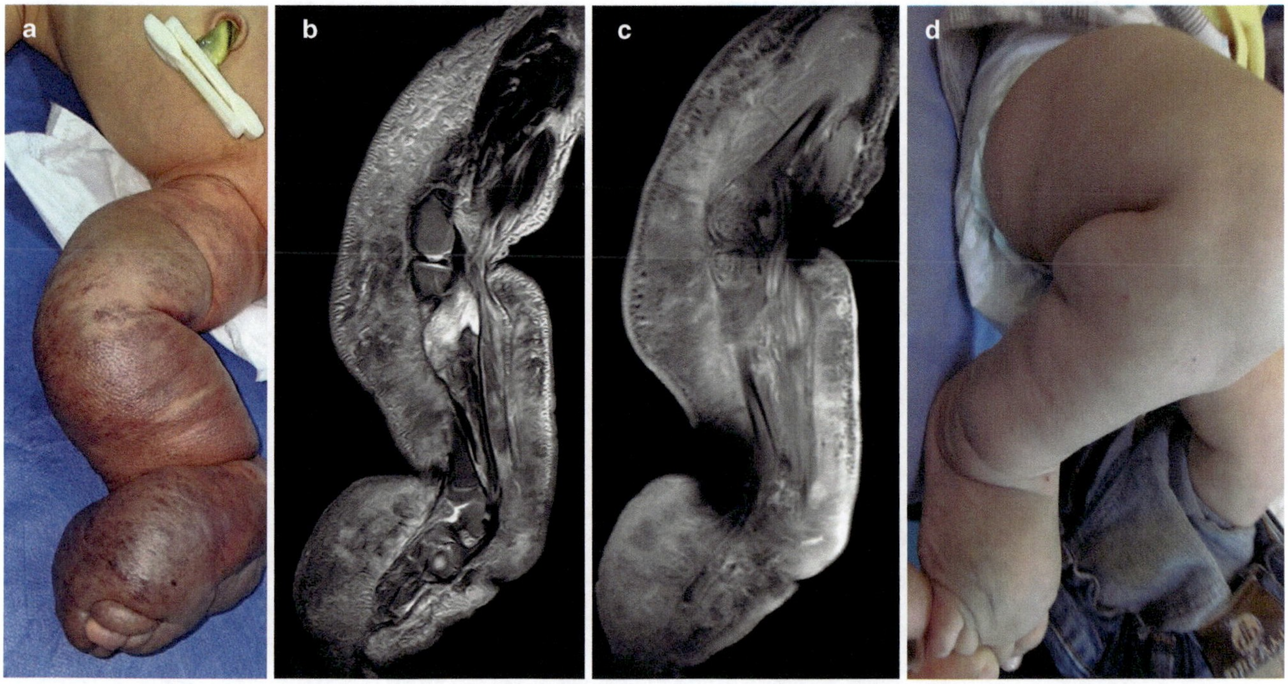

Fig. 7.7 Kaposiform hemangioendothelioma of the right lower limb in a 3-day-old boy. (**a**) Clinical photograph at presentation. (**b**) Sagittal T2-WI MRI showing cutaneous thickening and subcutaneous reticular stranding. (**c**) Sagittal fat-suppressed contrast-enhanced T1-WI demonstrating post-contrast enhancement of the lesion. (**d**) Follow-up after 6 weeks of steroid and vincristine therapy showing significant regression

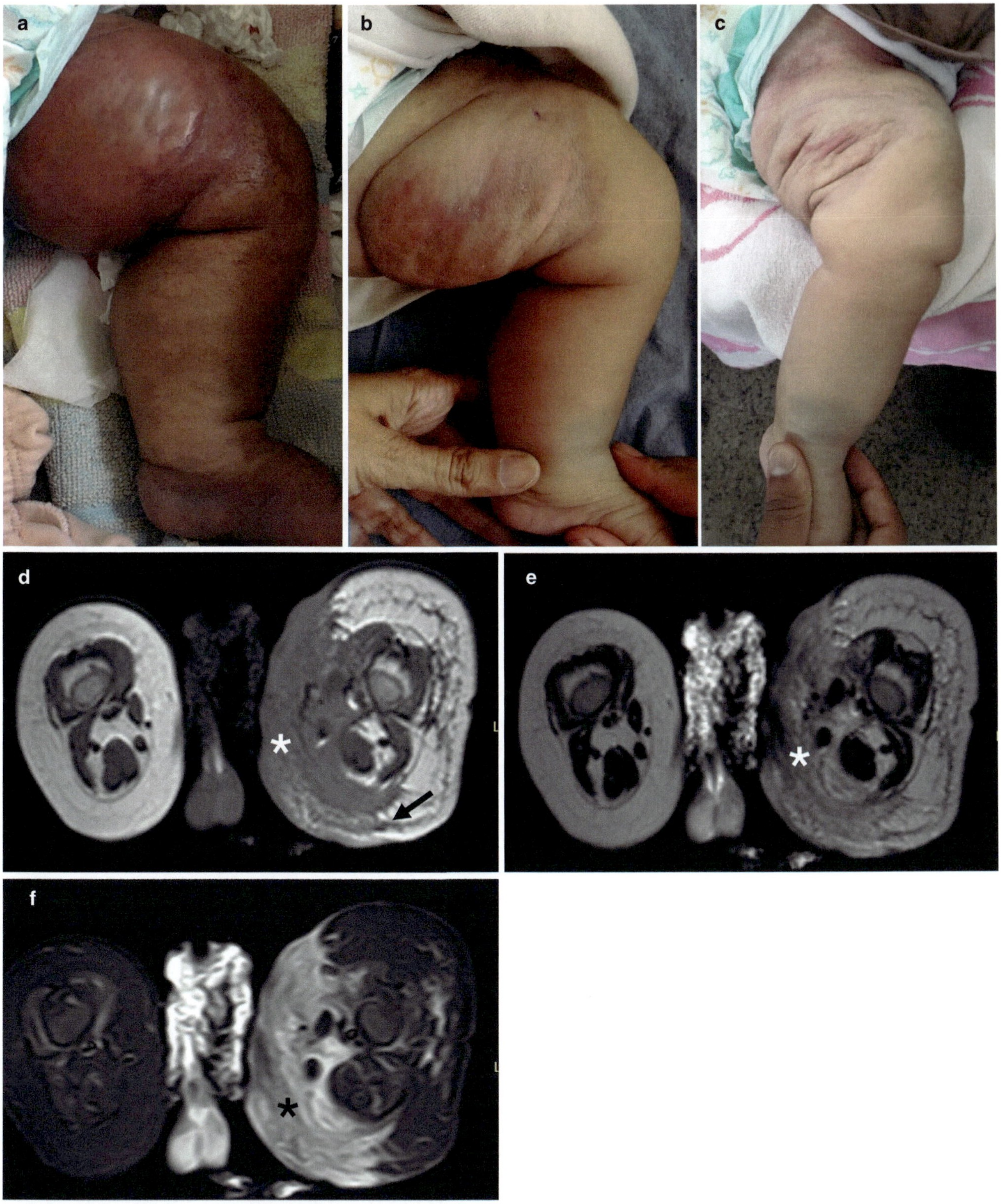

Fig. 7.8 Kaposiform hemangioendothelioma of the left lower limb in a 4-month-old boy. (**a**) Clinical photograph at presentation. (**b**) Photograph after initiation of steroid and vincristine therapy. (**c**) Follow-up at 6 months showing remarkable improvement. (**d–f**) MRI axial T1-WI, T2-WI, and STIR images demonstrating a soft tissue lesion (asterisk) with irregular infiltrative margins and transspatial extension. The lesion shows intermediate signal on T1-WI (**d**), hyperintense signal on T2-WI (**e**) and STIR (**f**). Abnormal subcutaneous stranding (arrow in **d**) and overlying cutaneous thickening are also evident

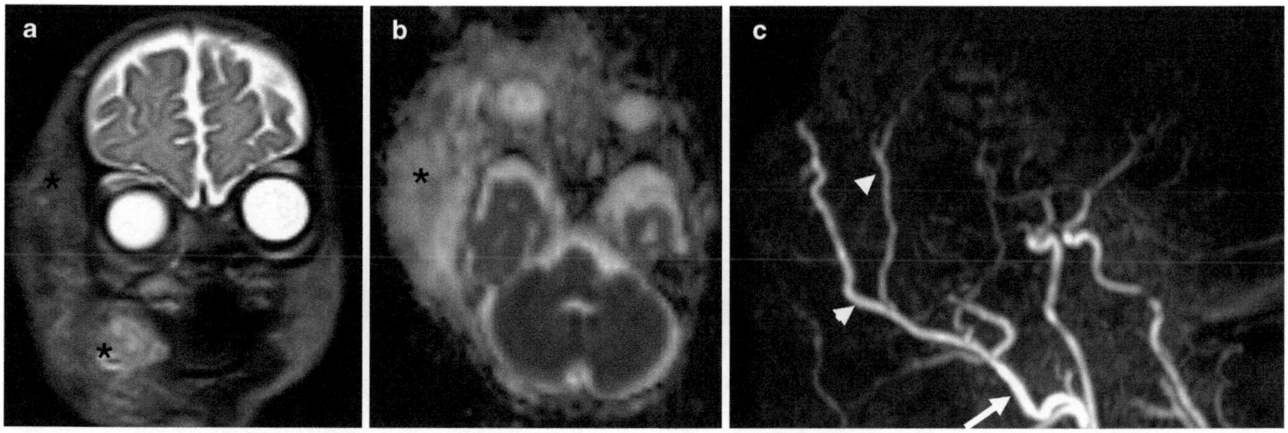

Fig. 7.9 Kaposiform hemangioendothelioma in a 4-week-old girl (same case as in Fig. 7.5). (**a**) Coronal T2-WI demonstrating right hemifacial swelling (asterisk) with heterogeneous signal. (**b**) Axial apparent diffusion coefficient (ADC) map showing bright signal consistent with facilitated diffusion. (**c**) Oblique coronal reformat from non-contrast MR angiography revealing increased vascularity (arrowheads) with an enlarged arterial feeder from the right external carotid artery (arrow)

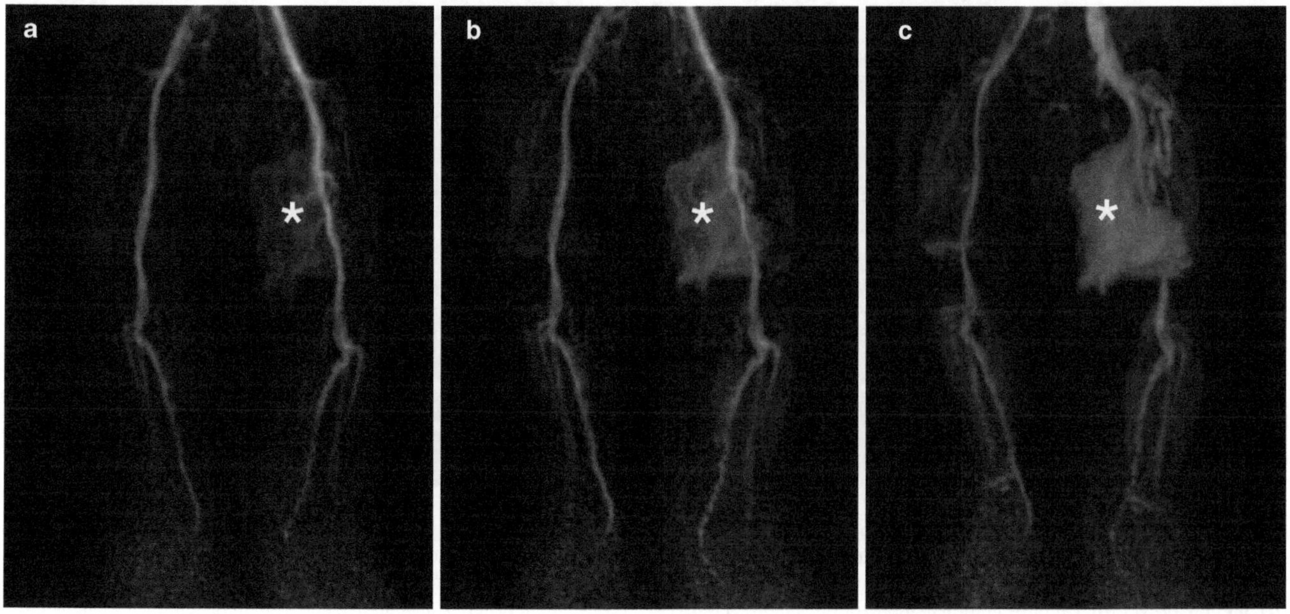

Fig. 7.10 Kaposiform hemangioendothelioma in a 4-month-old boy (same case as in Fig. 7.8). (**a–c**) Successive phases of dynamic contrast-enhanced MR angiography demonstrating an early enhancing soft tissue lesion (asterisk) in the arterial phase (**a**), with progressive contrast filling in the subsequent phases (**b**, **c**)

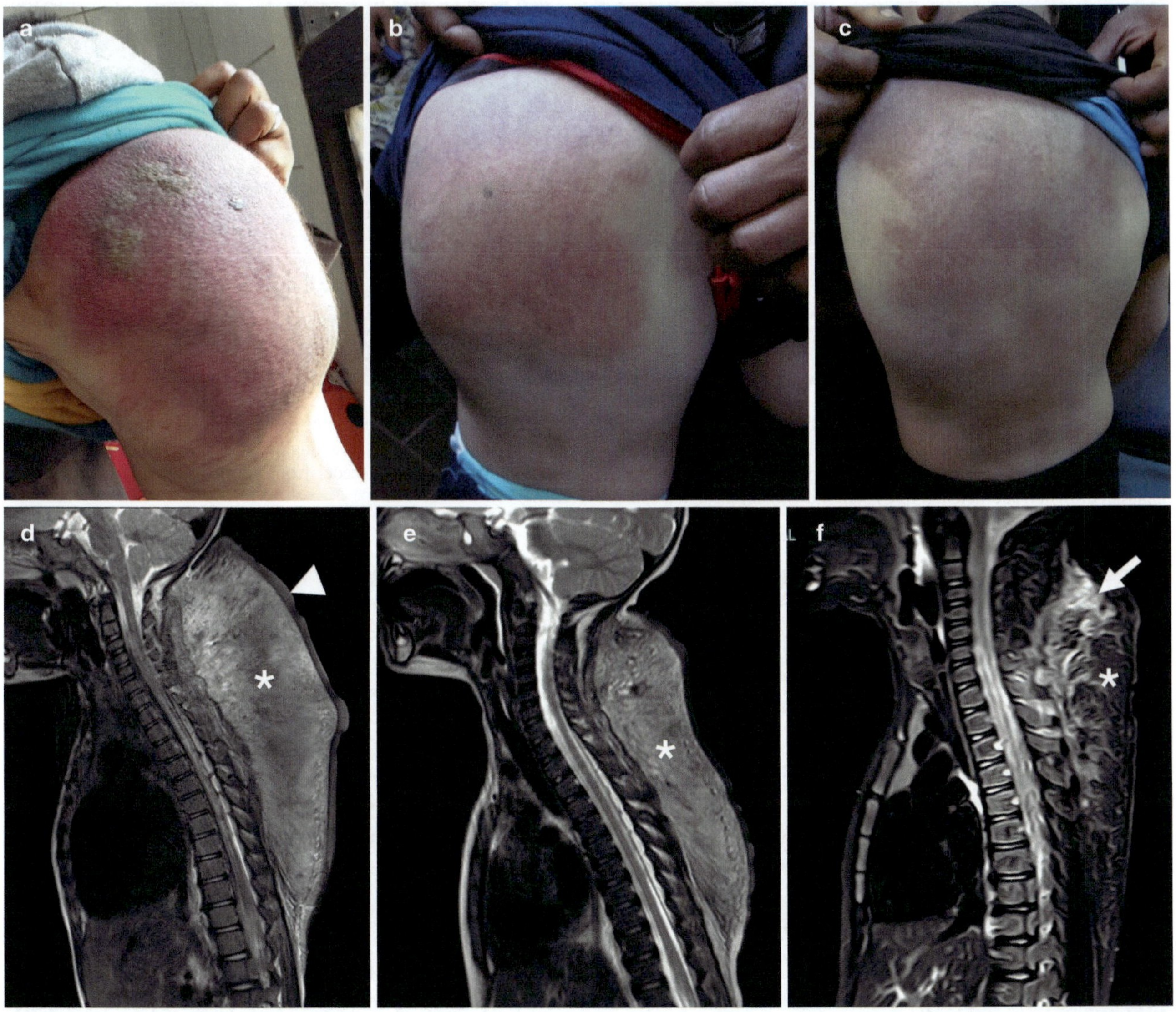

Fig. 7.11 Kaposiform hemangioendothelioma (same case as in Fig. 7.3). (**a–c**) Clinical photographs at presentation and during follow-up showing progressive reduction in tumor size with sirolimus therapy. (**d**) Sagittal T2-WI MRI at presentation demonstrating a large heterogeneous mass with overlying cutaneous thickening (arrowhead). (**e**) Sagittal T2-WI at 5 months' follow-up after initiation of treatment showing marked reduction in lesion size (asterisk). (**f**) Sagittal STIR at 19 months' follow-up demonstrating further size reduction with fatty replacement (asterisk, low signal) and a small residual component at the superior aspect (arrow)

Tufted Angioma (TA)

Tufted angioma (TA) is a rare benign cutaneous vascular neoplasm that predominantly affects children and young adults. Approximately half of all reported cases are diagnosed within the first year of life [14]. A male predominance has been noted, and the most common anatomical sites of involvement include the trunk (Fig. 7.12), neck, and extremities [15].

There is increasing consensus among vascular tumor specialists that TA and kaposiform hemangioendothelioma (KHE) are part of a spectrum.

TA most commonly presents in the form of a tumor or infiltrative plaque. The lesions are typically dusky red to violaceous in color (Fig. 7.12) and may be accompanied by local hyperhidrosis or hypertrichosis [16]. The clinical course is generally indolent, with lesions expanding gradually before stabilizing in size [17].

Although usually benign in behavior, TA can be complicated by Kasabach–Merritt phenomenon (KMP) or, less frequently, chronic coagulopathy [14]. KMP is a consumptive coagulopathy characterized by profound thrombocytopenia and hypofibrinogenemia, resulting from intralesional sequestration of platelets and subsequent activation of the coagula-

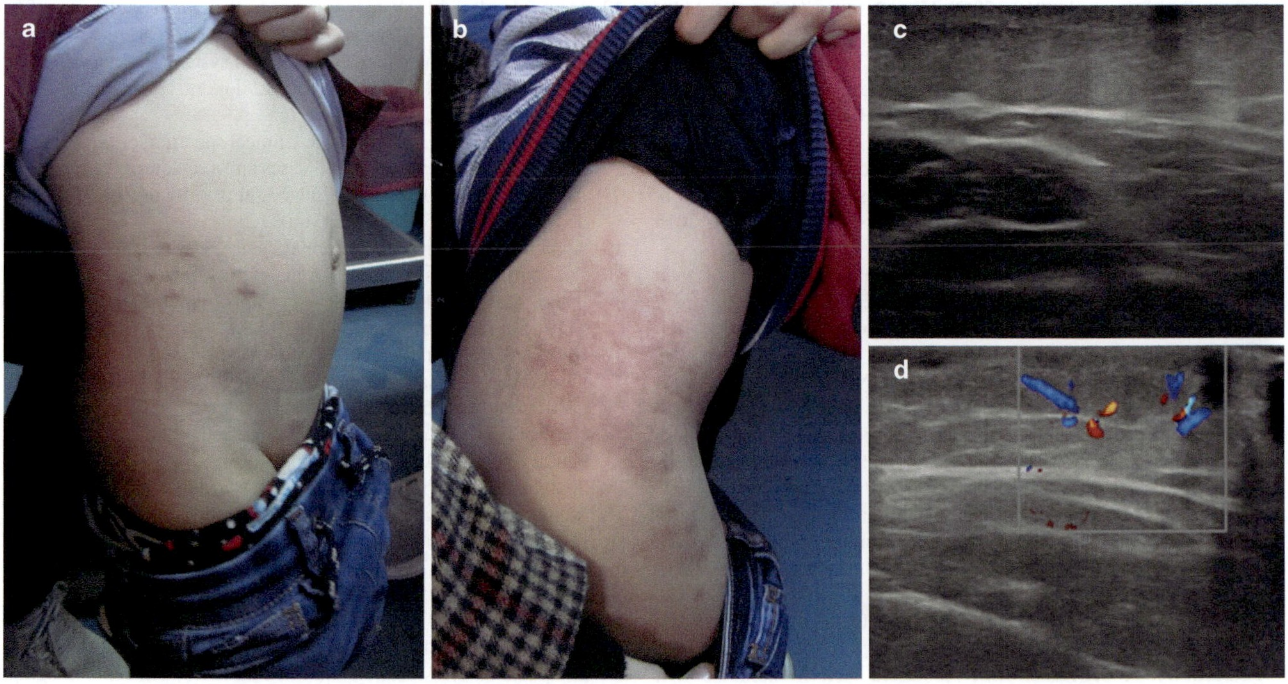

Fig. 7.12 Tufted angioma in a 3-year-old boy (histopathologically confirmed). (**a**, **b**) Clinical photographs showing cutaneous lesions on the trunk. (**c**) B-mode ultrasound demonstrating increased subcutaneous tissue thickness. (**d**) Color Doppler revealing increased vascularity with low-resistance arterial flow (waveform not shown)

tion cascade with fibrinogen consumption [18]. In this respect, TA is often regarded as a milder and more superficial counterpart of KHE.

Imaging Findings

Unlike KHE, imaging is rarely required in the diagnostic evaluation of TA [19]. When performed, imaging may reveal a localized vascular lesion, but the diagnosis is primarily clinical and histopathological.

Histopathology

The definitive diagnosis of TA relies on histological examination. Characteristic findings include multiple well-circumscribed tufts of capillaries distributed throughout the dermis in a distinctive "cannonball" pattern. These vascular tufts infiltrate the dermis in discrete nodules, separated by normal dermal collagen.

Management

Multiple therapeutic approaches have been employed in the management of TA. Options include surgical excision, systemic therapies, and laser modalities, particularly pulsed dye laser, which has demonstrated efficacy in selected cases [20].

References

1. Deraedt K, Poorten VV. Multifocal kaposiform haemangioendothelioma. Virchows Arch. 2006;448(6):843–6. https://doi.org/10.1007/s00428-006-0177-6. Epub 2006 Apr 5. PMID: 16596383.
2. Lyons LL, North PE. Kaposiform hemangioendothelioma: a study of 33 cases emphasizing its pathologic, immunophenotypic, and biologic uniqueness from juvenile hemangioma. Am J Surg Pathol. 2004;28(5):559–68. https://doi.org/10.1097/00000478-200405000-00001. PMID: 15105642.
3. Croteau SE, Liang MG. Kaposiform hemangioendothelioma: atypical features and risks of Kasabach–Merritt phenomenon in 107 referrals. J Pediatr. 2013;162(1):142–7.
4. Ji Y, Yang K. Kaposiform haemangioendothelioma: clinical features, complications and risk factors for Kasabach–Merritt phenom-

enon. Br J Dermatol. 2018;179(2):457–63. https://doi.org/10.1111/bjd.16601.
5. Gruman A, Liang MG. Kaposiform hemangioendothelioma without Kasabach-Merritt phenomenon. J Am Acad Dermatol. 2005;52(4):616–22. https://doi.org/10.1016/j.jaad.2004.10.880. PMID: 15793511.
6. Johnson CM, Navarro OM. Clinical and sonographic features of pediatric soft-tissue vascular anomalies part 1: classification, sonographic approach and vascular tumors. Pediatr Radiol. 2017 Aug;47(9):1184–95.
7. Calvo-Garcia MA, Kline-Fath BM. Imaging evaluation of fetal vascular anomalies. Pediatr Radiol. 2015;45(8):1218–29. https://doi.org/10.1007/s00247-014-3248-x. Epub 2014 Dec 10. PMID: 25492302.
8. AbouZeid AA, Mohammad SA, Aly NH, Elghandour MM, AbdelLatif M, Elsayed SM, El-Naggar O, Attia EA, Ragab IA. Differential diagnostic features between congenital haemangioma, KHE, and congenital fibrosarcoma: a single-centre experience. Eur J Pediatr. 2021;180(8):2581–9.
9. Ryu YJ, Choi YH. Imaging findings of Kaposiform Hemangioendothelioma in children. Eur J Radiol. 2017;86:198–205. https://doi.org/10.1016/j.ejrad.2016.11.015. Epub 2016 Nov 10. PMID: 28027747.
10. Hu PA, Zhou ZR. Clinical and imaging features of Kaposiform Hemangioendothelioma. Br J Radiol. 2018;91(1086):20170798.
11. Ragab IA, Abdel-Kader SM, AbouZeid AA, Mohammad SA, Raheem HG, Aly NH. A successful tale of sirolimus treatment in refractory vascular tumors. J Pediatr Surg Case Rep. 2022;78:102180.
12. Borst AJ, Eng W. Treatment practices and response in kaposiform hemangioendothelioma: a multicenter cohort study. Pediatr Blood Cancer. 2024;71(3):e30779. https://doi.org/10.1002/pbc.30779. Epub 2023 Dec 10. PMID: 38073018.
13. Maza-Morales M, Valdés-Loperena S, Durán-McKinster LC, García-Romero MT. The use of mTOR inhibitors for the treatment of kaposiform hemangioendothelioma. A systematic review. Pediatr Dermatol. 2023;40(3):440–5. https://doi.org/10.1111/pde.15262. Epub 2023 Jan 30. PMID: 36716766.
14. Osio A, Fraitag S, Hadj-Rabia S. Clinical spectrum of tufted angiomas in childhood: a report of 13 cases and a review of the literature. Arch Dermatol. 2010;146(7):758–63. https://doi.org/10.1001/archdermatol.2010.135. PMID: 20644037.
15. Bruder E, Alaggio R. Vascular and perivascular lesions of skin and soft tissues in children and adolescents. Pediatr Dev Pathol. 2012;15(1 Suppl):26–61. https://doi.org/10.2350/11-11-1119-PB.1. PMID: 22420724.
16. Herron MD, Coffin CM. Tufted angiomas: variability of the clinical morphology. Pediatr Dermatol. 2002;19(5):394–401. https://doi.org/10.1046/j.1525-1470.2002.00113.x. PMID: 12383094.
17. North PE. Pediatric vascular Tumors and malformations. Surg Pathol Clin. 2010;3(3):455–94. https://doi.org/10.1016/j.path.2010.07.002. Epub 2010 Oct 20. PMID: 26839221.
18. Mahajan P, Margolin J. Kasabach-Merritt phenomenon: classic presentation and management options. Clin Med Insights Blood Disord. 2017;16(10):1179545X17699849. https://doi.org/10.1177/1179545X17699849. PMID: 28579853; PMCID: PMC5428202.
19. Brahmbhatt AN, Skalski KA. Vascular lesions of the head and neck: an update on classification and imaging review. Insights Imaging. 2020;11(1):19. https://doi.org/10.1186/s13244-019-0818-3. PMID: 32034537; PMCID: PMC7007481.
20. Dwiyana RF, Lestari ER, Effendi RMRA, Gondokaryono SP, Diana IA, Usman HA, Suhada KU, Anandita R. Effectiveness of pulsed dye laser treatment in tufted angioma: a promising intervention. Clin Cosmet Investig Dermatol. 2023;16:2885–91. https://doi.org/10.2147/CCID.S428371.

Differential Diagnosis of Vascular Tumors

8

Introduction

Vascular tumors account for approximately 50% of cases attending the vascular anomaly clinic. Hemangiomas—whether infantile or, less commonly, congenital—are benign vascular tumors recognized for their favorable prognosis and tendency to regress spontaneously with few reported complications. Complications associated with hemangiomas typically arise when lesions are large or located in areas where they obstruct vital structures. Kaposiform Hemangioendothelioma (KHE) is a distinct type of vascular tumor described as benign but locally aggressive, often demonstrating initial invasive behavior before eventual regression. Malignant vascular tumors are extremely rare.

Not uncommonly, the term hemangioma is given as a generic diagnosis for various vascular and non-vascular neoplasms in infancy, which can lead to inappropriate treatment [1]. Moreover, vascular tumors may be confused with other high-flow vascular malformations such as arteriovenous malformations [2]. In this chapter, we will explore the differential diagnoses of vascular tumors and present real clinical cases that illustrate commonly encountered diagnostic challenges.

First: Malignant Soft Tissue Tumors in Infancy That Can Mimic Vascular Tumors

A subset of malignant tumors can appear during infancy, which are often initially misdiagnosed as vascular tumors (hemangiomas) even in tertiary care pediatric hospitals [2]. These malignant soft tissue tumors are characterized by high vascularity and typically appear as rapidly enlarging red or bluish lesions in the skin and subcutaneous tissue (Figs. 8.1 and 8.2). This presentation encourages the initial referral of such cases to a vascular anomaly clinic [3]. Unlike hemangiomas, which are soft and compressible, these malignant tumors are firm and often exhibit overlying skin changes, such as multiple dilated vessels and/or ulcerations (Figs. 8.3 and 8.4). Nevertheless, malignant tumors can mimic congenital vascular tumors on most imaging modalities, as both may exhibit similar high-flow vessels [4]. However, the feeding arteries in malignant neoplasms are typically irregular (Fig. 8.5) in contrast to the sharply demarcated homogenous lesions of hemangiomas with evenly distributed feeding arteries (Fig. 8.6) [2]. Malignant neoplasms often show deep tissue infiltration, bone invasion, and destruction—features that help distinguish them

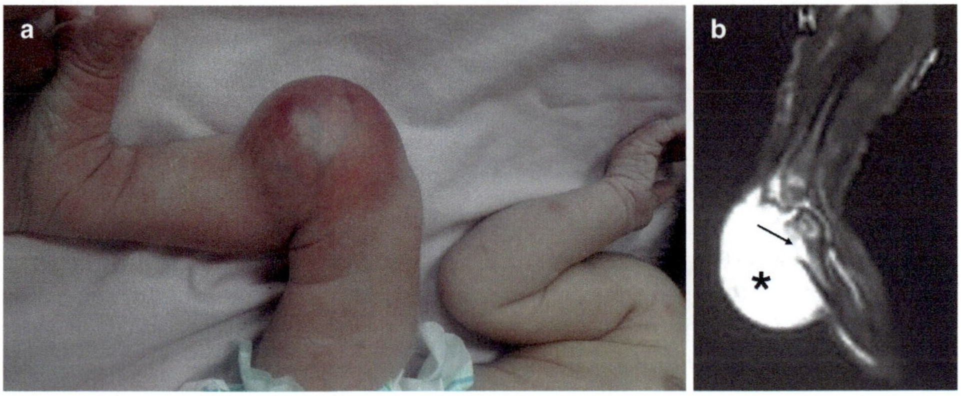

Fig. 8.1 Congenital fibrosarcoma. (**a**) Clinical photograph; (**b**) sagittal STIR MRI showing hyperintense soft-tissue mass (asterisk) with bone invasion (arrow). Initially misdiagnosed as hemangioma and referred to vascular anomaly clinic

A. A. AbouZeid et al., *Atlas of Pediatric Vascular Anomalies*, https://doi.org/10.1007/978-3-032-30866-5_8

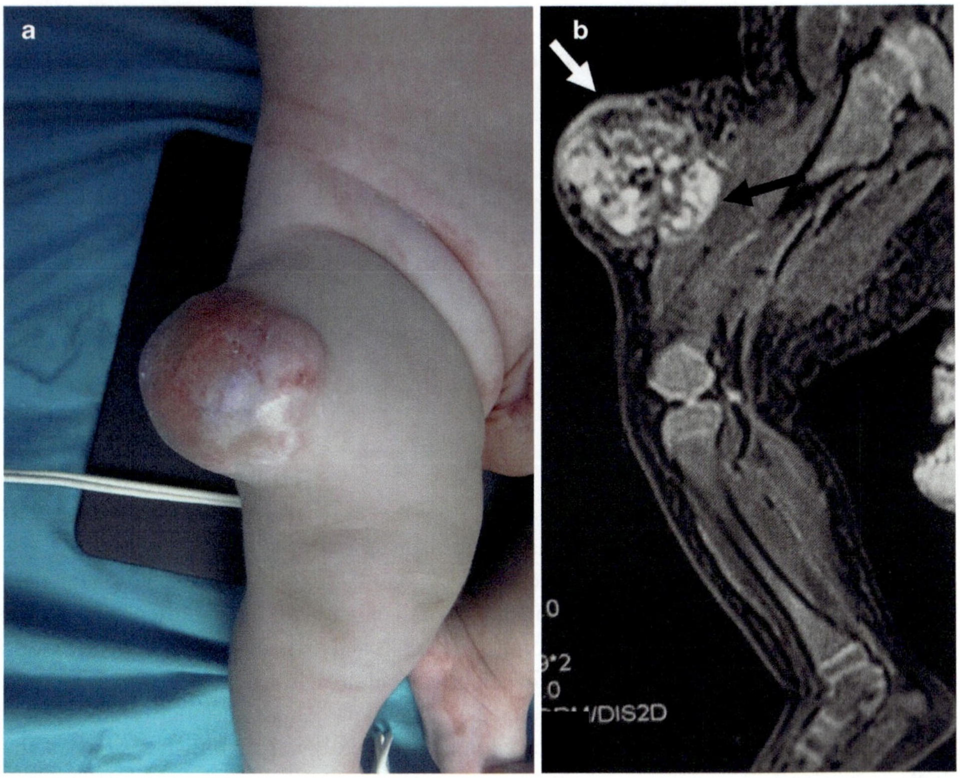

Fig. 8.2 (**a**) A 40-day-old boy presenting with a firm rapidly growing swelling in the right thigh, subsequently diagnosed as fibrosarcoma. (**b**) Sagittal STIR MRI of the lower limb demonstrates a heterogeneously hyperintense mass (white arrow) with flow voids and local invasion into the adjacent muscle (black arrow)

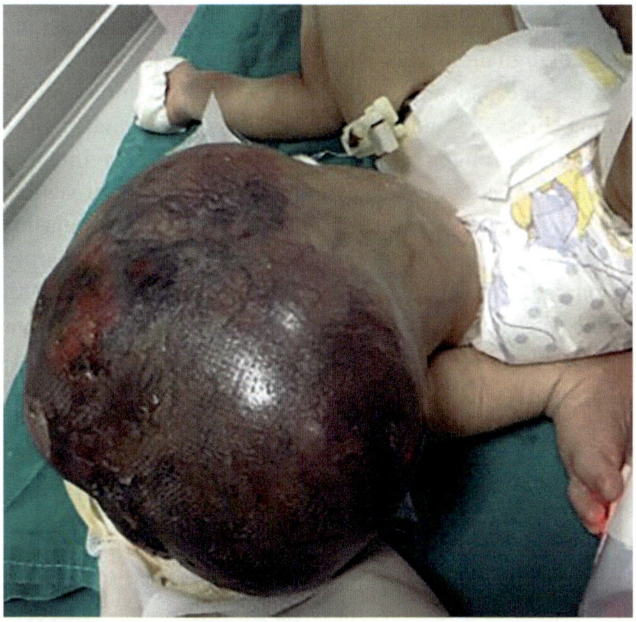

Fig. 8.3 Neonate with huge congenital fibrosarcoma

from hemangiomas (Fig. 8.7) [2]. As a rule, Burrows and Paltiel recommended that any growing mass in infancy not precisely matching the imaging characteristics of a vascular anomaly should be biopsied [2]. Here are some examples of cases that were initially misdiagnosed as hemangiomas and referred to the vascular anomaly clinic but were ultimately found to be malignant tumors.

(a) *Infantile fibrosarcoma:* Congenital fibrosarcoma (CFS) is a rare malignant mesenchymal tumor originating from fibroblasts, typically present at birth or developing in early childhood [3]. It is classified under the non-rhabdomyosarcoma group and commonly presents as a rapidly enlarging, vascularized mass—most frequently affecting the extremities (Fig. 8.8), followed by the head, neck, and trunk (Fig. 8.9) [5]. Given its generally favorable prognosis, primary surgical excision is recommended when the tumor can be completely removed without compromising vital structures or causing permanent disability. If complete resection is not initially feasible, neoadjuvant chemotherapy may be used to shrink the tumor and facilitate later surgical removal [3, 5].
(b) *Rhabdomyosarcoma:* This is a rapidly proliferating, highly aggressive malignant tumor characterized by invasion and destruction of underlying bone, often associated with a guarded prognosis (Fig. 8.10) [2]. Typically occurs after 3 months of age. Due to its high vascularity and infiltrative behavior, the mass may be mistaken for the locally aggressive vascular tumor kaposiform hemangioendothelioma (KHE) (Fig. 8.10). Kaposiform hemangioendothelioma (KHE) typically presents as diffuse, indurated skin lesions with a dusky red color, often extending deeply across tissue planes into the fascia and underlying muscles. The hallmark of KHE is platelet trapping, leading to marked throm-

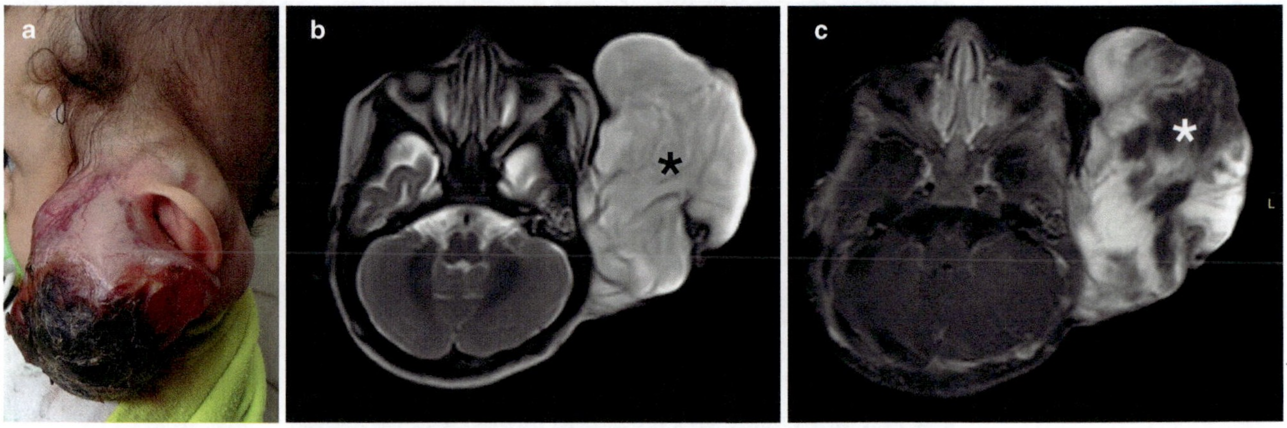

Fig. 8.4 Primary myxoid mesenchymal tumor: (**a**) Clinical photograph. (**b, c**) Axial T2-weighted image and fat-suppressed contrast-enhanced T1-weighted image demonstrate a soft tissue mass (asterisk), appearing hyperintense on T2-WI (**b**) with heterogeneous contrast enhancement (**c**)

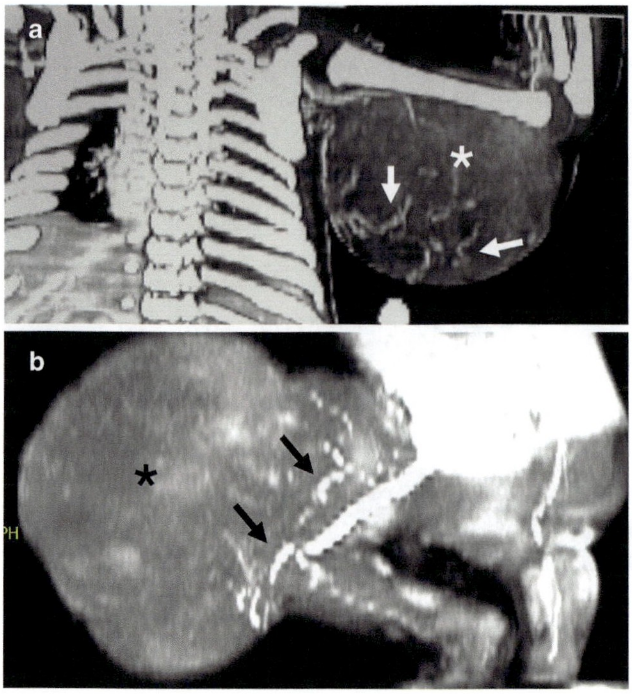

Fig. 8.5 Two patients with congenital fibrosarcoma:(**a, b**) Coronal maximum intensity projection (MIP) from contrast-enhanced CT (**a**) and sagittal MIP from non-contrast MR angiography (**b**) demonstrate disorganized vessels (arrow) within a large soft tissue mass (asterisk)

bocytopenia [2, 3]. Despite their aggressive appearance at presentation, KHEs generally respond well to medical therapy, with most cases showing significant tumor regression and minimal residual skin changes (Fig. 8.10d–g) (refer to Chap. 7).

(c) *Rhabdoid tumor:* This is another aggressive malignant tumor. It can present with fungating skin lesion with central ulceration and everted edges (Fig. 8.11a). This rare tumor may be confused with infantile hemangioma (Fig. 8.11c, d) that may also ulcerate during its proliferative phase, especially in certain anatomical locations (refer to Chap. 3). Examination of the mass away from the ulcerated area will reveal a soft compressible lesion in hemangiomas in contrast to malignant lesions. The latter are firm to hard and may show draining lymph node metastasis (Fig. 8.11b). Any atypical clinical or radiological features in a suspected hemangioma should raise suspicion and prompt biopsy of the lesion [2].

(d) *Leukemia cutis/neuroblastoma skin metastasis:* Leukemia cutis refers to the infiltration of the skin by malignant leukocytes in patients with leukemia, resulting in various cutaneous manifestations such as papules, nodules, or plaques that may appear violaceous or erythematous (Fig. 8.12). It is most commonly associated with acute myeloid leukemia and often indicates systemic disease progression or relapse. In contrast, neuroblastoma skin metastasis typically occurs in infants with disseminated neuroblastoma, presenting as multiple bluish subcutaneous nodules, sometimes described as a "blueberry muffin" appearance (Fig. 8.13). These lesions arise due to dermal infiltration by tumor cells and are usually a sign of advanced disease, although some cases in infants may show spontaneous regression, particularly in stage 4S neuroblastoma.

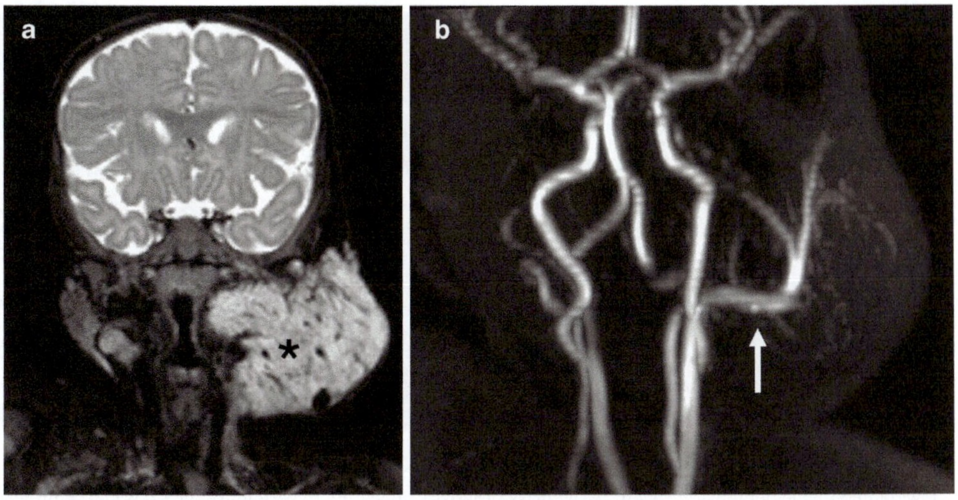

Fig. 8.6 Infant with parotid hemangioma: (**a**) MRI (Coronal STIR image) demonstrates parotid enlargement containing a well-demarcated, homogeneous hyperintense lesion (asterisk) with multiple flow voids. (**b**) Coronal maximum intensity projection from non-contrast MR angiography reveals an enlarged feeding vessel (arrow) with evenly distributed branches

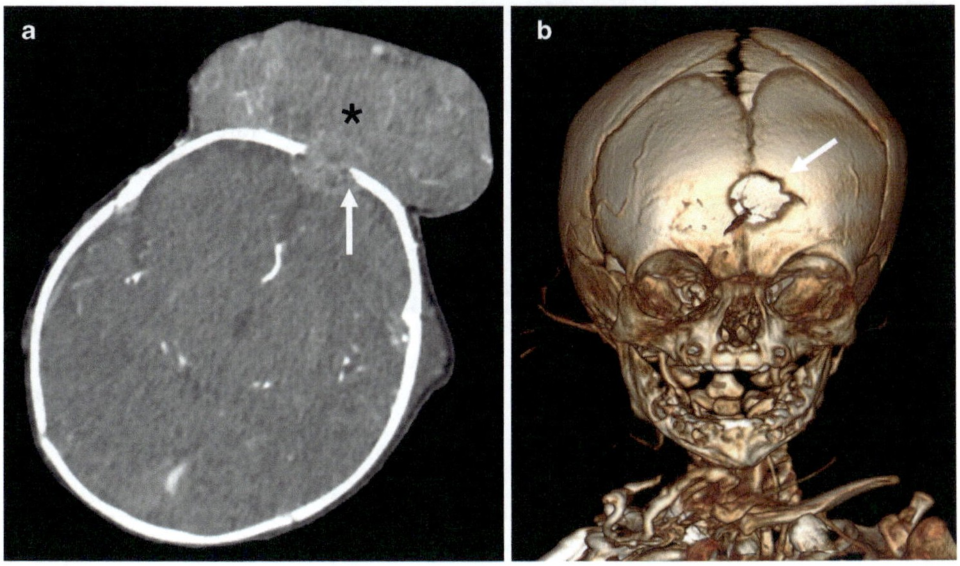

Fig. 8.7 Infant with round cell tumor: (**a**) Axial contrast-enhanced CT demonstrates an enhancing soft tissue mass (asterisk) with osseous invasion (arrow). (**b**) Three-dimensional reconstruction of skull CT depicts an osseous defect in the frontal bone (arrow)

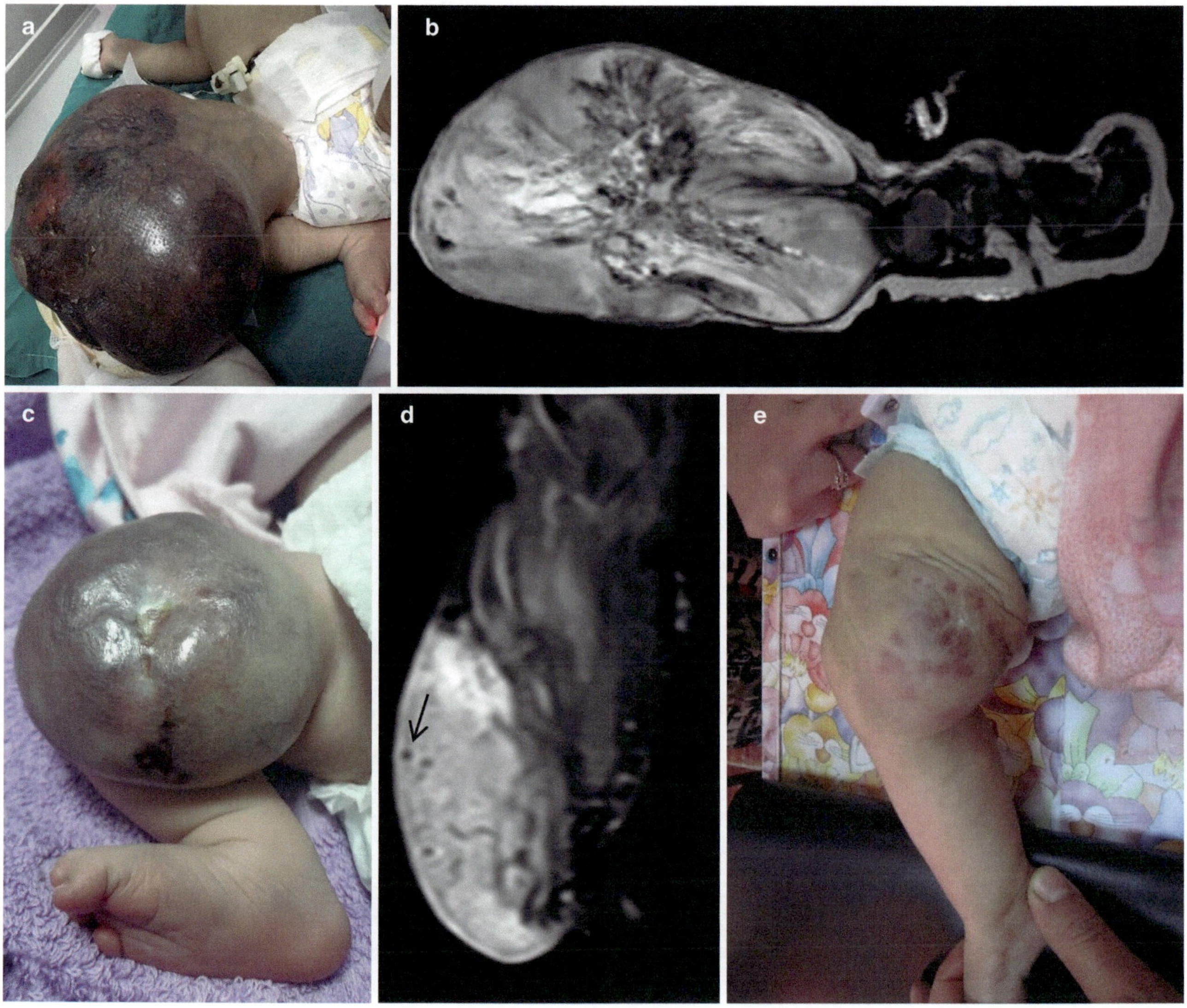

Fig. 8.8 Differential diagnosis of thigh swelling: Upper row (a,b) Congenital fibrosarcoma: (**a**) Male neonate with large left thigh mass; (**b**) MRI shows a heterogeneous soft tissue lesion. Lower row (**c**–**e**) Congenital hemangioma: (**c**) Female neonate with compressible left thigh mass; (**d**) MRI (T2WI with fat suppression) demonstrates a hyperintense lesion with intralesional flow voids (arrow); (**e**) Four-month follow-up reveals rapid involution (RICH)

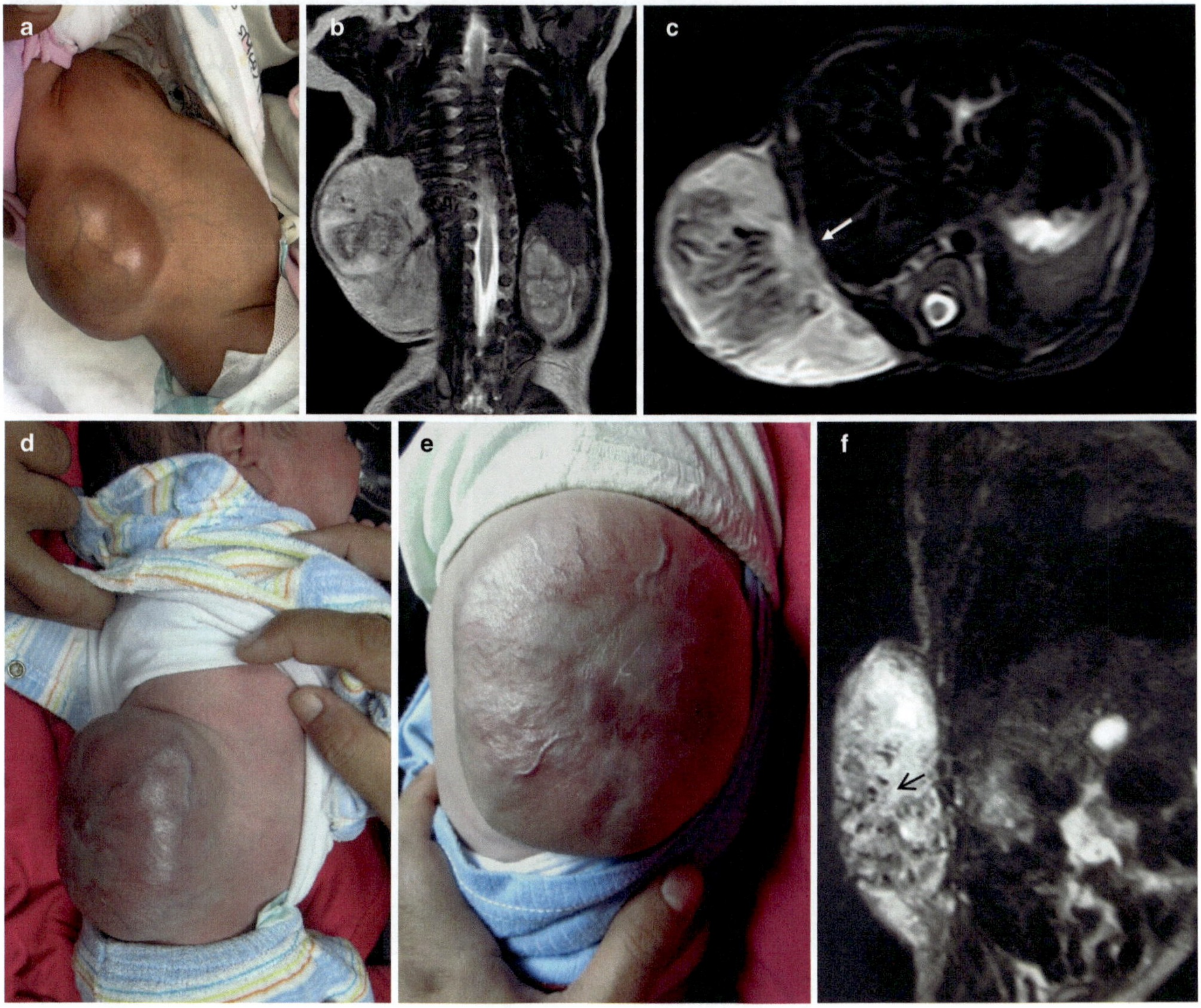

Fig. 8.9 Differential diagnosis of neonatal back swelling. Upper row (**a**–**c**): congenital fibrosarcoma—(**a**) large firm swelling; (**b**, **c**) MRI T2WI showing heterogeneous soft-tissue mass infiltrating chest wall muscles (white arrow). Lower row (**d**–**f**): congenital hemangioma—(**d**, **e**) large compressible swelling (~9 × 7 cm) with central pallor; (**f**) MRI T2WI (fat suppression) showing hyperintense mass with intralesional flow voids (black arrow)

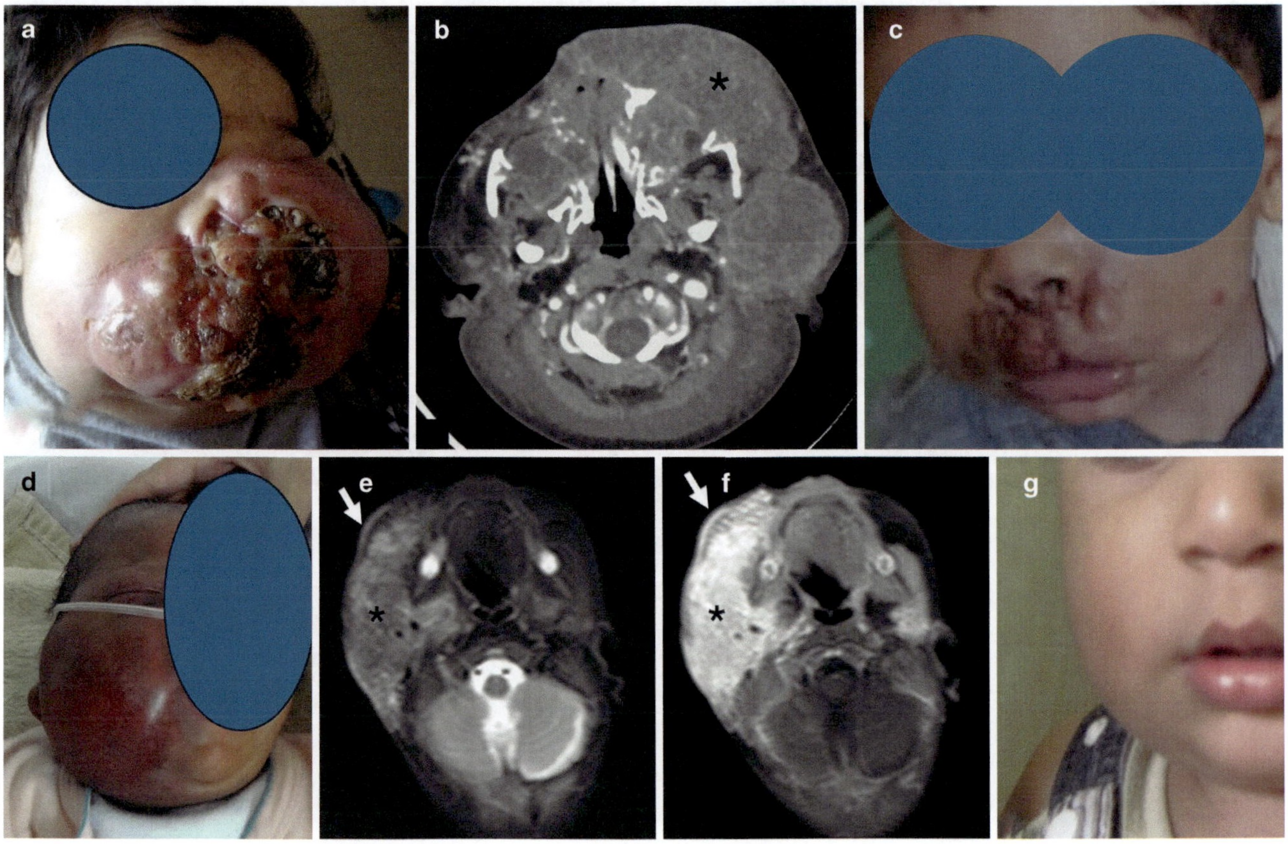

Fig. 8.10 Differential diagnosis of facial swelling. Upper row (**a**–**c**): rhabdomyosarcoma—(**a**) clinical photograph; (**b**) contrast-enhanced CT showing heterogeneously enhancing infiltrative mass invading maxillary sinus (asterisk); (**c**) initial improvement at follow up after chemotherapy. Lower row (d–g): kaposiform hemangioendothelioma (KHE)—(**d**) presentation at 1 month; (**e**, **f**) MRI (STIR and fat-suppressed contrast-enhanced) showing trans-spatial hyperintense lesion (asterisk) with surrounding stranding and skin thickening (arrow), without bone invasion; (**g**) Follow-up at 17 months after successful treatment

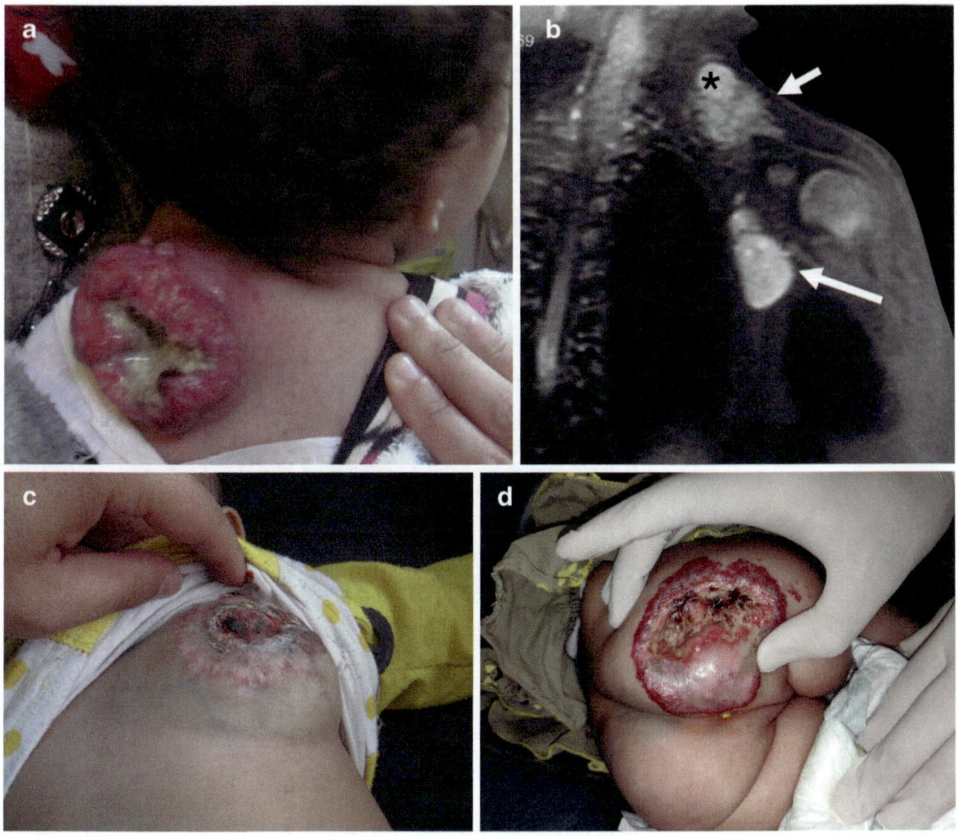

Fig. 8.11 Differential diagnosis of ulcerated lesions. Upper row (**a**, **b**): malignant rhabdoid tumor—(**a**) rapidly enlarging ulcerated back mass; (**b**) coronal contrast-enhanced fat-suppressed T1-WI showing enhancing mass (asterisk) with irregular spiculated margin (short arrow) and malignant lymph node (long arrow). Lower row (**c**, **d**): infantile hemangiomas with skin ulceration in the breast and gluteal regions, respectively

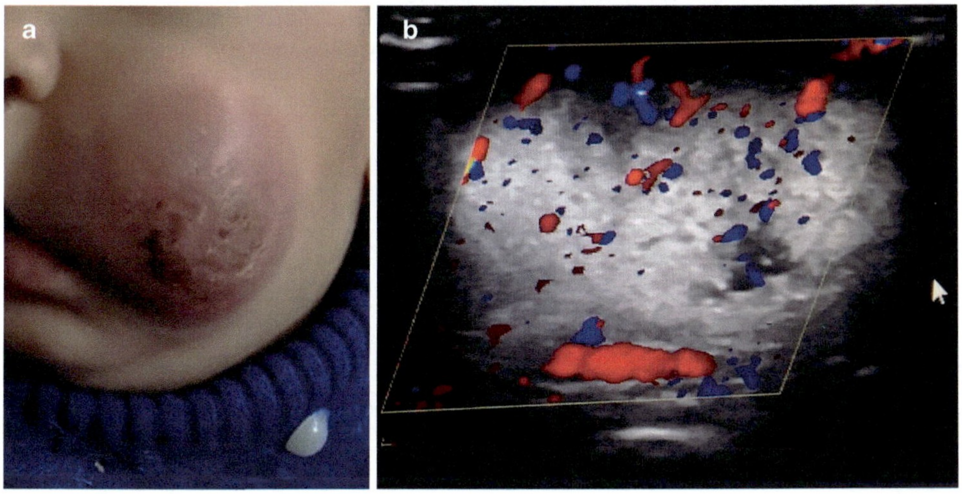

Fig. 8.12 Leukemia cutis in an infant. (**a**) Clinical photograph; (**b**) Color Doppler showing echogenic mass with internal vascularity

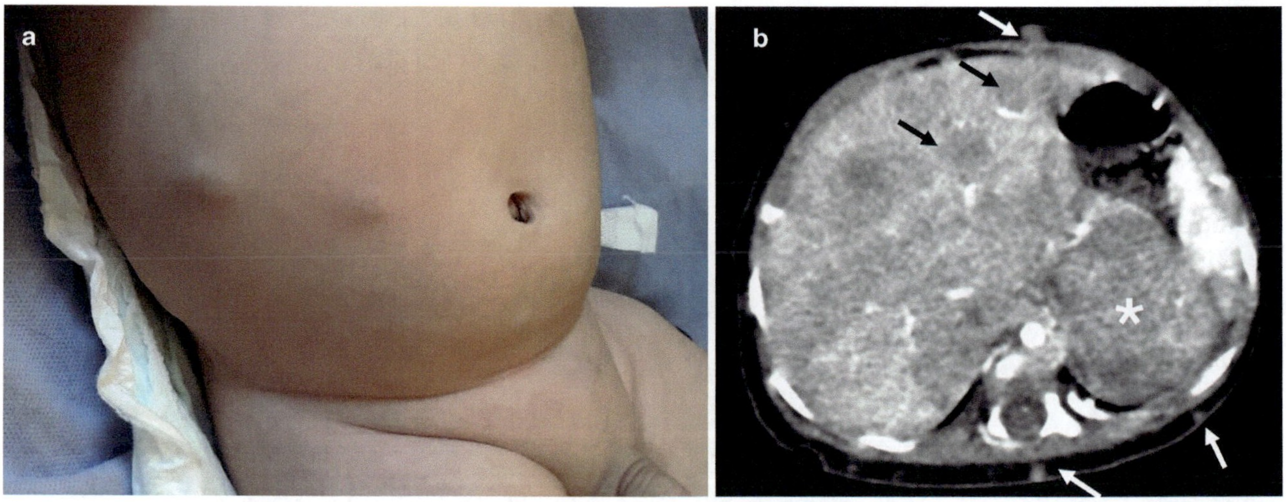

Fig. 8.13 (**a**) Five-month-old boy with multiple cutaneous "blueberry muffin" lesions, confirmed as metastatic neuroblastoma. (**b**) Contrast-enhanced CT showing abdominal mass (asterisk), liver metastases (black arrows), and skin nodules (white arrows)

Second: High Flow Vascular Malformations That May Be Mistaken for Vascular Tumors

Arteriovenous malformations (AVMs) are high-flow vascular malformations characterized by a central nidus of abnormal blood vessels that directly connect feeding arteries to draining veins without an intervening capillary bed (Fig. 8.14) [6, 7]. Typically, a pulsatile thrill can be palpated on AVMs, and a red-colored skin patch is commonly seen overlying the lesion (Fig. 8.15) [8]. On imaging, AVM appears as a highly enhancing lesion with multiple feeding arteries associated with early opacification of dilated draining veins, usually without a discrete soft tissue mass (Figs. 8.14, 8.15, 8.16 and 8.17) [9, 10]. The absence of a distinct soft tissue mass is the most reliable imaging feature for differentiating AVM from hemangioma (Fig. 8.18), which typically presents as a well-defined, homogeneous soft tissue mass with high-flow vessels crossing through it (Fig. 8.19) [2]. In contrast to hemangiomas, AVMs generally follow a progressive course, making embolization and/or surgical excision the preferred treatment options whenever feasible (refer to Chap. 17).

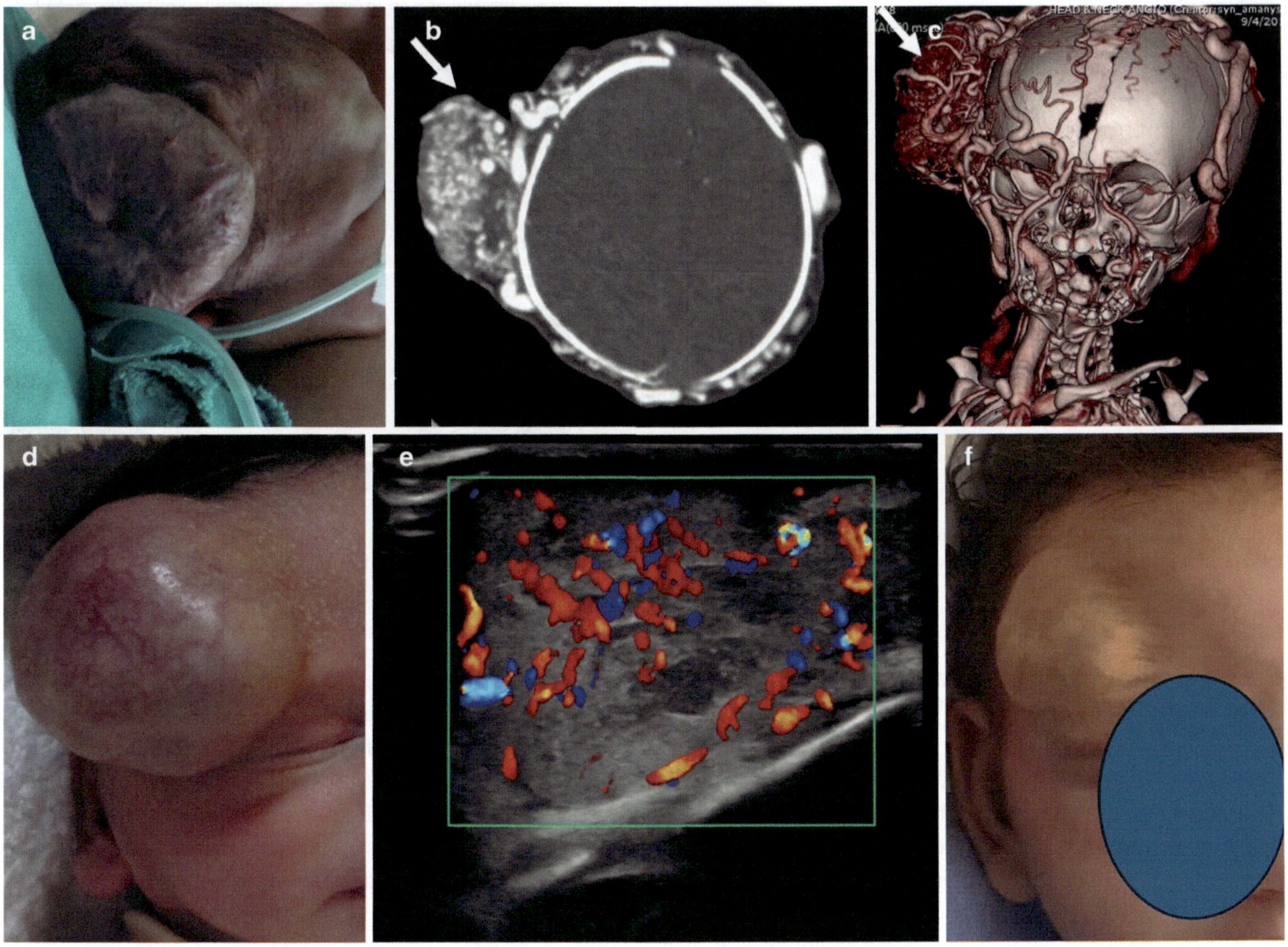

Fig. 8.14 Differential diagnosis of vascular swelling at birth. Upper row (**a–c**): arteriovenous malformation—(**a**) clinical photograph; (**b**, **c**) axial CT angiography and 3D reconstruction showing large nidus (arrow) with tangled feeding arteries and draining veins. Lower row (**d–f**): congenital hemangioma—(**d**) clinical photograph; (**e**) Color Doppler showing echogenic soft tissue mass with increased vascularity; (**f**) follow-up photograph demonstrating spontaneous regression (RICH)

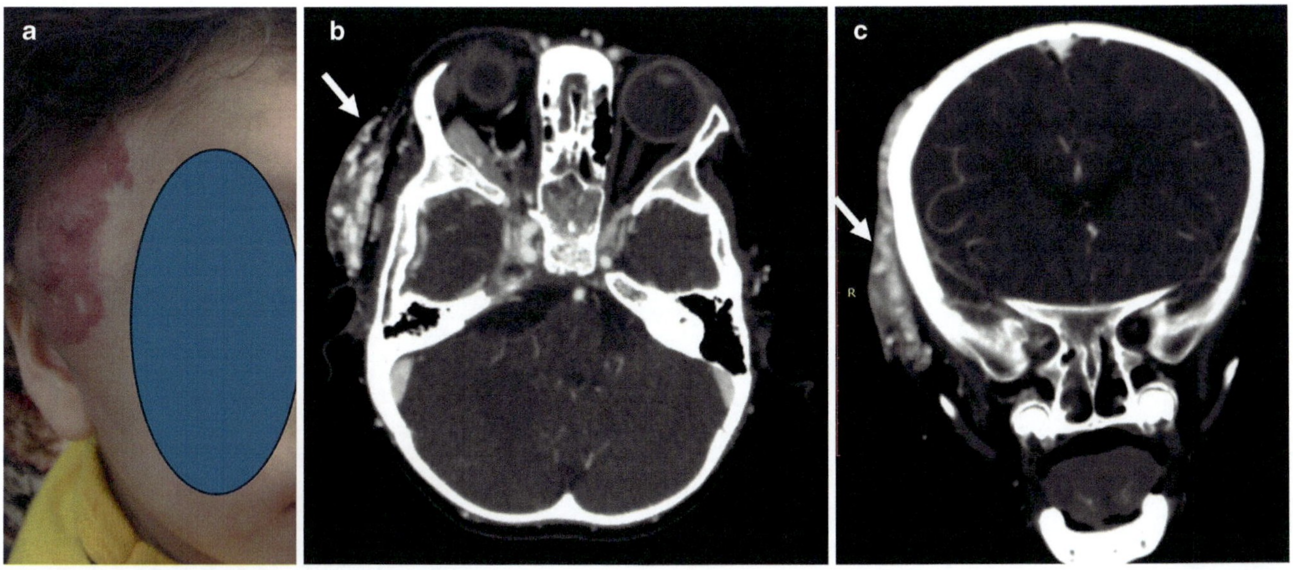

Fig. 8.15 (**a**) Arteriovenous malformation in a one-year-old boy. (**b**, **c**) Axial and coronal CT angiography showing subcutaneous nidus in the right temporal region

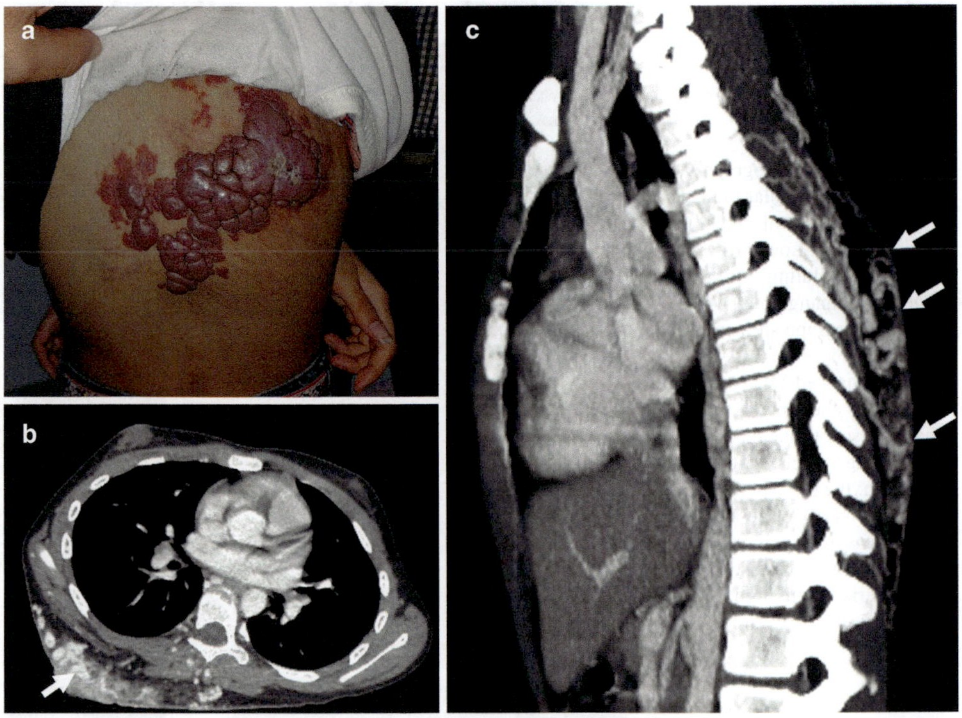

Fig. 8.16 Nine-year-old girl with arteriovenous malformation of the back. (**a**) Clinical photograph; (**b, c**) axial and sagittal contrast-enhanced CT showing large nidus (arrows) involving skin and subcutaneous tissue. Initially misdiagnosed as hemangioma and observed for spontaneous regression until referral with bleeding

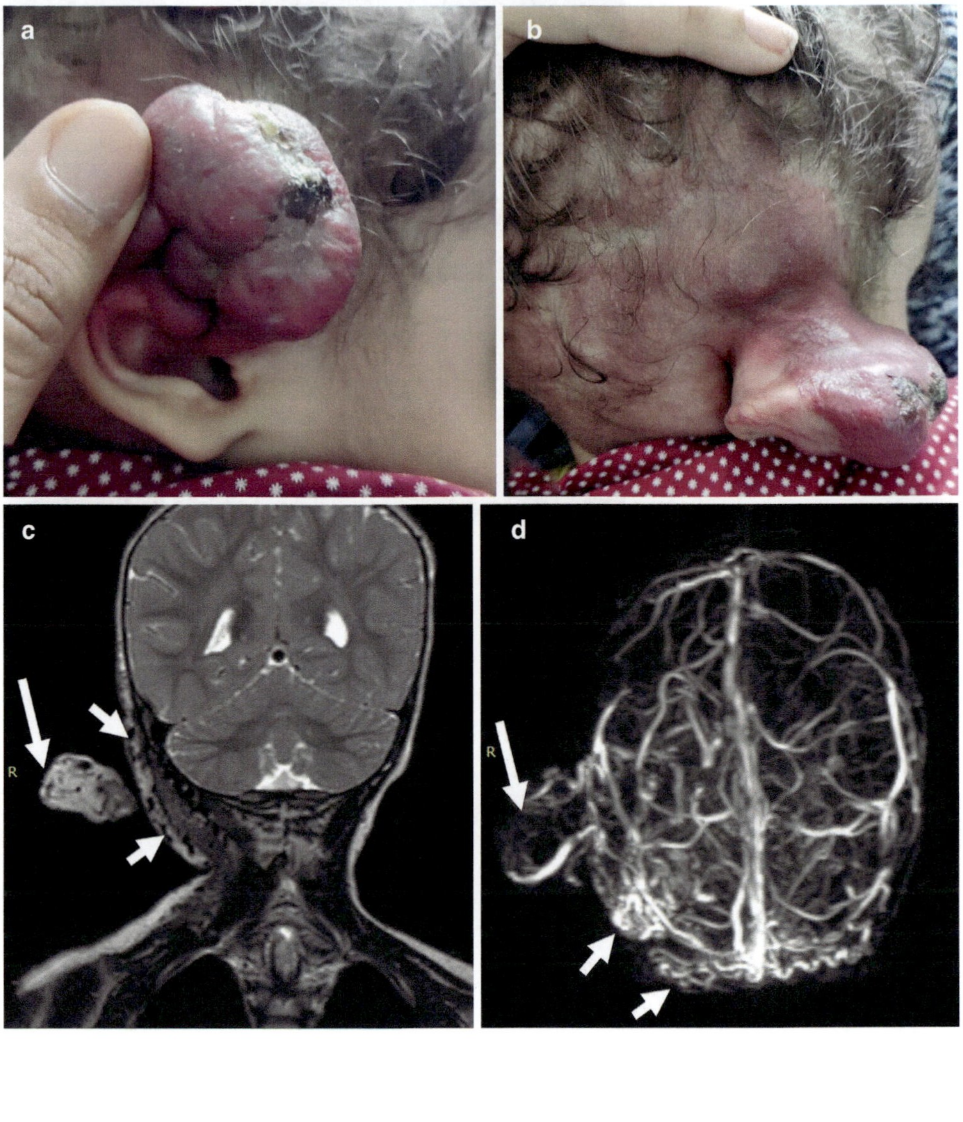

Fig. 8.17 Infant with auricular arteriovenous malformation. (**a, b**) Clinical photographs showing soft-tissue mass; (**c**) coronal T2-WI showing hyperintense mass (long arrow) with multiple flow voids in adjacent tissues (short arrows); (**d**) axial MR venography showing abnormal vessels in the auricle (long arrow) and surrounding tissues (short arrow). Exceptionally, AVMs may appear mass-like when infiltrating muscle or organs, as in this case

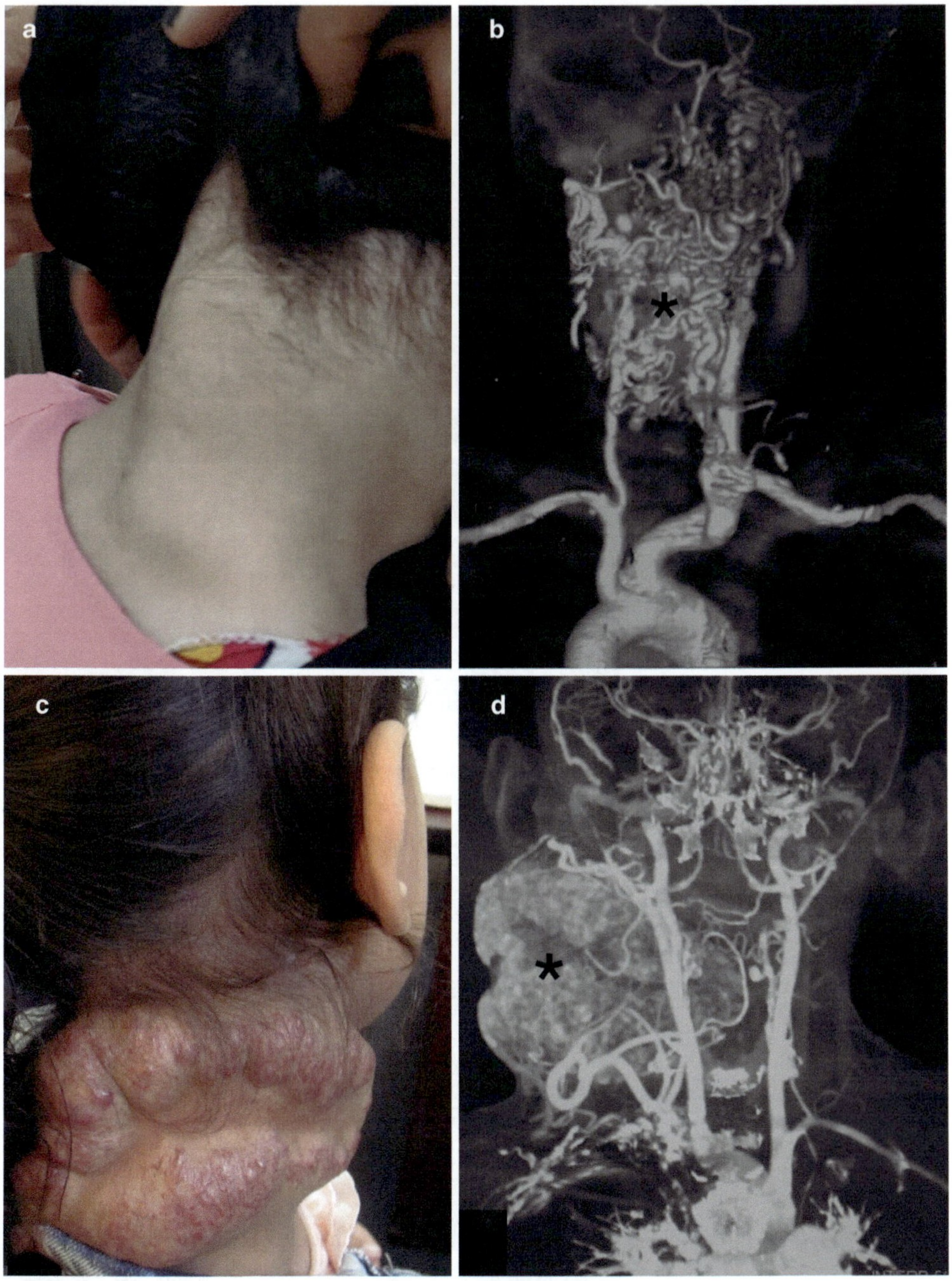

Fig. 8.18 Differential diagnosis of vascular swelling. Upper row (a, b): arteriovenous malformation—(**a**) clinical photograph showing subcutaneous swelling; (**b**) CT angiography revealing large vascular nidus (asterisk) without a discrete soft-tissue mass. Lower row (c, d): non-involuting congenital hemangioma—(**c**) clinical photograph showing large reddish swelling; (**d**) contrast-enhanced MR angiography showing enhancing soft-tissue mass with feeding vessels. Note the distinction: the mass in AVM consists primarily of vessels (**b**), whereas hemangioma shows a distinct soft tissue mass (asterisk) with high vascularity (**d**)

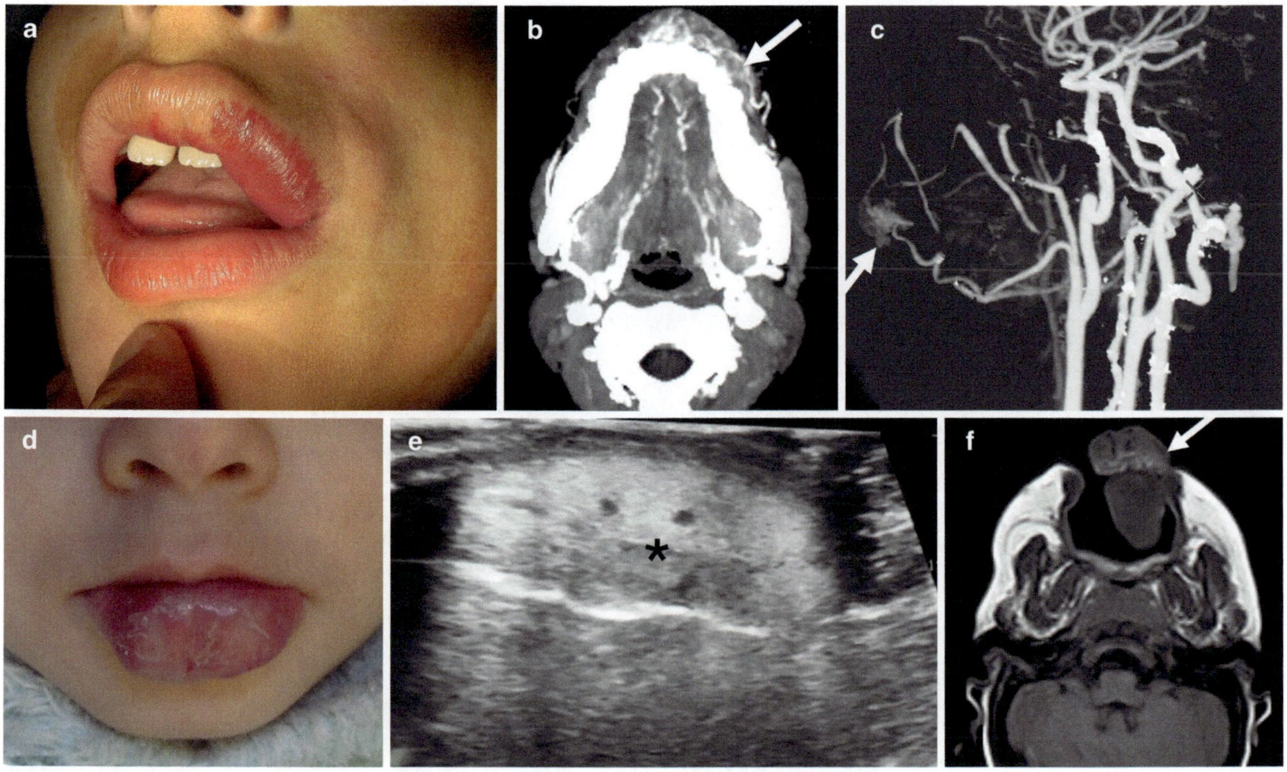

Fig. 8.19 Differential diagnosis of lip swelling. Upper row (**a–c**): arteriovenous malformation —(**a**) clinical photograph showing red swelling of the upper lip; (**b**, **c**) axial and sagittal CT angiography (MIP) demonstrating nidus (arrow) with feeding artery and draining vein. Lower row (**d–f**): hemangioma—(**d**) clinical photograph showing lower lip swelling; (**e**) B-mode ultrasound showing echogenic soft tissue mass (asterisk); (**f**) MRI (axial T1-WI) showing soft-tissue mass (arrow) with internal flow voids

Third: Other Benign Lesions That Can Masquerade as Common Hemangioma

(a) *Pyogenic granuloma (lobular capillary hemangioma):* Pyogenic granulomas (PGs), also referred to as lobular capillary hemangiomas, are acquired benign vascular tumors that can develop in both children and adults [11]. PGs are usually solitary and most commonly seen on the head and neck in children [12]. Although the exact cause and pathogenesis remain unclear, PGs are classified as benign vascular tumors by the International Society for the Study of Vascular Anomalies (ISSVA) [13]. Immunohistochemical staining for endothelial markers is negative for GLUT-1, which differentiates PGs from infantile hemangiomas. PGs typically present as rapidly growing, exophytic, pedunculated red papules (Fig. 8.20). They are prone to ulceration, profuse easily bleeding, and rarely undergo spontaneous regression [12]. A variety of treatment options exist for PG, including surgical excision, cryotherapy, laser therapy, or topical agents such as silver nitrate. However, the most definitive treatment is surgical excision of the entire lesion, which also provides tissue for histopathological confirmation of the diagnosis (Fig. 8.20d) [12].

(b) *Juvenile xanthogranuloma (JXG):* JXG is a rare, generally benign, non-Langerhans cell histiocytosis, primarily affecting infants and young children. JXG typically presents as a solitary, self-limiting reddish-yellow skin nodule on the head, neck, or trunk [14, 15] (Fig. 8.21).

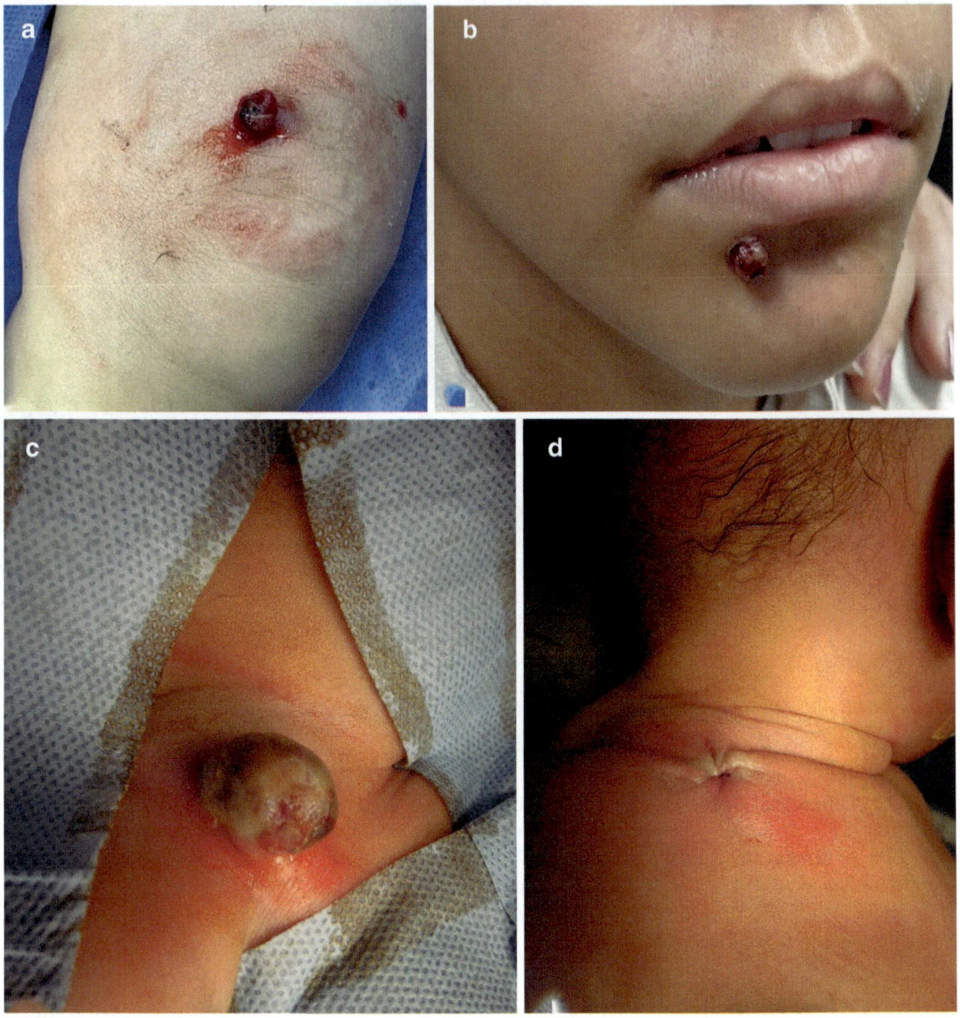

Fig. 8.20 Pyogenic granuloma. (**a–c**) Clinical photographs from three cases involving the knee, lower mandible, and supraclavicular regions. (**d**) Excision with purse-string wound closure

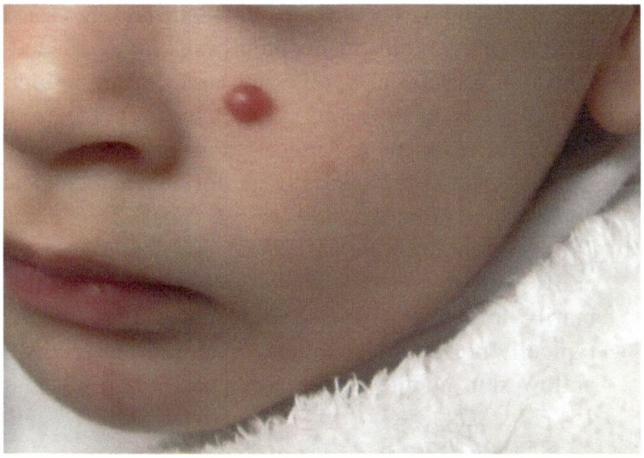

Fig. 8.21 Juvenile xanthogranuloma (JXG) in a 15-month-old boy, presenting as an acquired lesion that developed at 1 year of age. The atypical timing of onset served as a key feature in excluding the more common diagnosis of hemangioma

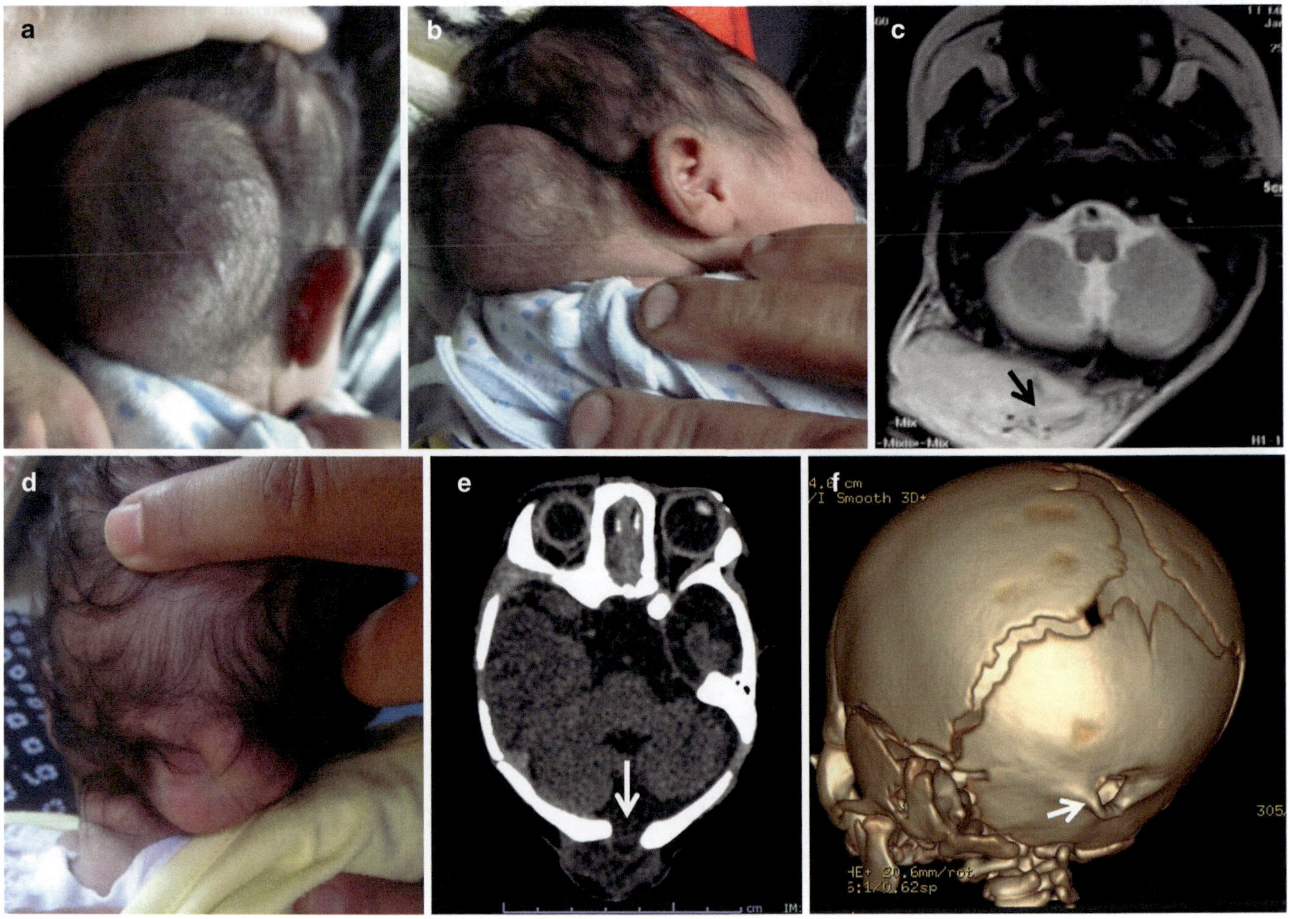

Fig. 8.22 Differential diagnosis of occipital swelling. Upper row (**a**–**c**): congenital haemangioma—(**a**, **b**) clinical photographs; (**c**) MRI showing soft-tissue mass with T2 hyperintensity and intralesional flow voids (arrow). Lower row (**d**–**f**): occipital meningocele—(**d**) clinical photograph; (**e**, **f**) non-contrast CT and 3D reconstruction showing underlying osseous defect (arrow)

Fourth: Occipital Meningocele

The skull and the back of the neck are common sites for congenital hemangiomas. When presenting in the occipital region, we must exclude other swellings that can occur in this particular location, like occipital meningoceles (Fig. 8.22).

References

1. Enjolras O, Mulliken JB, Kozakewich HPW. Vascular tumors and tumor-like lesions. In: Mulliken JB, Burrows PE, Fishman SJ, editors. Mulliken & Young's vascular anomalies: hemangiomas and malformations. Oxford University Press; 2013. p. 259–324.
2. Burrows PE, Paltiel HJ. Radiological imaging of Hemangiomas and related vascular Tumors. In: Mulliken JB, Burrows PE, Fishman SJ, editors. Mulliken & Young's vascular anomalies: hemangiomas and malformations. Oxford University Press; 2013. p. 111–60.
3. AbouZeid AA, Mohammad SA, Aly NH, et al. Differential diagnostic features between congenital haemangioma, KHE, and congenital fibrosarcoma: a single-centre experience. Eur J Pediatr. 2021;180:2581–9. https://doi.org/10.1007/s00431-021-04119-7.
4. Boon LM, Fishman SJ, Lund DP, Mulliken JB. Congenital fibrosarcoma masquerading as congenital hemangioma: report of two cases. J Pediatr Surg. 1995;30:1378–81.
5. Dasgupta R, Rodeberg D. Non-rhabdomyosarcoma. Semin Pediatr Surg. 2016;25:284–9.
6. Uller W, Alomari AI, Richter GT. Arteriovenous malformations. Semin Pediatr Surg. 2014;23:203–7. https://doi.org/10.1053/j.sempedsurg.2014.07.005.
7. Flors L, Park AW, Norton PT, Hagspiel KD, Leiva-Salinas C. Soft-tissue vascular malformations and tumors. Part 1: Classification, role of imaging and high-flow lesions. Radiologia (English edition). 2019;61:4–15.
8. Do YS, Kim YW, Lee BB, Yakes WF. Arteriovenous malformations (AVMs): clinical features and evaluation. In: Kim YW, Lee BB, Yakes WF, Do YS, editors. Congenital vascular malformations. Springer-Verlag Berlin Heidelberg; 2017. p. 105–12.
9. Vaghi M, Ianniello A. CT and CT angiogram in the diagnosis of congenital vascular malformations. In: Kim YW, Lee BB, Yakes WF, Do YS, editors. Congenital vascular malformations. Berlin/Heidelberg: Springer-Verlag; 2017. p. 161–4.
10. Park KB, Do YS. Angiographic classification: arteriovenous malformation and venous malformation. In: Kim YW, Lee BB, Yakes

WF, Do YS, editors. Congenital vascular malformations. Berlin/Heidelberg: Springer-Verlag; 2017. p. 55–62.
11. Mills SE, Cooper PH, Fechner RE. Lobular capillary hemangioma, the underlying lesion of pyogenic granuloma: a study of 73 cases from the oral and nasal mucous membranes. Am J Surg Pathol. 1980;4:471–9.
12. Khorsand K, Gupta D. Pyogenic Granuloma (Lobular Capillary Hemangioma). In: Perkins JA, Balakrishnan K, editors. Evidence-based management of head and neck vascular anomalies. Springer Nature Switzerland; 2018. p. 52–7.
13. ISSVA Classification of Vascular Anomalies. International Society for the Study of Vascular Anomalies. 2014. Available at: "issva.org/classification."
14. Mulliken JB. Diagnosis and natural history of Hemangiomas. In: Mulliken JB, Burrows PE, Fishman SJ, editors. Mulliken & Young's vascular anomalies: Hemangiomas and malformations. Oxford University Press; 2013. p. 68–110.
15. Zou T, Wei A, Ma H, Lian H, Liu Y, Wang D, Zhao Y, Cui L, Li Z, Zhang R, Wang T. Systemic juvenile xanthogranuloma: a systematic review. Pediatr Blood Cancer. 2023;70(5):e30232.

Part III

Lymphatic Malformations

Cervicofacial Lymphatic Malformations

9

Introduction

Lymphatic malformations (LMs) are classified as slow-flow vascular malformations and represent the second most common vascular malformation following the venous anomalies [1, 2]. LMs typically consist of lymph-filled cysts that do not connect with normal lymphatic vessels (Fig. 9.1) [3]. Based on their size, LMs are generally categorized as macrocystic, microcystic (Fig. 9.2), or, more often, the lesion consists of a combination of both types [4, 5]. LMs frequently develop in the areas of major lymphatic channels such as the neck and axilla (Fig. 9.1), but they may also involve any other part of the body—excluding the central nervous system, which does not have lymphatics [1, 5]. In this chapter, we will focus on lymphatic malformations occurring in one of their most common locations—the head and neck region, also known as cervicofacial LMs. The complex cervicofacial anatomy, along with the potential cosmetic consequences, makes the management of LMs in this region especially challenging [5].

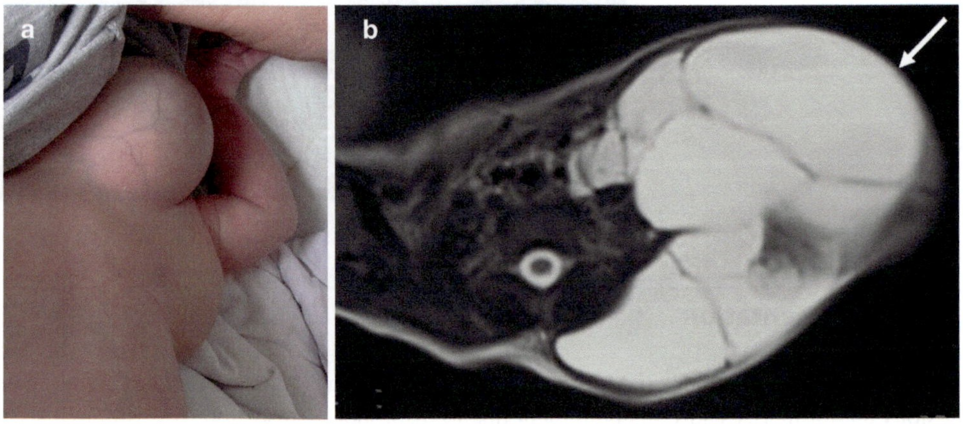

Fig. 9.1 Neonate with macrocystic lymphatic malformation. (**a**) Clinical photograph demonstrating swelling involving the neck and extending to axilla. (**b**) Axial T2-weighted MRI showing trans-spatial, multilocular cystic lesions exhibiting hyperintense signal (arrow)

A. A. AbouZeid et al., *Atlas of Pediatric Vascular Anomalies*, https://doi.org/10.1007/978-3-032-30866-5_9

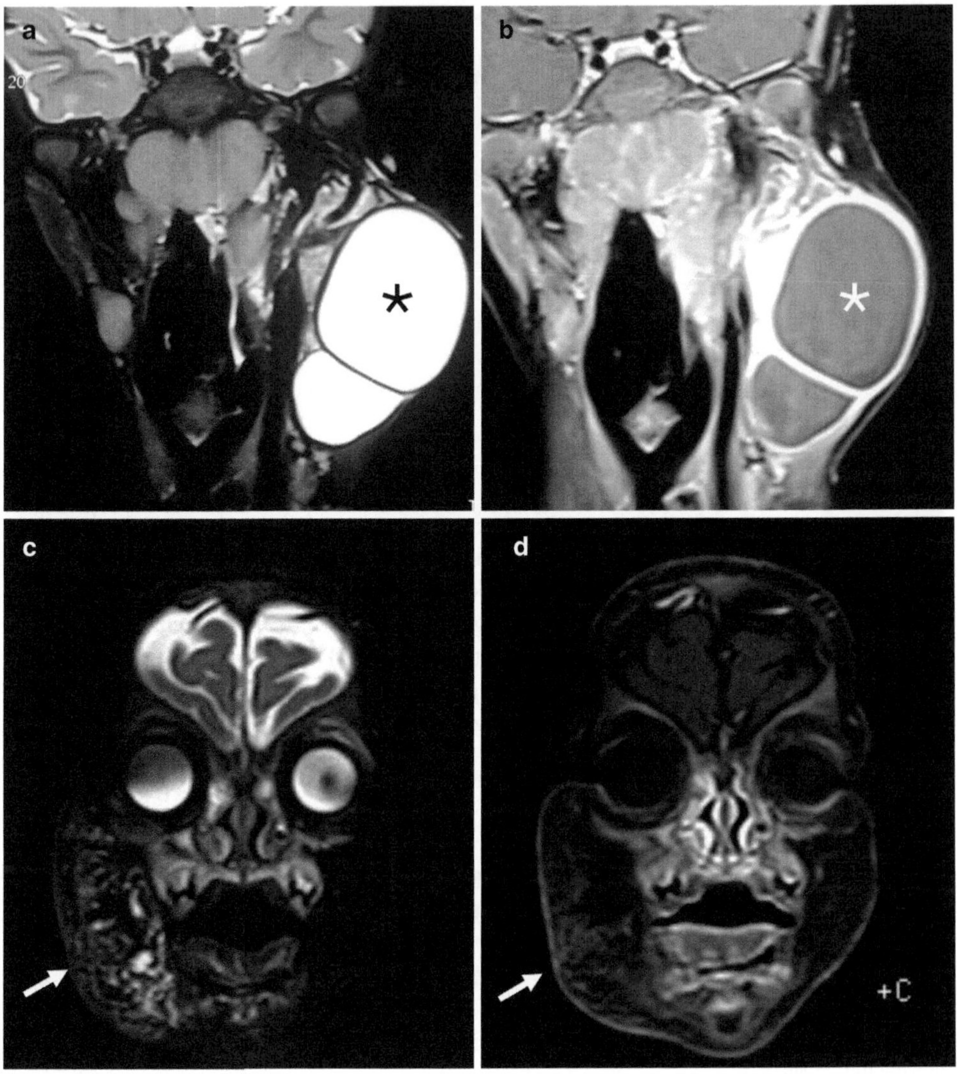

Fig. 9.2 MRI of different types of lymphatic malformation. (**a**, **b**) Macrocystic lymphatic malformation with large cystic spaces (asterisk) showing hyperintense signal on STIR (**a**) and smooth marginal post-contrast enhancement (**b**). (**c**, **d**) Microcystic lymphatic malformation with tiny cysts (arrow) demonstrating hyperintense signal on STIR (**c**) and absence of post-contrast enhancement (**d**)

Clinical Presentation

Lymphatic malformations (LMs) are generally benign lesions that primarily cause disfigurement due to disproportionate growth (Fig. 9.3). However, in certain anatomical locations—such as the submandibular (Fig. 9.4), or retro-orbital region (Fig. 9.5)—they may lead to additional complications due to compressive effects [6]. Most LMs are apparent at birth, with approximately 80% becoming evident within the first year of life [5]. LMs usually grow in proportion to the growth of the child. Cervicofacial LMs may expand in association with viral upper respiratory tract infections due to reactive lymphocytic hyperplasia [5]. Rapid expansion may indicate superadded bacterial infection or intralesional bleeding (Fig. 9.6). The latter may indicate combined veno-lymphatic malformations, which are not uncommon due to common embryonic origin (Fig. 9.7). Bleeding into lymphatic cysts may occur spontaneously or more commonly after attempts of aspiration or surgical resection [5]. Although spontaneous regression of LMs has been reported in the literature, it has not been observed in our clinical practice [6].

Cystic LMs can be diagnosed in utero (Fig. 9.8). When a large cervicofacial LM is identified antenatally, special preparations for delivery are required. This may include planning for an EXIT procedure (Ex Utero Intrapartum Treatment), which involves evaluating and, if necessary, securing the newborn's airway while the infant is still attached to the placenta before the umbilical cord is clamped [5]. However, clinical experience has shown that cervical LMs are usually soft and externally protruding, allowing the newborn to breathe spontaneously in most cases [5, 6].

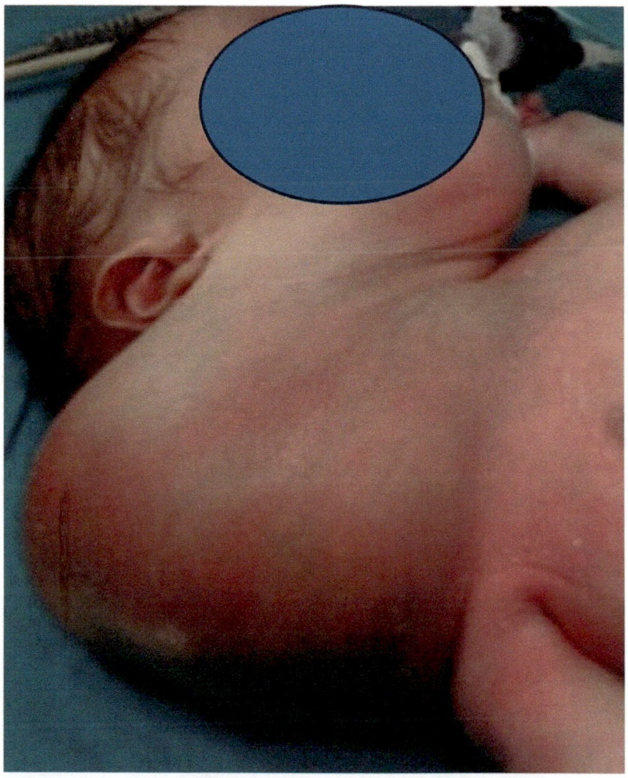

Fig. 9.3 Neonate with large cervical lymphatic malformation

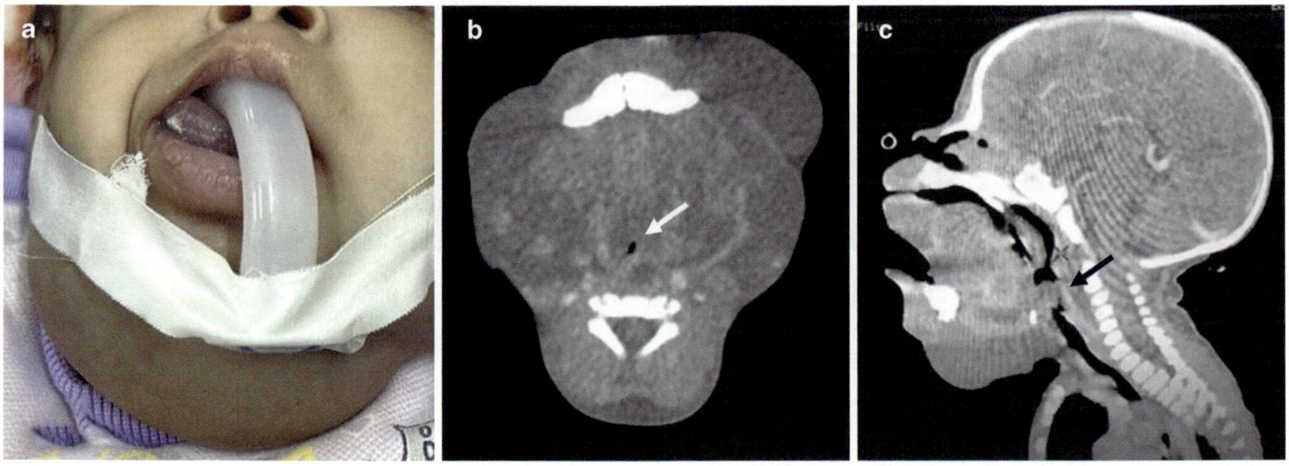

Fig. 9.4 Neonate with submandibular lymphatic malformation presenting with respiratory stridor. (**a**) Clinical photograph. (**b**, **c**) Axial and sagittal reconstructions of contrast-enhanced CT demonstrating a non-enhancing cystic lesion with trans-spatial extension through the neck spaces and larynx, causing marked airway compromise (arrow)

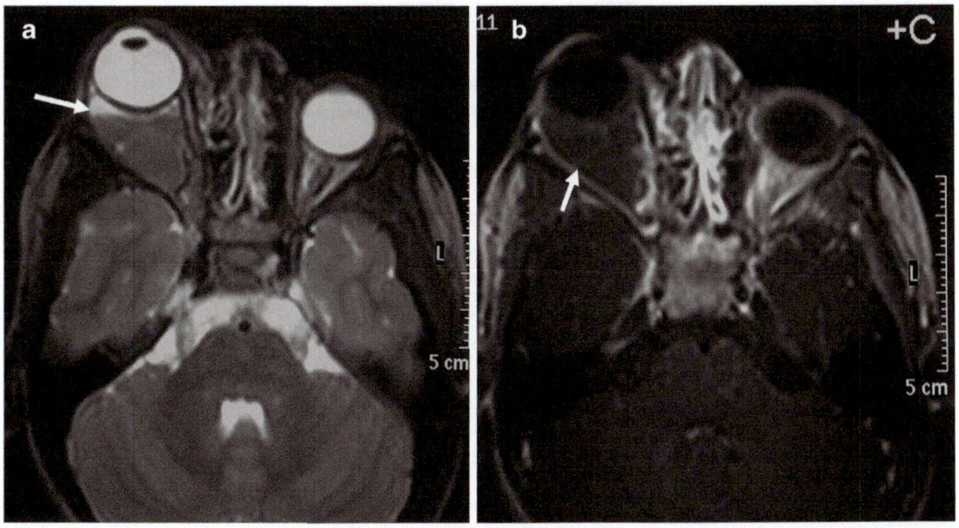

Fig. 9.5 Lymphatic malformation of the right orbit causing proptosis. (**a**) Axial STIR MRI showing intraconal multilocular cystic spaces with fluid–fluid levels (arrow) due to intralesional hemorrhage. (**b**) Axial contrast-enhanced fat-suppressed T1-weighted MRI demonstrating thin, smooth marginal enhancement (arrow) of the cystic spaces

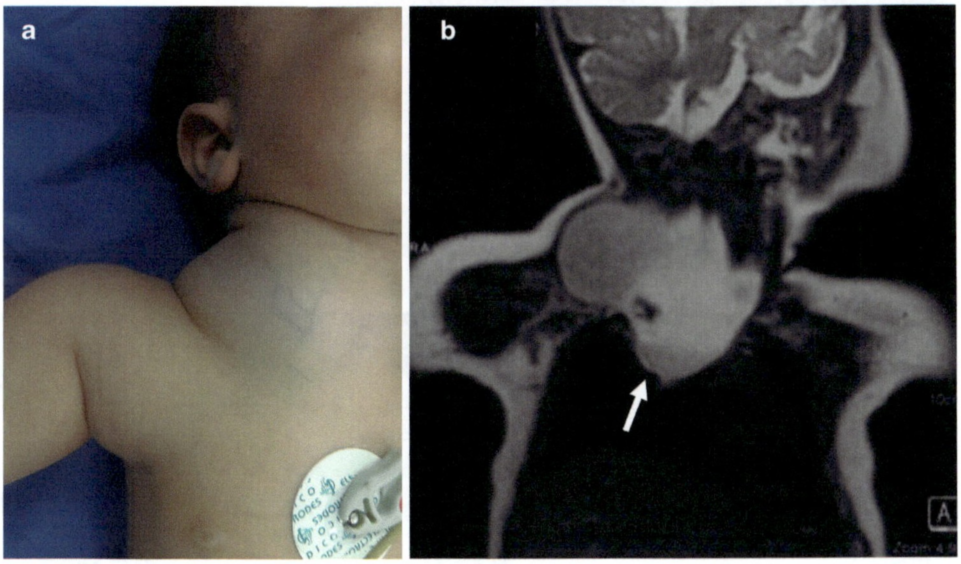

Fig. 9.6 Five-month-old girl with lymphatic malformation at root of the neck presenting with sudden rapid increase in lesion size and stridor. (**a**) Clinical photograph. (**b**) Coronal T2-weighted MRI showing a hyperintense lesion with areas of intermediate and low signal intensity due to hemorrhage and high protein content, extending into the superior mediastinum (arrow)

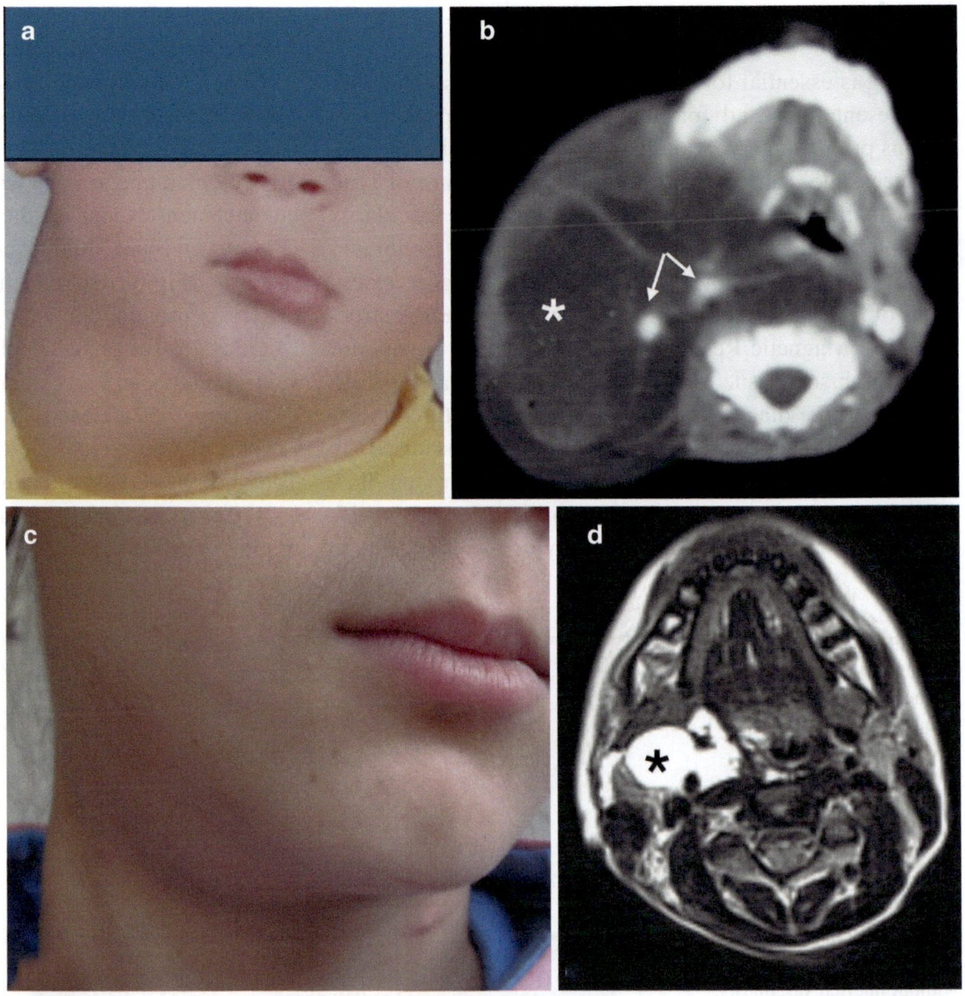

Fig. 9.7 Macrocystic lymphatic malformation of the neck before (**a**, **b**) and after sclerotherapy (**c**, **d**). (**a**) Clinical photograph at presentation. (**b**) Axial contrast-enhanced CT showing a multilocular cystic lesion with thin, smooth marginal enhancement (asterisk) extending deeply through several neck spaces. Note the cystic lesion encircling major neck vessels (arrows). (**c**) Clinical photograph after injection sclerotherapy. (**d**) Axial T2-weighted MRI demonstrating a small residual cystic lesion (asterisk) in the carotid and parapharyngeal spaces

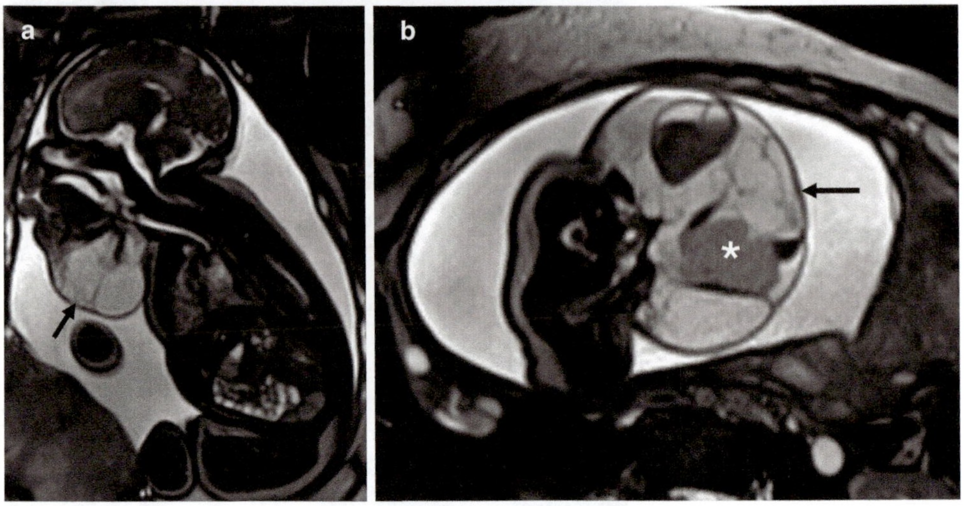

Fig. 9.8 Fetal MRI demonstrating cervical lymphatic malformation. (**a**) Sagittal view. (**b**) Axial view. The lesion shows the typical appearance of a multilocular cystic mass (arrow) with intralesional hemorrhage (asterisk) and fluid–fluid levels

Imaging

Imaging is essential for confirming the diagnosis in atypical presentations and for delineating the deep extent of lesions prior to intervention [5, 6]. Ultrasound, being readily accessible, can confirm the multicystic nature of lymphatic malformations and the absence of internal vascularity (Fig. 9.9). Advanced cross-sectional imaging techniques (CT/MRI) are superior for demonstrating deeper extensions of LMs as well as relations to important nearby structures [6]. Magnetic Resonance Imaging (MRI) is superior for its high soft tissue resolution and multiplanar capabilities. When the diagnosis is uncertain, MRI with contrast-enhanced T1-weighted images (Fig. 9.2) is used to distinguish lymphatic malformations from other slow-flow vascular malformations, such as venous malformations [7, 8]; otherwise, non-contrast MRI is typically sufficient to assess lesion extent prior to intervention (Fig. 9.1). The MRI technique for evaluating vascular anomalies is detailed in Chap. 2. Lymphatic malformations typically appear as multiple cysts of variable size (Fig. 9.10). The cysts are usually hyperintense on T2-weighted images, isointense on T1-weighted images, and with no appreciable post-contrast enhancement except for the capsule and intervening septa (Fig. 9.11). Fluid–fluid levels may also be observed within the cysts (Fig. 9.10), reflecting sedimentation of fluid with differing protein content, possibly due to hemorrhage. Microcystic lymphatic malformations represent a distinct subtype characterized by numerous tiny, often microscopic, cysts (Fig. 9.12). Despite its higher radiation exposure and lower soft tissue resolution compared to MRI, Computed Tomography (CT) is often more readily available and easier to perform, especially in emergency situations (does not require anesthesia) (Fig. 9.4) [6].

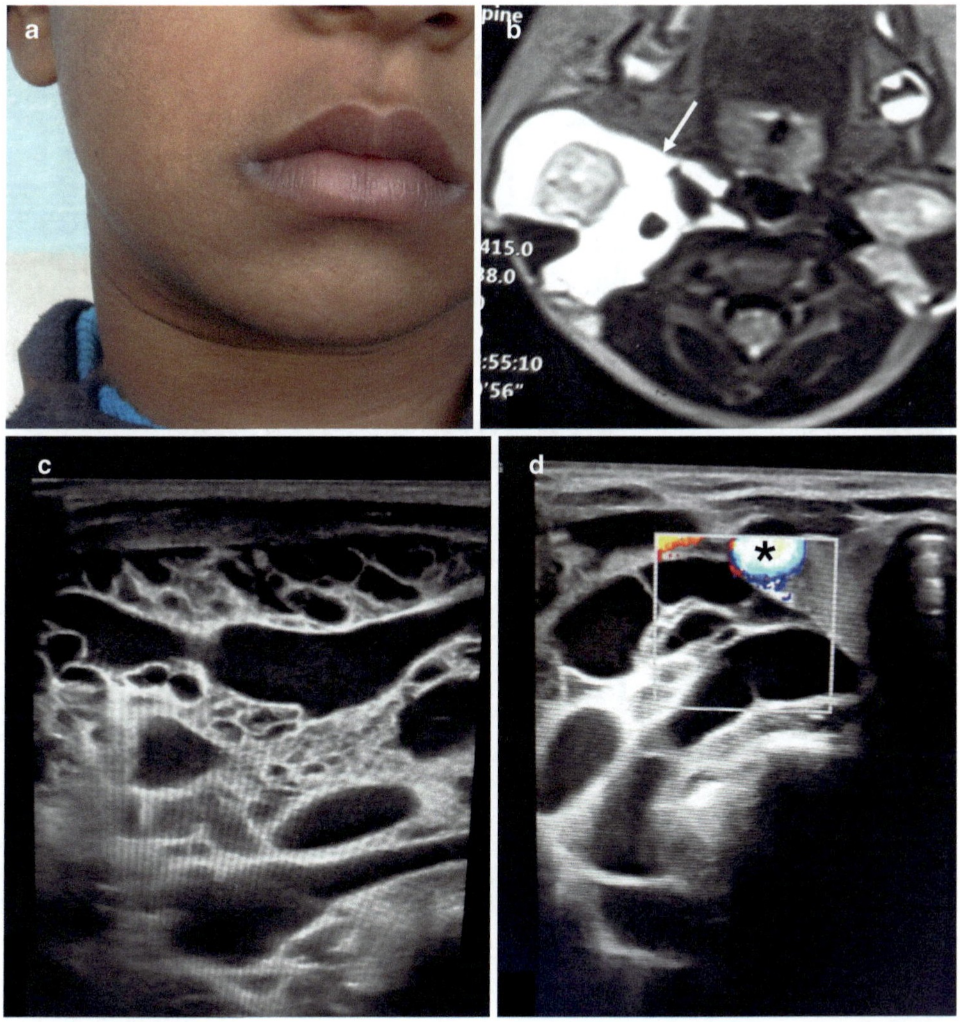

Fig. 9.9 Lymphatic malformation (right side of the neck). (**a**) clinical photograph (**b**) Axial T2-WI MRI shows hyperintense cystic lesion (arrow) with trans-spatial extension through the parapharyngeal, carotid and posterior cervical neck spaces. (**c, d**) B-mode ultrasound and color Doppler show variable-sized multilocular cystic lesion without internal vascularity. (asterisk: carotid artery)

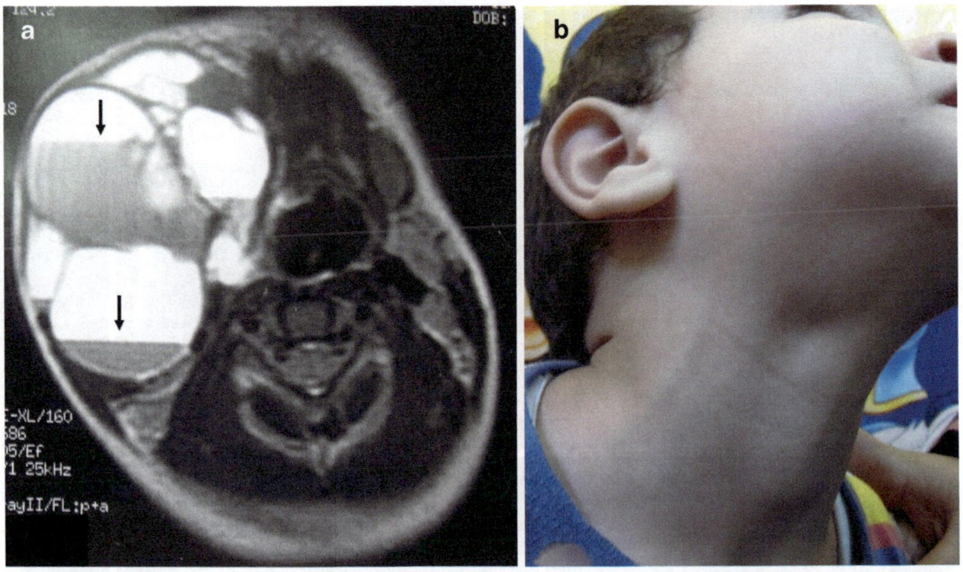

Fig. 9.10 Eleven-month-old boy with right submandibular lymphatic malformation. (**a**) Axial T2-weighted MRI showing characteristic fluid–fluid levels within the cysts (arrows). (**b**) Follow-up demonstrating marked reduction in lesion size after bleomycin injection. (Reproduced from AbouZeid et al. [6])

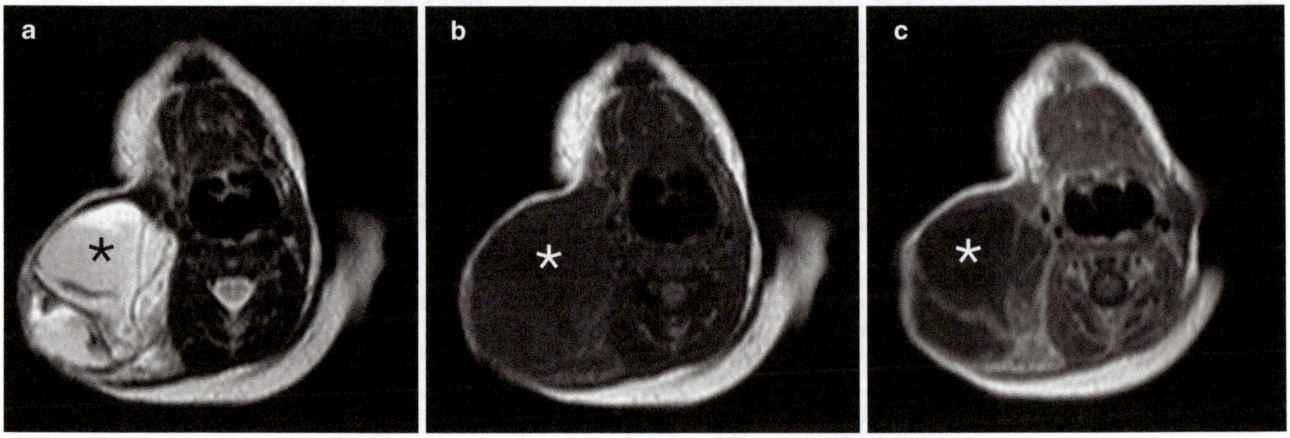

Fig. 9.11 Typical MRI appearance of lymphatic malformation. (**a**) Multilocular cystic lesion (asterisk) with hyperintense signal on T2-weighted imaging. (**b**) Hypointense signal on T1-weighted imaging. (**c**) Smooth marginal post-contrast enhancement

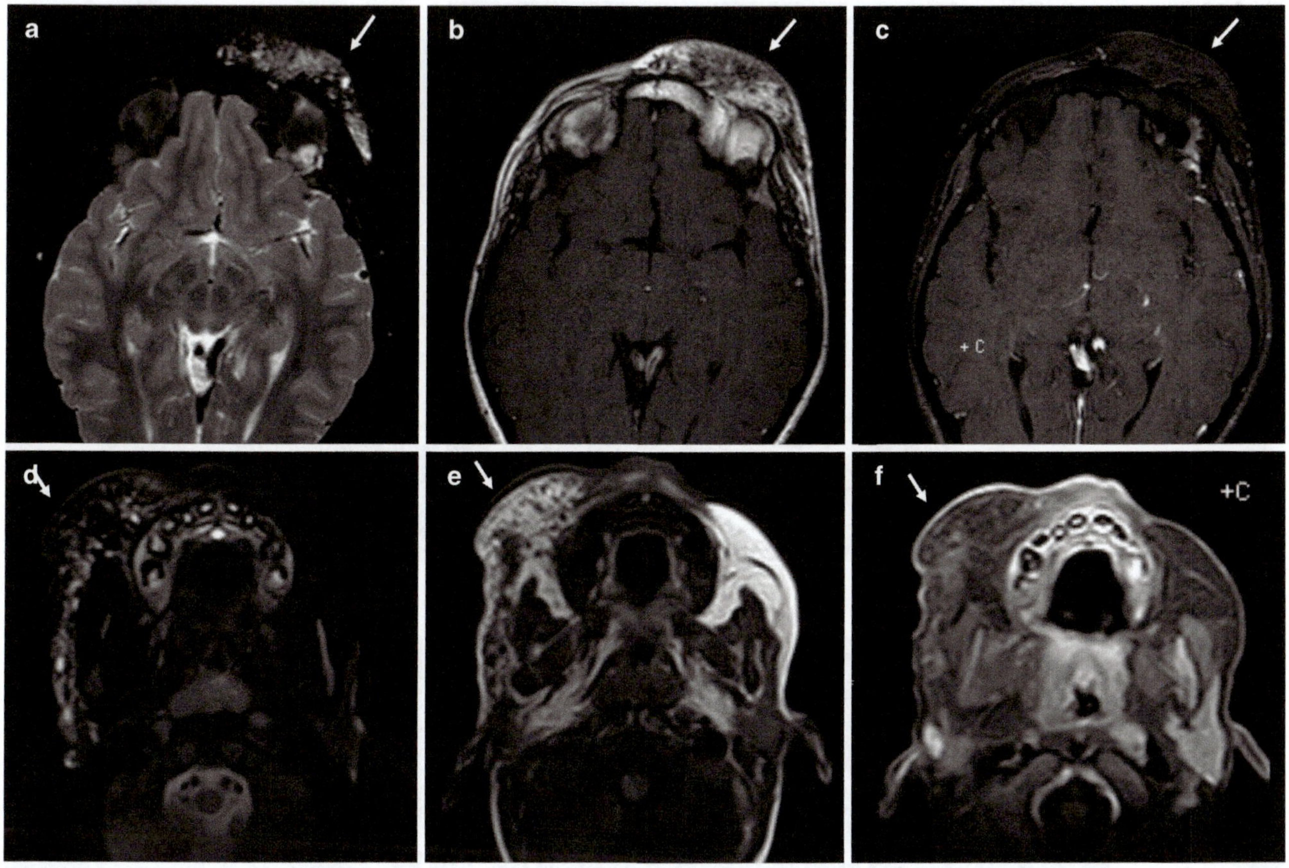

Fig. 9.12 MRI appearance of Microcystic lymphatic malformations (arrow) in the forehead (**a–c**) and right cheek (**d–f**). (**a, d**) Fat-suppressed T2-weighted MRI demonstrating rounded and tubular tiny lesions (arrow) with hyperintense signal. Lesions demonstrate hypointense signal on T1-weighted MRI (**b, e**); and absence of post-contrast enhancement in (**c, f**)

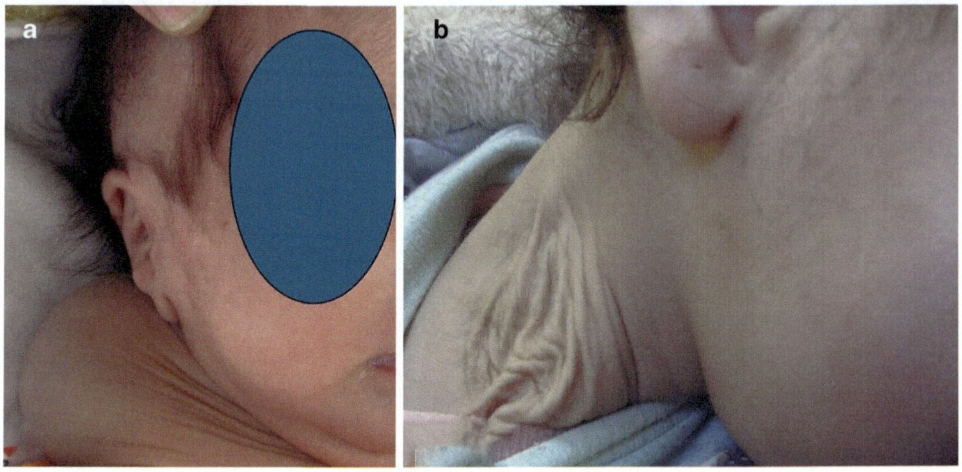

Fig. 9.13 Macrocystic lymphatic malformation before (**a**) and after (**b**) bleomycin sclerotherapy, showing reduction in size

Treatment

When discussing treatment options with parents, it's important to emphasize that lymphatic malformations (LMs) are benign lesions. Complete eradication is often unnecessary and may not be always feasible; instead, the primary goal is to minimize the impact of the lesions as much as possible [9]. This can be accomplished through various approaches, including sclerotherapy, surgical intervention, medical therapy, or a combination of all of these [6].

Injection sclerotherapy: Macrocystic lymphatic malformations generally show a favorable, though variable, response to sclerotherapy, often leading to significant reduction in lesion size (Figs. 9.7, 9.10 and 9.13). At our center, bleomycin is the sclerosing agent of choice for LMs. The procedure is conducted under general anesthesia. Initially, cyst aspiration is performed, followed by the injection of bleomycin at a dose of 0.2–0.5 mg/kg body weight, using an aqueous solution with a concentration of 1 mg/ml [6, 10]. For large or diffuse lesions, the procedure may need to be repeated once or twice at intervals of 3–6 months. It is crucial to document the bleomycin dose administered each time to ensure the total cumulative dose does not exceed the recommended lifetime maximum of 5 mg/kg [6, 10].

Surgical treatment: Surgical excision remains a valuable treatment option for lymphatic malformations, particularly for microcystic lesions, which typically show limited response to sclerotherapy (Fig. 9.14.). The location of

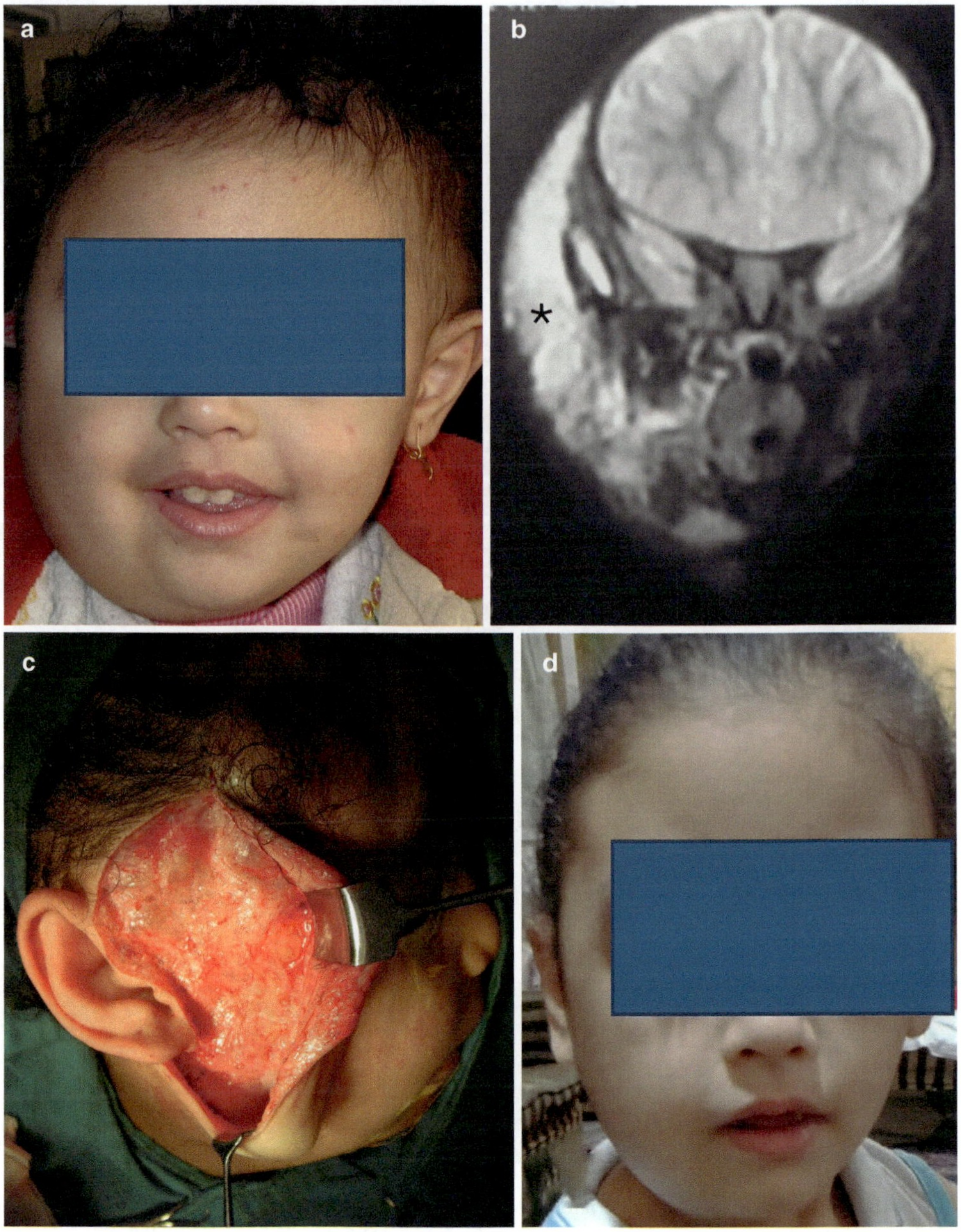

Fig. 9.14. (**a**) One-year-old girl with microcystic lymphatic malformation in the right face. (**b**) Coronal fat-suppressed T2-weighted MRI showing lesion extent (asterisk). (**c**) Surgical excision through pre-auricular incision. (**d**) Follow-up after surgery. (Reproduced from AbouZeid et al. [6])

LMs and degree of trans-spatial and deep extension are one major decisive factor on the feasibility of surgical excision. Considering the benign nature of LMs, surgical excision should not leave disfiguring scars nor functional disability resulting from injury to important structures and nearby nerves [5]. Partial excision (debulking) may be the only feasible solution for large lesions with deep trans-spatial extensions [6]. Postoperative fluid collections and surgical site wound infections are not uncommon after excision of LMs [11]; it is recommended to leave drains in the surgical wounds for several days postoperatively [12].

Drug therapy: Medical treatment may involve antibiotics and anti-inflammatory drugs to control acute lesion enlargement secondary to bacterial infection [6]. Sirolimus, a more recent therapeutic option, represents a promising advancement in biomedical genetic therapy, particularly for extensive or complicated cases of LMs (Fig. 9.15) [13, 14]. The dosage of sirolimus is calculated based on body surface area and is subsequently adjusted according to blood trough levels. It is administered orally on a continuous schedule, starting at 0.8 mg/m^2, with therapeutic levels maintained between 5 and 15 ng/ml.

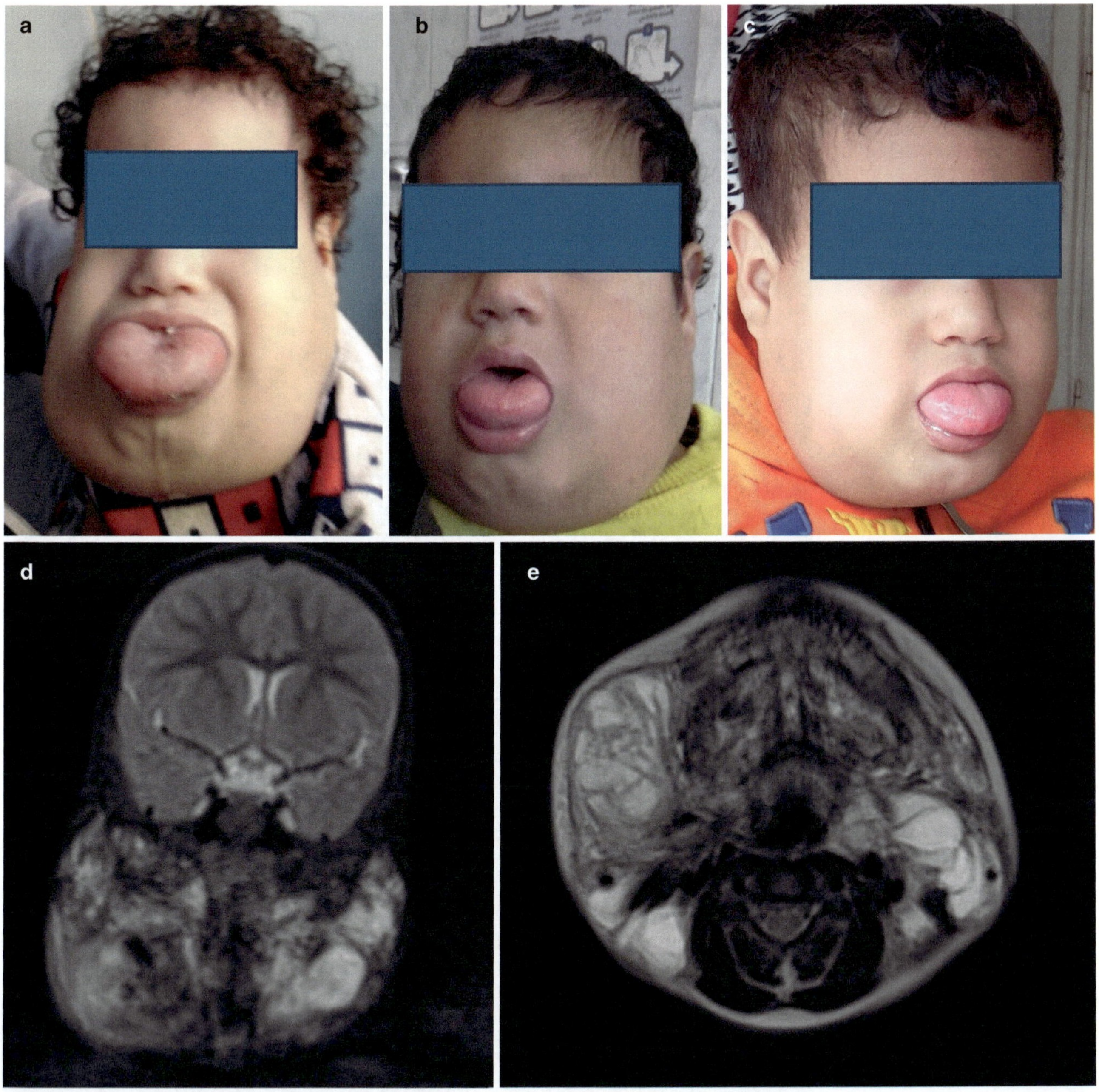

Fig. 9.15 One-year-old boy with bilateral submandibular lymphatic malformation and macroglossia. The lesion was resistant to repeated sclerotherapy but showed marked improvement after 15 months of sirolimus therapy (**a**–**c**). Coronal and axial MRI demonstrate deep extension (**d**, **e**). (Reproduced from AbouZeid et al. [6])

Special Considerations in Managing LMs According to Its Location

(a) Cervical LMs: It may be useful to categorize cervical LMs based on their location, whether in the anterior or posterior cervical triangles. In the posterior cervical triangle, LMs are mostly macrocystic, unilateral, and externally protruding. Even when large, they rarely cause significant airway compromise (Fig. 9.16). They typically respond well to injection sclerotherapy, and when surgery is pursued, near-complete resection is often attainable [5, 6]. On the other hand, LMs in the anterior cervical triangle (submandibular region) usually contain significant microcystic components encroaching on midline structures and posing a higher risk of airway compromise (Fig. 9.17) [5, 6]. Anterior triangle LMs may be bilateral and are generally more difficult to excise (Fig. 9.15), often resulting in incomplete resections, higher recurrence rates, and episodes of intermittent swelling [5]. Careful dissection is required to preserve adjacent nerves, such as the mandibular branch of the facial nerve, while removal of the submandibular salivary gland is often unavoidable (Fig. 9.17) [5].

(b) Facial LMs: Facial LMs are predominantly microcystic (Fig. 9.12) and may affect various regions of the face, including the forehead, cheeks, lips, and temporal areas. Injection sclerotherapy usually results in suboptimal response, and surgery represents the mainstay. Lateral facial lesions are typically accessed via a preauricular incision (Fig. 9.14.), which may be extended into the cervical region if needed. When feasible, medial lesions are best resected using a transoral approach (Fig. 9.18) [5]. Lesions in the cheek may be accompanied by soft tissue and bony hypertrophy of the malar eminence, leading to facial asymmetry with ptosis of the upper lip (Fig. 9.19).

(c) Periorbital: Retro-orbital LMs present with proptosis (Figs. 9.5 and 9.20). Injection sclerotherapy (bleomycin) is the main stay. More recently, mTOR inhibitors such as sirolimus have been introduced in the management of LMs, demonstrating excellent therapeutic response, particularly for lesions situated in deep, inaccessible regions.

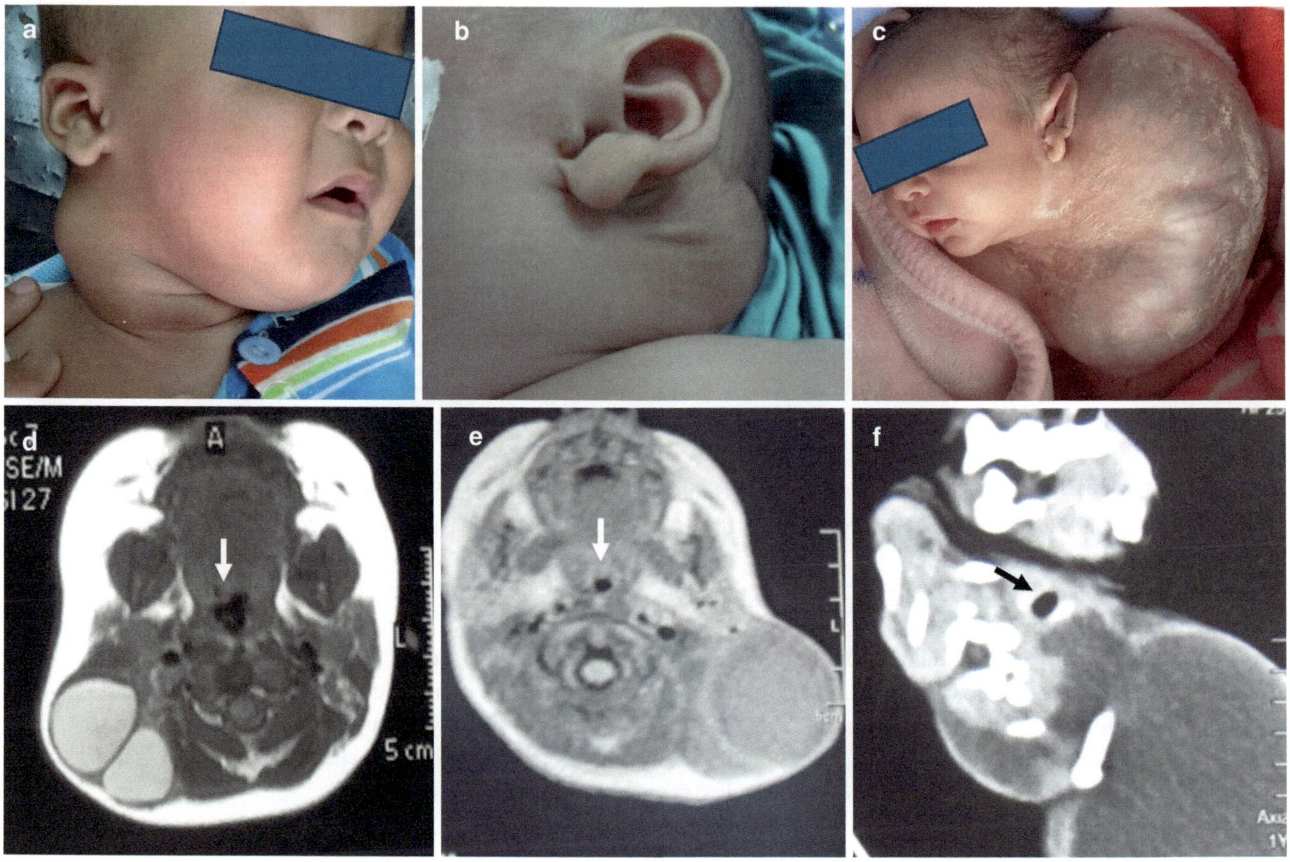

Fig. 9.16 Lymphatic malformations (LMs) in the posterior triangle of the neck in three different cases (**a**, **b**, **c**), and their corresponding cross-sectional imaging (**d**, **e**, **f**), respectively. Note that in this type of LMs there is no compromise to the airway (arrow) even when lesions are very large in size (**c**, **f**). (Reproduced from AbouZeid et al. [6])

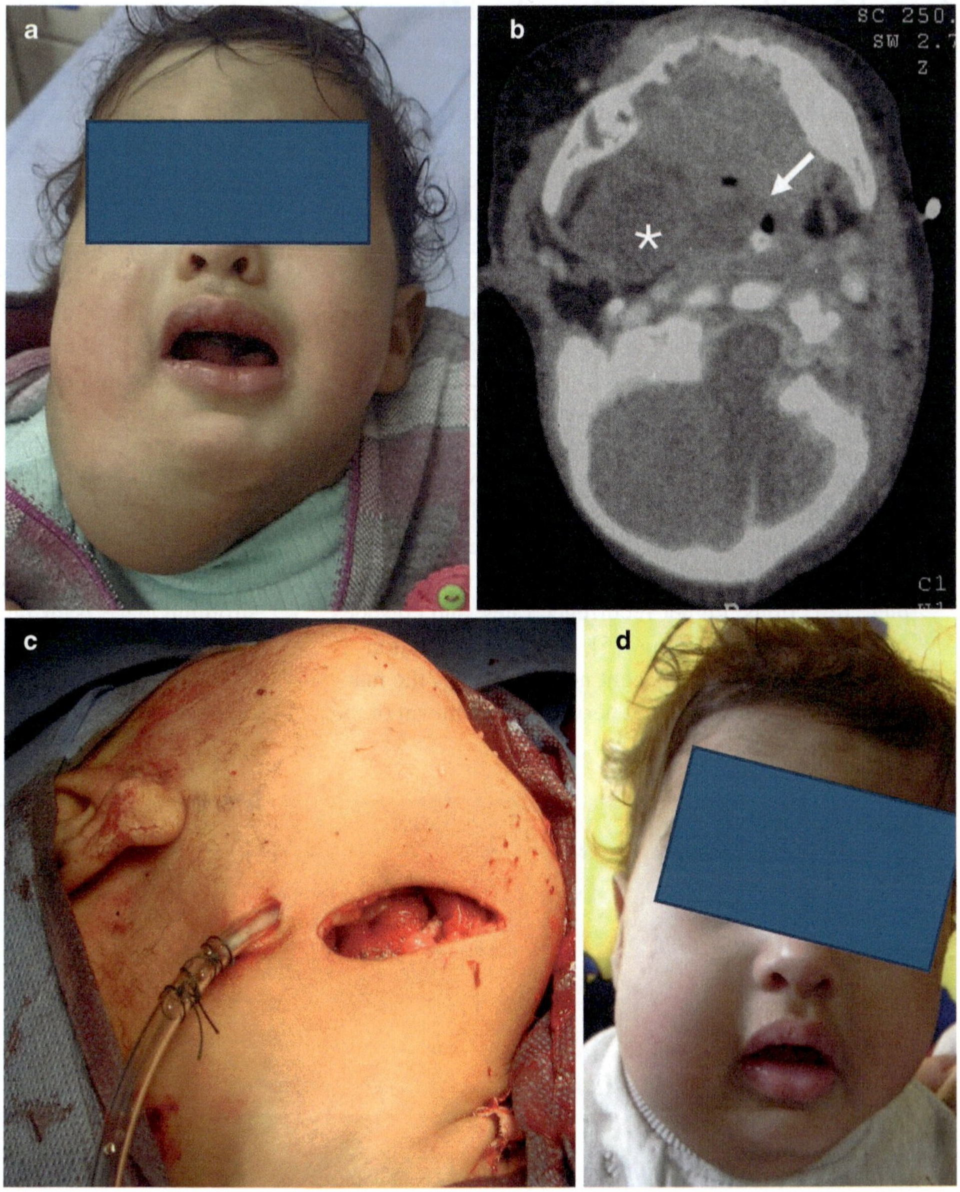

Fig. 9.17 An eleven-month-old girl with a submandibular lymphatic malformation. (**a**) Clinical presentation with upper airway obstruction. (**b**) CT scan demonstrating a cystic lesion (asterisk) extending to the deep midline and encroaching on the airway (arrow). (**c**) Intraoperative view during surgical excision. (**d**) Postoperative recovery with successful discharge. (Reproduced from AbouZeid et al. [6])

(d) Parotid: Parotid surgery poses an inherent risk of facial nerve injury and demands special surgical expertise. As a safer alternative, sclerotherapy for lymphatic malformations in the parotid region (Fig. 9.21) may be preferable to avoid surgical risks.

(e) Tongue: Lymphatic malformations of the tongue may appear as localized lesions (Fig. 9.22) but more commonly manifest as diffuse lesions that also involve the neck and the floor of the mouth (Figs. 9.15 and 9.23). Affected tongues are typically enlarged (macroglossia), may protrude outside the mouth, and often exhibit numerous vesicles on the dorsal surface, sometimes containing hemorrhagic fluid (Fig. 9.22). Management is usually multimodal, including sclerotherapy and medical therapy. Sirolimus has demonstrated efficacy in treating these vesicular eruptions (Fig. 9.24) and has shown some success in reducing tongue enlargement (Fig. 9.15). In cases of significant residual macroglossia, reduction glossoplasty is often necessary to allow the child to achieve oral closure.

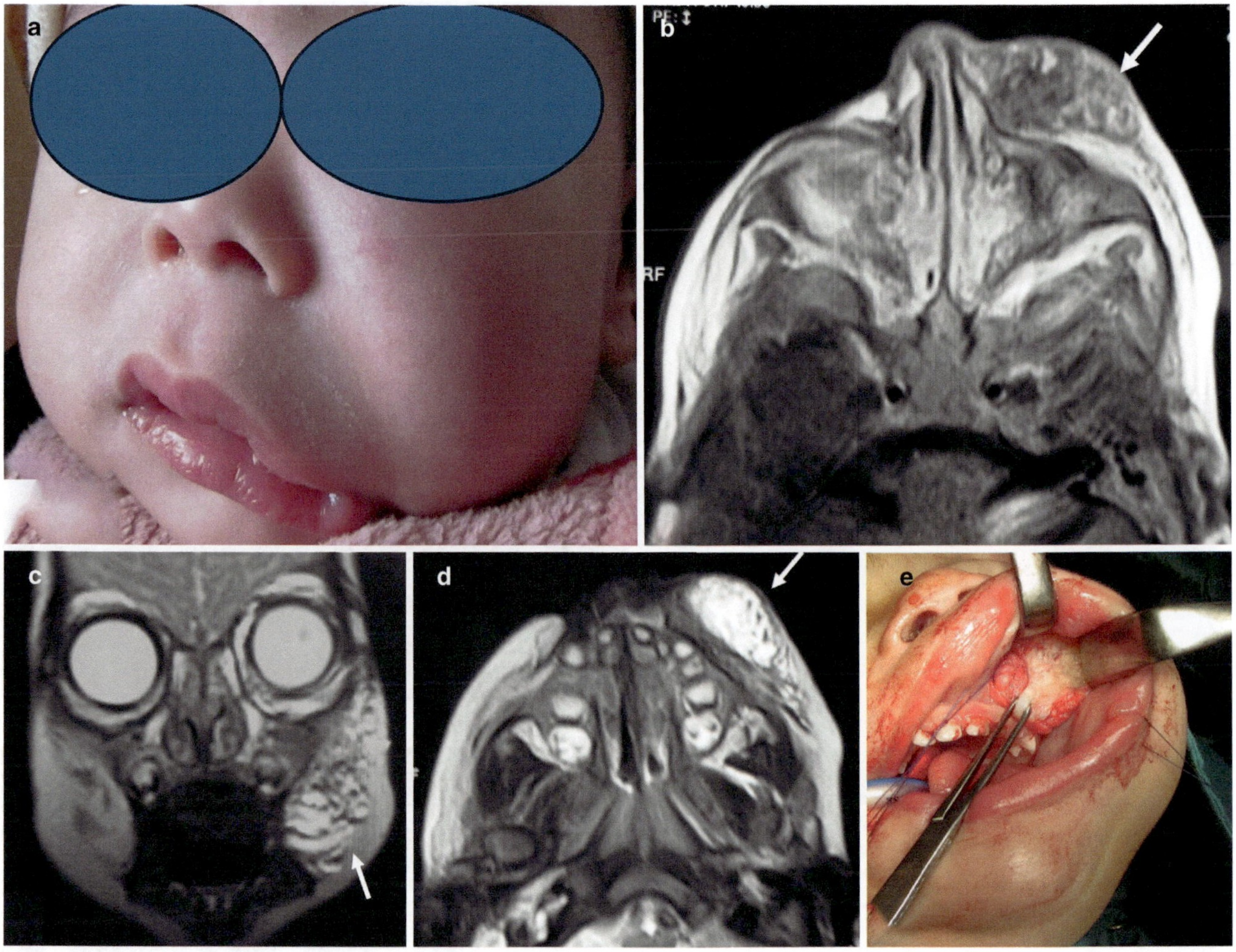

Fig. 9.18 Microcystic lymphatic malformation of the left cheek. (**a**) Clinical photograph. (**b–d**) MRI showing multiple tiny rounded and tubular lesions (arrow), hypointense on T1-WI (**b**) and hyperintense on T2-WI (**c**, **d**). (**e**) Surgical excision via a transoral approach

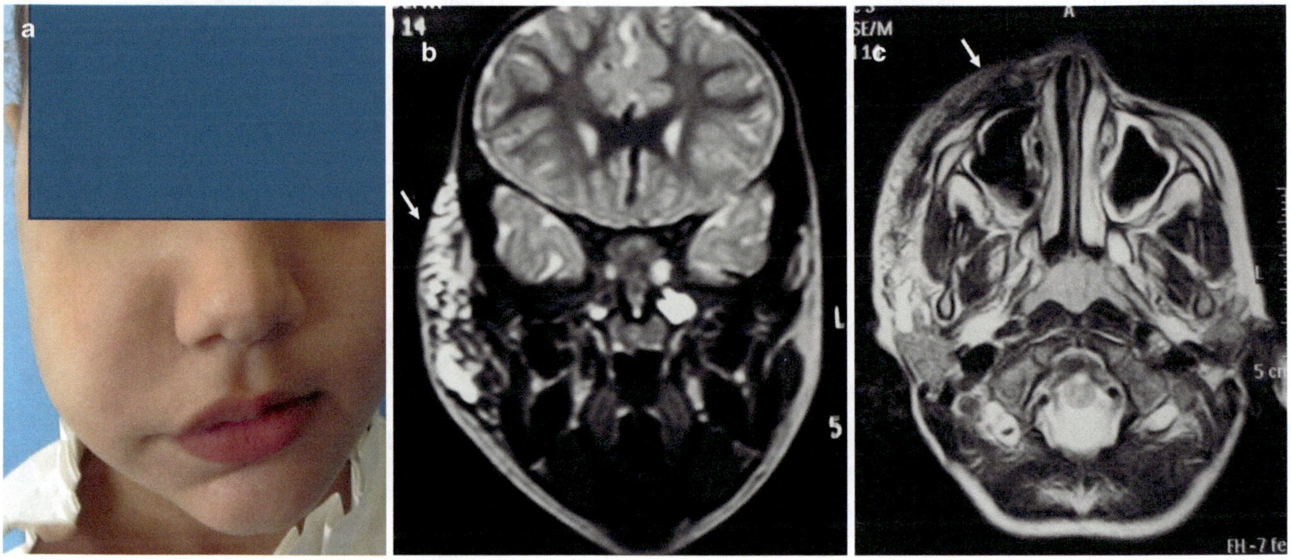

Fig. 9.19 Microcystic lymphatic malformation of the right face. (**a**) Clinical photograph. (**b**, **c**) Coronal and axial T2-WI MRI demonstrating extent of the subcutaneous lesion (arrow). Note the facial asymmetry caused by the prominent bone beneath the lesion compared with the unaffected left side (**c**)

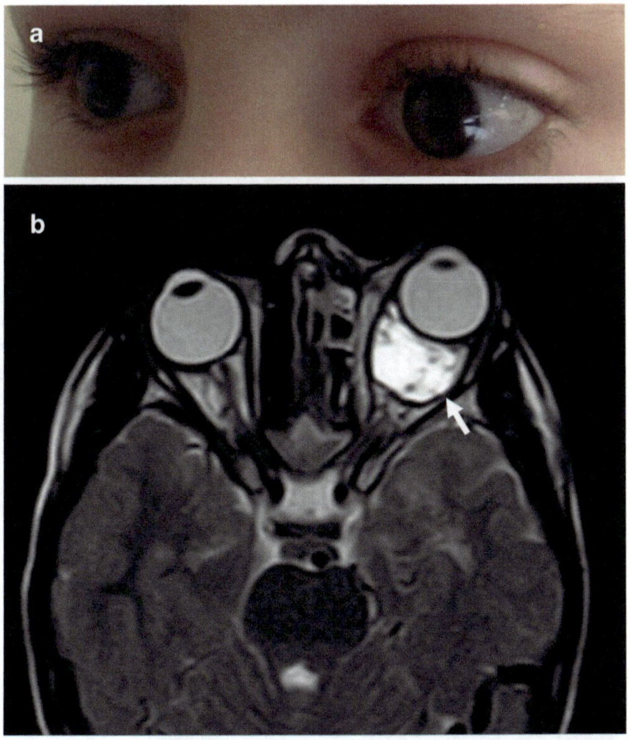

Fig. 9.20 Intra-orbital lymphatic malformation presenting with proptosis (**a**). (**b**) Axial T2-WI MRI demonstrating the intraconal cystic lesion (arrow)

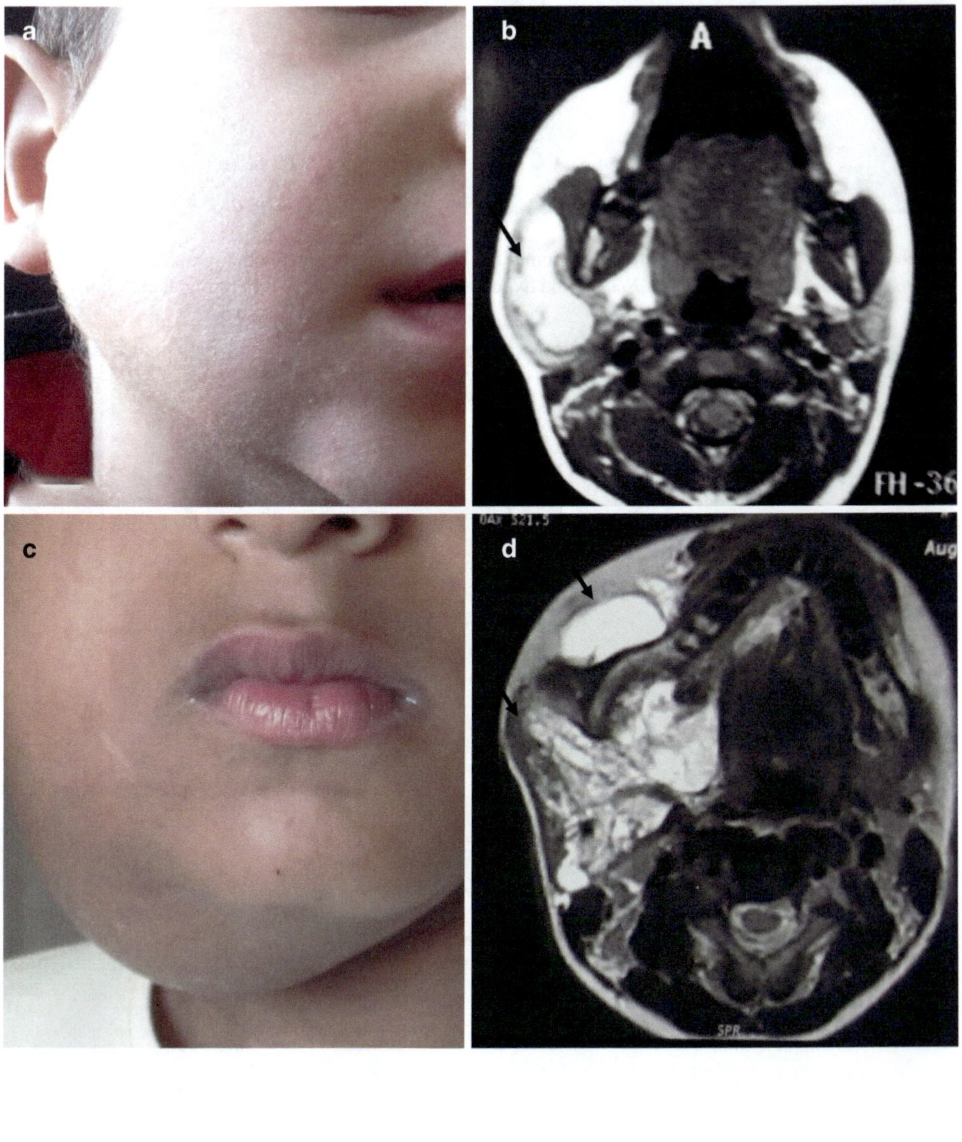

Fig. 9.21 Lymphatic malformation in the parotid gland of two cases. (**a**, **c**) Clinical photographs. (**b**) Axial T2-weighted MRI demonstrates a hyperintense cystic lesion (arrow) confined to the right parotid gland in the first case. (**d**) Axial T2-weighted MRI of the other case (**c**) shows a similar cystic lesion (arrows) with trans-spatial extension involving the masticator, parapharyngeal, carotid, and buccal spaces

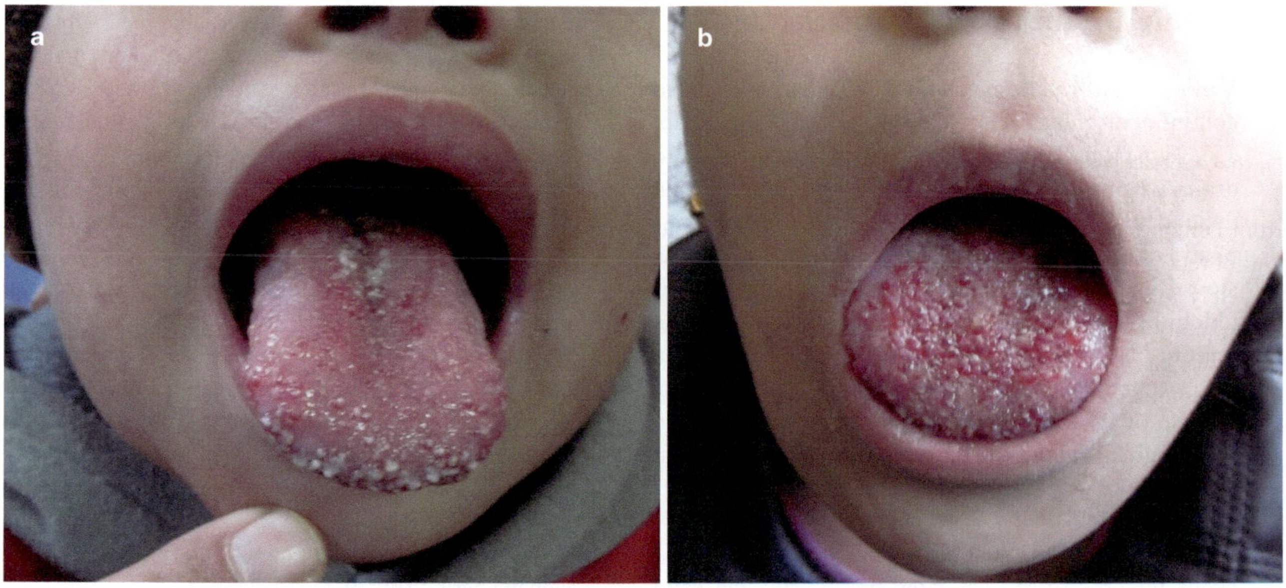

Fig. 9.22 Lymphatic malformations of the tongue with numerous vesicles in two different cases **a** and **b**

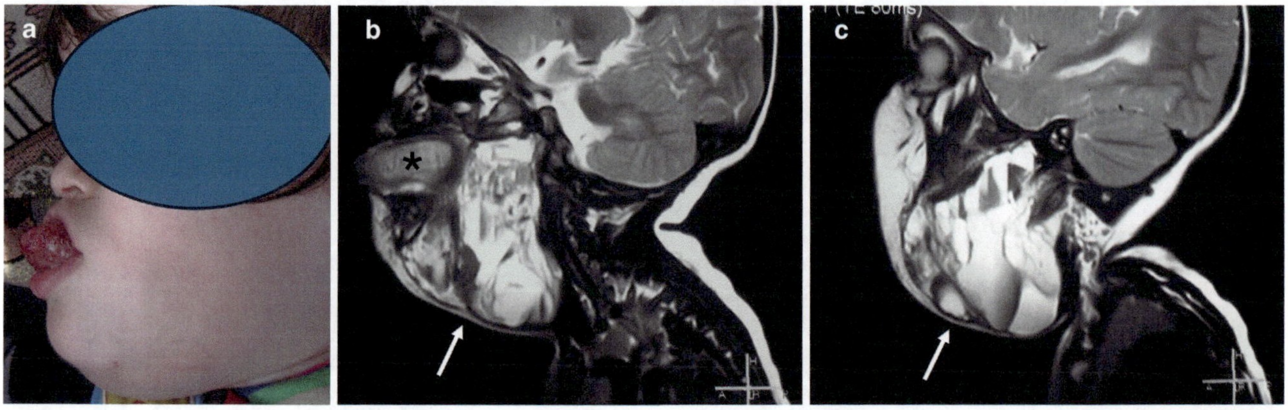

Fig. 9.23 Lymphatic malformation involving the neck and tongue. (**a**) Clinical photograph showing tongue protrusion (macroglossia). (**b**, **c**) Sagittal T2-weighted MRI demonstrates a multilocular cystic lesion in the submandibular space (arrow) with fluid–fluid levels. The tongue is enlarged (asterisk) and shows high signal intensity

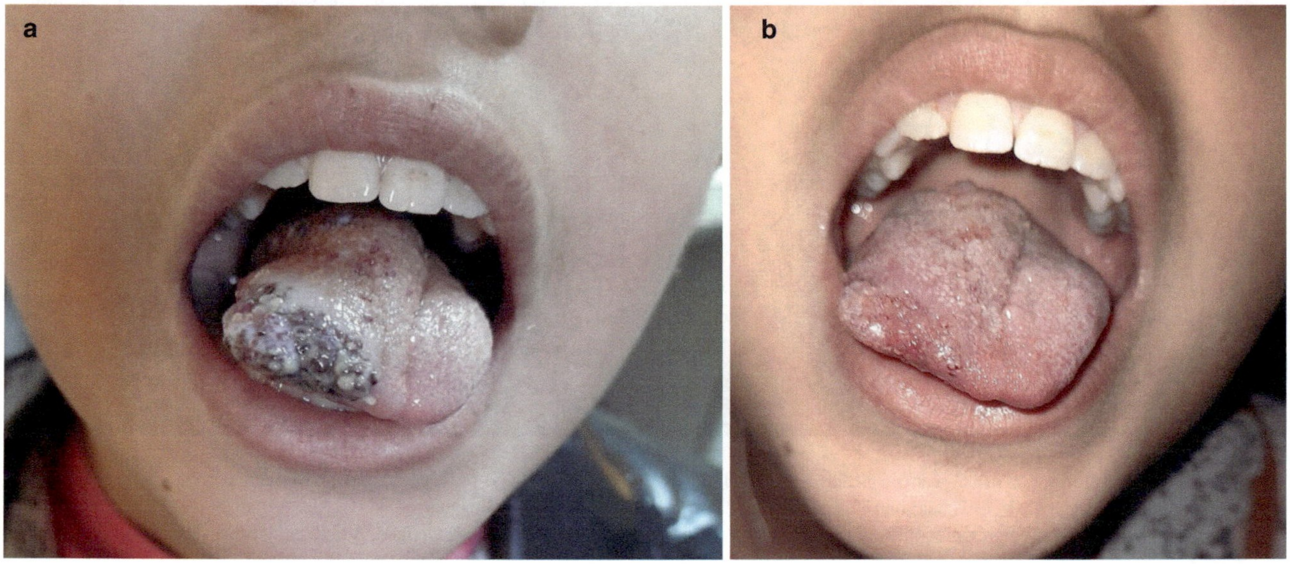

Fig. 9.24 Lymphatic malformations of the tongue showing the effect of sirolimus treatment on vesicular eruptions. (**a**) Before treatment. (**b**) After treatment, demonstrating improvement

Differential Diagnosis of Cervicofacial LMs

(a) Venous malformations (VMs): VMs are the most common vascular malformations [9, 15] (see Chap. 13). Typical lesions are bluish, compressible, tend to drain when elevated, and become engorged when dependent. [2, 9]. VMs can be mistaken for lymphatic malformations, as both are categorized as slow-flow vascular anomalies. The presence of phleboliths (calcified thrombi) is a distinguishing feature of venous malformations (Fig. 9.25) [2]. On MRI, venous malformations typically appear hyperintense on T2-weighted images and hypointense on T1-weighted images, with post-gadolinium contrast scans showing delayed, gradual, and patchy enhancement (Fig. 9.25).

(b) Cervical teratoma: Teratomas are complex, heterogeneous tumors—often containing both cystic and solid elements—that can develop in the neck region. Teratomas are usually present at birth and may be detected prenatally. Because of their size and location, they can lead to respiratory distress at birth, often requiring preparation for an EXIT procedure (Ex Utero Intrapartum Treatment) to manage potential airway obstruction [15]. Predominantly cystic teratomas are easily confused with cervical LMs. In contrast to cervical lymphatic malformations, teratomas tend to appear more aggressive, often presenting with irregular borders and prominent dilated veins over the skin (Figs. 9.26 and 9.27). MRI is typically the preferred imaging modality for assessing the extent of cervical teratomas and identifying any solid components or fat within the tumor, which can help to differentiate it from lymphatic malformations (Figs. 9.26 and 9.27). Cervical teratomas are typically treated through surgical excision during the neonatal period (Fig. 9.27).

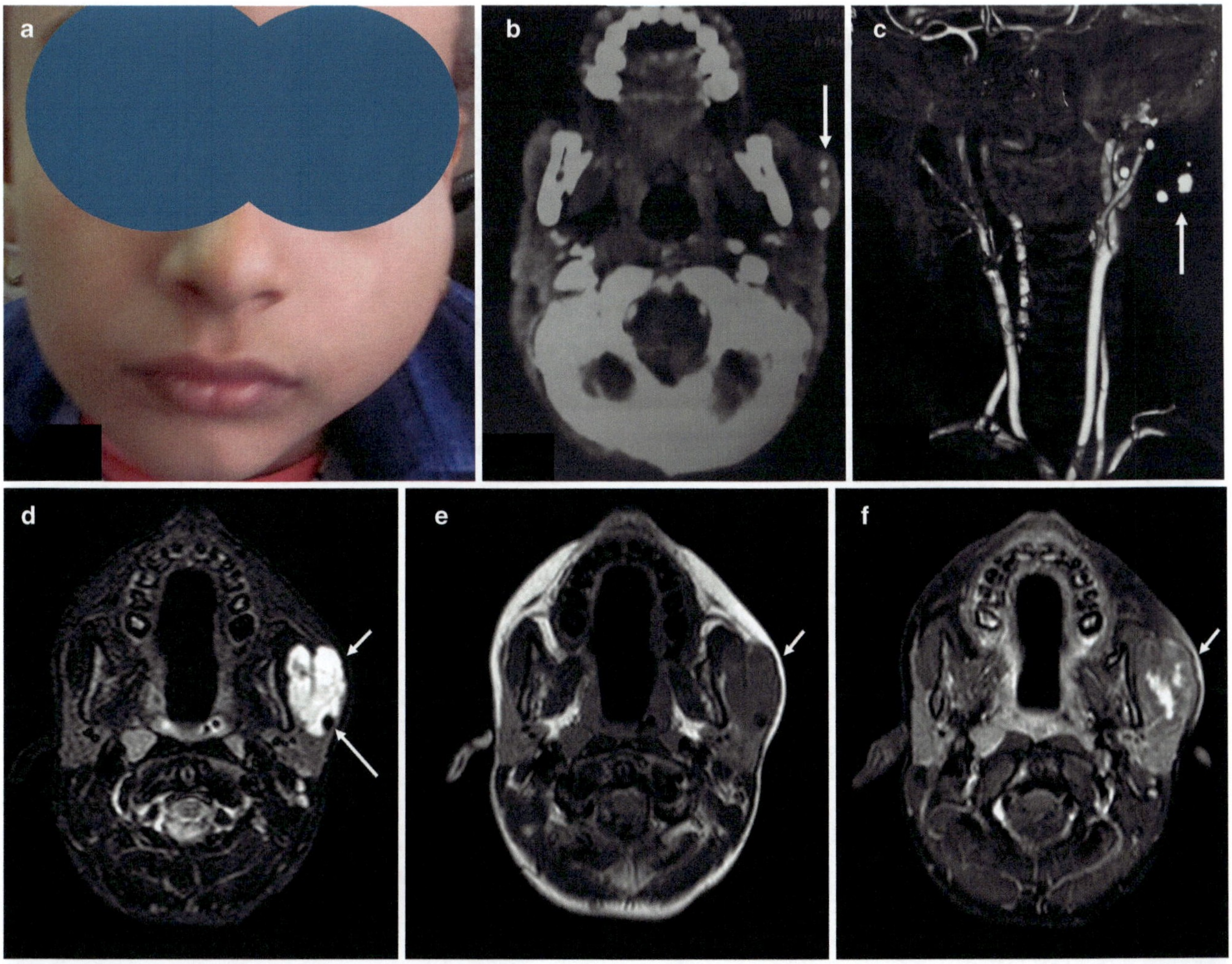

Fig. 9.25 Venous malformation in a 6-year-old girl involving the left masseter. (**a**) Clinical photograph. (**b, c**) Axial contrast-enhanced CT and 3D reconstruction demonstrate multiple phleboliths within the lesion (arrow). (**d–f**) MRI shows the lesion (short arrow) with hyperintense signal on STIR (**d**), intermediate signal on T1-weighted images (**e**), and delayed patchy post-contrast enhancement (**f**). A phlebolith is also seen (long arrow) in (**d**)

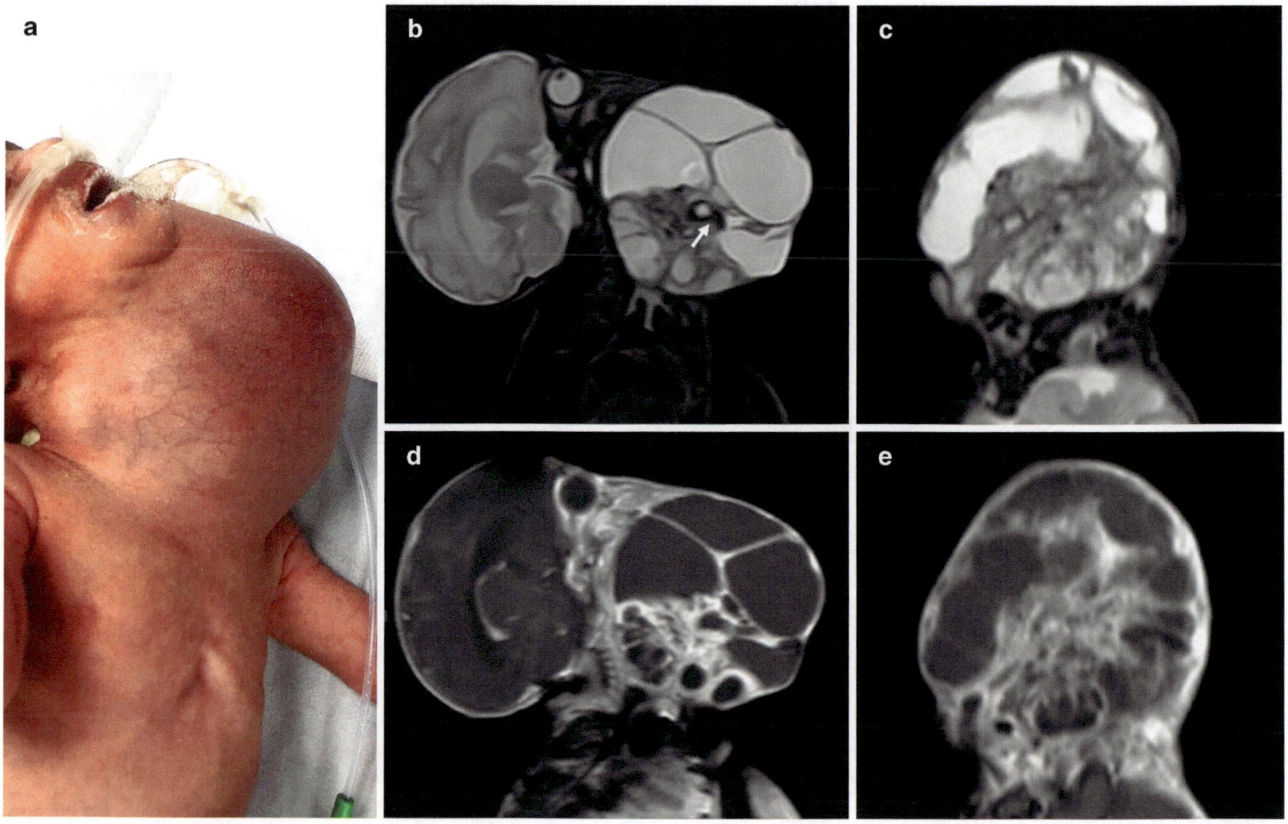

Fig. 9.26 Neonate with cervical teratoma (**a**) Clinical photograph, (**b**, **c**) Sagittal and axial STIR shows a complex lesion having mixed cystic and solid areas. Areas of low signal intensity (short arrow) represents hemorrhage/ calcification. (**d**, **e**) Sagittal and axial contrast-enhanced fat suppressed T1-WI show that the marginal enhancement of the cystic spaces is of variable thickness with solid enhancing areas

(c) Developmental cystic lesions in the neck: Several developmental cysts can present in the neck and may mimic cervical lymphatic malformations. These include branchial cleft cysts (Fig. 9.28), thyroglossal duct cysts (Fig. 9.29), and thymic cysts (Fig. 9.30)—typically unilocular, occurring in characteristic locations, and presenting in older children.

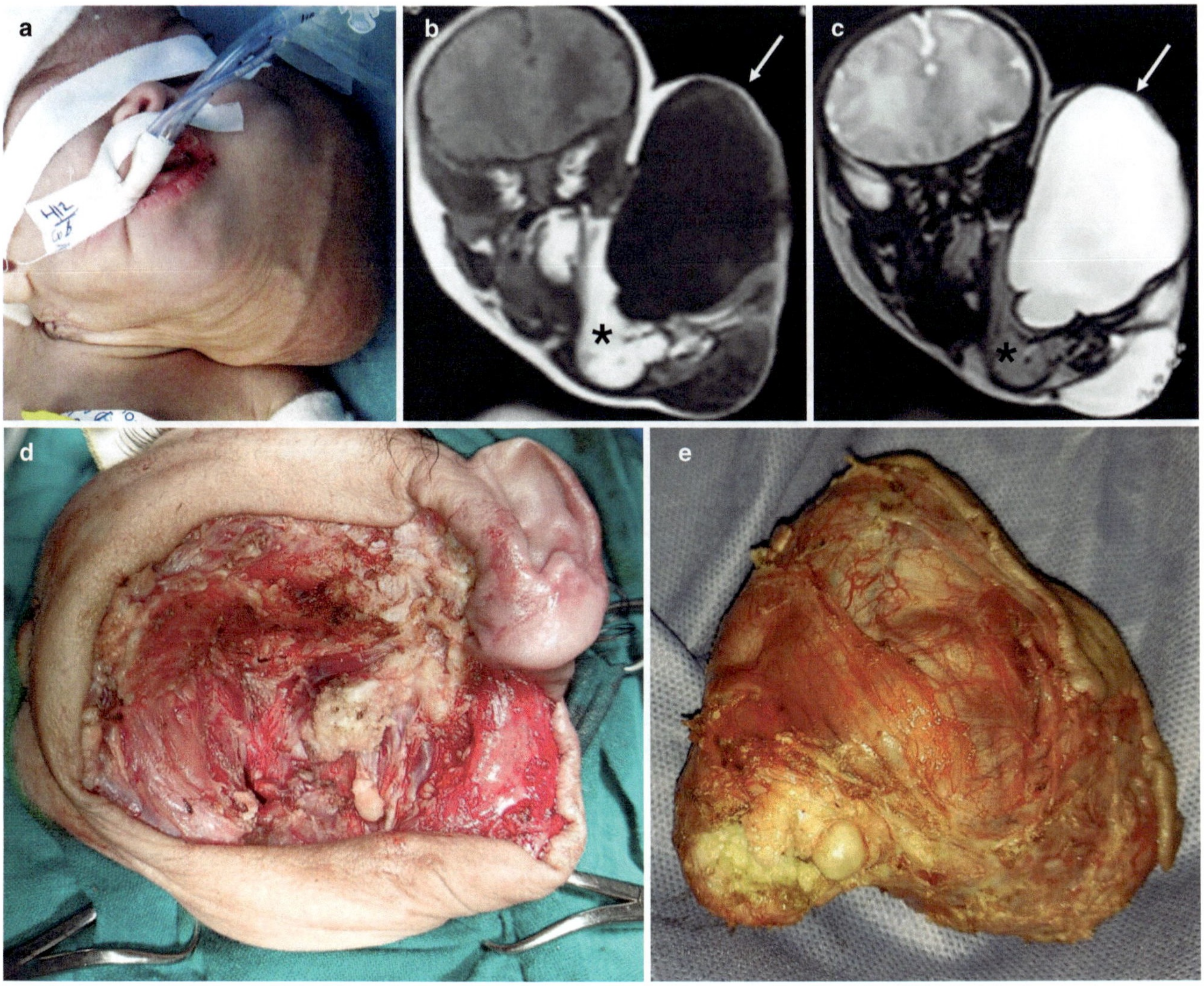

Fig. 9.27 Cervical mature cystic teratoma. (**a**) Clinical photograph. (**b**, **c**) Coronal T1-WI and T2-WI demonstrating a complex lesion with cystic areas appearing hypointense on T1-WI and hyperintense on T2-WI (arrow), along with a mixed fatty component (asterisk). (**d**, **e**) Intraoperative photographs

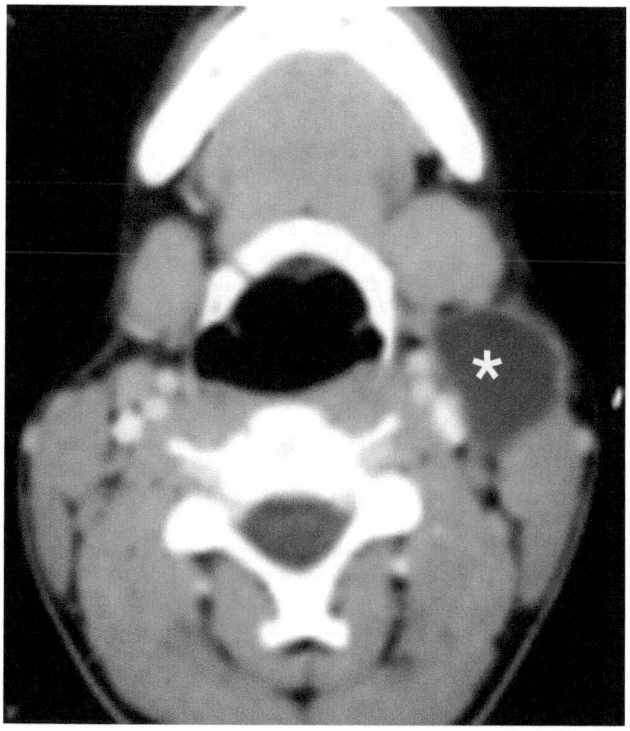

Fig. 9.28 Branchial cyst: Axial contrast-enhanced CT shows non-enhancing cystic lesion (asterisk)

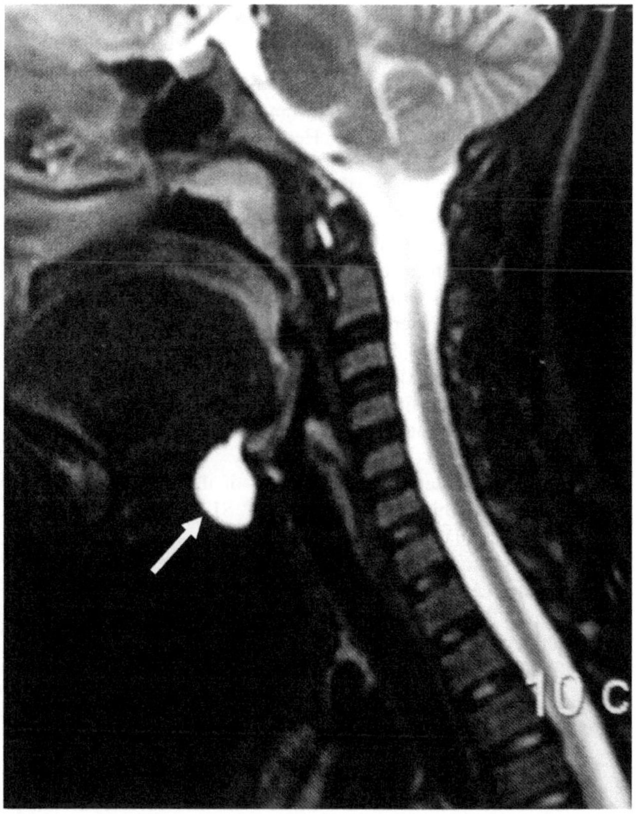

Fig. 9.29 Thyroglossal duct cyst. Sagittal STIR MRI demonstrating a hyperintense, thin-walled cystic lesion (arrow) located in the visceral space of the neck at the level of the hyoid bone, extending superiorly toward the foramen cecum

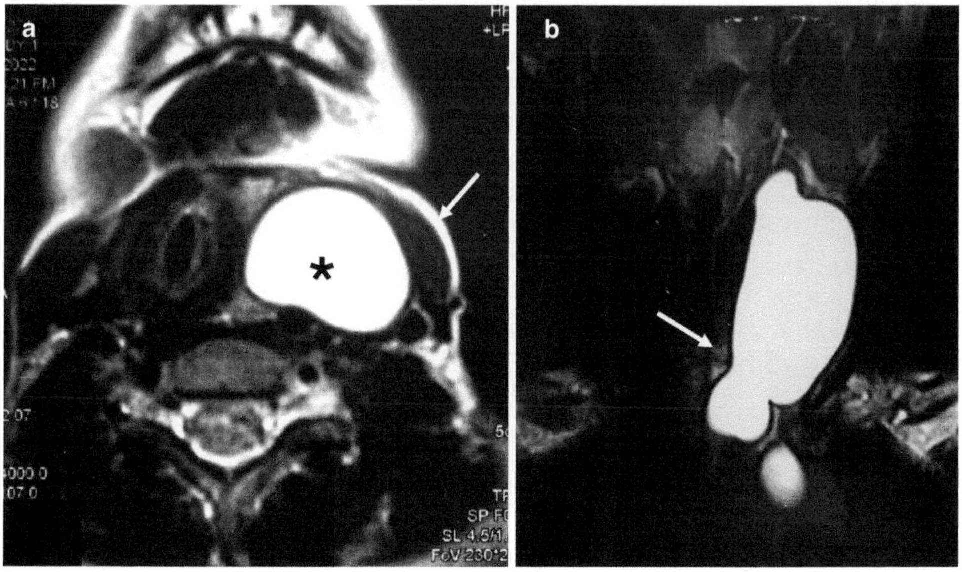

Fig. 9.30 Thymic cyst. (**a**) Axial T2-WI MRI showing a large unilocular cystic lesion (asterisk) displacing the airway, located deep to the sternomastoid muscle (arrow) and superficial to the carotid sheath. (**b**) Coronal STIR image demonstrating an ovoid cystic lesion extending into the superior mediastinum with a dumbbell-shaped morphology (arrow)

References

1. Fishman SJ, Young AE. Slow-flow vascular malformations. In: Mulliken JB, Burrows PE, Fishman SJ, editors. Mulliken & Young's vascular anomalies: Hemangiomas and malformations. Oxford University Press; 2013. p. 562–94.
2. Flors L, Hagspiel KD, Park AW, Norton PT, Leiva-Salinas C. Vascular malformations and tumors. Part 2: Low-flow lesions. Radiologia (English edition). 2019;61:124–33.
3. Parsi K. Management of lymphatic malformations. In: Kim YW, Lee BB, Yakes WF, Do YS, editors. Congenital vascular malformations. Berlin/Heidelberg: Springer-Verlag; 2017. p. 241–56.
4. Perkins JA, Monroe EJ, Bly RA, Shivaram G. Head and neck lymphatic malformation diagnosis and treatment. In: Perkins JA, Balakrishnan K, editors. Evidence-based management of head and neck vascular anomalies. Springer Nature Switzerland; 2018. p. 161–70.
5. Mulliken JB. Vascular malformations of the head and neck. In: Mulliken JB, Burrows PE, Fishman SJ, editors. Mulliken & Young's vascular anomalies: hemangiomas and malformations. Oxford University Press; 2013. p. 839–904.
6. AbouZeid AA, Mohammad SA, Aly NH, et al. Lymphatic malformations: a 9-year experience at the vascular anomaly clinic. Egypt Pediatric Association Gaz. 2023;71:88. https://doi.org/10.1186/s43054-023-00236-0.
7. Mamlouk MD, Nicholson AD, Cooke DL, Hess CP. Tips and tricks to optimize MRI protocols for cutaneous vascular anomalies. Clin Imaging. 2017;45:71–80.
8. Mohammad SA, AbouZeid AA, Fawzi AM, et al. Magnetic resonance imaging of head and neck vascular anomalies: pearls and pitfalls. Ann Pediatr Surg. 2017;13:116–24.
9. Gokani VJ, Sivakumar B, Kangesu L. Vascular anomalies. Surgery (Oxford). 2018;36:314–23.
10. Bhatnagar A, Upadhyaya VD, Kumar B, Neyaz Z, Kushwaha A. Aqueous intralesional bleomycin sclerotherapy in lymphatic malformation: our experience with children and adult. Natl J Maxillofac Surg. 2017;8(2):130–5. https://doi.org/10.4103/njms.NJMS_6_17. PMID: 29386816; PMCID: PMC5773987.
11. Chute C, Stein B, Sylvia MB, Spera E. Perioperative care of the vascular anomaly patient. Semin Pediatr Surg. 2014;23:233–7.
12. Johnson AB, Richter GT. Surgical considerations in vascular malformations. Tech Vasc Interv Radiol. 2019;22:100635. https://doi.org/10.1016/j.tvir.2019.100635.
13. Adams DM, Fishman SJ. Late sequelae and long-term outcomes of vascular anomalies. Semin Pediatr Surg. 2017;26:317–21.
14. Adams DM. Practical genetic and biologic therapeutic considerations in vascular anomalies. Tech Vasc Interve Rad. 2019;22:Article 100629.
15. Rollins N, et al. Head and neck. In: Esposito G, et al., editors. Pediatric surgical diseases. Berlin/Heidelberg: Springer; 2009. https://doi.org/10.1007/978-3-540-71516-0_1.

Lymphatic Malformations of the Extremities

10

Introduction

Lymphatic malformations (LMs) of the extremities often result in disfigurement, characterized by abnormal enlargement and a bulky contour of the affected limb. A combination of macro- and microcysts often coexist (Fig. 10.1) [1, 2]. Macrocystic lesions tend to be more prevalent in the proximal regions of the limbs, whereas microcystic malformations are commonly found in distal areas such as the hands and feet (Fig. 10.2) [1]. Due to the shared embryological origin of the lymphatic and venous systems, extensive lymphatic malformations in the extremities are often accompanied by localized venous anomalies in the same region (Fig. 10.1) [1]. LMs of the extremities are predominantly in the subcutaneous planes and are often accompanied by increased amounts of fibroadipose tissue (Figs. 10.3 and 10.4). Extensive LMs of the upper extremity frequently extend into the ipsilateral axilla and chest wall (Fig. 10.1). Likewise, LMs of the lower extremities—commonly found in the groin and gluteal regions—can also extend into the pelvis (Fig. 10.5). LMs may be associated with tissue overgrowth (both soft tissue and bone), particularly when combined with other types of vascular malformations such as capillary and/or venous malformations (see Chap. 20).

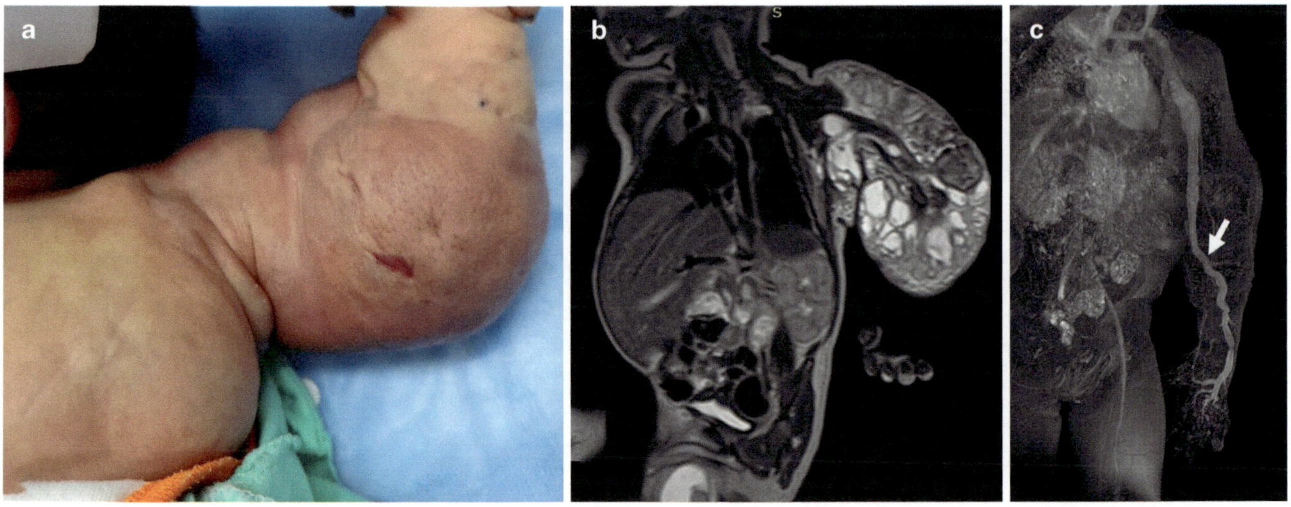

Fig. 10.1 Lymphatic malformation (combined macro- and micro-cysts) in the upper extremity of a neonate (**a**) Clinical photograph showing bulky appearance. (**b**) Coronal STIR MRI shows multilocular cystic lesion exhibiting hyperintense signal with trans-spatial spread in axilla, and lateral chest wall. (**c**) Venous phase of the dynamic contrast enhanced MR angiography shows anomalous ectatic draining vein (arrow)

A. A. AbouZeid et al., *Atlas of Pediatric Vascular Anomalies*, https://doi.org/10.1007/978-3-032-30866-5_10

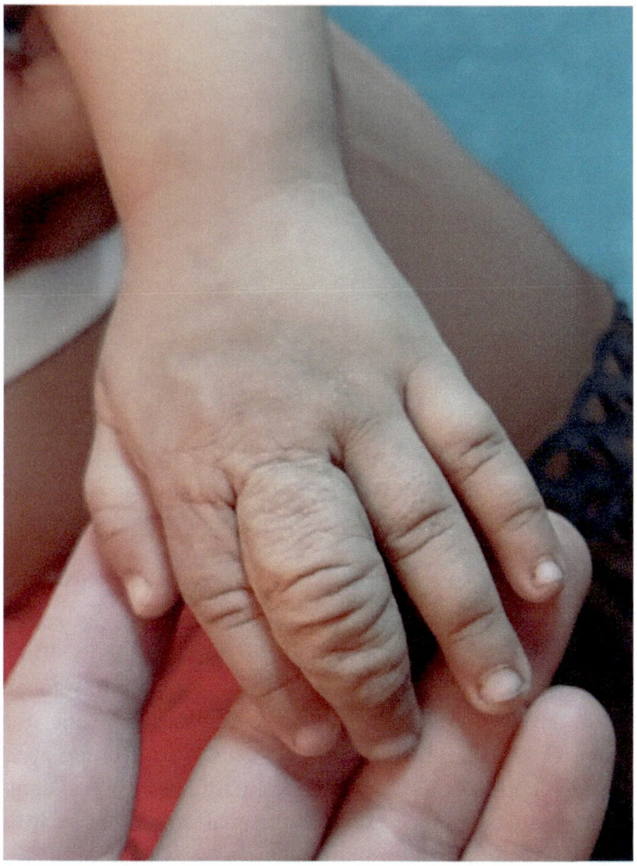

Fig. 10.2 Lymphatic malformation of middle finger

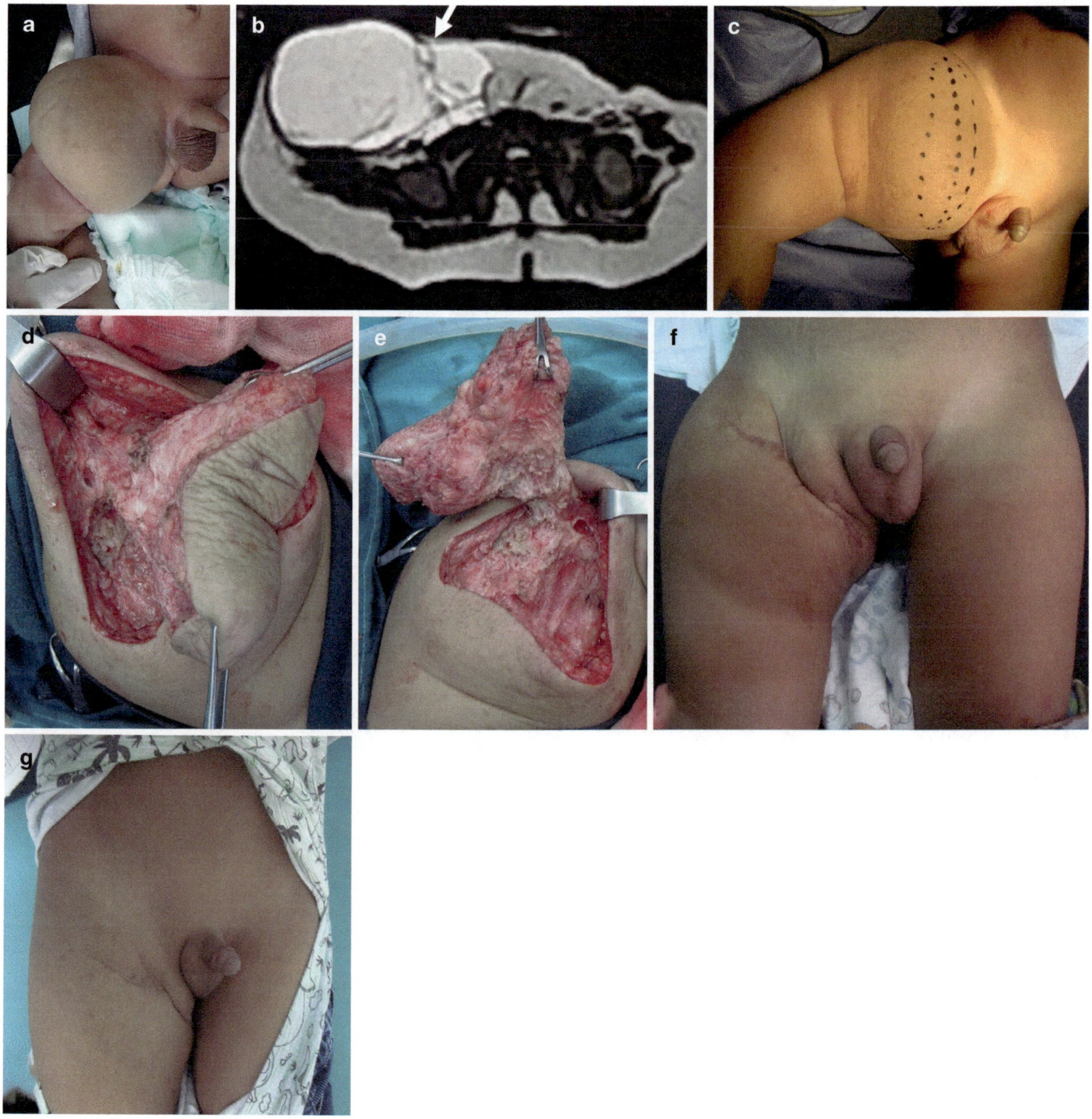

Fig. 10.3 Lymphatic malformation of the right groin. (**a**) Clinical photograph at presentation (1 month of age). (**b**) Axial T2-weighted MRI demonstrating a multilocular cystic lesion (arrow) with hyperintense signal. (**c**–**e**) Intraoperative views during surgical excision at 2 years of age. (**f**, **g**) Postoperative follow-up at 3 months and 7 years, respectively

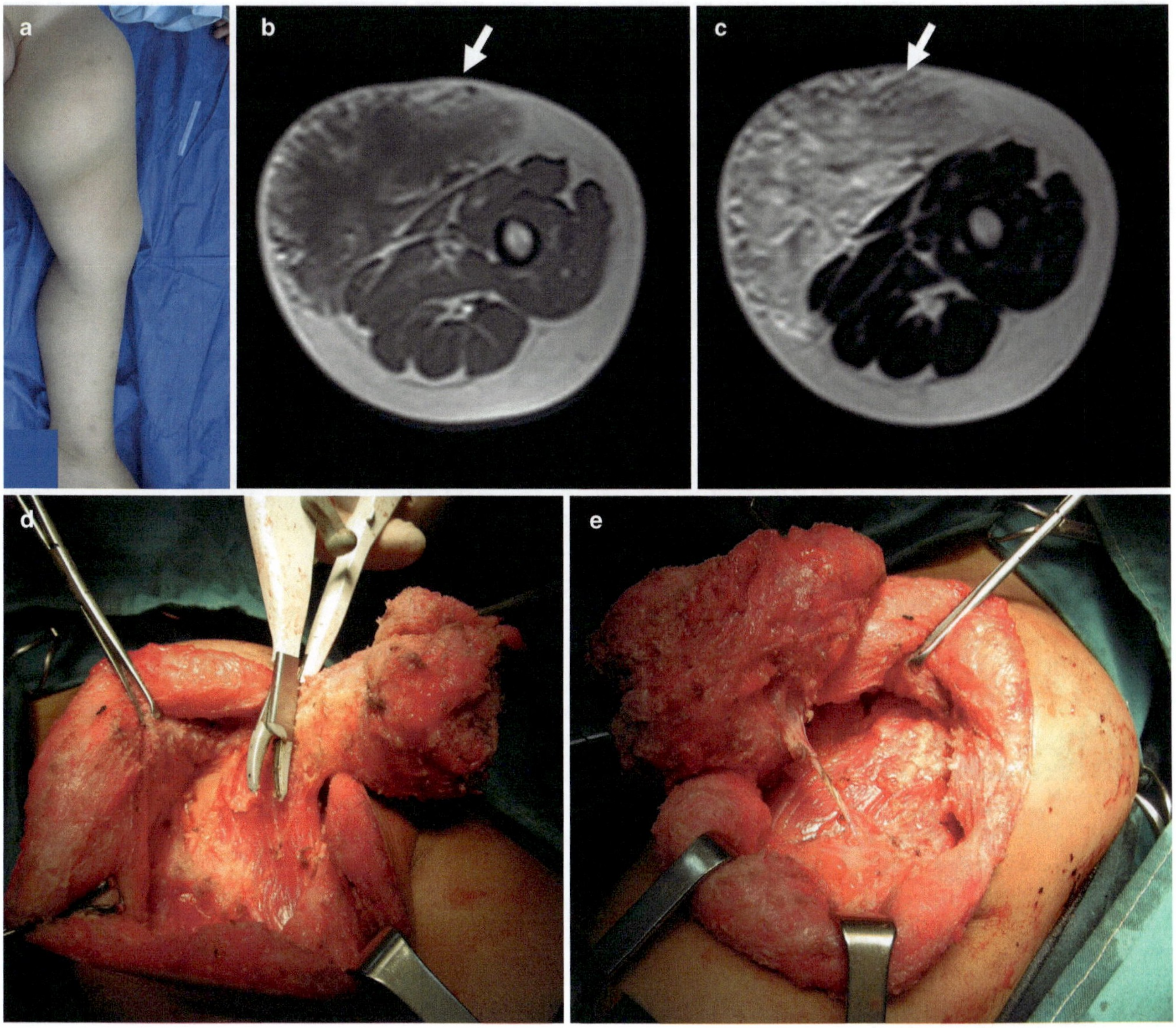

Fig. 10.4 Lymphatic malformation of the left upper thigh in a 3-year-old boy. (**a**) Clinical photograph. (**b**, **c**) MRI of the lesion (arrow) showing hypointense signal on T1-weighted imaging (**b**) and hyperintense signal on T2-weighted imaging (**c**). (**d**, **e**) Intraoperative views during surgical excision, demonstrating abnormal fibroadipose tissue

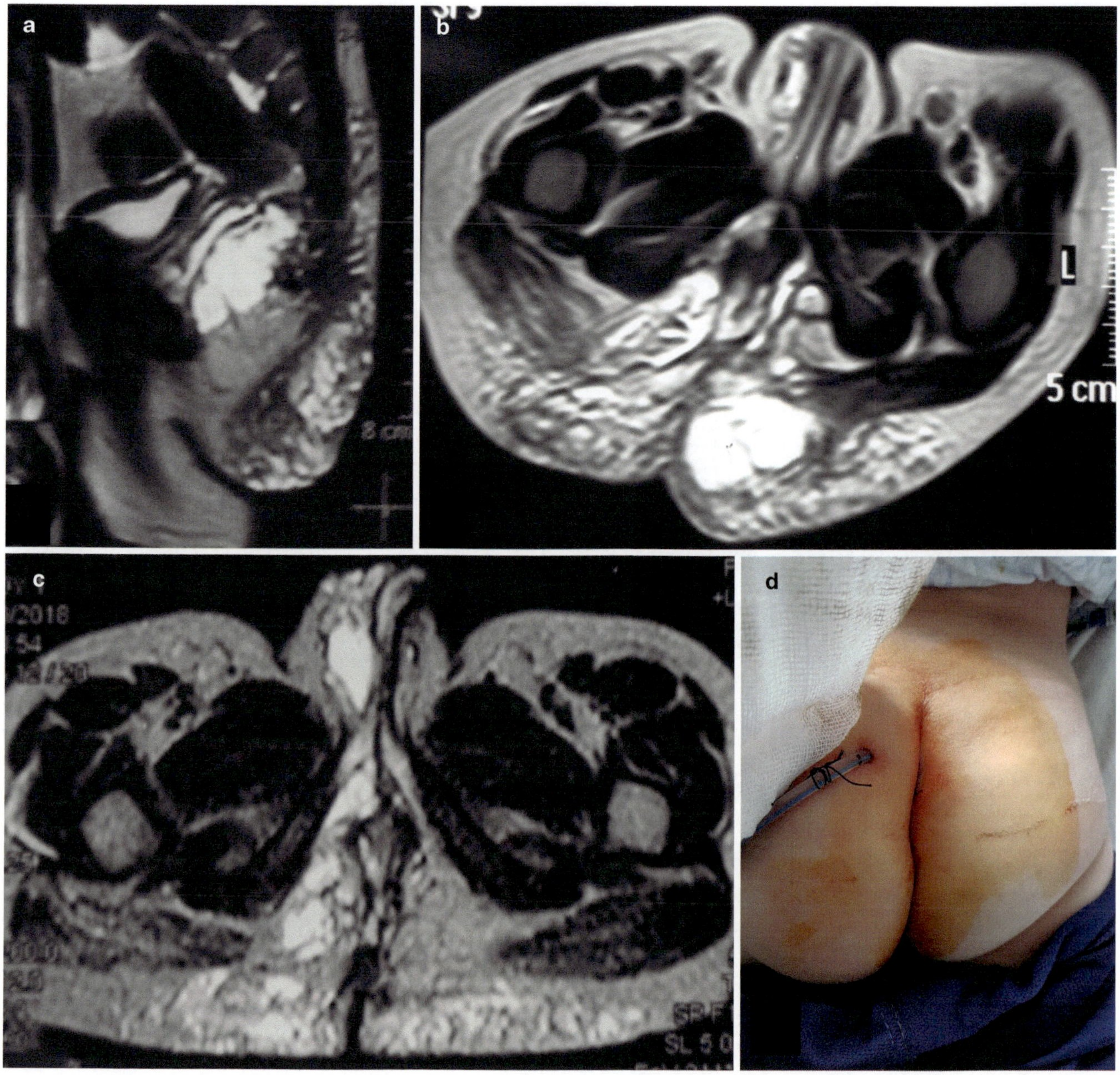

Fig. 10.5 Lymphatic malformation of the gluteal region in a 2-year-old boy. (**a**) Sagittal and (**b**, **c**) axial T2-weighted MRI showing a multilocular cystic lesion extending into the ischiorectal fossa, ischioanal space, and perineum. (**d**) Bilateral gluteal lesions excised via a midline natal cleft incision, resulting in a concealed scar

Diagnosis

Lymphatic malformations (LMs) of the extremities are usually present at birth. Unlike venous malformations, LMs do not reduce in size with elevation or direct compression. Pain is generally uncommon in LMs, unless complicated by secondary infection (Fig. 10.6). In such cases, prompt treatment with broad-spectrum antibiotics is essential to prevent potentially serious progression (Fig. 10.7) [1, 2]. The presence of epidermal vesicles filled with serous fluid is pathognomonic for underlying lymphatic lesions (Fig. 10.8). These cutaneous vesicles may also contain hemorrhagic fluid and can appear along surgical incision scars following the excision of lymphatic malformations (Fig. 10.7c).

MRI is the preferred imaging modality for confirming the diagnosis and delineating the extent of LMs—an essential step in treatment planning (Fig. 10.9). Characteristic findings include fluid-filled spaces that may be macrocystic, microcystic, or a combination of both (Fig. 10.1). Large cysts often display fluid-fluid levels and multiple septations (Fig. 10.10) [3].

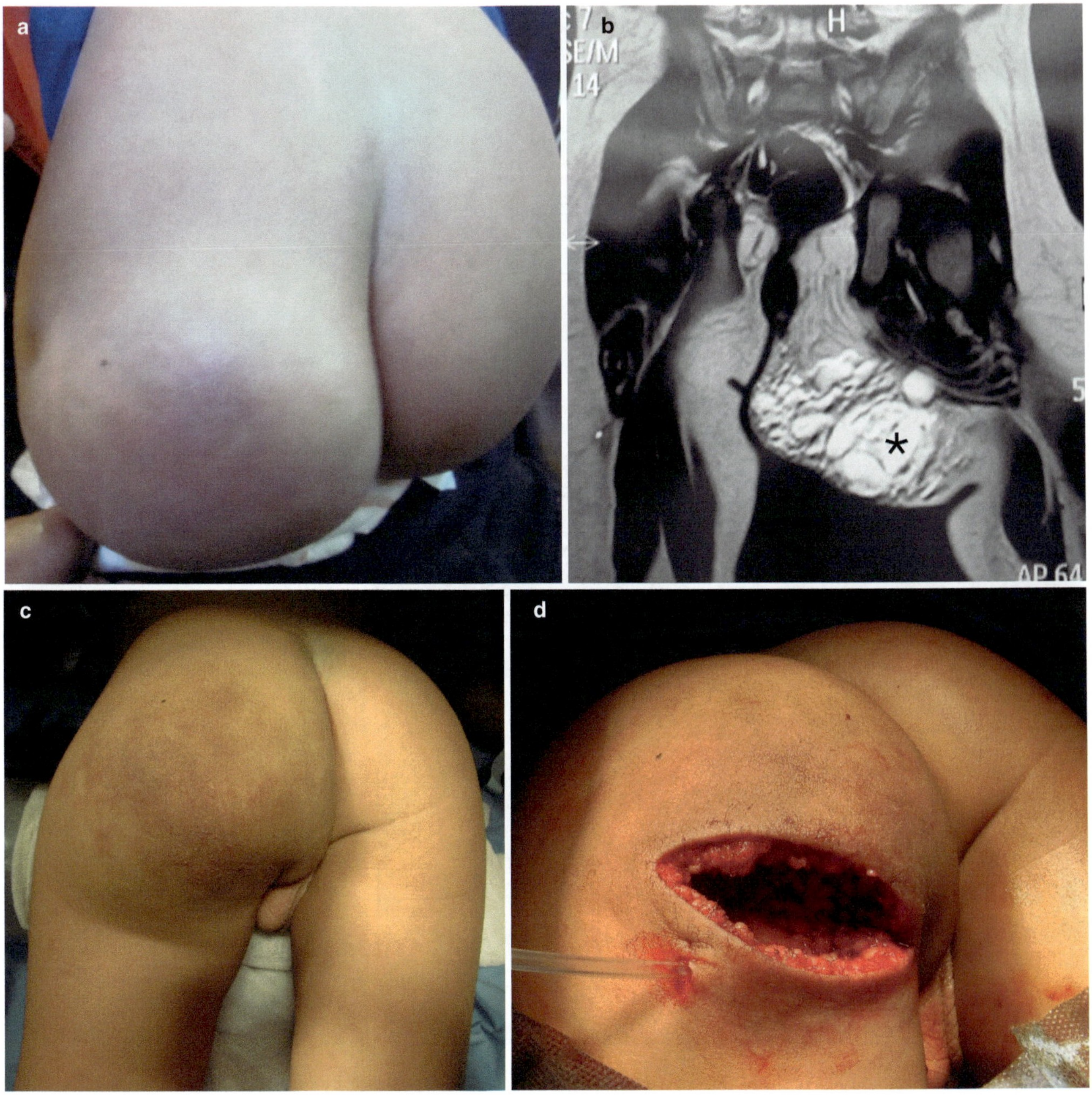

Fig. 10.6 Lymphatic malformation of the left gluteal region in a 20-month-old boy. (**a**) Clinical photograph at presentation, showing sudden increase in size of a congenital lesion due to superadded infection. (**b**) Coronal T2-weighted MRI demonstrating the subcutaneous lesion composed of multiple small cysts (asterisk). (**c**, **d**) Surgical excision performed after resolution of infection. (Reproduced from AbouZeid et al. [2])

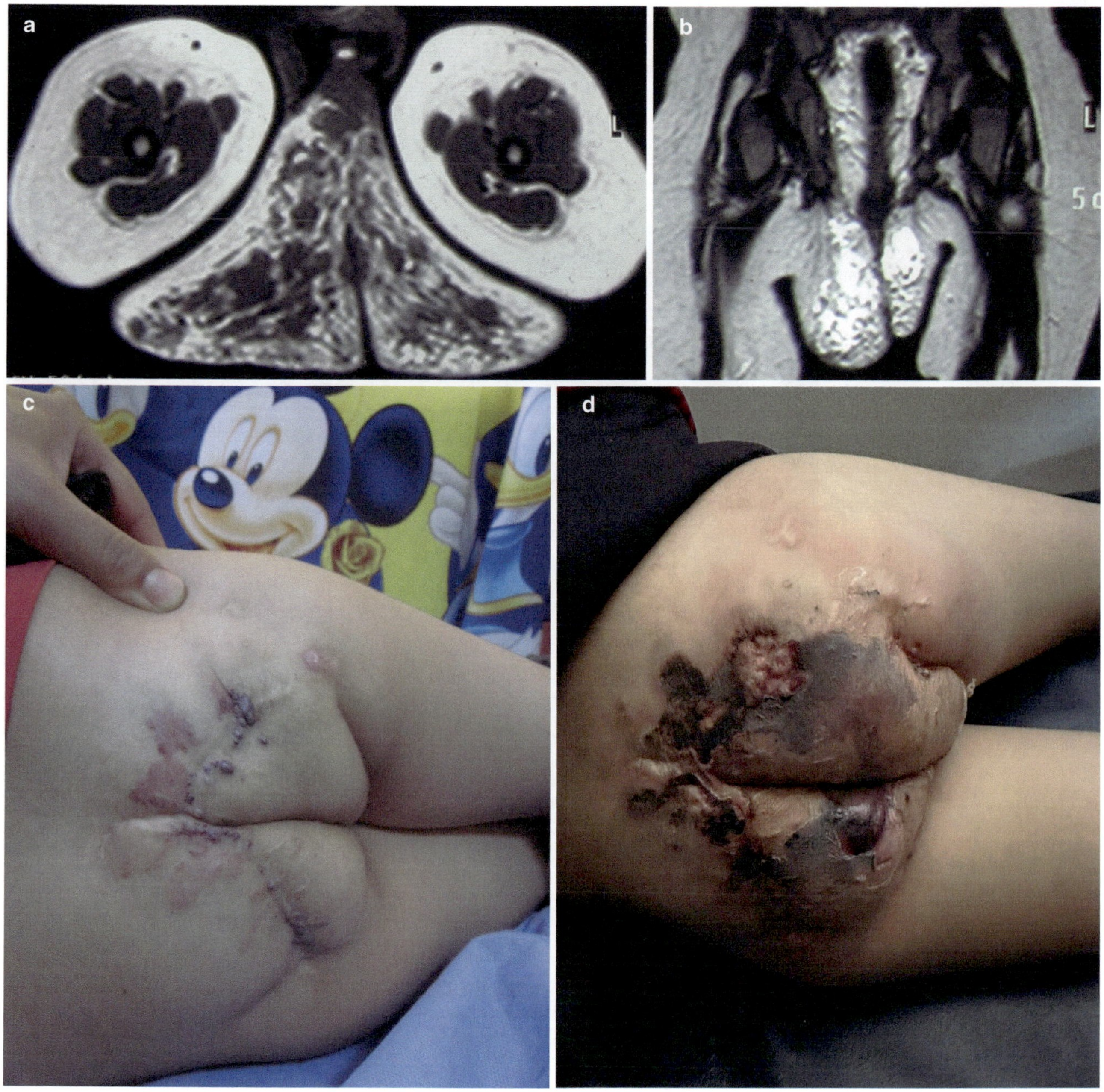

Fig. 10.7 Lymphatic malformation of the perineum and gluteal region (arrow). (**a**) Axial T1-weighted MRI showing hypointense signal. (**b**) Coronal T2-weighted MRI showing hyperintense signal. (**c**) Excision of gluteal lesions through a transverse incision resulted in a disfiguring scar, whereas a vertical incision within the natal cleft is preferable for cosmetic outcome. (**d**) Three years postoperatively, the patient developed necrotizing fasciitis at the scar site and within residual lymphatic malformation

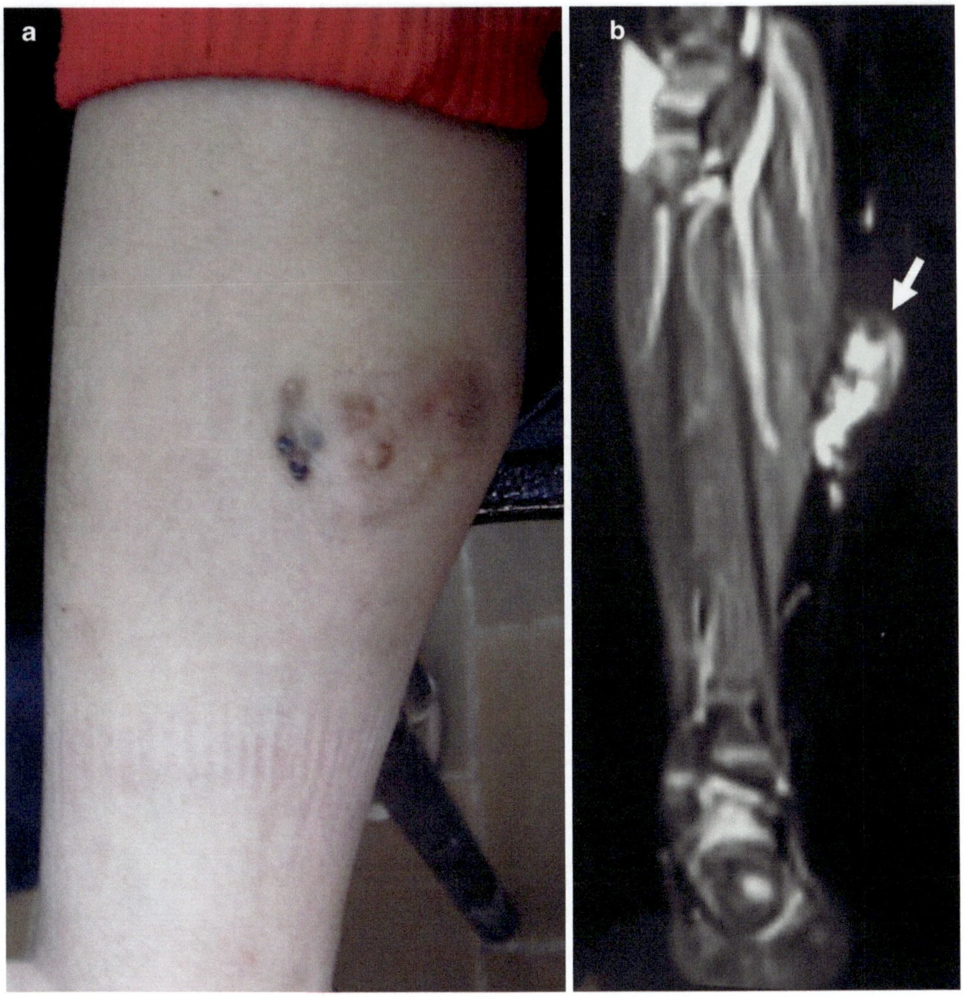

Fig. 10.8 Lymphatic malformation in the leg. (**a**) Clinical photograph shows characteristic epidermal vesicles. (**b**) Sagittal STIR MRI demonstrates a bright signal from the lymphatic malformation (arrow)

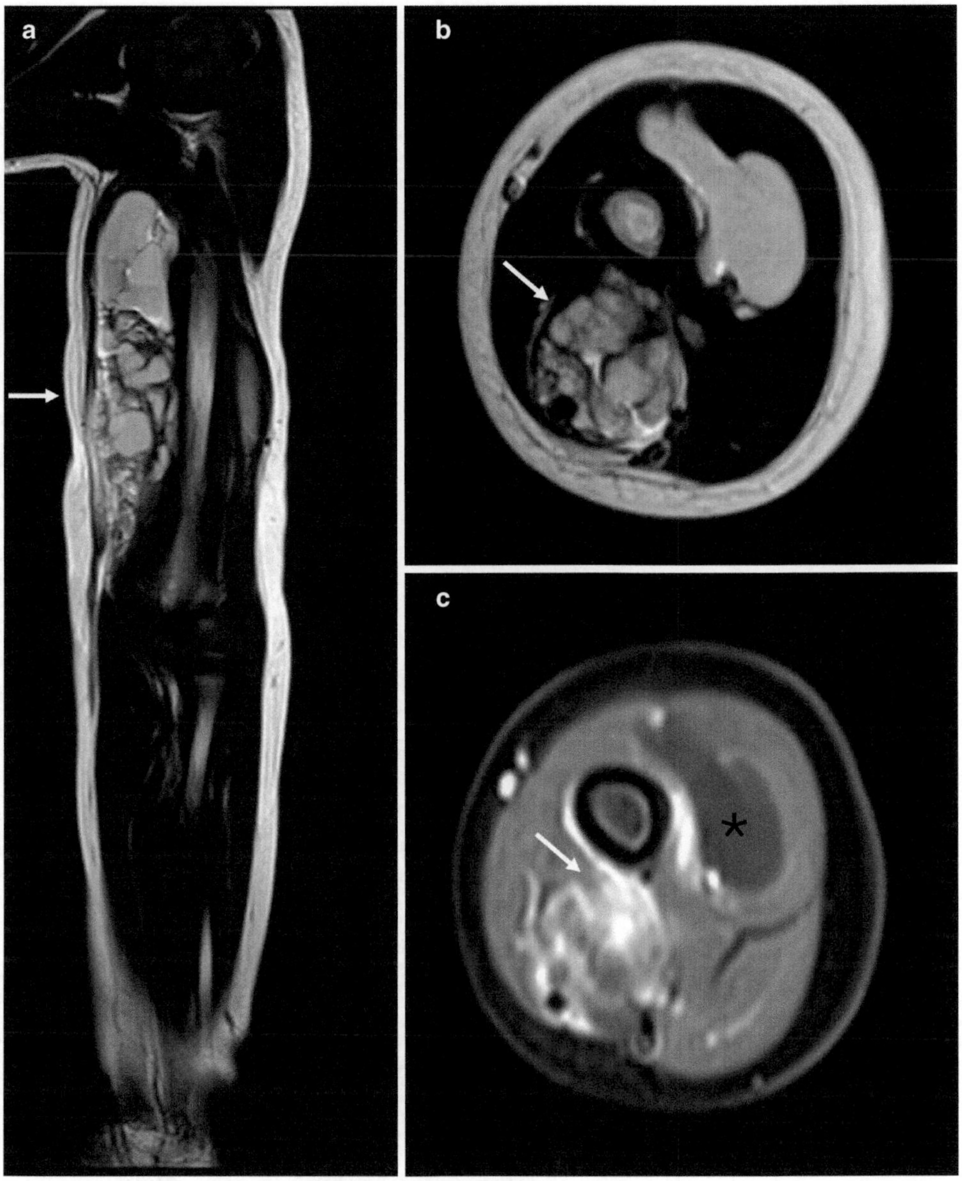

Fig. 10.9 Combined veno-lymphatic malformation of the upper extremity in a 2-year-old boy. (**a**, **b**) Coronal and axial T2-weighted MRI demonstrating an intramuscular multicystic hyperintense lesion. (**c**) Contrast-enhanced fat-suppressed T1-weighted MRI showing a non-enhancing lymphatic malformation (asterisk) with an associated patchy enhancing venous malformation (arrow)

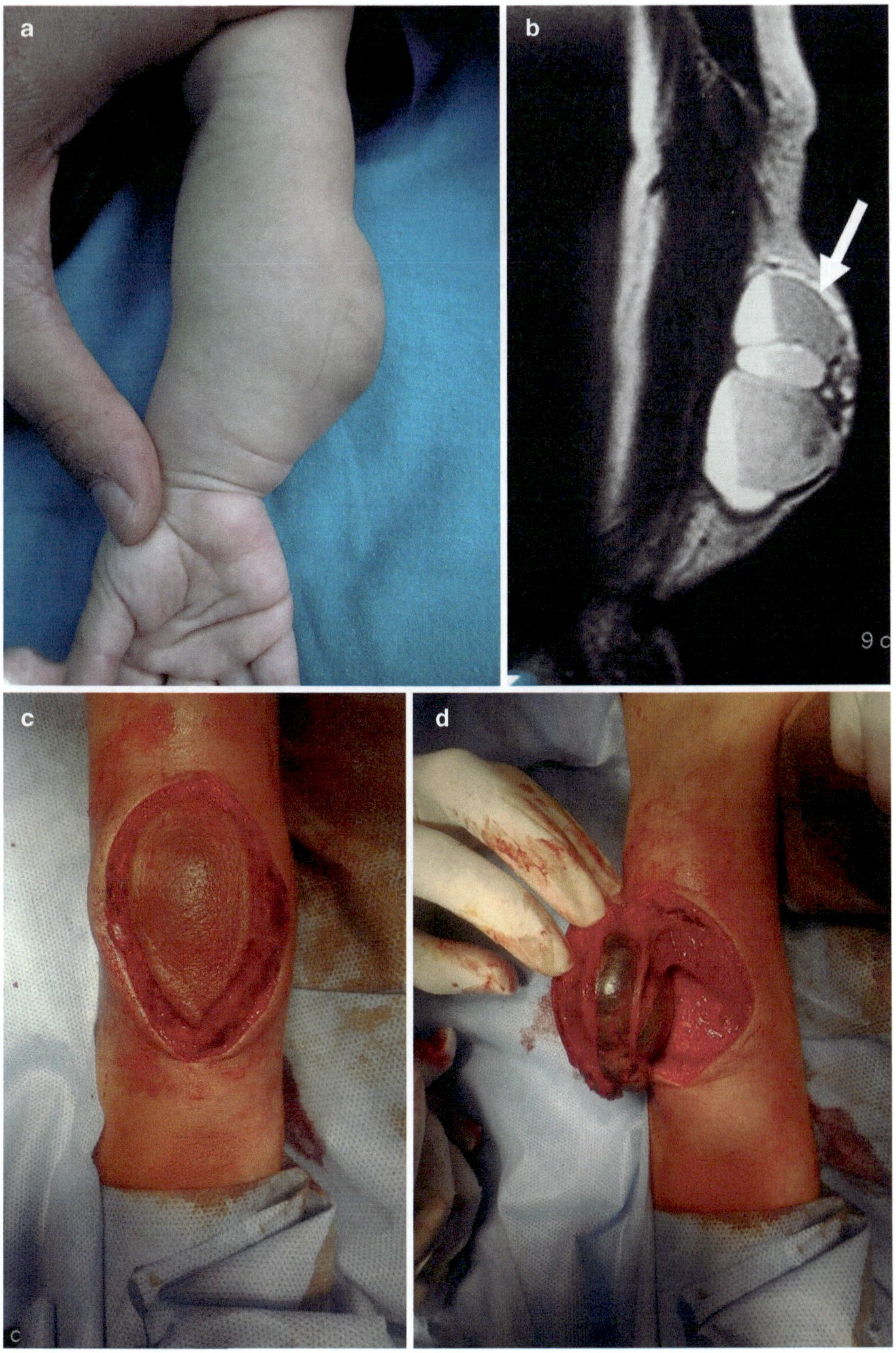

Fig. 10.10 Lymphatic malformation of the forearm. (**a**) Clinical photograph. (**b**) Sagittal T2-weighted MRI demonstrating a multilocular cystic lesion with fluid–fluid levels (arrow). (**c**, **d**) Intraoperative views during surgical excision

Due to their high-water content, these lesions appear hyperintense on T2-weighted sequences, with mild post-contrast enhancement primarily seen in the capsule and internal septa. Notably, significant internal enhancement suggests the presence of a coexisting venous malformation (Fig. 10.9).

Histological examination of excised specimens demonstrates abnormal dilated vascular channels with endothelial lining, protein-rich fluid, and collections of lymphocytes. Immunostaining with lymphatic markers (D2-40) is positive [1, 4].

Treatment

Lymphatic malformations are benign lesions, and management is guided by the presence and severity of symptoms. The primary clinical concerns typically relate to the size and bulky contour of the affected area. For macrocystic lesions, sclerotherapy may be considered as an initial treatment option. However, since most extremity LMs are located within subcutaneous planes, surgical resection may be generally preferred (Fig. 10.11)—especially for microcystic lesions, which tend to respond poorly to sclerotherapy (Fig. 10.4). Preoperative planning is mandatory with careful placement of the incisions to avoid visible scars (Figs. 10.5 and 10.6). Drains are essential to avoid expected postoperative fluid collections. Regular follow-up is essential for early detection and management of delayed complications such as keloids and contractures; otherwise, we risk merely trading tissue bulk for unsightly scarring (Fig. 10.12).

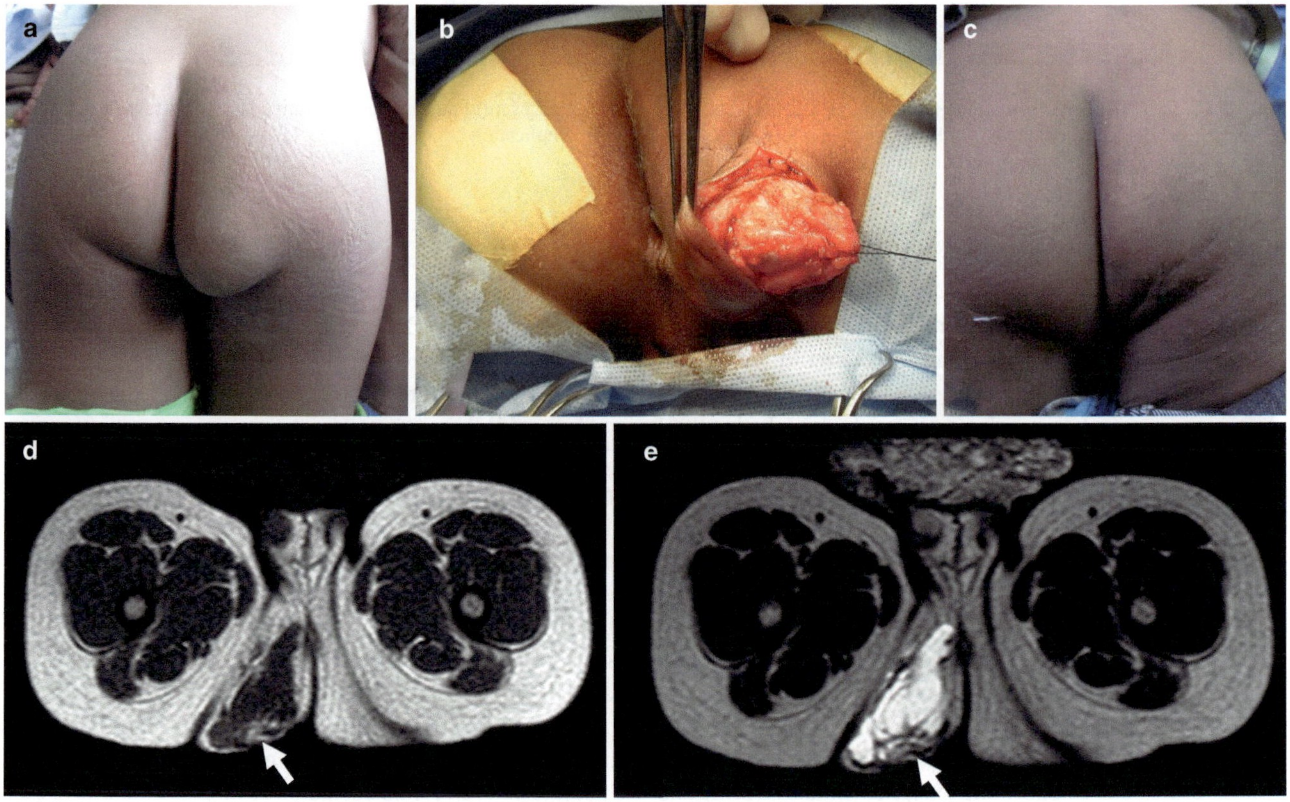

Fig. 10.11 Lymphatic malformation of the right gluteal region in a 3-year-old boy. (**a**) Clinical photograph demonstrating a gluteal bulge. (**b**) Intraoperative view during surgical excision. (**c**) Postoperative appearance with healed scar at 2-month follow-up. (**d, e**) MRI depicting a multilocular cystic lesion (arrow), showing hypointense signal on T1-weighted imaging (d) and hyperintense signal on T2-weighted imaging (**e**)

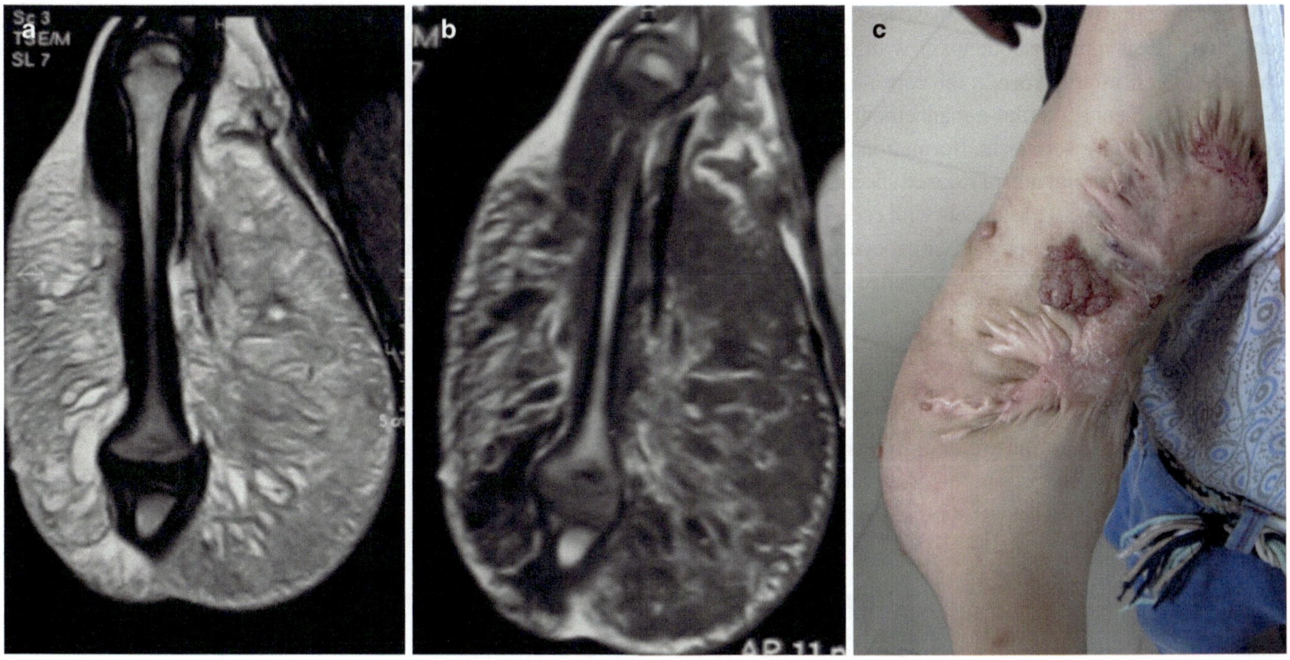

Fig. 10.12 Lymphatic malformation of the arm in a 4-year-old boy. (**a**) T2-weighted MRI showing a multilocular hyperintense lesion. (**b**) Post-contrast T1-weighted MRI demonstrating marginal enhancement of the cystic spaces. (**c**) Four-year postoperative follow-up revealing a keloid scar complication

Lymphedema

Lymphedema is rare disorder with estimated prevalence of 1.2 per 100,000 patients less than 20 years old with equal male and female distribution. Lymphedema refers to the abnormal accumulation of protein-rich lymphatic fluid within the interstitial tissues as a result of impaired lymphatic drainage. Lymphedema is considered a special form of lymphatic malformation that commonly affects the extremities. The lower extremities are most frequently involved in 91.7% of patients, being unilateral in 50% (Fig. 10.13). Genitals and upper extremities are less frequently involved (Fig. 10.14). It may be classified as primary or secondary. Traditionally, primary lymphedema has been divided into congenital, praecox, and tarda; however, this system has proven confusing. A developmental classification is now preferred, categorizing onset as infancy (birth-one year), childhood (1–9 years), adolescence (10–21 years), or adulthood (more than 21 years). This standardized terminology improves clarity in clinical communication and facilitates progress in lymphedema research [5]. Chronic lymphedema leads to inflammatory alterations to the skin and interstitium, with 19% of children developing cellulitis and 15% developing hyperkeratosis or lymphorrhea. Angiosarcoma may develop in long-standing lymphedema.

Several mutations have been implicated in the development of primary lymphedema. Mutation in vascular endothelial growth factor receptor-3 (VEGFR3) is found in infants with Milroy disease. Forkhead transcription factor C2 (FOXC2) is related to lymphedema distichiasis; SRY-related HMG-box 18 (SOX18) is related to hypotrichosis-telangiectasia-lymphedema, while collagen- and calcium-binding EGF-like domains 1(CCBE1) is related to Hennekam syndrome [5].

Imaging of lymphedema: Imaging plays a key role not only in assessing the extent of lymphedema but also in identifying lymphatic vessels. Ultrasound can demonstrate skin and subcutaneous thickening as well as increased echogenicity of the subcutaneous tissue. Differentiation of lymphatic vessels from veins on ultrasound can be achieved using the D-CUPS criteria (Doppler, Crossing, Uncollapsible, Parallel, Superficial fascia): 1.Lymphatic vessels show no color flow on Doppler, unlike veins. 2. Crossing: lymphatic channels cross veins, while veins join nearby veins. 3. Uncollapsible: In lymphedematous limbs, lymphatic vessels remain uncollapsible. 4. Parallel: lymphatic vessels may run in parallel without merging (seen in ~20%). 5. Superficial fascia: lymphatic channels lie parallel and just beneath it [6]. Lymphoscintigraphy and indocyanine green lymphography are imaging modalities used to visualize lymphatic vessels and detect dermal backflow [7].

Owing to its excellent soft tissue contrast, MRI is able to delineate the extent of lymphedema. The STIR sequence is useful for identifying soft tissue edema, typically showing a honeycomb pattern, dermal thickening, and epifascial fluid (Fig. 10.15). It can also demonstrate fluid accumulation, adi-

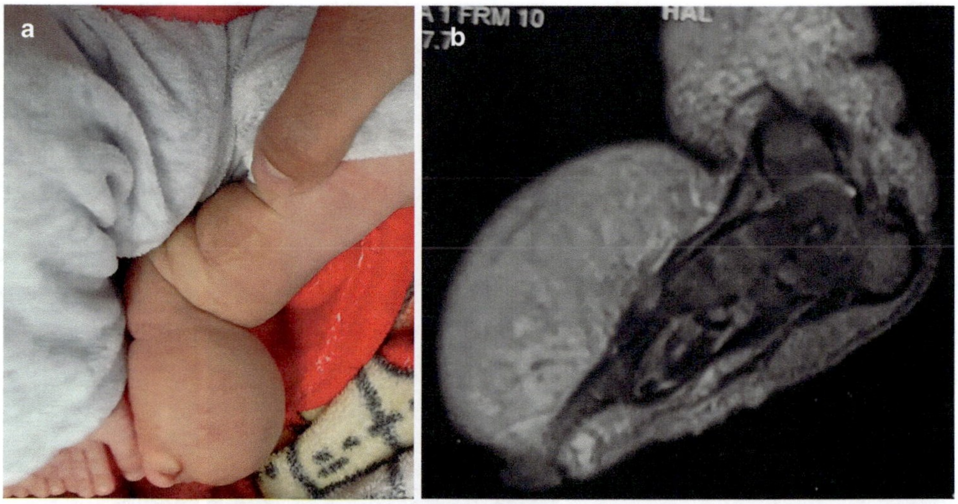

Fig. 10.13 Unilateral lymphedema of the left foot and leg. (**a**) Clinical photograph demonstrates swelling, most pronounced at the dorsum of the foot. (**b**) Sagittal T2-weighted image shows epifascial edema with sparing of the underlying muscles

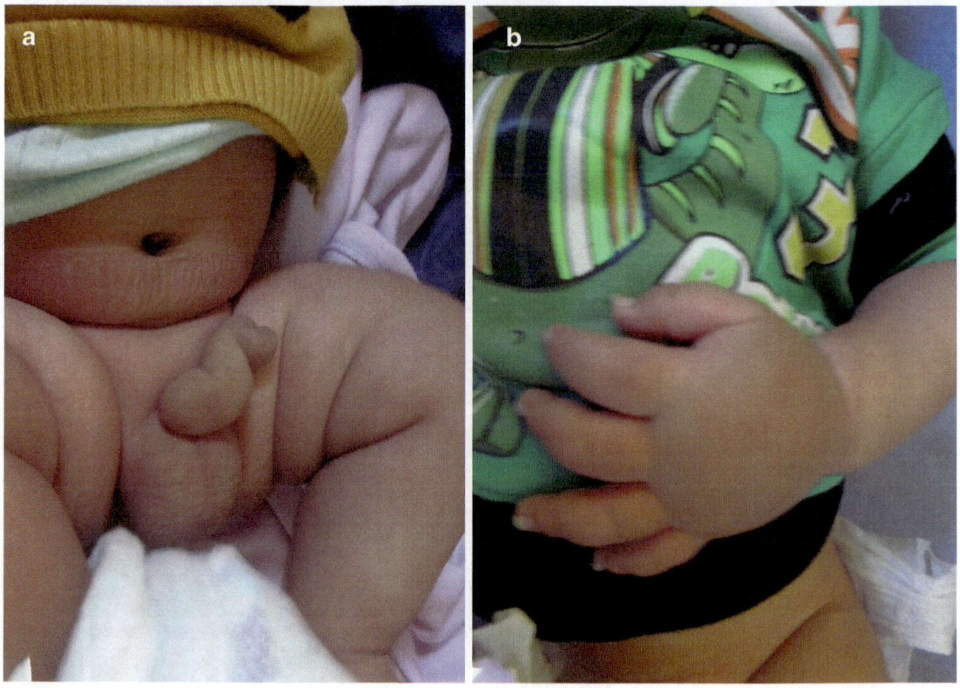

Fig. 10.14 Different sites of lymphedema: (**a**) genitals; (**b**) upper extremity

pose tissue hypertrophy, skin thickening, and dilated lymphatic vessels (Fig. 10.16). In addition, non-contrast MR lymphangiography can be performed using heavily T2-weighted sequences. For more detailed evaluation, contrast-enhanced MR lymphangiography is achieved via intradermal, subcutaneous, or intranodal injection of a gadolinium-based agent, enabling visualization of abnormal lymphatic vessels and dermal backflow [8].

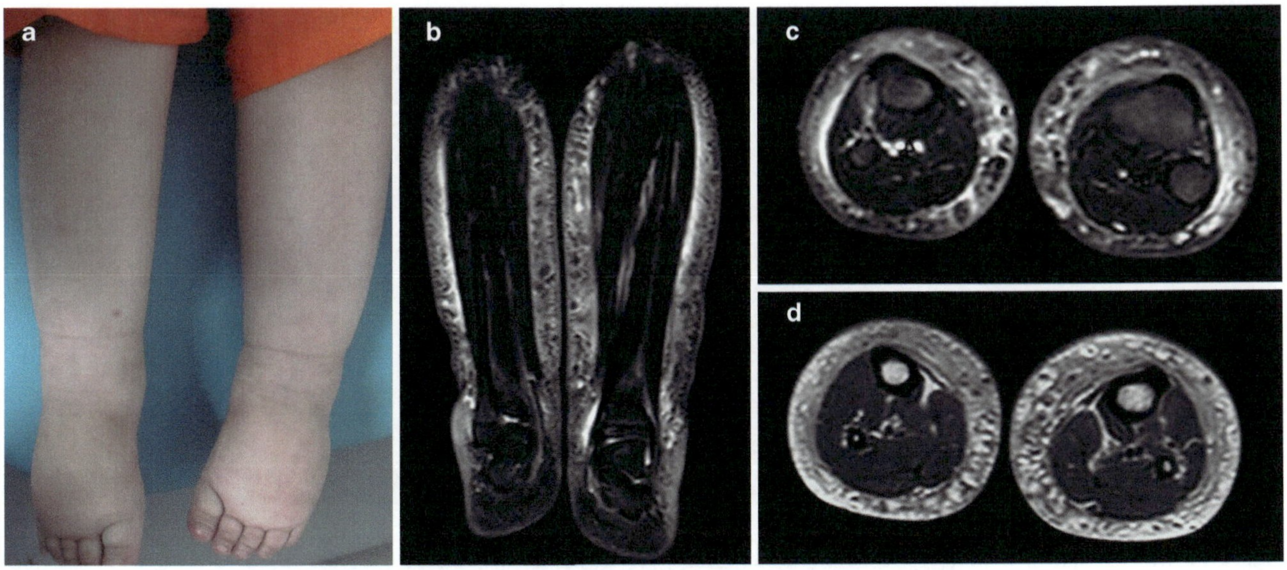

Fig. 10.15 Primary lymphedema of both legs in a 5-year-old girl. (**a**) Clinical photograph shows swelling of both legs. (**b**, **c**) Coronal and axial STIR images demonstrate the characteristic features of lymphedema: epifascial distribution with muscle sparing, honeycombing, and cutaneous thickening, best appreciated on STIR sequence. (**d**) Axial T1-weighted image shows epifascial edema with relative preservation of muscle signal

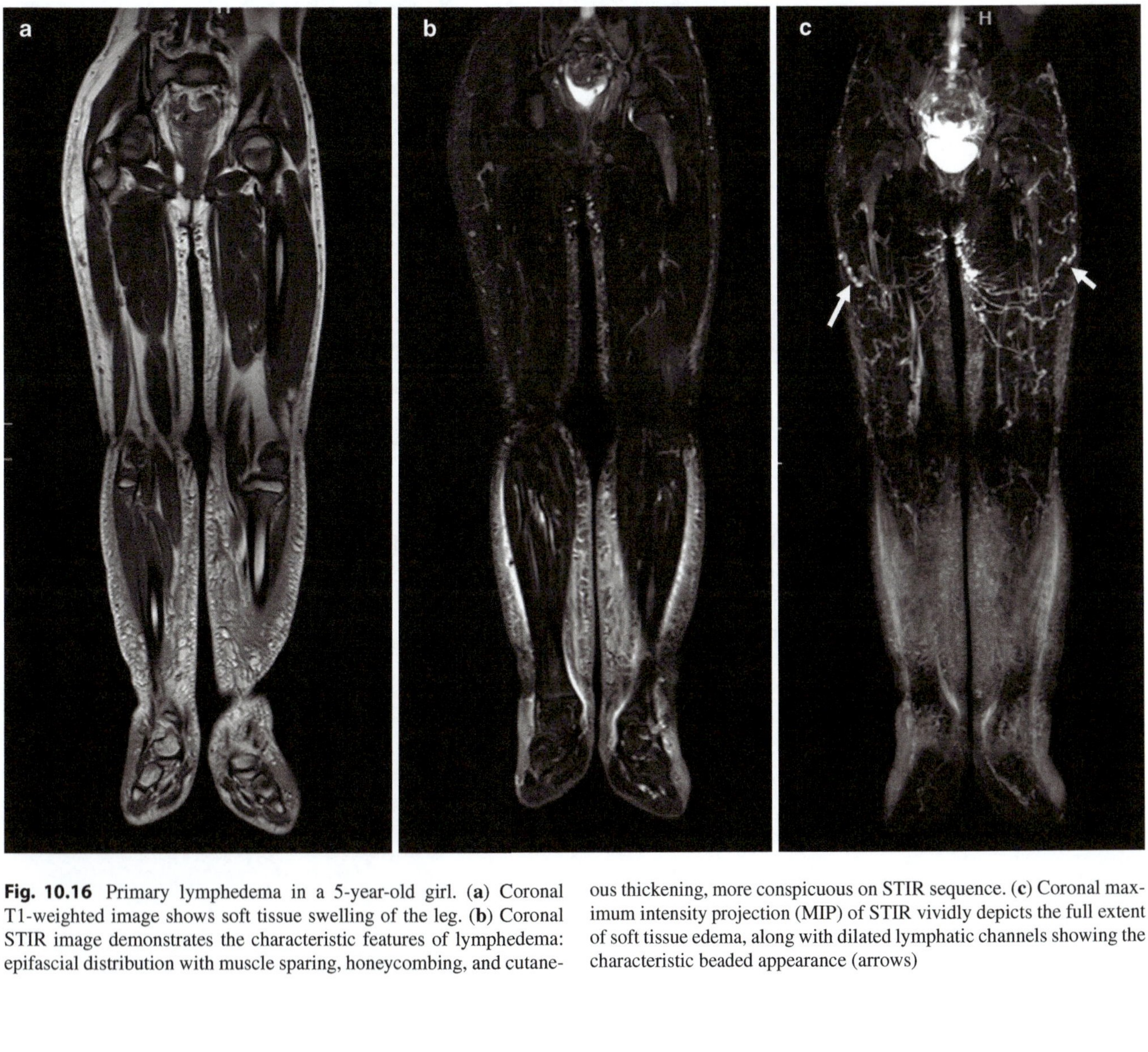

Fig. 10.16 Primary lymphedema in a 5-year-old girl. (**a**) Coronal T1-weighted image shows soft tissue swelling of the leg. (**b**) Coronal STIR image demonstrates the characteristic features of lymphedema: epifascial distribution with muscle sparing, honeycombing, and cutaneous thickening, more conspicuous on STIR sequence. (**c**) Coronal maximum intensity projection (MIP) of STIR vividly depicts the full extent of soft tissue edema, along with dilated lymphatic channels showing the characteristic beaded appearance (arrows)

References

1. Upton IIIJ. Vascular malformations of the extremities. In: Mulliken JB, Burrows PE, Fishman SJ, editors. Mulliken & Young's vascular anomalies: hemangiomas and malformations. Oxford University Press; 2013. p. 905–65.
2. AbouZeid AA, Mohammad SA, Aly NH, et al. Lymphatic malformations: a 9-year experience at the vascular anomaly clinic. Egypt Pediatric Association Gaz. 2023;71:88. https://doi.org/10.1186/s43054-023-00236-0.
3. Mohammad SA, AbouZeid AA, Fawzi AM, et al. Magnetic resonance imaging of head and neck vascular anomalies: pearls and pitfalls. Ann Pediatr Surg. 2017;13:116–24.
4. Flors L, Hagspiel KD, Park AW, Norton PT, Leiva-Salinas C. Vascular malformations and tumors. Part 2: Low-flow lesions. Radiologia (English edition). 2019;61:124–33.
5. Feins NR, Greene AK. Primary lymphedema. In: Mulliken JB, Burrows PE, Fishman SJ, editors. Mulliken & Young's vascular anomalies: hemangiomas and malformations. Oxford University Press; 2013. p. 1056–76.
6. Hara H, Mihara M. Screening lymphatic ultrasound to detect lymphatic dysfunction. Lymphat Res Biol. 2025;23(2):64–70.
7. Nagy BI, Mohos B, Tzou CH. Imaging modalities for evaluating lymphedema. Medicina. 2023;59(11):2016.
8. Salehi BP, Sibley RC, Friedman R, Kim G, Singhal D, Loening AM, Tsai LL. MRI of lymphedema. J Magn Reson Imaging. 2023;57(4):977–91.

11 Truncal and Visceral Lymphatic Malformations

Introduction

Lymphatic malformations (LMs) consist of abnormal lymph-filled cysts of variable size, which are lacking communication with the normal lymphatic system. These benign lesions, classified as slow-flow vascular malformations, often lead to disfigurement due to their disproportionate growth and may exert compressive effects depending on their anatomical location. In the preceding chapters, we discussed the manifestations of LMs in the head and neck region as well as in the extremities. In this section, we will focus on truncal and visceral LMs. Truncal LMs generally resemble those found in the head, neck, and extremities, sharing similar clinical presentations and treatment plans [1]. In contrast, visceral LMs are less frequently identified, as they are typically asymptomatic and often discovered incidentally during routine imaging or upon the occurrence of complications [1, 2].

Truncal Lymphatic Malformations (LMs)

Truncal LMs can arise anywhere along the thoracic or abdominal wall, including specific regions such as the breast or axilla (Fig. 11.1). Following the neck, the axilla is the second most frequent site for LMs [3, 4]. Lesions in the axilla often extend into adjacent regions, such as the neck (Fig. 11.2) and upper limb (Fig. 11.3). Most truncal LMs are noticed at birth and grow proportionate to the growth of the child. Different imaging modalities (ultrasound, CT, and MRI) can be used to confirm diagnosis and delineate the deep extent of lesions before intervention [5]. LMs typically appear as multiple cysts of varying sizes (Figs. 11.4 and 11.5), lacking internal vascularity and with no appreciable post-contrast enhancement except for the capsule and intervening septa (Fig. 11.1) (refer to Chap. 2).

Like LMs in other parts of the body, management may include sclerotherapy, surgical excision, medical therapy, or a combination of these approaches. Apart from axillary LMs, truncal lesions are typically subcutaneous and do not significantly involve the skin, muscle, or major neurovascular structures, making their surgical removal relatively straightforward [1]. Following resection, skin flaps should be closed over suction drains to effectively manage the expected postoperative lymphatic leakage (Fig. 11.6). Lesions with a substantial microcystic component may manifest with prominent cutaneous vesicles spreading over extensive skin areas, posing greater challenges for surgical excision (Fig. 11.7). The emergence of novel agents, such as mTOR inhibitors, has shown promise in the medical treatment of such complex and extensive lymphatic malformations [5].

Axillary lesions are typically more challenging to resect because of their proximity to critical neurovascular structures: the axillary vessels and brachial plexus [1]. While complete excision of the lymphatic malformation is not always required, it is essential to remove as much of the lesion as safely possible to minimize the need for reoperations, which may be even more complex (Fig. 11.8) [1]. Injection sclerotherapy may be a good alternative that may be used as a first line for treating axillary LMs with deep extensions.

Lymphatic malformations (LMs) may occur in association with other vascular anomalies, including venous and capillary malformations, as well as segmental tissue overgrowth (Fig. 11.9). This combination of findings is typical of tissue overgrowth syndromes such as CLOVES syndrome (Chap. 21) and Klippel-Trénaunay syndrome (Chap. 20), the latter of which more frequently involves the lower limbs.

A. A. AbouZeid et al., *Atlas of Pediatric Vascular Anomalies*, https://doi.org/10.1007/978-3-032-30866-5_11

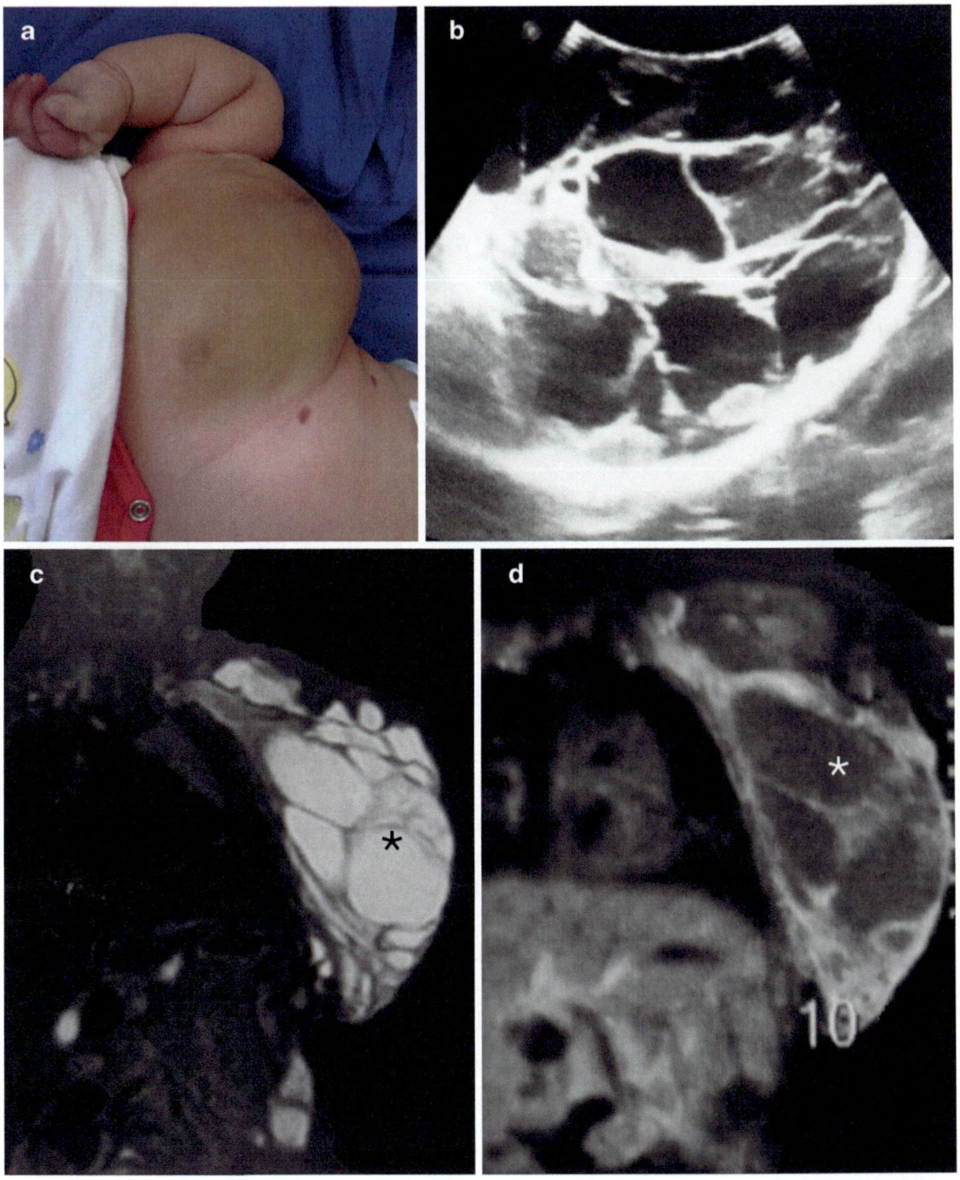

Fig. 11.1 Lymphatic malformation of the chest wall. (**a**) Clinical photograph. (**b**) B-mode ultrasound showing multilocular cystic spaces. (**c**, **d**) Coronal STIR MRI and contrast-enhanced T1-weighted images demonstrate a multilocular cystic lesion (asterisk), hyperintense on STIR (**c**) with marginal post-contrast enhancement (**d**)

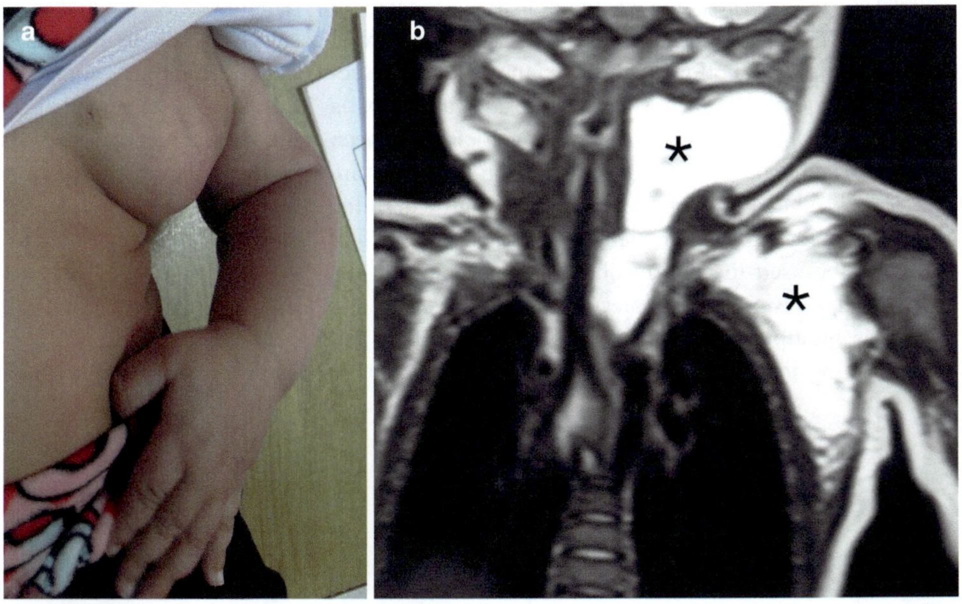

Fig. 11.2 Lymphatic malformation of the axilla. (**a**) Clinical photograph. (**b**) T2-weighted MRI shows a multilocular cystic lesion with hyperintense signal extending across the neck, mediastinum, and axilla (asterisk)

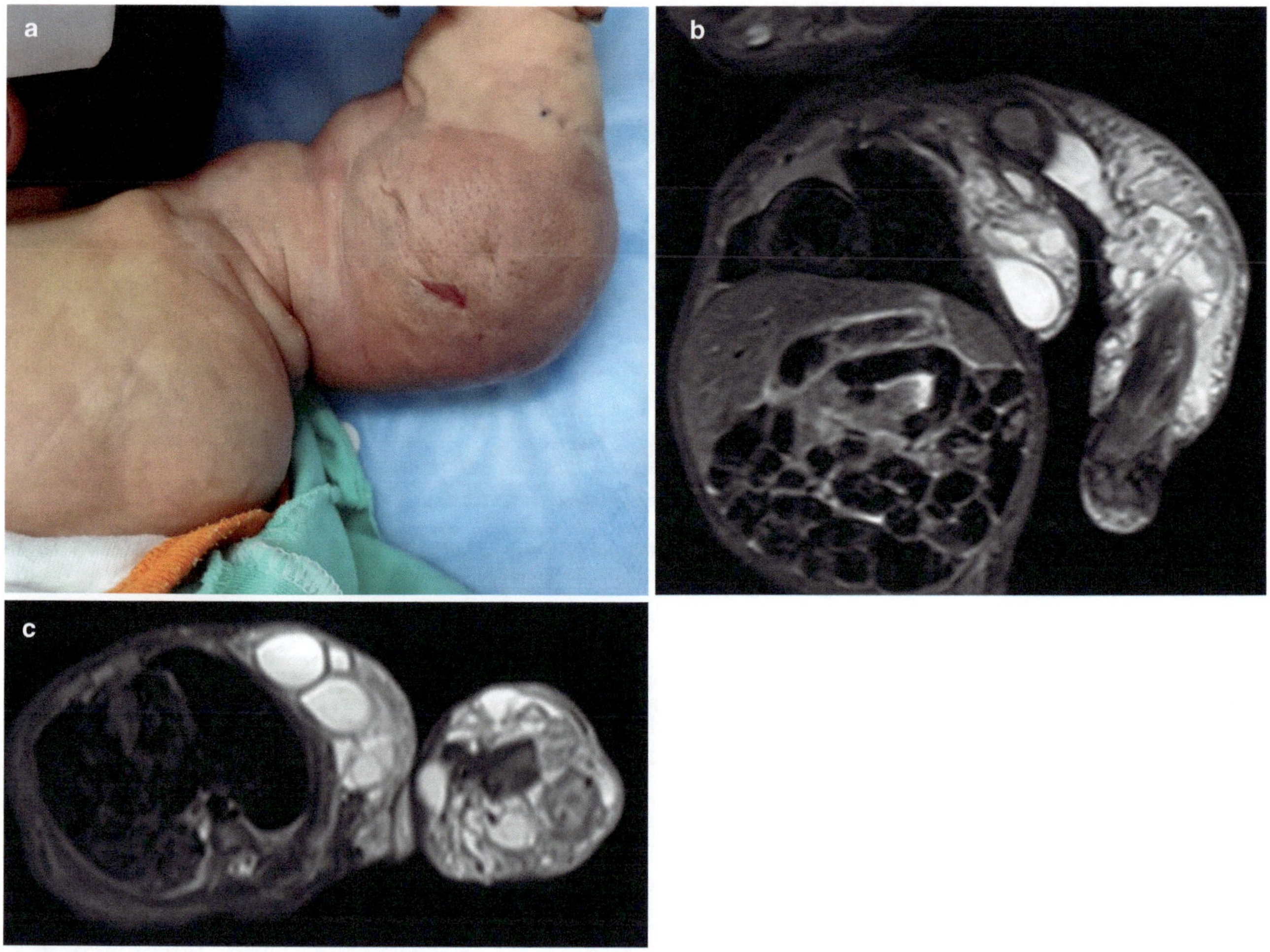

Fig. 11.3 Lymphatic malformation of the left arm and axilla. (**a**) Clinical photograph. (**b**, **c**) Coronal and axial STIR MRI show a multilocular cystic lesion with hyperintense signal extending into the axilla, lateral chest wall, and left upper limb

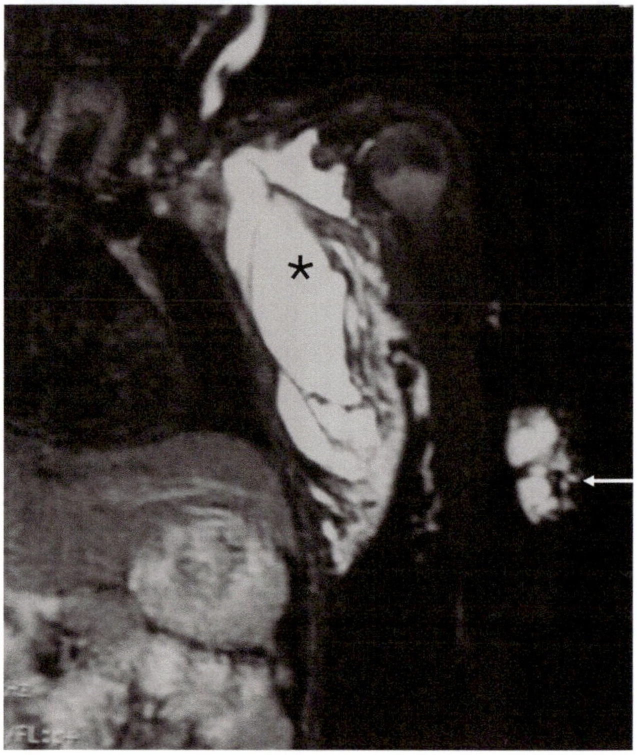

Fig. 11.4 Lymphatic malformation of the chest wall. Coronal STIR MRI shows a multilocular cystic lesion (asterisk) with hyperintense signal extending into the axilla, neck, and left upper limb (arrow)

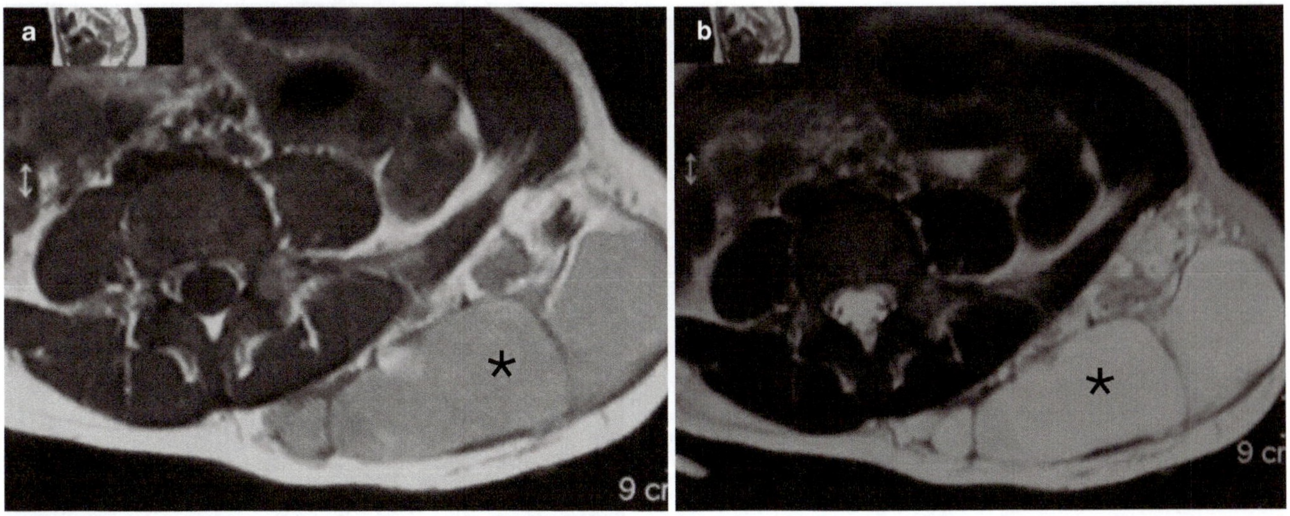

Fig. 11.5 Lymphatic malformation of the back. (**a**, **b**) Axial T1-weighted and T2-weighted MRI demonstrate a multilocular cystic lesion (asterisk) with hyperintense signal on both sequences, suggesting internal hemorrhage or high protein content

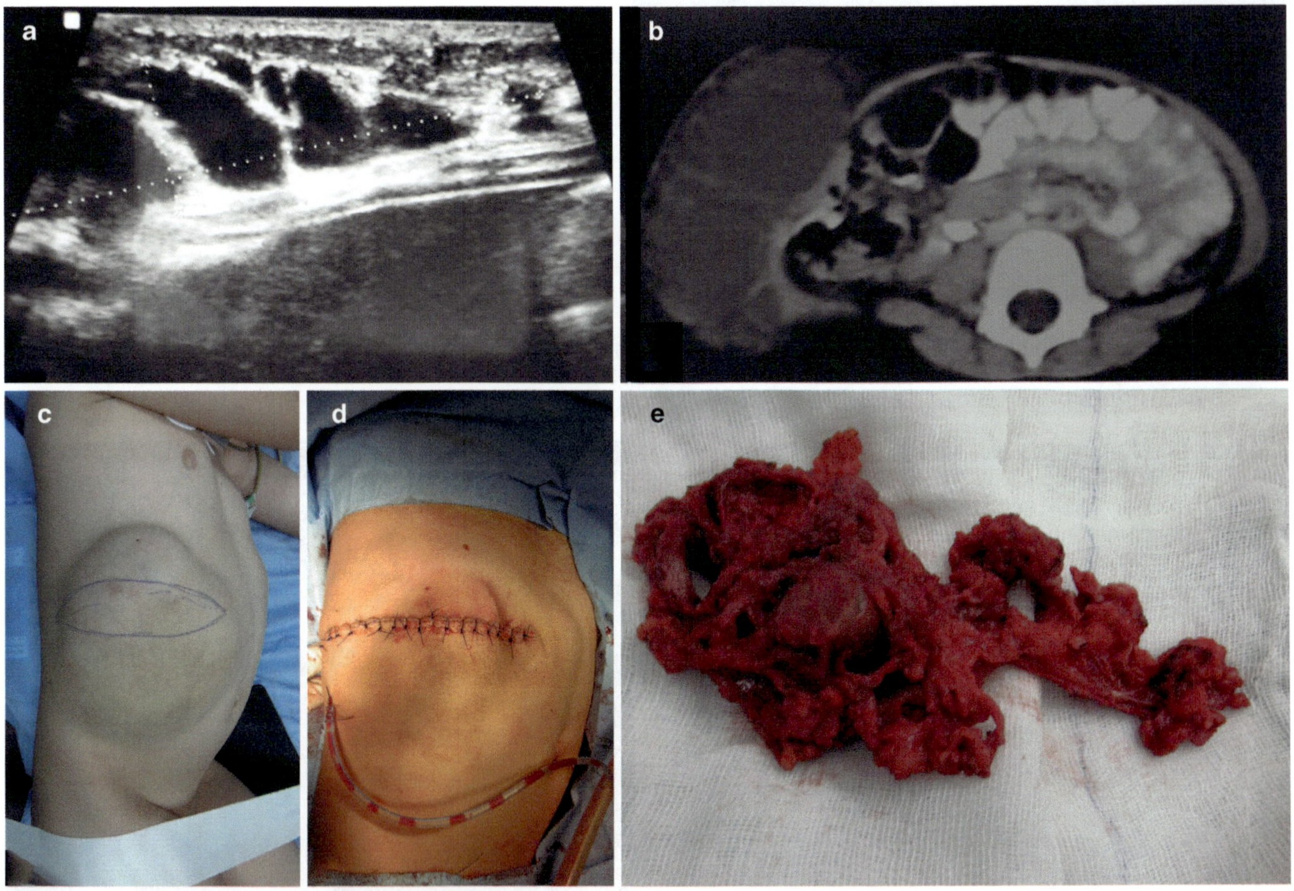

Fig. 11.6 Lymphatic malformation of the abdominal wall. (**a**) B-mode ultrasound shows multilocular cystic spaces. (**b**) Axial contrast-enhanced CT demonstrates a large multilocular cystic lesion with marginal enhancement. (**c**–**e**) Excision of the multi-cystic mass; note the skin incision design from lenticular to linear closure over a suction drain

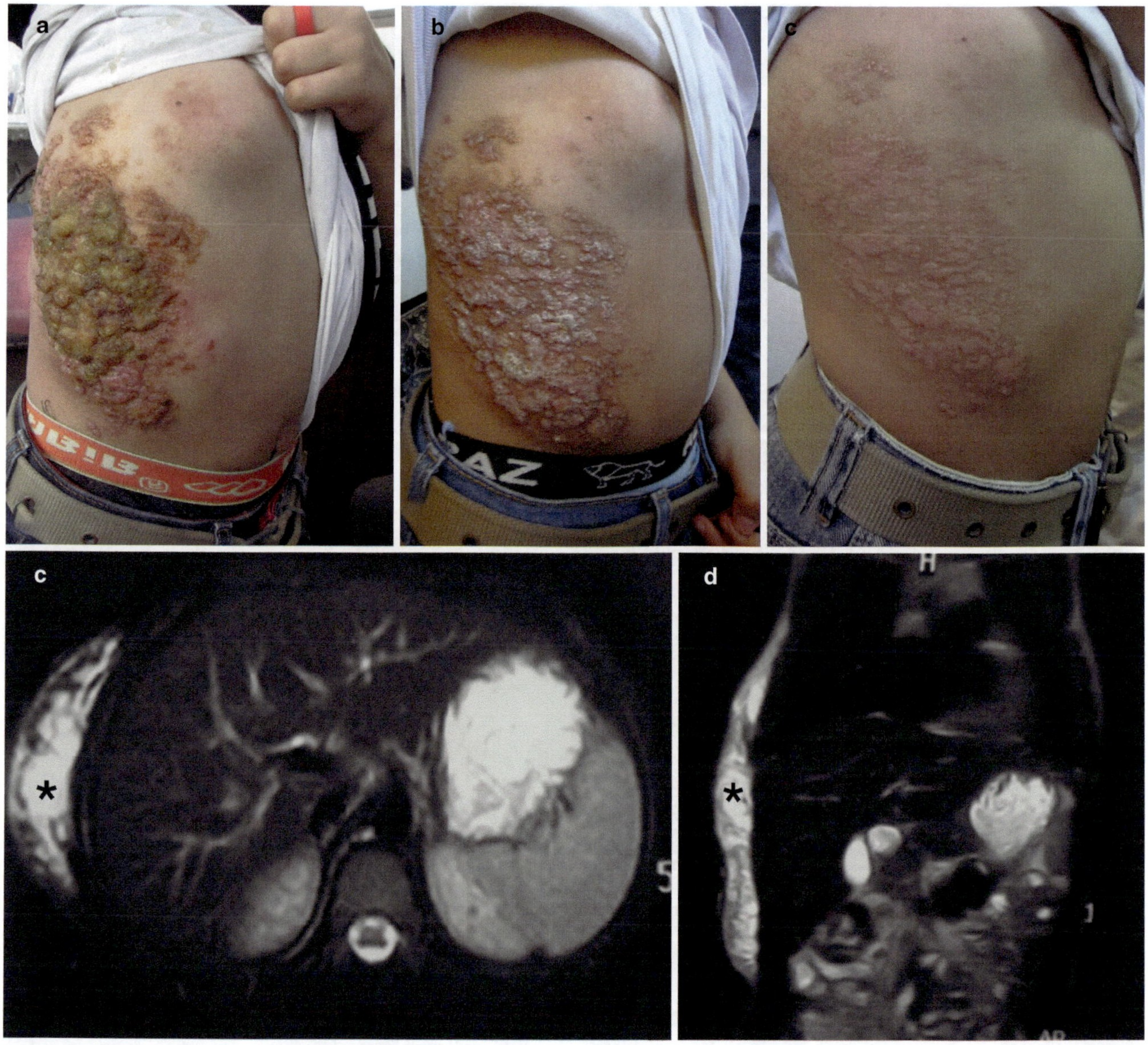

Fig. 11.7 Lymphatic malformation in an 11-year-old boy involving the right side of the trunk with cutaneous vesicles (raised fluid-filled blebs). Sequential clinical images show the lesion at presentation (**a**), two weeks after initiation of sirolimus therapy (**b**), and at 8-month follow-up while still on sirolimus (**c**). (**d**, **e**) Axial and coronal fat-saturated T2-weighted MRI demonstrate a hyperintense multilocular cystic lesion (asterisk). (Reproduced from AbouZeid et al. [5])

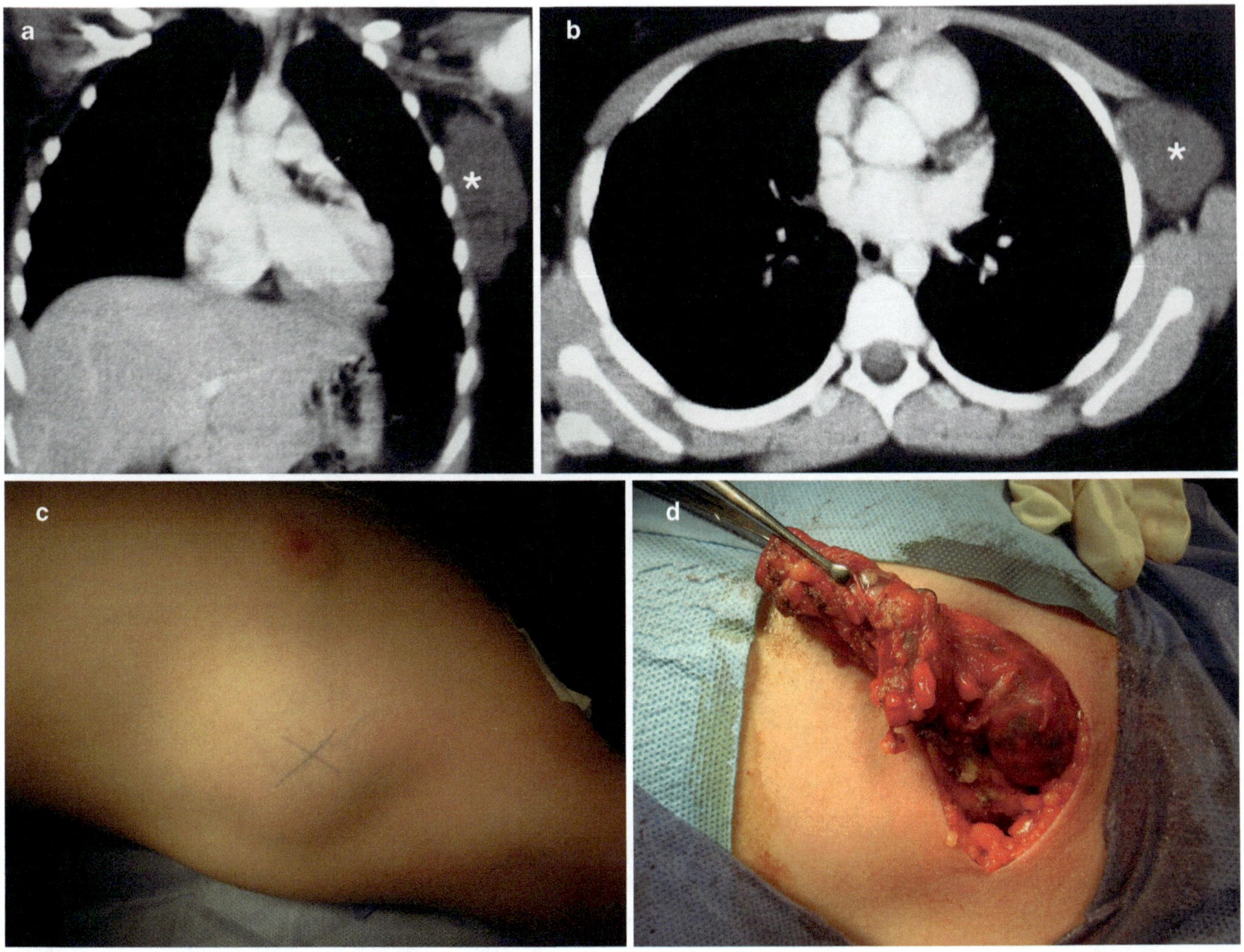

Fig. 11.8 Lymphatic malformation of chest wall. (**a**, **b**) Coronal and axial contrast-enhanced CT show a cystic swelling in the left axilla (asterisk). (**c**, **d**) Intraoperative views of surgical excision

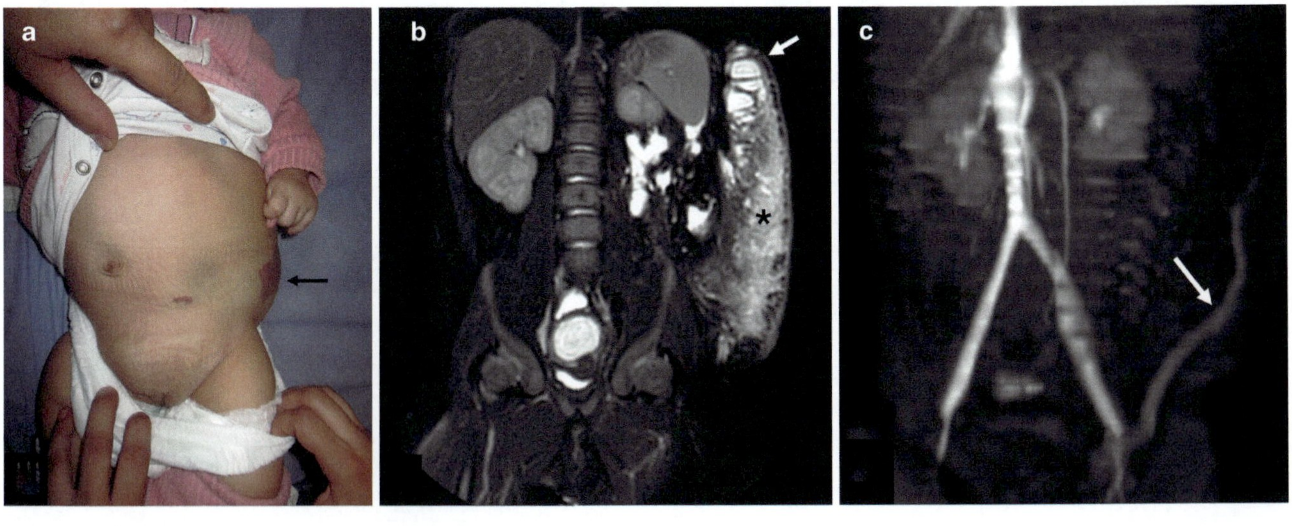

Fig. 11.9 Combined vascular malformations in the trunk. (**a**) Clinical photograph showing cutaneous capillary malformation associated with asymmetric tissue hypertrophy (black arrow). (**b**) Coronal STIR MRI demonstrates lymphatic malformation formed of variable-sized cystic spaces (arrow) with associated soft tissue overgrowth (asterisk). (**c**) Non-contrast MR venography reveals an anomalous vein (arrow)

Visceral Lymphatic Malformations (LMs)

Visceral LMs account for approximately 3–9% of all lymphatic malformations [2]. Most visceral LMs present during childhood as cystic abdominal lesions originating from the mesentery (Fig. 11.10), omentum, or retroperitoneum (Fig. 11.11) [2]. Visceral lymphatic malformations (LMs) may be diagnosed incidentally during routine imaging (Fig. 11.12) or may present with complications such as infection or cyst torsion. In neonates, visceral lymphatic malformations can manifest with marked abdominal distension and signs of intestinal obstruction (Fig. 11.13), often requiring prompt medical or surgical intervention (Fig. 11.14). The differential diagnosis includes other abdominal cystic masses. MRI is the imaging modality of choice for accurately identifying the anatomical location and characteristic features of lymphatic malformations, which typically appear as cysts of varying sizes without internal vascularity and show no significant post-contrast enhancement, except for the internal septations (Fig. 11.15). Management of visceral lymphatic malformations is primarily symptom-driven. Asymptomatic and relatively small lesions may be managed with watchful waiting, while symptomatic cases may require surgical resection or sclerotherapy [2]. For extensive lesions, Sirolimus—an mTOR inhibitor—has emerged as a promising therapeutic option.

A distinctive presentation of visceral lymphatic malformations is hypoproteinemia and failure to thrive, resulting from protein-losing enteropathy associated with diffuse microcystic lesions affecting the mesentery and/or bowel mucosa (Fig. 11.10). When the disease is localized, surgical resection of the affected bowel can be curative. In more extensive cases, lifelong dietary management with a low-fat, high-protein regimen supplemented by medium-chain triglycerides is required, as these are absorbed directly into the portal system, bypassing the lymphatics and reducing lymphatic engorgement [2].

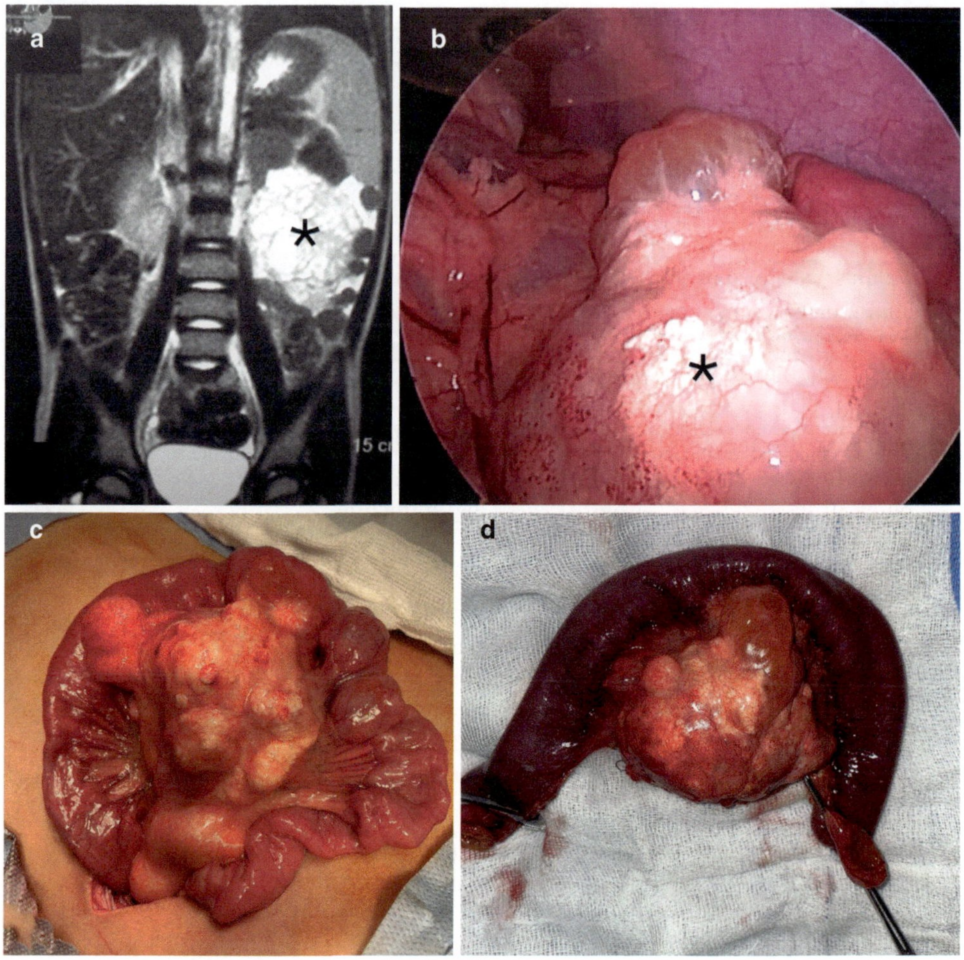

Fig. 11.10 Mesenteric lymphatic malformation in a 6-year-old girl. (**a**) Coronal T2-WI MRI shows a well-defined multilocular cystic lesion (asterisk). (**b**) The mass at laparoscopic exploration (asterisk). (**c, d**) Delivery of the mass and resection with attached bowel segment

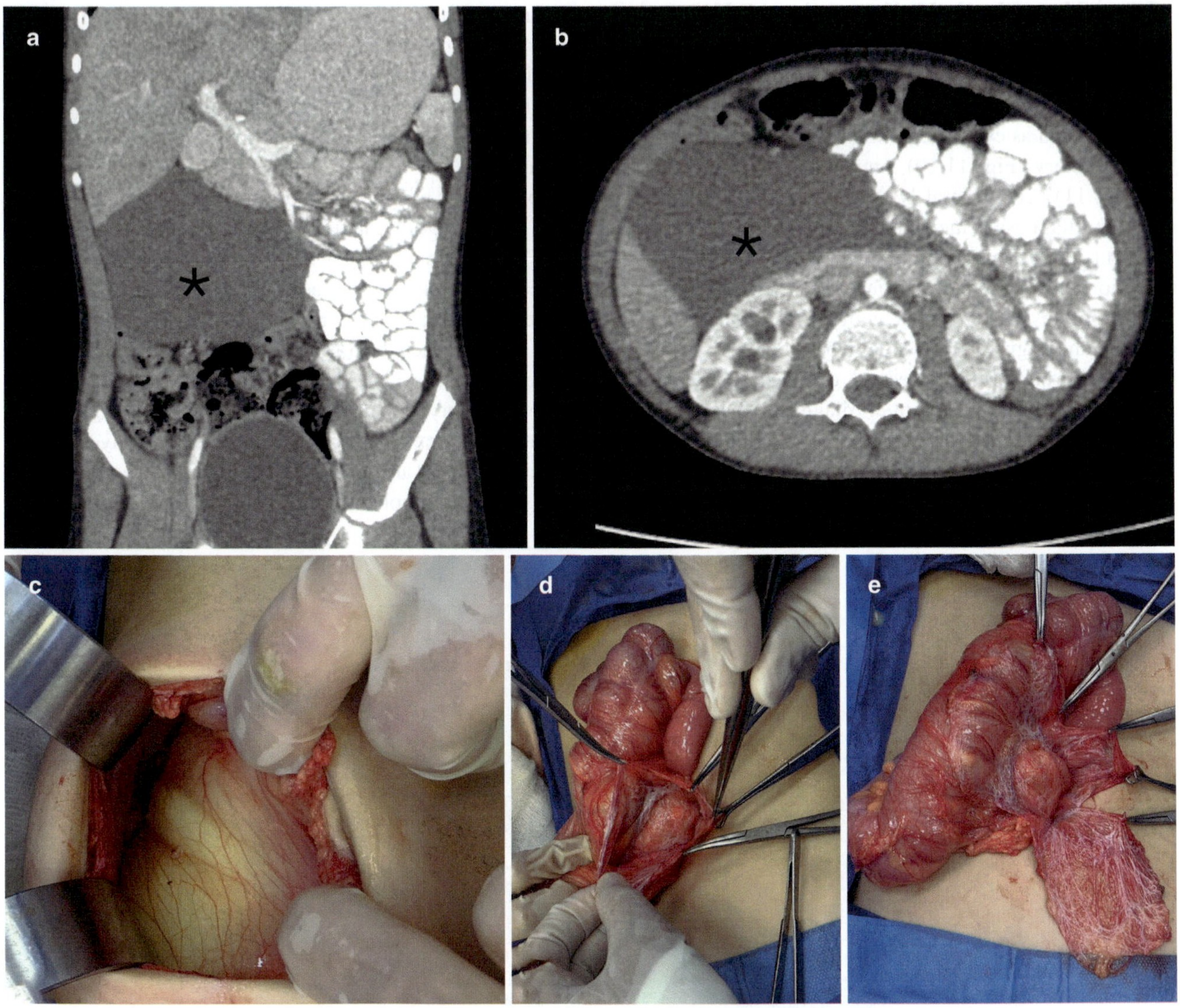

Fig. 11.11 Retroperitoneal lymphatic malformation in a 7-year-old girl. (**a**, **b**) Coronal and axial contrast-enhanced CT demonstrate a retroperitoneal cystic lesion (asterisk) displacing bowel loops anteriorly. (**c**–**e**) Intraoperative findings show a retrocolic cyst containing yellowish fluid and subsequent excision of the cyst wall

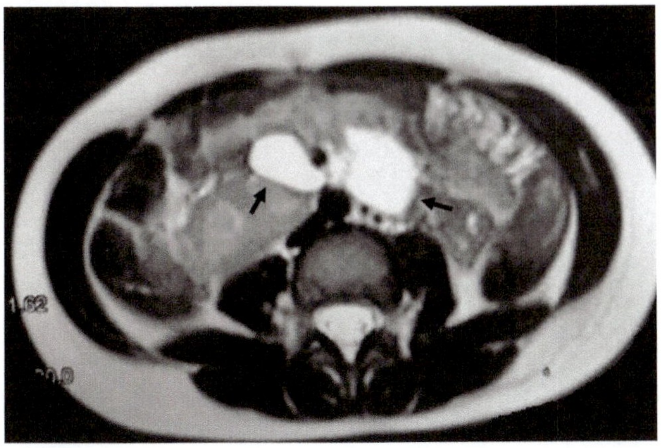

Fig. 11.12 Retro peritoneal Lymphatic malformation in a 13-year-old boy. The cystic lesion was discovered accidentally during MRI examination of the abdomen. Note the hyperintense signal of the lesions in T2 weighted images (arrows). (Reproduced from AbouZeid et al. [5])

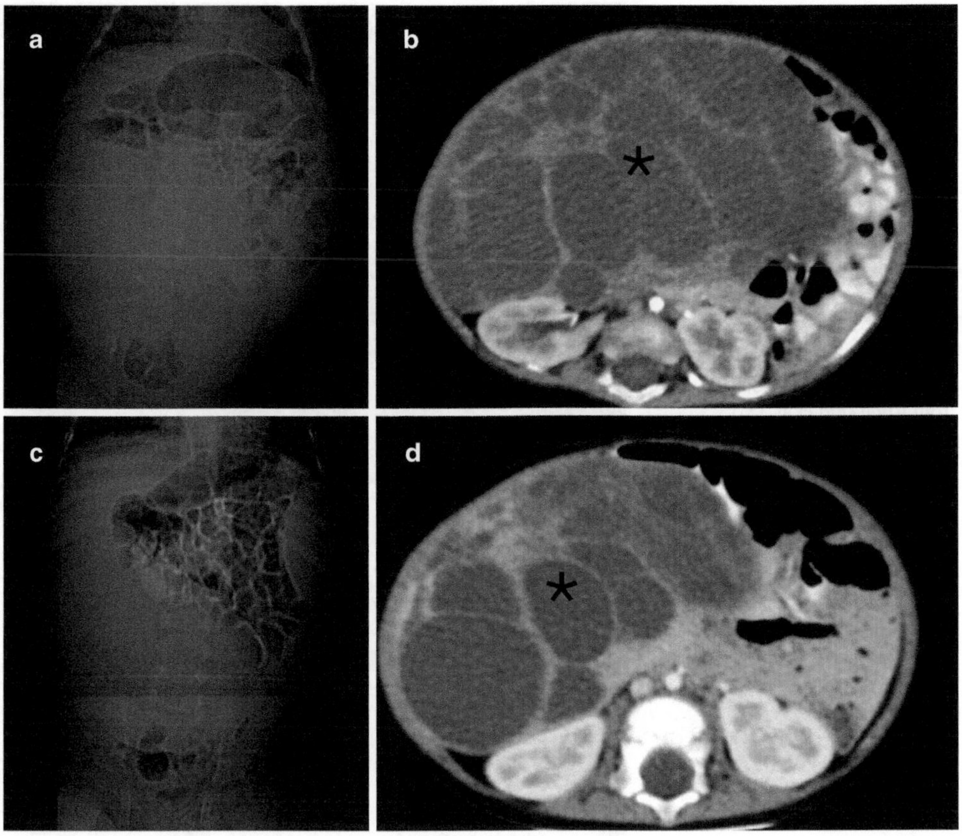

Fig. 11.13 Mesenteric lymphatic malformation in a neonate presenting with abdominal distension. (**a**, **b**) Initial imaging: coronal CT scout and contrast-enhanced CT demonstrating a large multilocular cystic lesion (asterisk). (**c**, **d**) Follow-up after 6 months of sirolimus therapy: coronal scout and axial contrast-enhanced CT show a reduction in lesion size

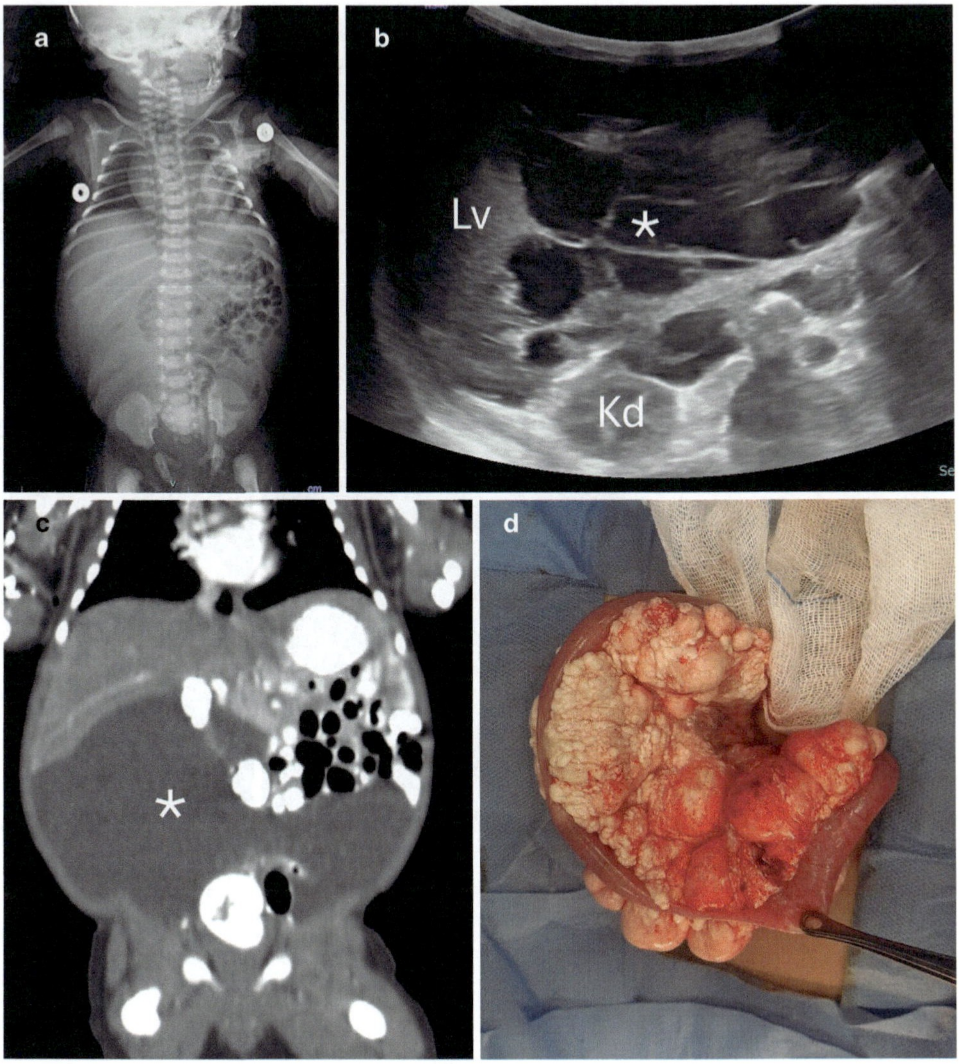

Fig. 11.14 Mesenteric lymphatic malformation in a neonate presenting with marked abdominal distension and vomiting. (**a**) Plain X-ray showing displacement of bowel to left side. (**b**) Abdominal ultrasound showing intra-abdominal multi-cystic lesion (asterisk) (LV: liver, Kd: kidney). (**c**) Same findings at CT. (**d**) Intraoperative findings: mesenteric lymphatic malformation. (Reproduced from AbouZeid et al. [5])

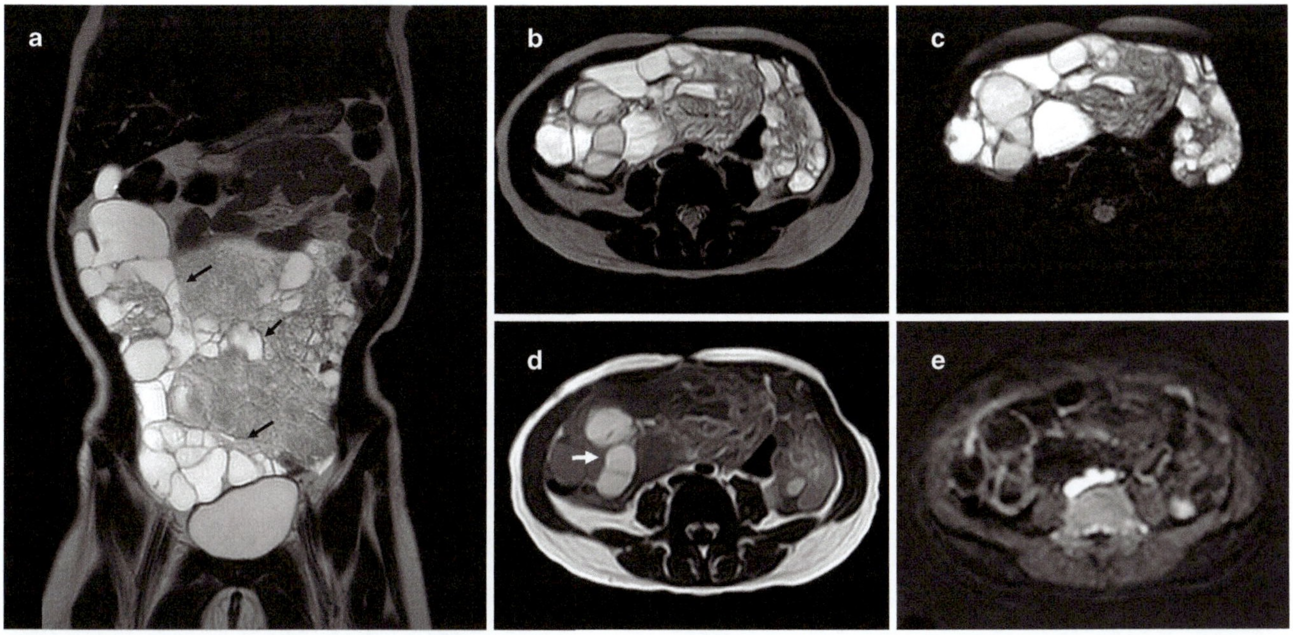

Fig. 11.15 MRI of mesenteric lymphatic malformation. Variable-sized cystic spaces (black arrows) show high signal intensity on T2-WI (**a**, **b**) and STIR (**c**), and low signal on T1-WI (**d**). A few cystic spaces (white arrow) demonstrate high T1 signal due to hemorrhage or proteinaceous content. (**e**) Post-contrast images reveal marginal enhancement of the cyst walls

References

1. Fishman SJ. Truncal, visceral, and genital vascular malformations. In: Mulliken JB, Burrows PE, Fishman SJ, editors. Mulliken & Young's vascular anomalies: hemangiomas and malformations. Oxford University Press; 2013. p. 966–1016.
2. Ghaffarpour N. Vascular malformations in the viscera. In: Mattassi R, Loose D, Vaghi M, editors. Hemangiomas and vascular malformations. Milano: Springer; 2015. https://doi.org/10.1007/978-88-470-5673-2_46.
3. Fishman SJ, Young AE. Slow-flow vascular malformations. In: Mulliken JB, Burrows PE, Fishman SJ, editors. Mulliken & Young's vascular anomalies: Hemangiomas and malformations. Oxford University Press; 2013. p. 562–94.
4. Flors L, Hagspiel KD, Park AW, Norton PT, Leiva-Salinas C. Vascular malformations and tumors. Part 2: low-flow lesions. Radiologia (English edition). 2019;61:124–33.
5. AbouZeid AA, Mohammad SA, Aly NH, et al. Lymphatic malformations: a 9-year experience at the vascular anomaly clinic. Egypt Pediatric Association Gaz. 2023;71:88. https://doi.org/10.1186/s43054-023-00236-0.

12 Complex Lymphatic Anomalies

Introduction

Complex lymphatic anomalies (CLAs) represent a recently identified group of intractable lymphatic disorders characterized by multifocal proliferation of lymphatic vessels affecting soft tissues, bones, and visceral organs [1]. There are 4 main types of complex lymphatic malformations: generalized lymphatic anomaly, kaposiform lymphangiomatosis, Gorham-Stout disease and central conducting lymphatic anomalies. Sometimes, proper diagnosis is challenging because their clinical features overlap (Fig. 12.1).

Recent advances in imaging of the lymphatic system hold great promise for improving the diagnosis and differentiation of complex lymphatic anomalies. Whole-body MRI can be utilized to assess multifocal lesions, particularly in cases involving multiple bone sites or combined bone and soft tissue abnormalities. MR lymphangiography is increasingly employed to evaluate the integrity of the central conducting lymphatic pathways. This imaging technique relies heavily on T2-weighted sequences to visualize fluid-filled lymphatic channels, allowing for detailed anatomical assessment. Additionally, dynamic post-contrast images obtained after the injection of gadolinium-based contrast material into the inguinal lymph nodes enhance visualization and diagnostic accuracy [2].

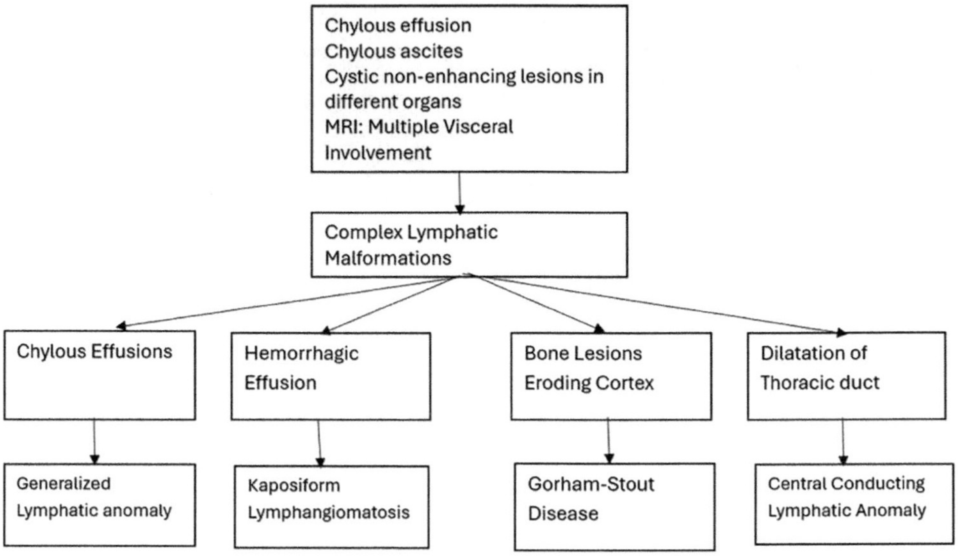

Fig. 12.1 Approach to diagnosis of complex lymphatic malformations

A. A. AbouZeid et al., *Atlas of Pediatric Vascular Anomalies*, https://doi.org/10.1007/978-3-032-30866-5_12

Generalized Lymphatic Anomaly (GLA)

Generalized lymphatic anomaly (GLA) is a multifocal lymphatic disorder characterized by the proliferation of abnormal lymphatic vessels within soft tissues, bones, and visceral organs. The lesions typically consist of thin-walled cystic spaces that expand but are generally non-destructive. Although they do not aggressively invade adjacent structures, they may cause clinical manifestations such as soft tissue swelling, pain, and pathological fractures due to bone involvement [3, 4].

GLA commonly affects intrathoracic (Fig. 12.2) and intra-abdominal (Fig. 12.3) regions. Imaging—particularly MRI—is essential for evaluation, typically revealing multiorgan lymphatic malformations involving the spleen, mediastinum, and bones, as well as pleural and pericardial effusions (Fig. 12.2). Vertebral body involvement is also common. Bone lesions usually affect the medullary cavity while sparing the cortex (Fig. 12.4), distinguishing GLA from Gorham–Stout disease. Diagnosis is primarily based on clinical history and the pattern and extent of lesions. Clinical presentation and disease course vary widely, but patients with extensive or central involvement tend to experience greater morbidity and poorer outcomes [3, 4].

Most patients with GLA harbor pathogenic somatic mutations in the PIK3CA gene, leading to overactivation of the PI3K/AKT/mTOR signaling pathway and abnormal lymphatic growth and development. Treatment is typically medical, with the mTOR inhibitor rapamycin—which acts downstream of the PIK3CA pathway—showing moderate clinical benefit [5].

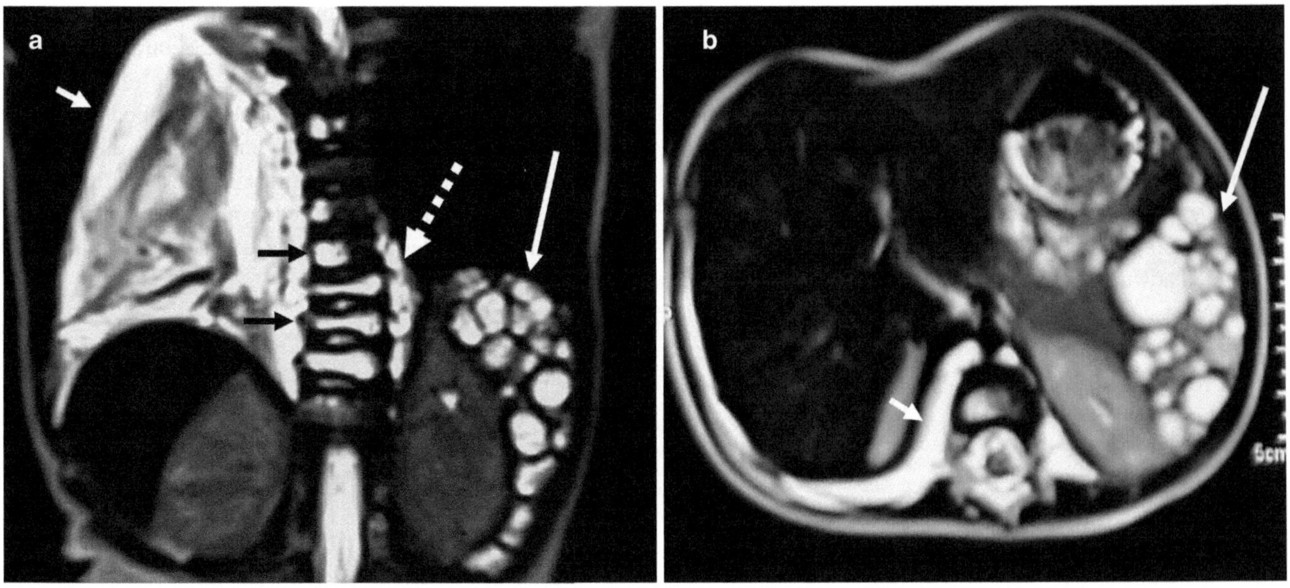

Fig. 12.2 MRI findings in a 17-month-old girl with generalized lymphatic anomaly. (**a**) Coronal T2-weighted image of the chest and upper abdomen. (**b**) Axial T2-weighted image of the upper abdomen. Both (**a**) and (**b**) demonstrate right-sided pleural effusion (short white arrow), multiple splenic cysts (long white arrow), and multilevel vertebral involvement (black arrows) without cortical destruction. Left paravertebral cysts are also visible (dashed arrow)

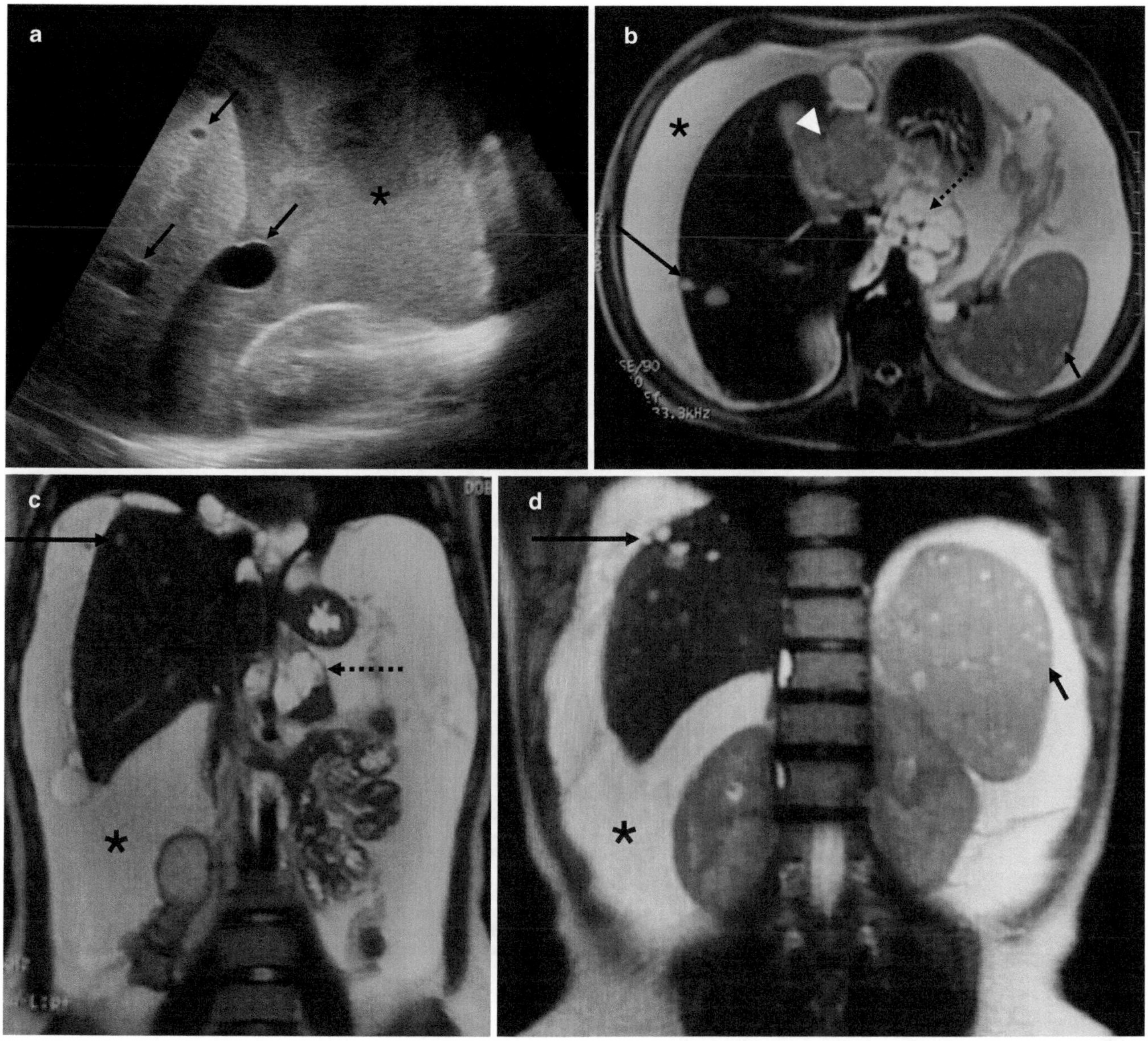

Fig. 12.3 Imaging findings in a 16-year-old girl with generalized lymphatic anomaly. (**a**) Abdominal ultrasound (longitudinal plane) shows turbid ascites (asterisk) and multiple intraparenchymal and capsular hepatic cysts (arrows). (**b**) Axial T2-weighted MRI of the abdomen. (**c**, **d**) Coronal T2-weighted MRI images of the abdomen. The MRI study (**b**–**d**) demonstrates ascites (asterisk), multiple hepatic cysts (long arrow), multiple splenic cysts (short arrow), and multiple preaortic cysts (dashed arrow). An associated hepatic hemangioma (arrowhead) is also observed in (**b**)

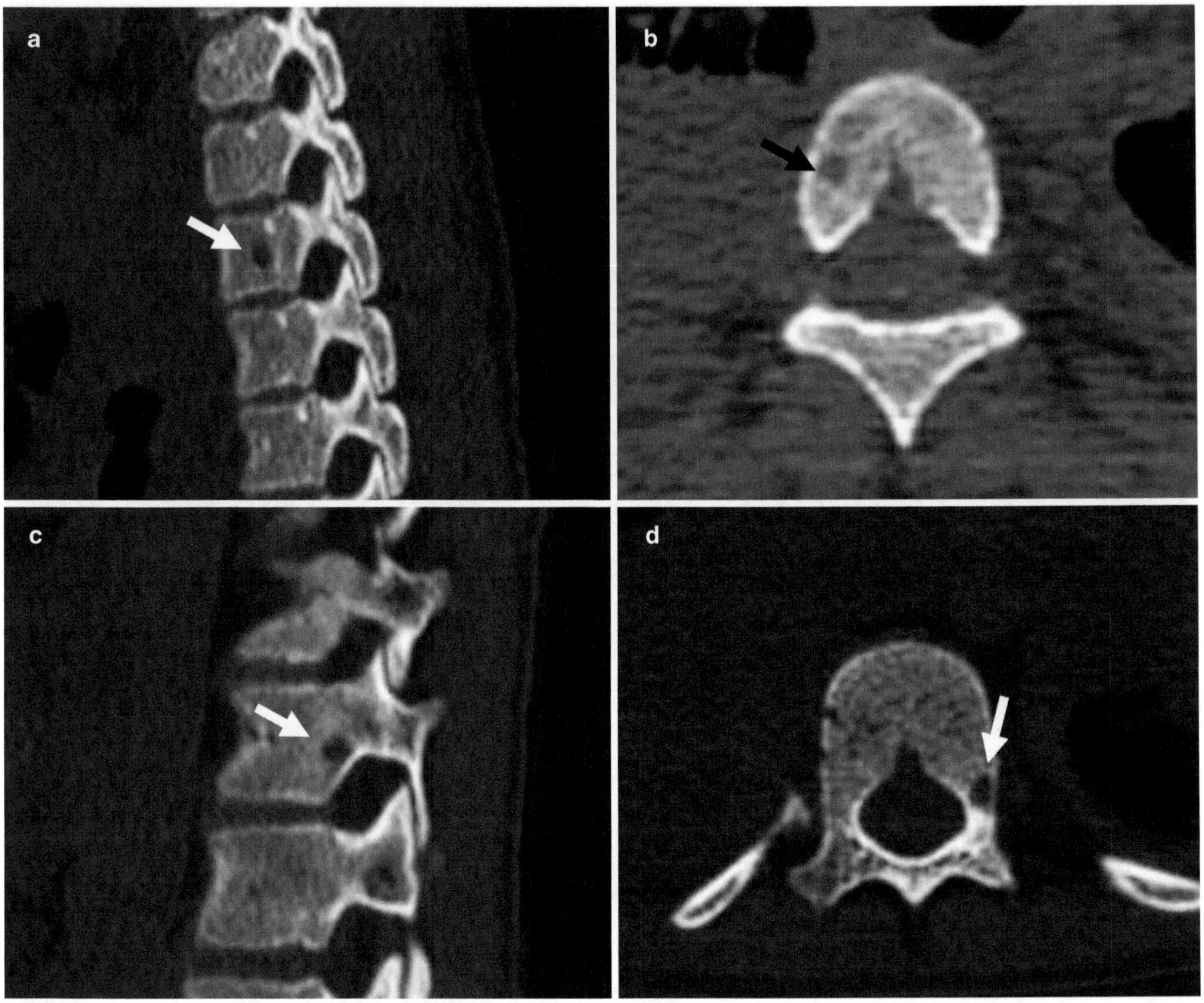

Fig. 12.4 A 13-year-old girl with a complex lymphatic anomaly. Non-contrast CT images of the spine: (**a**, **c**) sagittal and (**b**, **d**) axial views demonstrate multiple vertebral osteolytic lesions (arrows) with preservation of the cortical outline

Kaposiform Lymphangiomatosis

Kaposiform lymphangiomatosis (KLA) is a more aggressive variant of the complex lymphatic anomalies, most commonly involving the mediastinum and lungs (Fig. 12.5), and often resulting in serious complications such as respiratory distress and consumptive coagulopathy, characterized by thrombocytopenia and bleeding tendencies.

Clinically, patients often present with fatigue, dyspnea, cough, and fever [6–8]. Thoracic involvement is most common—affecting the mediastinum, lungs, and heart—and is frequently accompanied by pleural and pericardial effusions (Fig. 12.6), which may be hemorrhagic even in the absence of coagulopathy (Fig. 12.7). Hepatic and splenic involvement may occur (Fig. 12.8), and in some cases, pelvic involvement can lead to genital swelling that resembles a hernia. Skeletal lesions may also develop, presenting with bone pain (Fig. 12.9) [4]. Consumptive coagulopathy of unclear mechanism may occur, typically showing elevated D-dimer, reduced fibrinogen, and thrombocytopenia of variable severity [9].

Imaging typically begins with chest radiography (Figs. 12.5a and 12.6a), which may reveal mediastinal widening, pulmonary abnormalities, pleural effusions, or bone lesions. Chest CT typically reveals pleural and pericardial effusions, smooth thickening of the peribronchovascular and interlobular interstitium (Figs. 12.5 and 12.6), and infiltration of mediastinal fat by ill-defined, fluid-attenuation lesions lacking distinct macrocysts (Fig. 12.8) [4]. Osteolytic bone lesions may also be detected (Fig. 12.6). MRI provides supe-

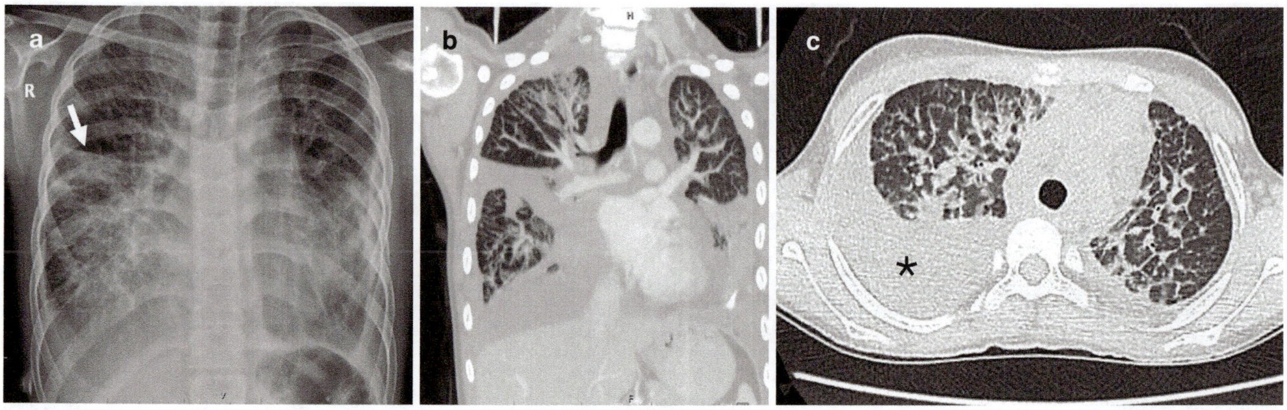

Fig. 12.5 A 13-year-old girl with kaposiform lymphangiomatosis. (**a**) Plain chest radiograph demonstrates semi-homogeneous opacities involving the middle and lower lung zones, with reticular densities extending into the upper zones. Bilateral pleural effusions are present, extending through the horizontal fissure (arrow). (**b**, **c**) Coronal and axial CT images of the chest (lung window) show interlobular septal thickening and bilateral pleural effusions, more prominent on the right side (asterisk)

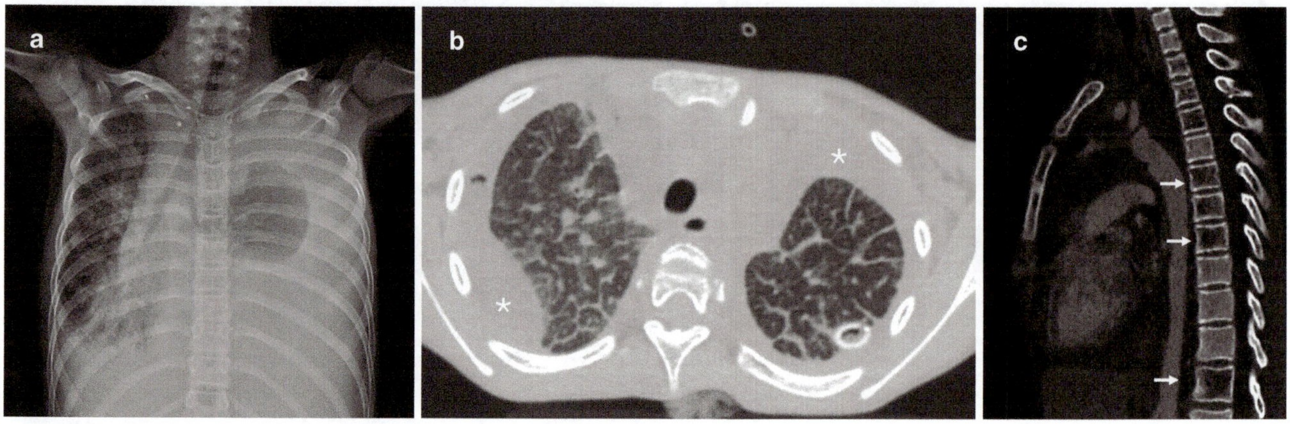

Fig. 12.6 Imaging findings in an 11-year-old girl with kaposiform lymphangiomatosis. (**a**) Chest X-ray at presentation shows massive left-sided pleural effusion with mediastinal shift, along with right-sided pleural effusion, consolidation, and linear opacities. (**b**) Axial chest CT obtained after intercostal tube insertion demonstrates interlobular septal thickening and bilateral pleural effusions (asterisk). (**c**) Sagittal chest CT (bone window) reveals multilevel vertebral involvement without cortical destruction (arrows)

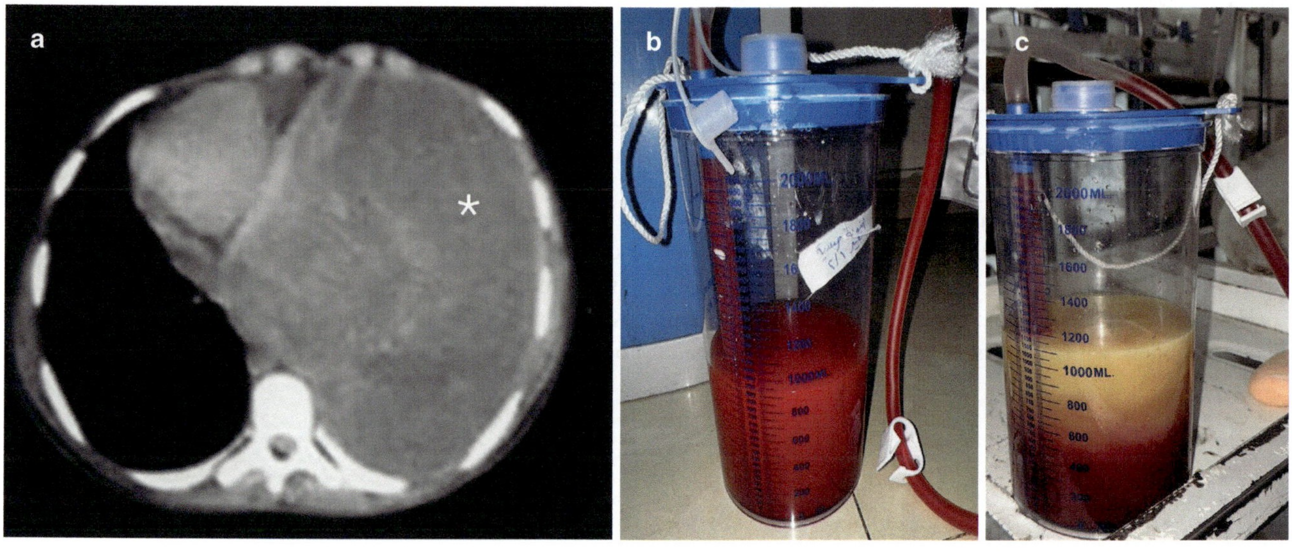

Fig. 12.7 12-year-old child with kaposiform lymphangiomatosis. (**a**) Axial chest CT shows massive left-sided pleural effusion (asterisk) with mediastinal shift to the contralateral side. (**b**, **c**) The pleural aspirate was hemorrhagic, and upon standing, demonstrated separation into two layers: a lower sedimented blood layer and an upper chylous layer

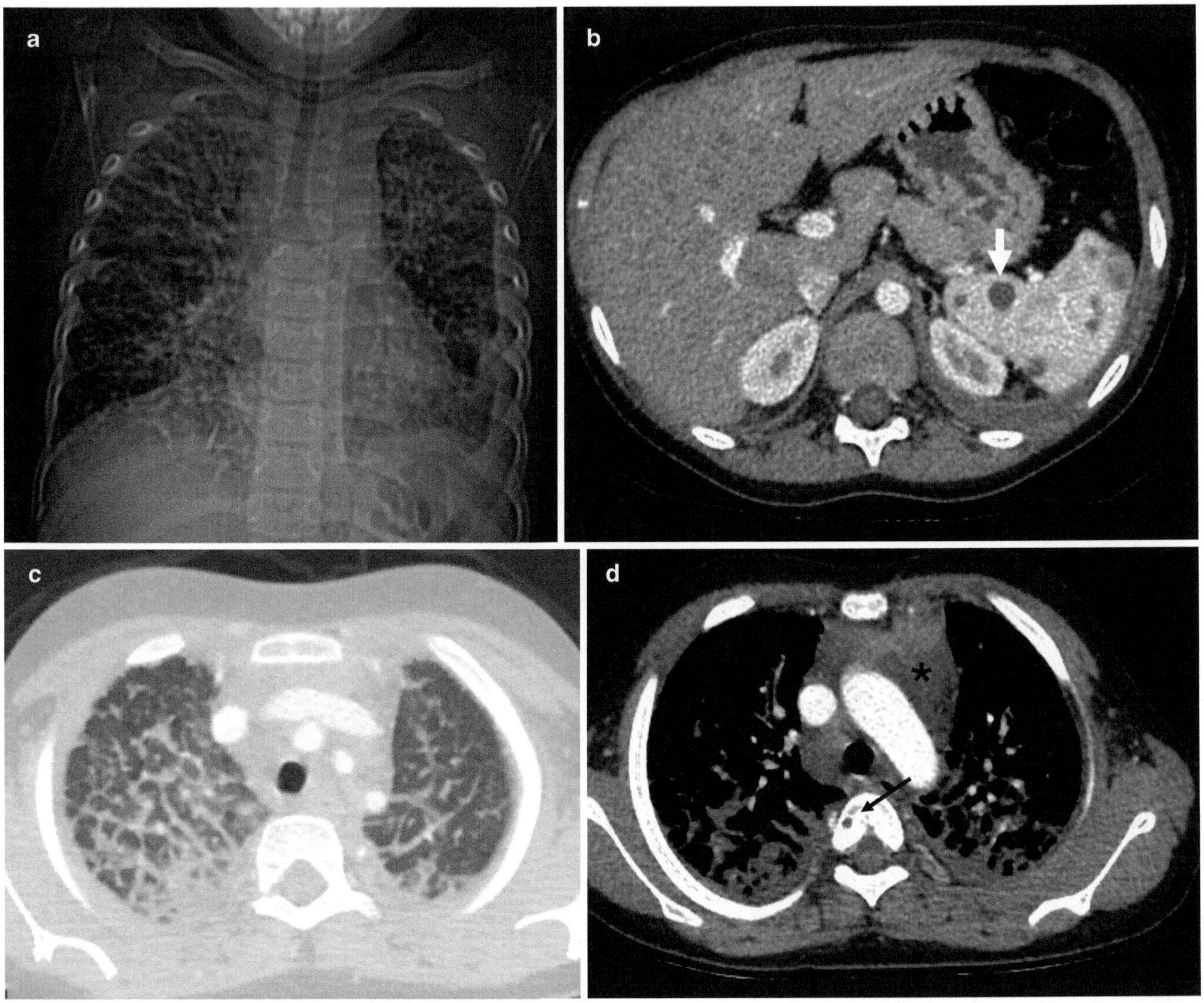

Fig. 12.8 A 6-year-old girl with kaposiform lymphangiomatosis. (**a**) Scout view of chest CT shows reticular and linear infiltrates involving both lungs. (**b**) Axial contrast enhanced CT of the abdomen shows multiple splenic cysts (arrow). (**c, d**) Axial CT of the chest lung window (**b**) and mediastinal window (**c**) show interlobular septal thickening and bilateral pleural effusion, mediastinal soft tissue thickening (asterisk). Note is made to associated vertebral involvement (arrow)

rior delineation of KLA lesions across the thorax, abdomen, pelvis, and skeleton (Fig. 12.9), with findings paralleling CT: interstitial thickening, mediastinal infiltration, and effusions that appear hyperintense on T2-weighted images. Splenic lesions, when present, appear cystic. Bone marrow lesions may be well-defined and cystic or ill-defined with increased fat deposition.

Histopathologically, KLA lesions show malformed lymphatic channels with clusters of spindle-shaped lymphatic endothelial cells (LECs) positive for lymphatic markers D2–40, LYVE1, and PROX1 [10]. Somatic RAS mutations have been identified in affected tissues [10].

KLA should be differentiated from kaposiform hemangioendothelioma (KHE), as both may present with coagulopathy. However, KHE typically occurs in infancy as a single indurated purpuric skin lesion (see Chap. 7), whereas KLA manifests with multifocal involvement of soft tissues, bones, and effusions [11].

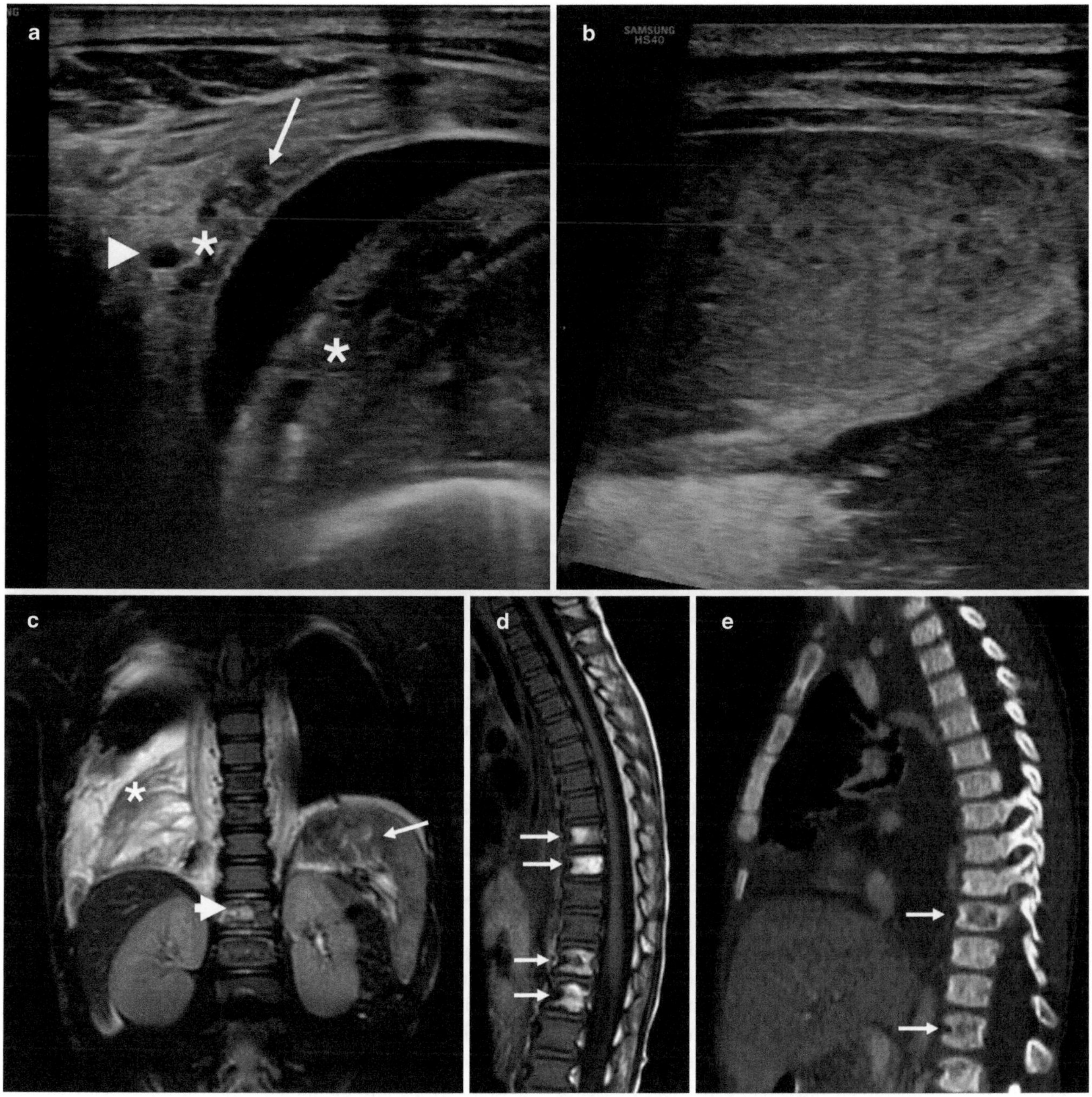

Fig. 12.9 A 25-month-old girl with kaposiform lymphangiomatosis. (**a**) Axial chest ultrasound demonstrates pleural thickening (asterisk) with associated cystic areas (arrowhead) and vascular channels (arrow). (**b**) Splenic ultrasound reveals multiple hypoechoic splenic lesions. (**c**) Coronal STIR image shows right-sided pleural effusion (asterisk); the spleen displays abnormal signal intensity (long arrow), and multiple vertebral levels exhibit abnormal signal (short arrow). (**d**) Sagittal T1-weighted image demonstrates abnormal signal intensity within several dorsal and lumbar vertebrae (arrows). (**e**) Sagittal chest CT (bone window) shows osteolytic vertebral lesions (arrows)

Gorham Stout Disease

Gorham–Stout disease (GSD) is a rare, progressive osteolytic disorder often referred to in the literature as "vanishing bone disease" or "phantom bone disease." It is characterized by spontaneous, progressive osteolysis affecting one or more bones simultaneously [12]. The underlying pathology involves abnormal proliferation of lymphatic and vascular channels within the bone, leading to progressive osteolysis and loss of cortical bone. The most commonly affected sites include the mandible, scapula, ribs, and pelvis (Fig. 12.10). Clinical manifestations typically consist of pain and pathological fractures [13].

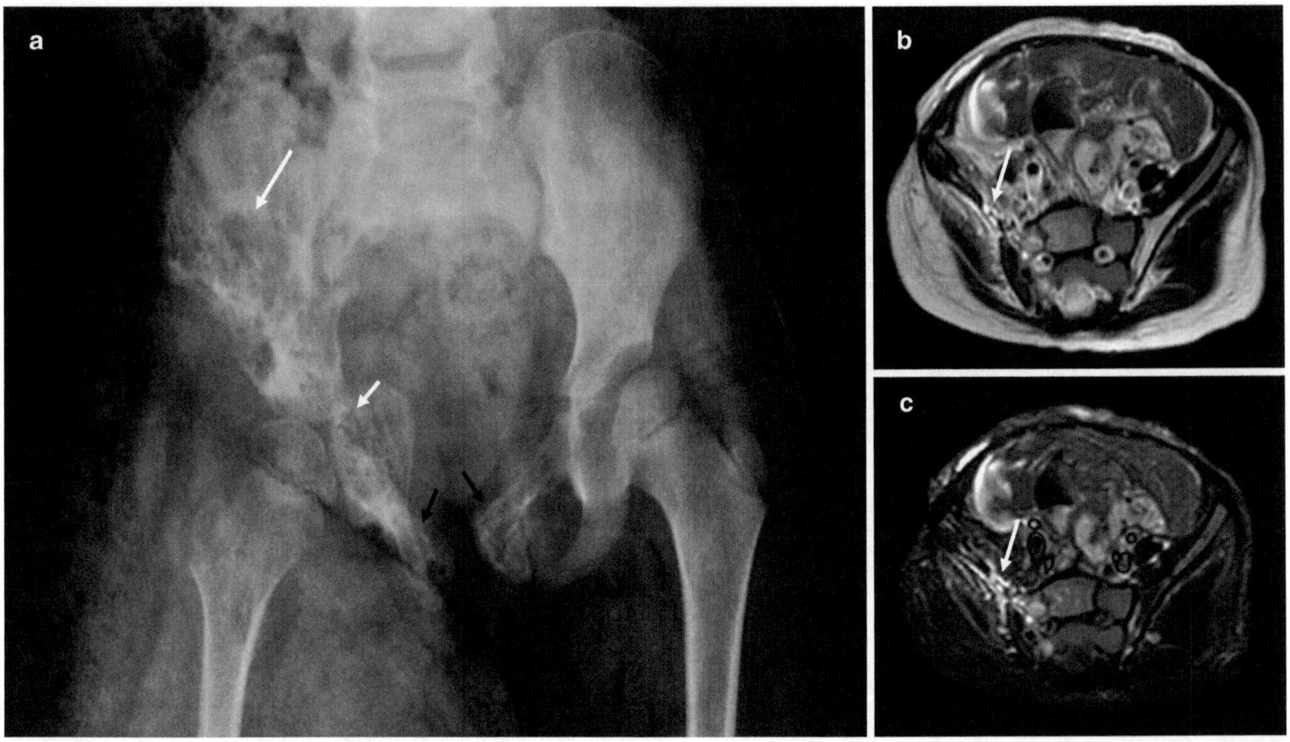

Fig. 12.10 A 4-year-old girl presenting with pain and swelling of the right hip region. (**a**) Plain radiograph shows multiple osteolytic lesions involving the right iliac bone (long white arrow), acetabulum (short white arrow), and both pubic bones (black arrows), with disappearance of the right inferior pubic ramus. (**b**, **c**) Pelvic MRI: Axial T2-weighted (**b**) and STIR (**c**) images demonstrate thinning and focal osteolysis (arrow) of the right iliac bone with associated fibrovascular infiltrate exhibiting hyperintense signal intensity

Plain radiographs initially show subcortical and intramedullary radiolucent areas; in later stages, they demonstrate progressive osteolysis without accompanying osteosclerosis, often associated with pathological fractures [14].

Several osteolytic conditions should be considered in the differential diagnosis of Gorham–Stout disease (GSD), including fibrous dysplasia, Langerhans cell histiocytosis, and multicentric osteolysis with nephropathy [14]. Heffez et al. proposed eight diagnostic criteria for GSD, which include a positive biopsy demonstrating angiomatous tissue with abnormal lymphatic channels and osteoclasts, absence of cellular atypia, minimal or no osteoblastic response with no dystrophic calcifications, evidence of locally progressive bone resorption, non-expansile and non-ulcerative lesions, absence of visceral involvement, an osteolytic radiographic pattern, and exclusion of hereditary, metabolic, neoplastic, immunologic, or infectious etiologies [15].

Several treatment approaches have been proposed for Gorham–Stout disease (GSD), including surgical intervention, supportive therapy with calcium, vitamin D, and bisphosphonates, as well as medical treatments such as sirolimus, anti-VEGF agents, and various chemotherapeutic drugs. Radiotherapy has also been used, with variable therapeutic outcomes reported [14].

Central Conducting Lymphatic Anomaly

Central conducting lymphatic anomaly (CCLA) is caused by dysfunction of the thoracic duct and/or cisternae chylae with reflux and leakage of lymphatic fluid, most commonly into the lungs and/or abdomen [16]. Pleural and pericardial effusions, ascites, and generalized edema are common and can result in organ dysfunction, protein loss, and infections. Definitive diagnosis requires lymphangiography demonstrating lymphangiectasia, lymphatic fluid reflux, and/or inability to drain lymph into the thoracic duct or the subclavian vein at the thoracic duct outlet. Dynamic magnetic resonance lymphangiography may also be used for diagnosis and to guide treatment [17].

Evaluation of central lymphatic flow patterns demonstrated distinct features in individuals with various genetic disorders, such as RASopathies, Down syndrome, and PIEZO1 generalized lymphatic dysplasia. RASopathies tend to have abnormalities of the thoracic duct and intercostal flow; children with Down syndrome have dilation of the lymphatics of the head and neck, while those with PIEZO1–generalized lymphatic dysplasia show connections between the hepatic and peribronchial lymphatics [18].

Treatment is largely surgical, such as re-implantation of the thoracic duct or embolization of refluxing channels, which may be attempted to lessen complications and improve symptoms [19].

References

1. Ozeki M, Fukao T. Generalized lymphatic anomaly and Gorham-stout disease: overview and recent insights. Adv Wound Care (New Rochelle). 2019;8(6):230–45.
2. Snyder EJ, Sarma A, Borst AJ, Tekes A. Lymphatic anomalies in children: update on imaging diagnosis, genetics, and treatment. AJR Am J Roentgenol. 2022;218(6):1089–101.
3. Lal A, Gupta P, Singhal M, Sinha SK, Lal S, Rana S, et al. Abdominal lymphatic malformation: spectrum of imaging findings. Indian J Radiol Imaging. 2016;26(4):423–8.
4. Ozeki M, Fujino A, Matsuoka K, Nosaka S, Kuroda T, Fukao T. Clinical features and prognosis of generalized lymphatic anomaly, Kaposiform lymphangiomatosis, and Gorham-stout disease. Pediatr Blood Cancer. 2016;63(5):832–8.
5. Ozeki M, Endo S, Yasue S, Nozawa A, Asada R, Saito AM, et al. Sirolimus treatment for intractable lymphatic anomalies: an open-label, single-arm, multicenter, prospective trial. Front Med (Lausanne). 2024;11:1335469.
6. Adams DM, Brandão LR, Peterman CM, Gupta A, Patel M, Fishman S, et al. Vascular anomaly cases for the pediatric hematologist oncologists-an interdisciplinary review. Pediatr Blood Cancer. 2018;65(1). https://doi.org/10.1002/pbc.26716.
7. Glaser K, Dickie P, Dickie BH. Proliferative cells from Kaposiform lymphangiomatosis lesions resemble mesenchyme stem cell-like pericytes defective in vessel formation. J Pediatr Hematol Oncol. 2018;40(8):e495–504.
8. Croteau SE, Kozakewich HPW, Perez-Atayde AR, Fishman SJ, Alomari AI, Chaudry G, et al. Kaposiform lymphangiomatosis: a distinct aggressive lymphatic anomaly. J Pediatr. 2014;164(2):383–8.
9. Crane J, Manfredo J, Boscolo E, Coyan M, Takemoto C, Itkin M, et al. Kaposiform lymphangiomatosis treated with multimodal therapy improves coagulopathy and reduces blood angiopoietin-2 levels. Pediatr Blood Cancer. 2020;67(9):e28529.
10. Barclay SF, Inman KW, Luks VL, McIntyre JB, Al-Ibraheemi A, Church AJ, et al. A somatic activating NRAS variant associated with kaposiform lymphangiomatosis. Genet Med. 2019;21(7):1517–24.
11. Ji Y, Chen S, Peng S, Xia C, Li L. Kaposiform lymphangiomatosis and kaposiform hemangioendothelioma: similarities and differences. Orphanet J Rare Dis. 2019;14(1):165.
12. Zhang C, Liu J, Wang Y, Zheng Y, Malashicheva A, Qi L, et al. Lymphatic malformation: classification, pathogenesis, and therapeutic strategies. Ann Vasc Surg. 2025;121:35–46.
13. Liang Y, Tian R, Wang J, Shan Y, Gao H, Xie C, et al. Gorham-Stout disease successfully treated with sirolimus (rapamycin): a case report and review of the literature. BMC Musculoskelet Disord. 2020;21(1):577.
14. Angelini A, Mosele N, Pagliarini E, Ruggieri P. Current concepts from diagnosis to management in Gorham-Stout disease: a systematic narrative review of about 350 cases. EFORT Open Rev. 2022;7(1):35–48.
15. Heffez L, Doku HC, Carter BL, Feeney JE. Perspectives on massive osteolysis. Report of a case and review of the literature. Oral Surg Oral Med Oral Pathol. 1983;55(4):331–43.
16. Trenor CC, Chaudry G. Complex lymphatic anomalies. Semin Pediatr Surg. 2014;23(4):186–90.
17. Krishnamurthy R, Hernandez A, Kavuk S, Annam A, Pimpalwar S. Imaging the central conducting lymphatics: initial experience with dynamic MR lymphangiography. Radiology. 2015;274(3):871–8.
18. Liu M, Smith CL, Biko DM, Li D, Pinto E, O'Connor N, et al. Genetics etiologies and genotype phenotype correlations in a cohort of individuals with central conducting lymphatic anomaly. Eur J Hum Genet. 2022;30(9):1022–8.
19. Taghinia AH, Upton J, Trenor CC, Alomari AI, Lillis AP, Shaikh R, et al. Lymphaticovenous bypass of the thoracic duct for the treatment of chylous leak in central conducting lymphatic anomalies. J Pediatr Surg. 2019;54(3):562–8.

Part IV

Venous Malformations

Cervicofacial Venous Malformations

13

Introduction

Venous malformations (VMs) are the most prevalent form of vascular malformations and are categorized as slow-flow lesions [1, 2]. VMs consist of thin-walled, valveless vascular channels that exhibit areas with deficient smooth muscle and elastic layer [1, 3]. The smooth muscle deficiency is probably responsible for their gradual and eccentric expansion. VMs present in various forms, ranging from the dilation of a single vascular channel to multiple sponge-like venous lakes that typically drain into nearby normal veins through narrow tributaries [1]. VMs commonly appear in the skin causing disfigurement and aching pain, but also can develop in any tissue, including muscle, bone, as well as hollow and solid internal organs [2–5]. Most VMs undergo a continuous cycle of spontaneous thrombosis and thrombolysis; persistent thrombi may calcify forming phleboliths. In extensive lesions, localized intravascular coagulopathy can develop, leading to depletion of fibrinogen and platelets [6–8]. This chapter focuses on VMs of the head and neck, a region frequently affected by vascular anomalies.

Venous Malformations (VMs) of the Head and Neck

Head and neck venous malformations (VMs) present as a wide spectrum ranging from well-defined, localized lesions (Fig. 13.1) to complex forms that permeate across tissue planes and encompass entire anatomical regions (Fig. 13.2). About 50% of VMs are noticed at birth, while the rest may appear in childhood or adulthood (Fig. 13.3). VMs are typically soft, compressible, non-pulsatile masses. VMs characteristically become distended with dependency (Fig. 13.4) or upon straining (Valsalva maneuver) (Fig. 13.5) [7]. Overlying skin may be normal or bluish. Typically, VMs grow proportionate to the child and expand slowly, while rapid expansion may be noticed during puberty or pregnancy [6, 8]. In about 50% of cases, phleboliths are detectable by palpation or are visible on plain radiographs (Fig. 13.6) [5].

Craniofacial venous malformations (VMs) commonly involve cheeks and lips leading to noticeable facial asymmetry and disfigurement (Fig. 13.7) and may extend into the ipsilateral orbit (Figs. 13.8 and 13.9). Diffuse cervicofacial VMs are more often associated with intracranial cerebral venous anomalies [6]. VMs may also affect the mucosal membranes of the pharynx, palate, tongue, and upper airway (Fig. 13.10). Not uncommonly, VMs may develop within skeletal muscle without affecting the overlying skin or mucous membranes; the masseter muscle being a frequent site of involvement (Figs. 13.11 and 13.12). Intraosseous VMs represent a distinct subtype. When they expand within the orbital bones or maxilla, they may cause a slowly enlarging, painless swelling that can lead to proptosis, tooth loosening, and gingival bleeding (Fig. 13.13) [6].

Pain is a frequent symptom in patients with VMs, often resulting from congestion and stretching of the affected area. Morning pain is particularly common due to overnight blood stasis in the malformed ectatic vessels, which can promote thrombosis [4, 7].

Imaging

Phleboliths are considered a hallmark of VMs and are most clearly visualized on plain radiographs. However, MRI is the preferred imaging modality for assessing the anatomical extent and guiding treatment. Fluid-sensitive sequences (T2-weighted images with fat suppression) best demonstrate the extent of the lesion. Contrast-enhanced T1-weighted sequences assist in differentiating venous from lymphatic malformations, when VMs typically exhibit delayed, patchy post-contrast enhancement (Fig. 13.14) [3, 9, 10].

Generally, VMs can be classified as focal or diffuse. Focal lesions often have minimal communication with the adjacent conducting veins, when they are known as sequestrated

A. A. AbouZeid et al., *Atlas of Pediatric Vascular Anomalies*, https://doi.org/10.1007/978-3-032-30866-5_13

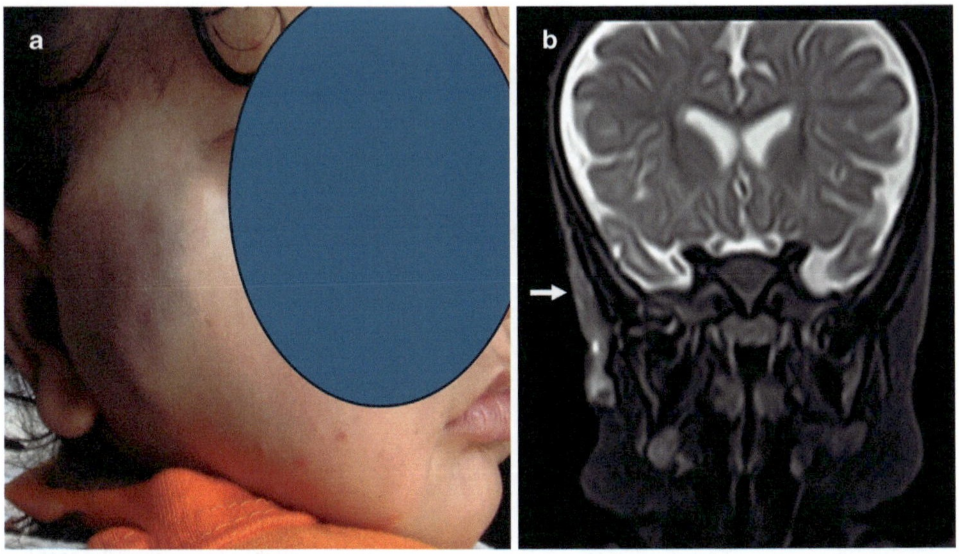

Fig. 13.1 Venous malformation in a 7-month-old girl. (**a**) Bluish compressible facial swelling. (**b**) Coronal STIR MRI showing hyperintense lesion (arrow)

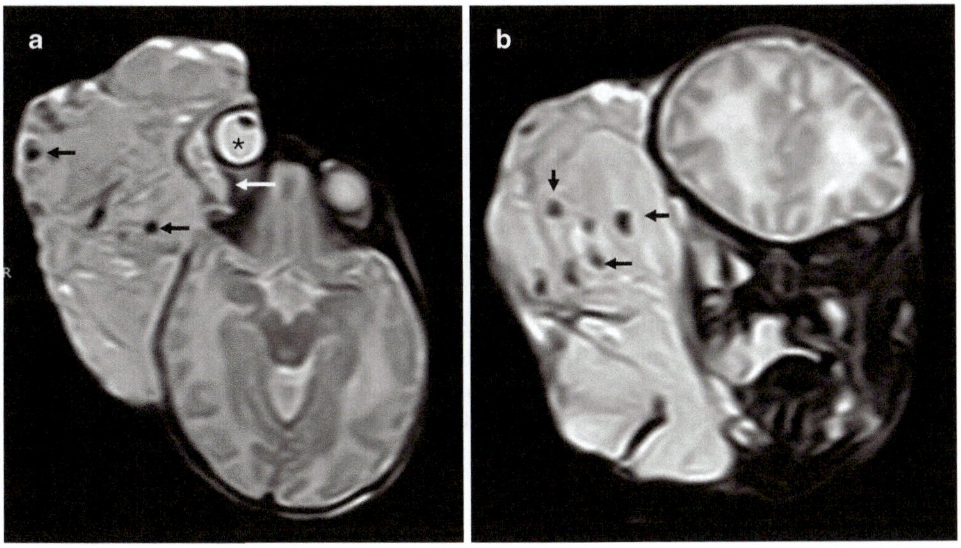

Fig. 13.2 MRI of a neonate demonstrating an extensive facial venous malformation. (**a**) Axial T2-weighted image and (**b**) coronal STIR image reveal a large right-sided facial lesion extending into the right orbit (white arrow) and causing protrusion of the right eyeball (asterisk). The lesion exhibits hyperintense signal with multiple phleboliths (black arrows), characteristic of venous malformations

lesions (Fig. 13.15) [11]. Diffuse lesions are non-sequestrated and communicate directly with the main conducting veins, which frequently are also abnormal (Fig. 13.5) [12]. Diffuse lesions are difficult to treat because injectant sclerosant can directly enter the circulation, potentially causing deep venous thrombosis, pulmonary embolisms, or cardiovascular effects. Recanalization also is more likely [6]. Multifocal lesions may suggest an underlying genetic disorder (familiar forms of VMs) [6] (see Chap. 16).

Treatment

The current management of VMs includes medical treatment, injection sclerotherapy, and surgical resection (Fig. 13.15) [3]. Laser therapy, particularly transcutaneous pulsed Nd:YAG laser, has been employed alongside sclerotherapy to aid in the shrinkage of venous malformations [6, 7]. Pharmacologic management may involve low-dose aspirin and/or anticoagulants to reduce thrombosis and localized intravascular coagulopathy. Symptom control can also be achieved with analgesics and, in extremity lesions, compression garments. In severe, treatment-resistant cases, sirolimus (an m-TOR inhibitor) has shown promising symptom relief; however, its role in VMs management is still being actively studied [7, 13].

Sclerotherapy: Direct injection of sclerosing agents results in gradual shrinkage of VMs and is considered the primary treatment in most vascular anomaly centers. Sclerotherapy is most effective when performed as a series of procedures, spaced 2–3 months apart, until there is no evidence of recanalization or residual swelling [3]. When planning sclerotherapy, careful consideration should be given to the patient's age, along with the num-

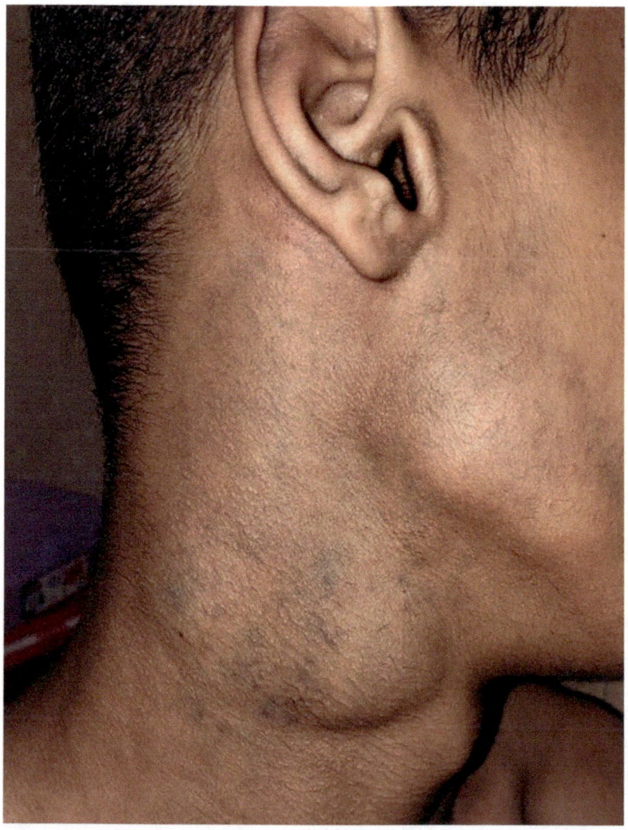

Fig. 13.3 Delayed presentation of a venous malformation in the neck of a teenager

ber and frequency of treatment sessions. Emerging evidence indicates that repeated exposure to general anesthesia in pediatric patients—especially those under 12 months of age—may carry a risk of long-term neurotoxic effects [14].

Sequestrated focal VMs with minimal communication with adjacent conducting veins can be safely injected with sclerosing agents, offering a high success rate and a low risk of recanalization. In contrast, diffuse VMs require occlusion of venous outflow prior to sclerosant injection to prevent systemic leakage. This is typically achieved by placing coils at the junction between the malformation and its draining veins to isolate/sequestrate the lesion. Before performing sclerotherapy on facial VMs, it is crucial to rule out sinus pericranii—a connection between extracranial veins and a dural venous sinus (see Chap. 19) [3].

Common sclerosing agents include bleomycin, surfactant-based sclerosants, and ethanol. Absolute ethanol (95–98%) is considered the most potent sclerosant, though it is also associated with the highest risk of serious side effects [3, 15]. Ethanol injection is associated not only with local complications—such as marked swelling, tissue necrosis, ulcer formation, and peripheral nerve injury—but also with potentially life-threatening systemic effects, including central nervous system depression, unpredictable pulmonary vasospasm, and acute cardiovascular collapse [3]. Therefore, ethanol should be used exclusively by skilled and experienced practitioners within a hospital setting equipped with appropriate supportive care facilities [3]. Bleomycin injection causes much less swelling and is the preferred sclerosant for use in sensitive areas such as the orbit and airway. Surfactant sclerosants, such as sodium tetradecyl sulfate, are gaining widespread acceptance in many vascular anomaly centers for treating VMs, due to their balanced combination of therapeutic efficacy and tolerable side effects [3].

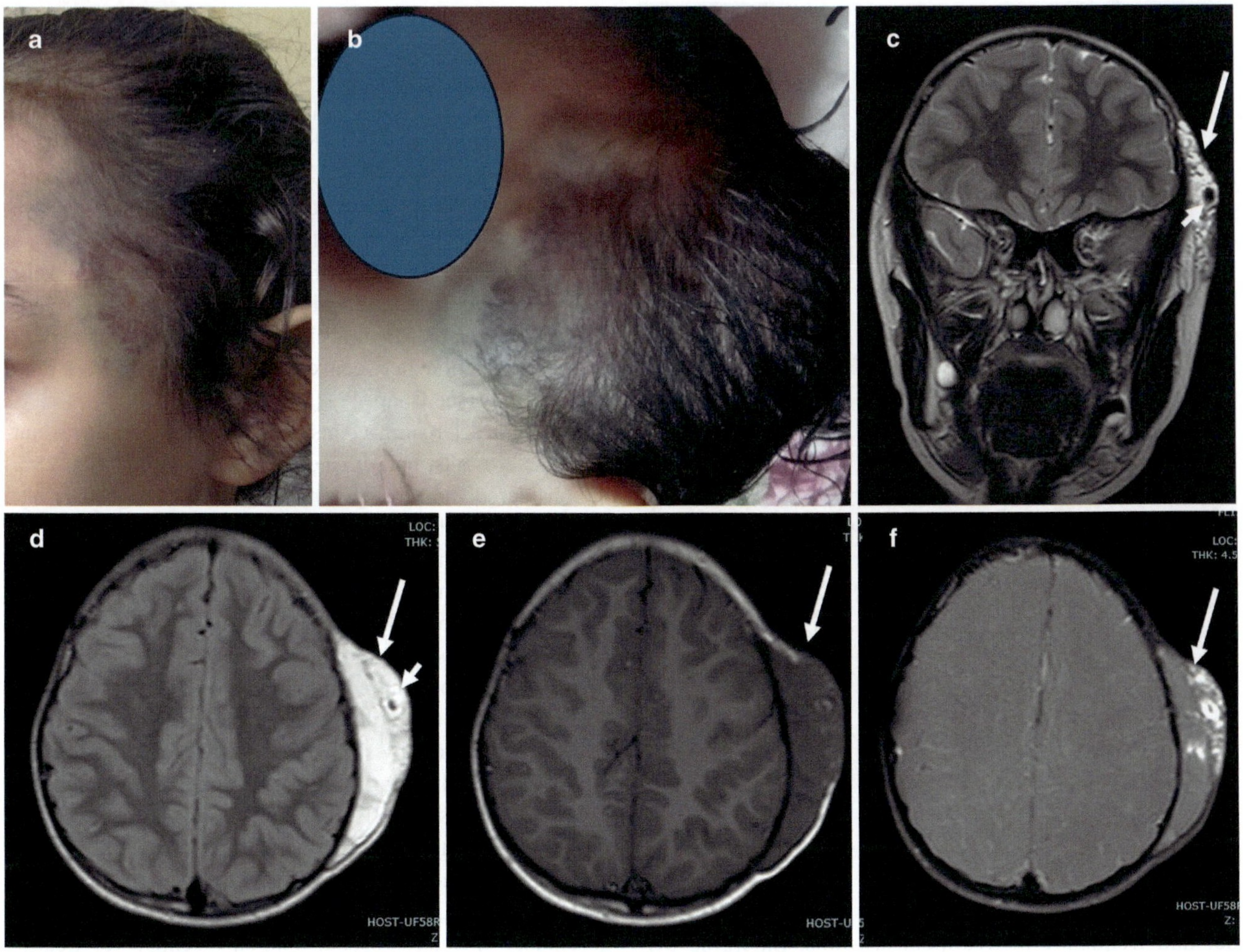

Fig. 13.4 Venous malformation in the temporal region of a 7-year-old girl. (**a**, **b**) The lesion shows distension upon dependency. (**c**) T2-weighted MRI and (**d**) FLAIR sequences demonstrate a hyperintense signal. Note the presence of phlebolith (short arrow). (**e**) T1-weighted MRI reveals a hypointense signal. (**f**) Contrast-enhanced T1-weighted MRI demonstrates patchy enhancement

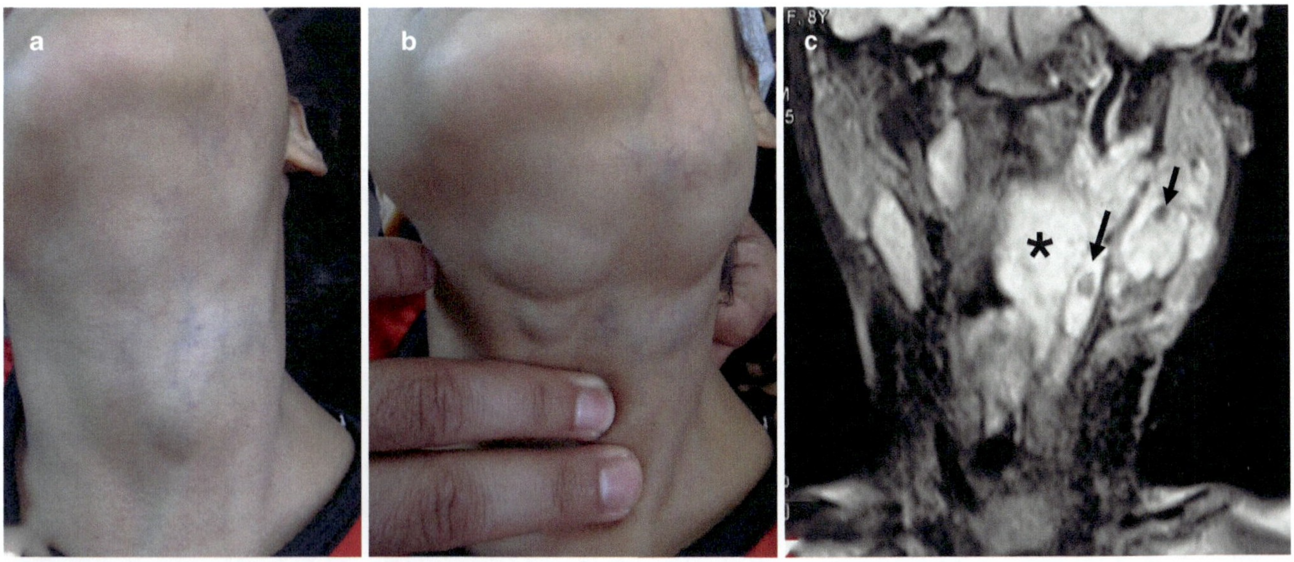

Fig. 13.5 Venous malformation (VM) in the neck of an 8-year-old girl. (**a**, **b**) Clinical photograph showing distension with compression at the root of the neck. (**c**) Coronal STIR MRI demonstrating a trans-spatial hyperintense lesion (asterisk) with multiple phleboliths (arrows)

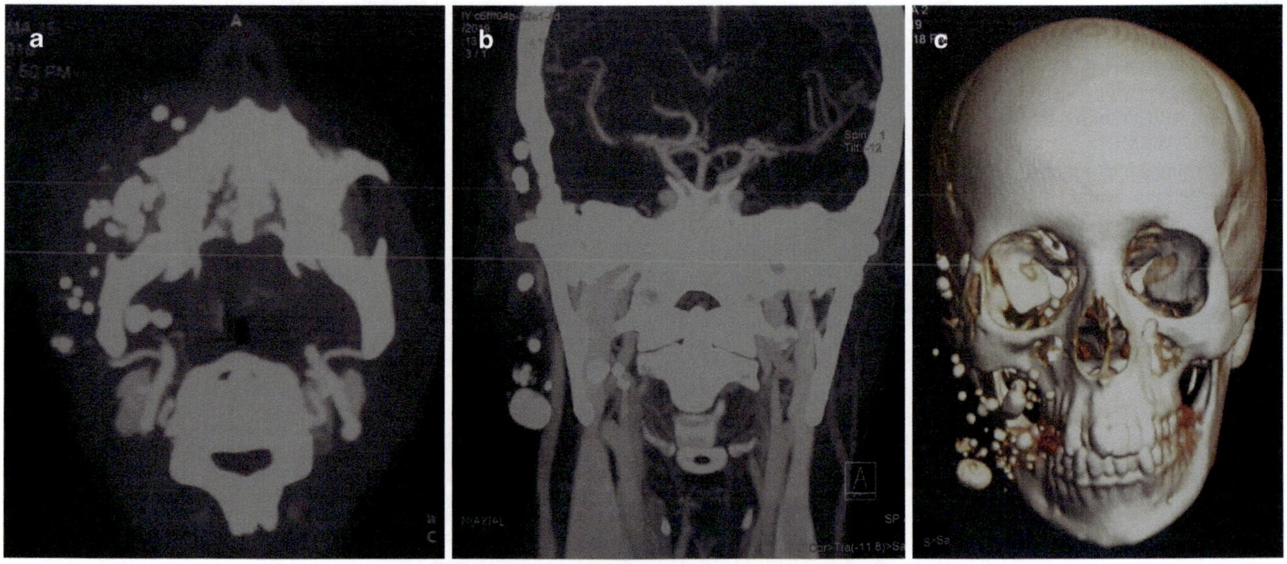

Fig. 13.6 Phleboliths in a venous malformation in a 20-year-old female. Contrast-enhanced CT in axial (**a**) and coronal (**b**) bone window views, along with 3D reconstruction (**c**), demonstrate multiple rounded calcifications (phleboliths) distributed within the lesion

Fig. 13.7 Facial venous malformations (VMs) involving the cheeks and lips, producing facial asymmetry. (**a–c**) Three different patient cases are shown

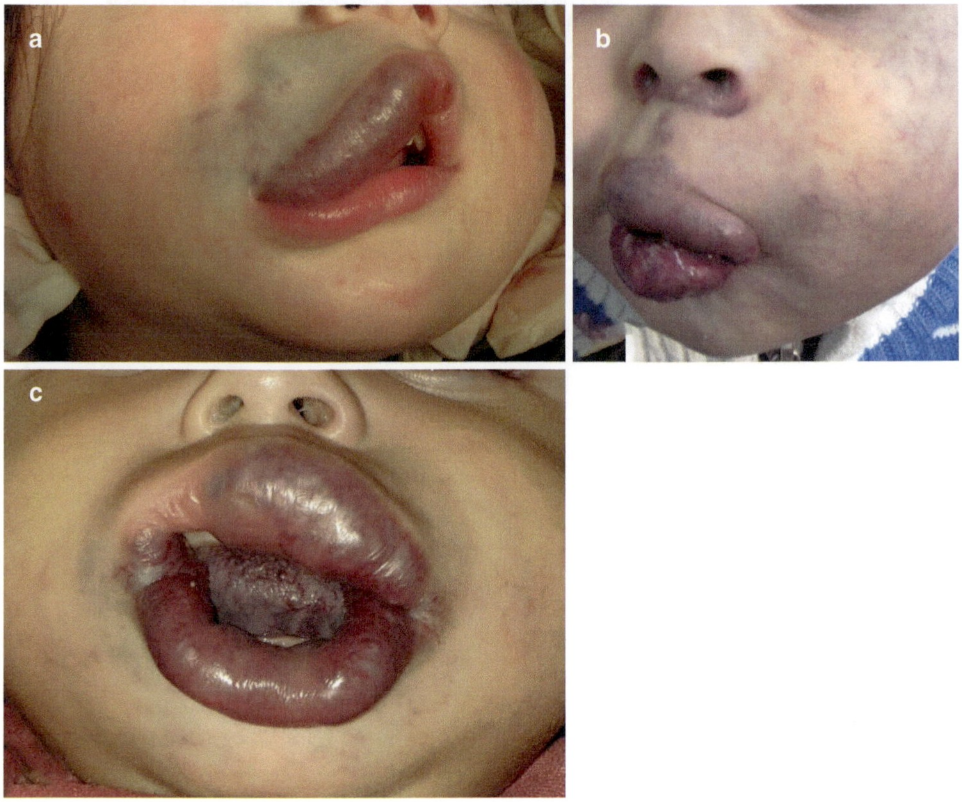

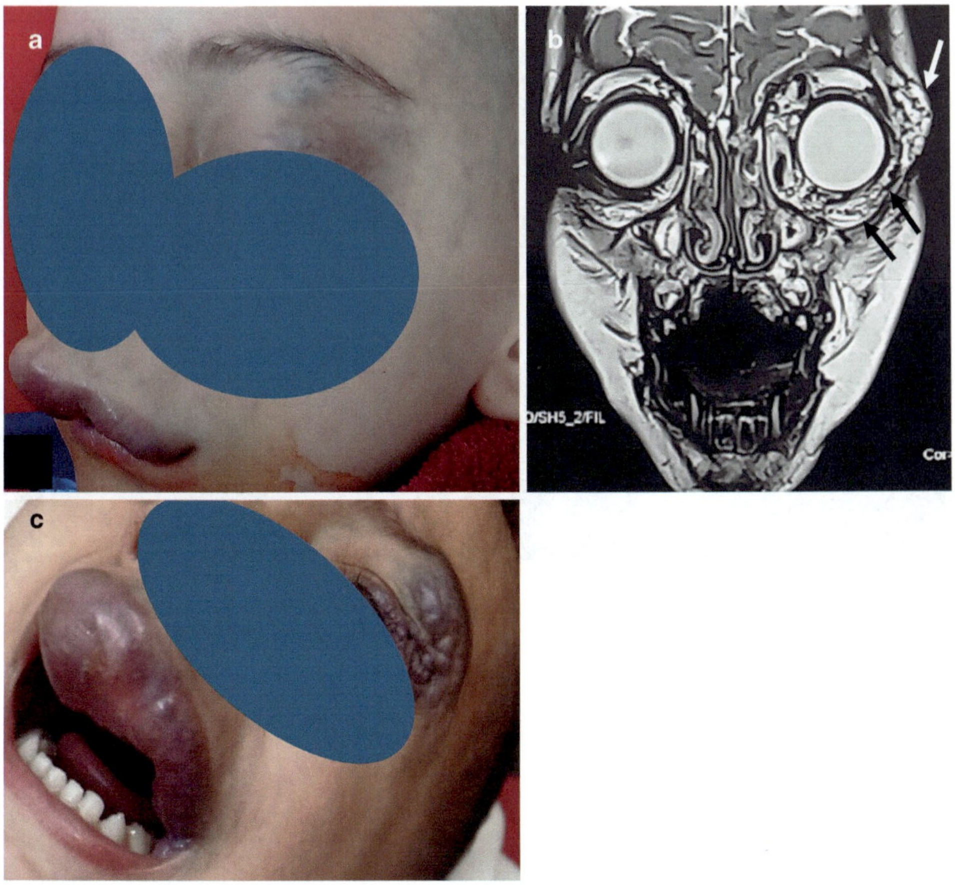

Fig. 13.8 Venous malformation (VM) in a 3-year-old boy. (**a**, **c**) Clinical photographs showing distension with straining. (**b**) Coronal T2-WI MRI demonstrating a hyperintense lesion with trans-spatial extension into the orbit (arrows)

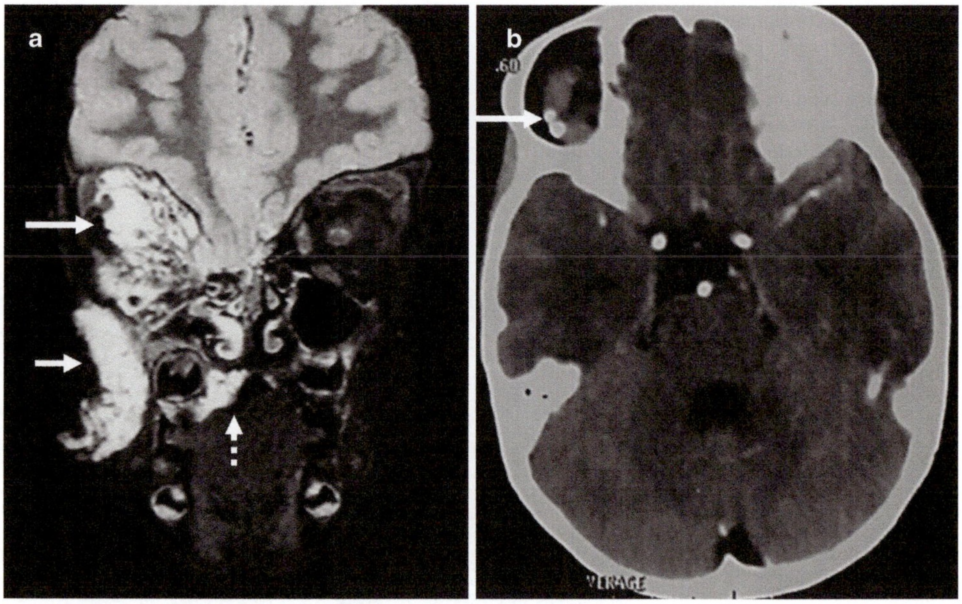

Fig. 13.9 Venous malformation demonstrating hyperintense signal on MRI STIR (**a**) with trans-spatial extension into the right cheek (short arrow), orbit (long arrow), and hard palate (dashed arrow). Axial CT (**b**) reveals a calcified phlebolith (arrow)

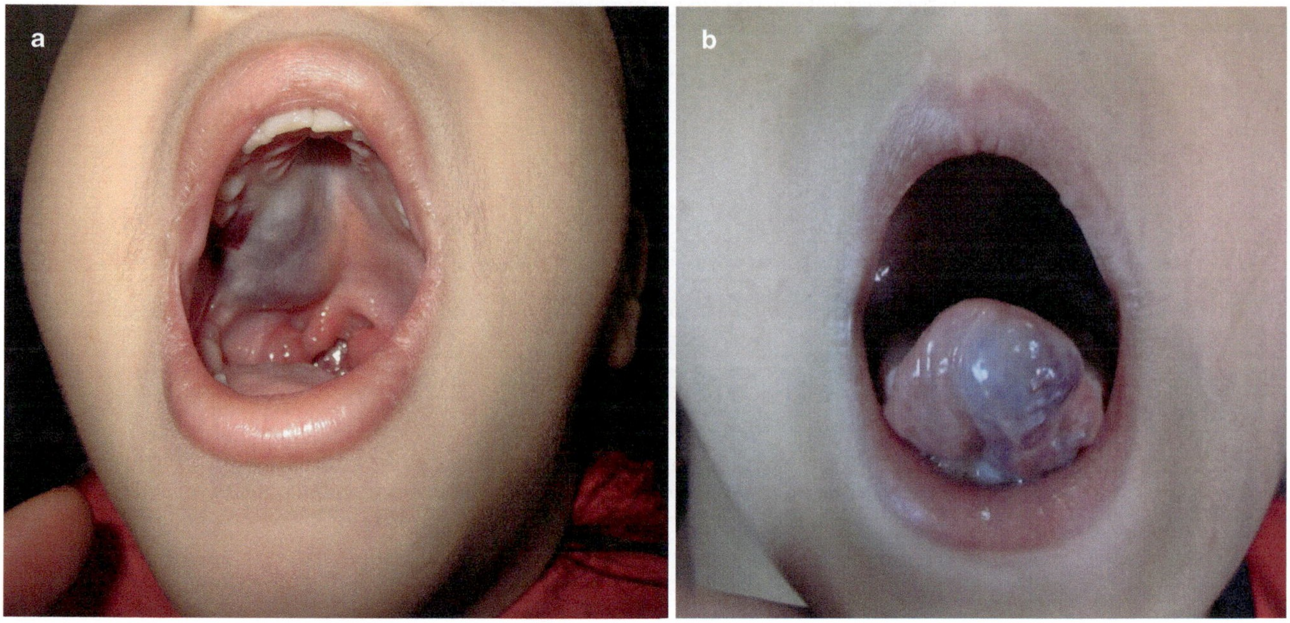

Fig. 13.10 Venous malformation involving the mucosa of the palate (**a**) and tongue (**b**)

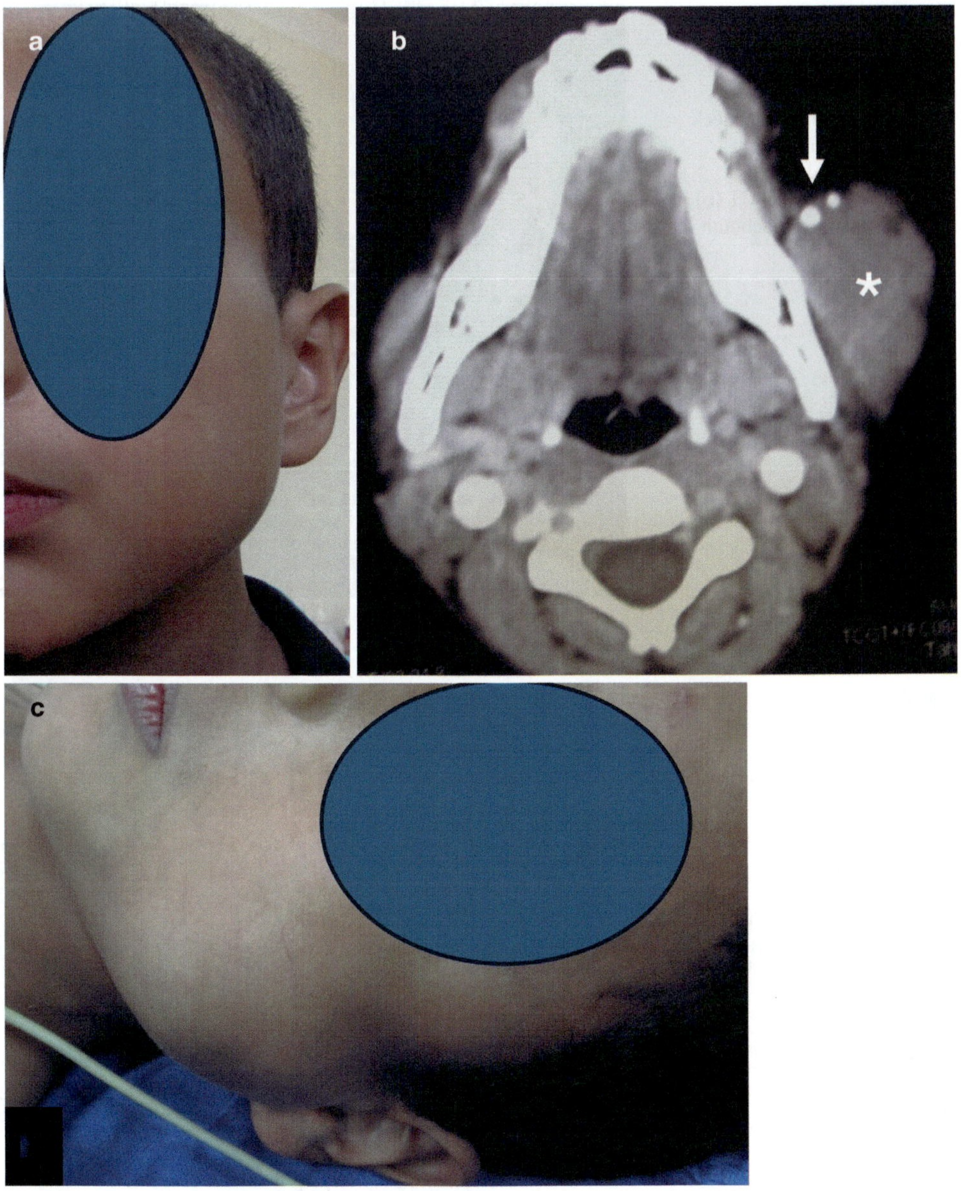

Fig. 13.11 (**a**) Intramuscular venous malformation of the left masseter in a 13-year-old boy. (**b**) Axial contrast-enhanced CT shows a hypo-enhancing lesion (asterisk) with phleboliths (arrow). (**c**) Swelling becomes distended with dependency

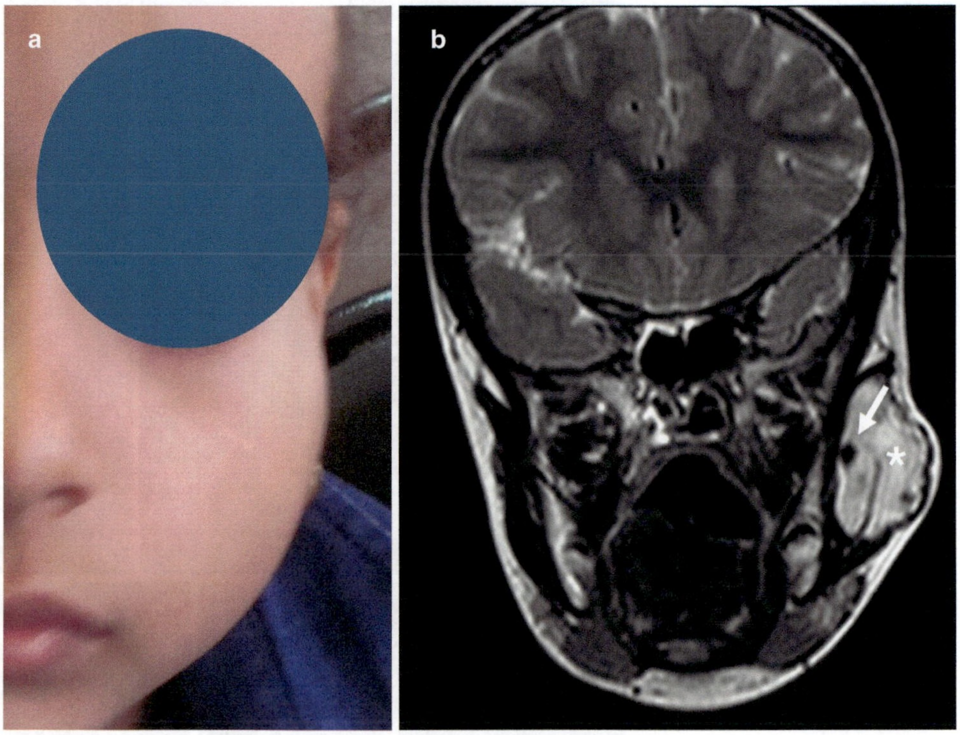

Fig. 13.12 (**a**) Intramuscular venous malformation of the left masseter in a 13-year-old girl. (**b**) Coronal T2-WI MRI shows a hyperintense lesion (asterisk) within the left masseter containing phleboliths (arrow)

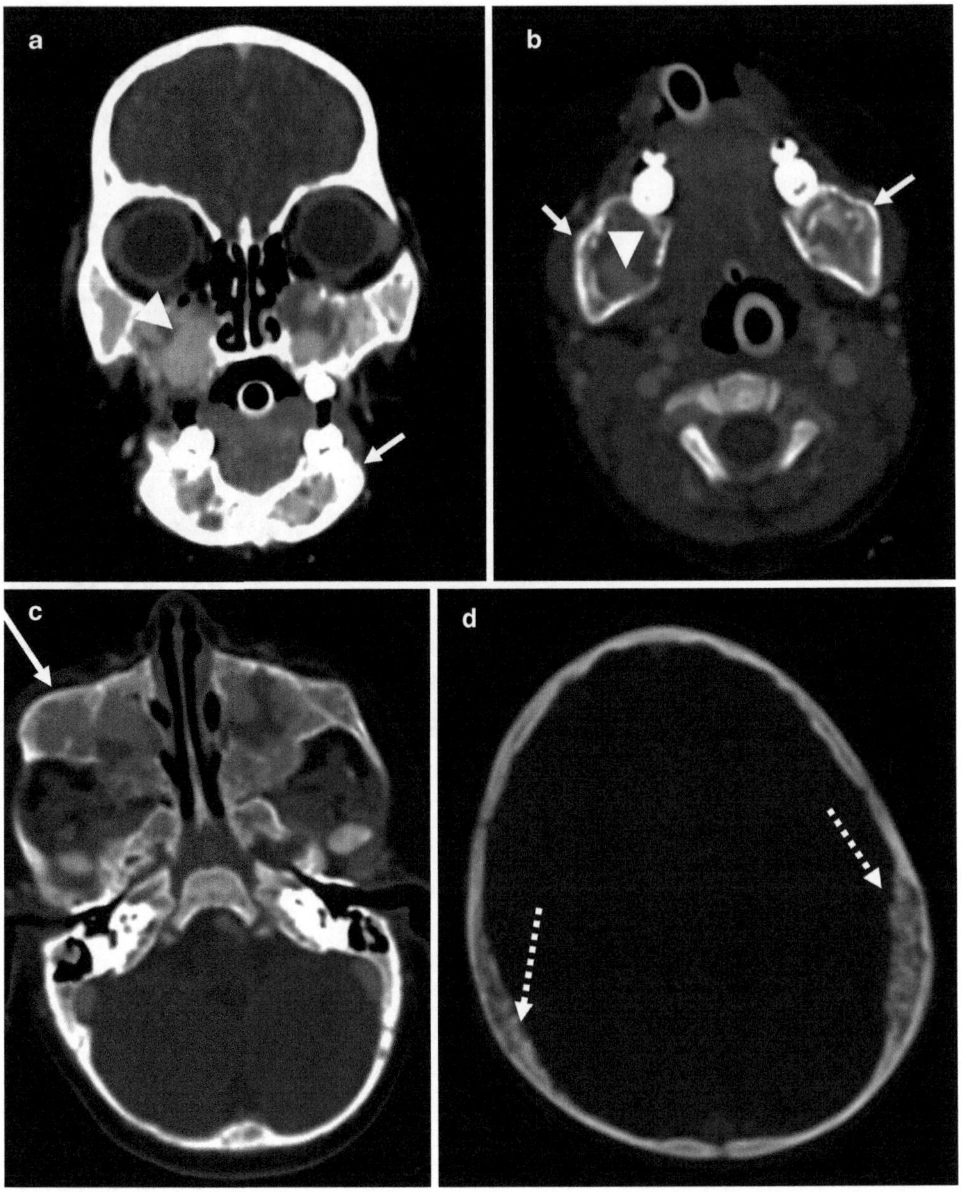

Fig. 13.13 Intra-osseous venous malformation in a two-year-old girl. Contrast-enhanced CT in coronal (**a**) and axial (**b–d**) sections demonstrates venous malformations causing osseous expansion in the mandible (short arrows), zygomatic bone (long arrow), and parietal bones of the skull (dashed arrows). Enhancing venous lakes are also observed (arrowheads)

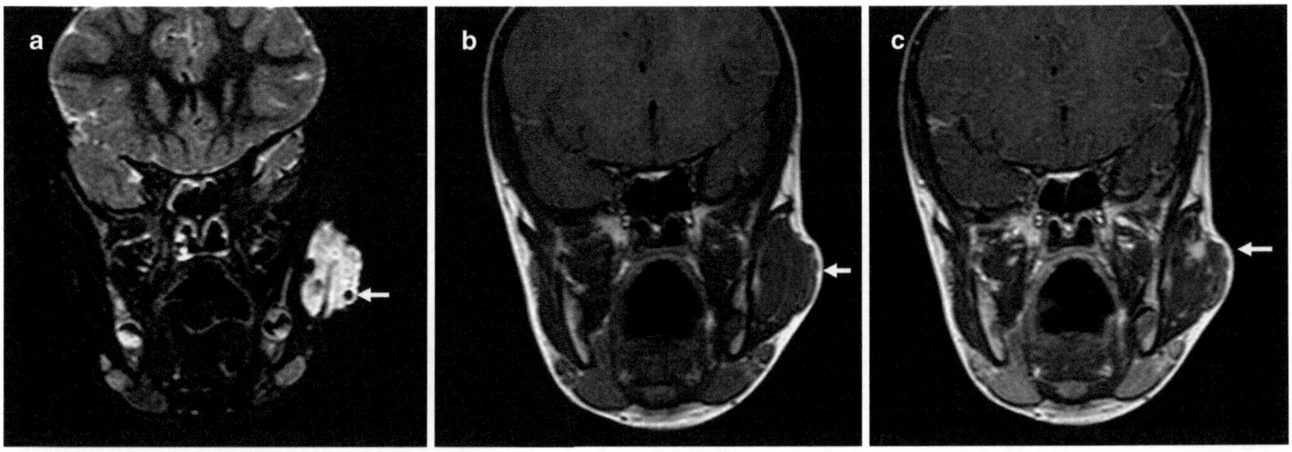

Fig. 13.14 MRI of venous malformation in the left masseter muscle. (**a**) Fat-suppressed STIR image shows a hyperintense lesion with phleboliths (arrow). (**b**) T1-WI shows hypointense signal. (**c**) Post-contrast T1-WI demonstrates faint patchy enhancement

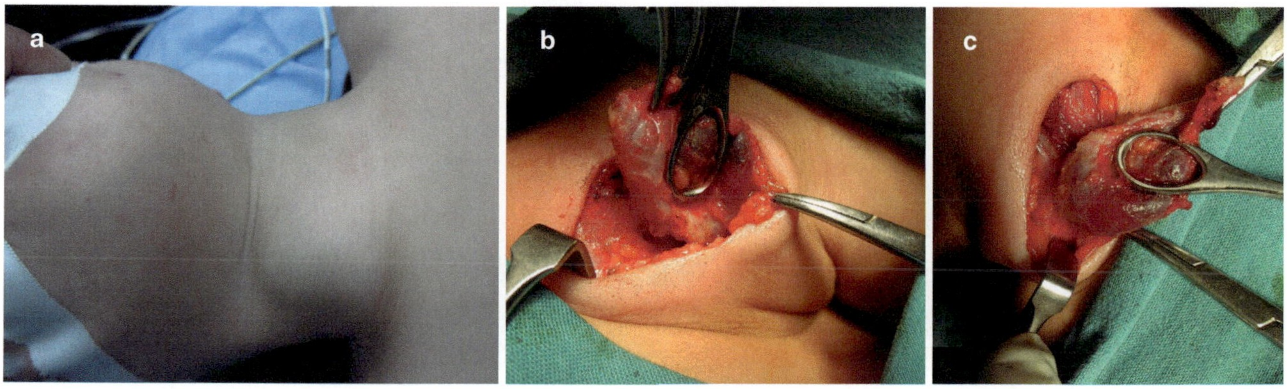

Fig. 13.15 Localized venous malformation in the neck (**a**), surgically excised (**b**, **c**)

References

1. Flors L, Hagspiel KD, Park AW, Norton PT, Leiva-Salinas C. Vascular malformations and tumors. Part 2: Low-flow lesions. Radiologia (English edition). 2019;61:124–33.
2. Gokani VJ, Sivakumar B, Kangesu L. Vascular anomalies. Surgery (Oxford). 2018;36:314–23.
3. Burrows PE. Percutaneous treatment of slow-flow vascular malformations. In: Mulliken JB, Burrows PE, Fishman SJ, editors. Mulliken & Young's vascular anomalies: Hemangiomas and malformations. Oxford University Press; 2013. p. 661–709.
4. Fishman SJ, Young AE. Clinical assessment of vascular malformations. In: Mulliken JB, Burrows PE, Fishman SJ, editors. Mulliken & Young's vascular anomalies: Hemangiomas and malformations. Oxford University Press; 2013. p. 376–91.
5. Fishman SJ, Young AE. Slow-flow vascular malformations. In: Mulliken JB, Burrows PE, Fishman SJ, editors. Mulliken & Young's vascular anomalies: Hemangiomas and malformations. Oxford University Press; 2013. p. 562–94.
6. Mulliken JB. Vascular malformations of the head and neck. In: Mulliken JB, Burrows PE, Fishman SJ, editors. Mulliken & Young's vascular anomalies: Hemangiomas and malformations. Oxford University Press; 2013. p. 839–904.
7. Bly RA, Shivaram G, Monroe EJ. Venous malformation. In: Perkins JA, Balakrishnan K, editors. Evidence-based management of head and neck vascular anomalies. Springer Nature Switzerland; 2018. p. 171–8.
8. Burrows PE. Venous malformation of the head and neck and extremities. In: Kim YW, Lee BB, Yakes WF, Do YS, editors. Congenital vascular malformations. Springer-Verlag Berlin Heidelberg; 2017. p. 83–90.
9. Mamlouk MD, Nicholson AD, Cooke DL, Hess CP. Tips and tricks to optimize MRI protocols for cutaneous vascular anomalies. Clin Imaging. 2017;45:71–80.
10. Mohammad SA, AA AZ, Fawzi AM, et al. Magnetic resonance imaging of head and neck vascular anomalies: pearls and pitfalls. Ann Pediatr Surg. 2017;13:116–24.
11. Puig S, Aref H, Chigot V, et al. Classification of venous malformations in children and implications for sclerotherapy. Pediatr Radiol. 2003;33:99.
12. Claudon M, Upton J, Burrows PE. Diffuse venous malformations of the upper limb: morphologic characterization by MRI and venography. Pediatr Radiol. 2001;31:507.
13. Adams DM. Practical Genetic and Biologic Therapeutic Considerations in Vascular Anomalies. Tech Vasc Interv Rad. 2019;22:Article 100629.
14. Bjur KA, Payne ET, Nemergut ME, Hu D, Flick RP. Anesthetic-related neurotoxicity and neuroimaging in children: a call for conversation. J Child Neurol. 2017;32(6):594–602.
15. Yakes WF, Haas DK, Parker SH, et al. Symptomatic vascular malformations: ethanol embolotherapy. Radiology. 1989;170:1059.

Venous Malformations of the Extremities

14

Introduction

Venous malformations (VMs) are the most common vascular anomaly affecting the extremities [1]. VMs are formed of dilated, thin-walled vascular channels with patchy deficiency of smooth muscle and elastic tissue, which contributes to their slow, progressive enlargement [2, 3]. Lesions typically exhibit engorgement when dependent and decompress upon elevation (Fig. 14.1). Their color ranges in various shades of blue, influenced by the lesion's depth beneath the skin [1]. Besides their prominent subcutaneous presentation, VMs of the extremities often involve deeper compartments, affecting muscles, nerves, and joints (Fig. 14.2) [1]. Phleboliths are a hallmark feature of VMs, which represent calcified thrombi within the lesion. They may be palpable within the lesion or visible on plain radiographs (Fig. 14.3) [4]. Extensive lesions may be associated with localized intravascular coagulopathy (Fig. 14.4). The latter is characterized by consumption of clotting factors manifested by reduced fibrinogen levels and elevated D-dimer concentrations [5, 6]; platelet counts usually remain within normal limits [1].

A. A. AbouZeid et al., *Atlas of Pediatric Vascular Anomalies*, https://doi.org/10.1007/978-3-032-30866-5_14

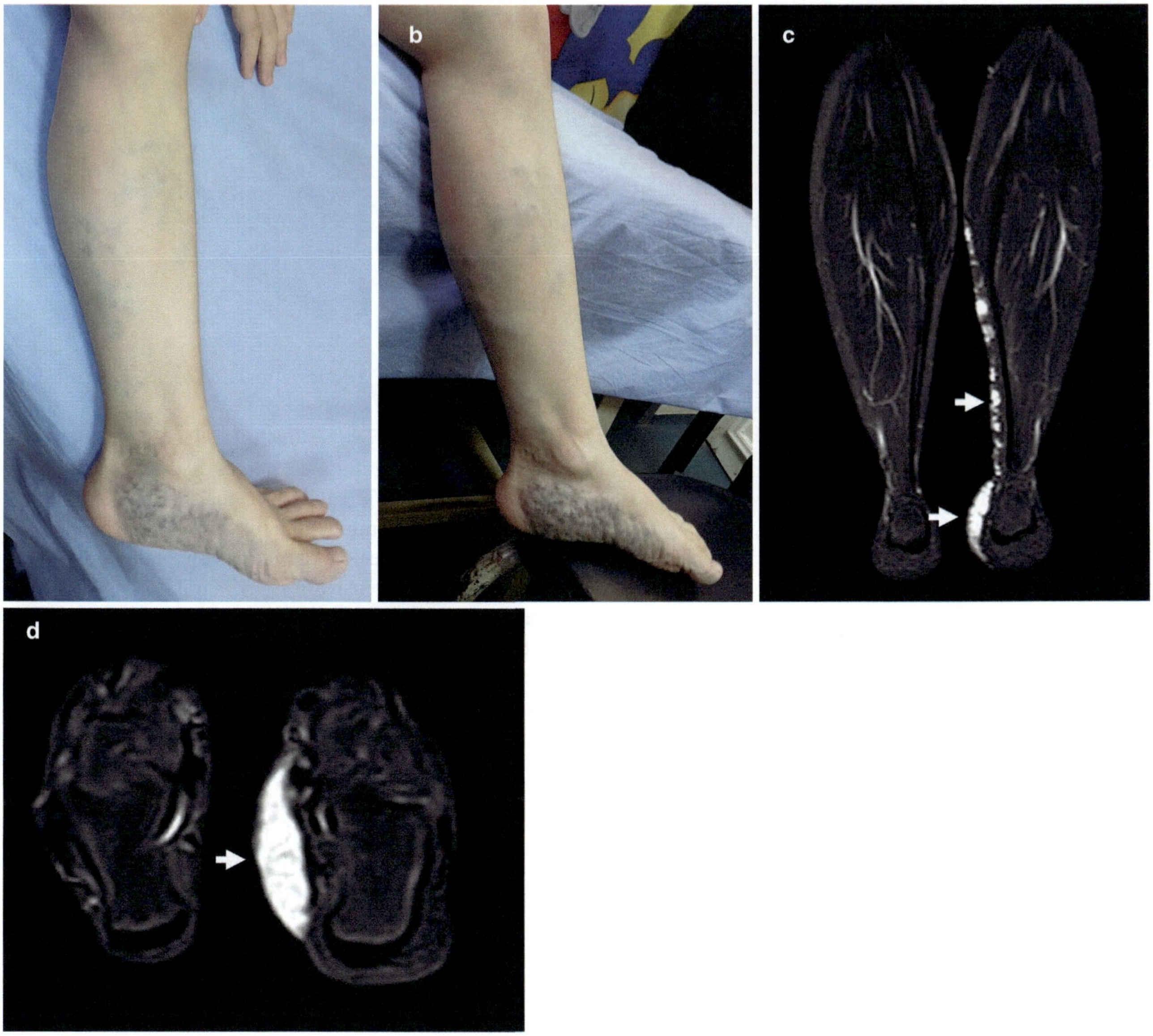

Fig. 14.1 (**a**) Venous malformation of the leg and foot, which becomes engorged in the dependent position (**b**). (**c**, **d**) MRI of the leg and foot (coronal and axial STIR sequences, respectively) demonstrates the venous malformation as a hyperintense lesion (arrows)

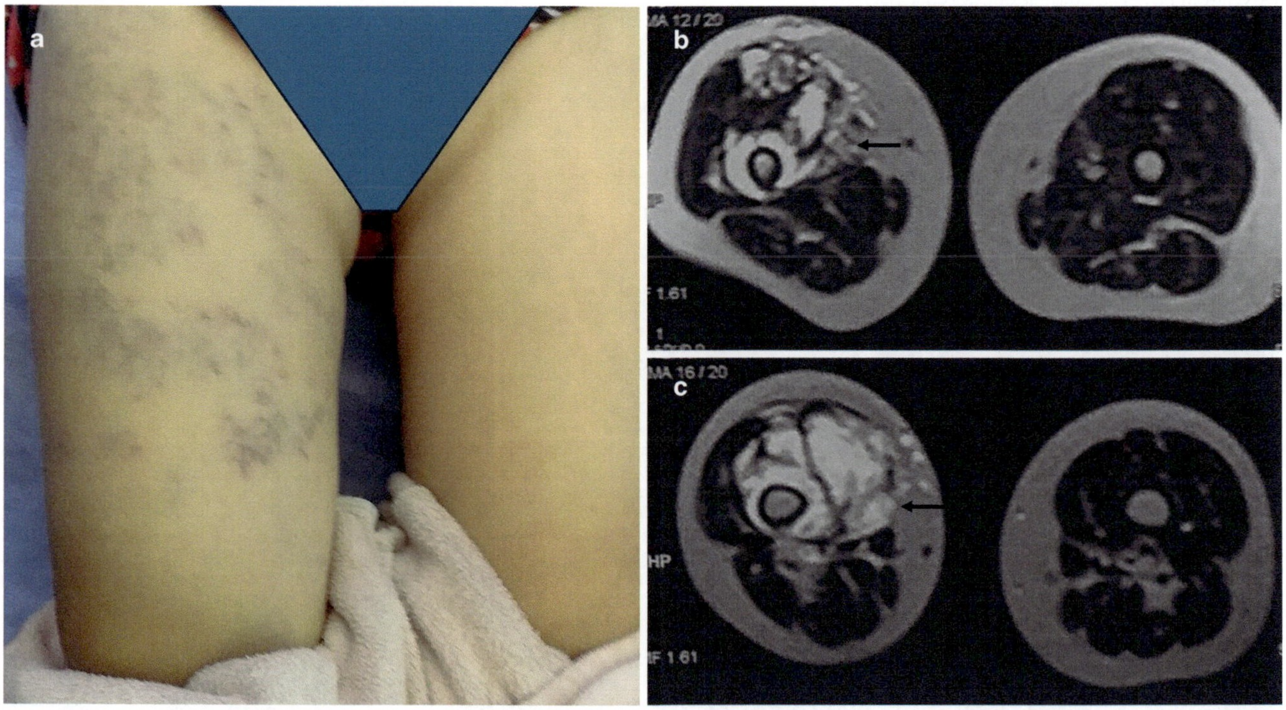

Fig. 14.2 Venous malformation of the right thigh in a 3-year-old girl. (**a**) Clinical photograph showing superficial lesions. (**b**, **c**) Axial T2-weighted MRI images reveal deeper extension of the malformation into the intramuscular compartment (arrow)

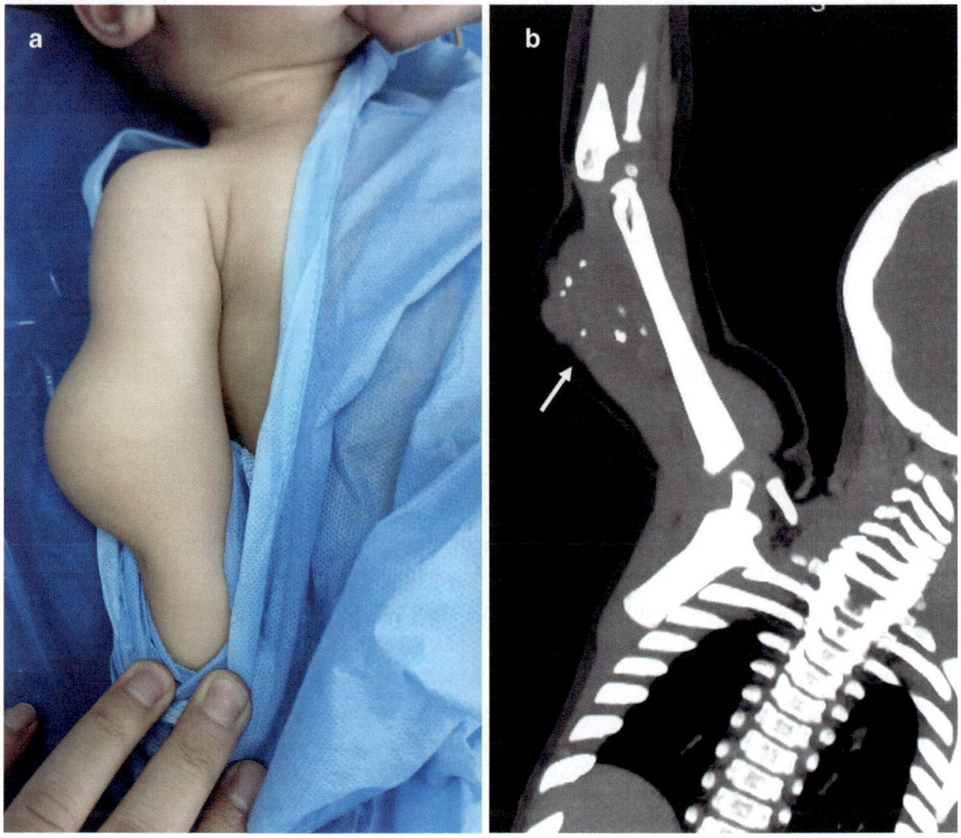

Fig. 14.3 (**a**) Venous malformation of the right arm in a 7-month-old boy. (**b**) Maximum intensity projection of non-contrast CT demonstrates characteristic phleboliths within the lesion (arrow)

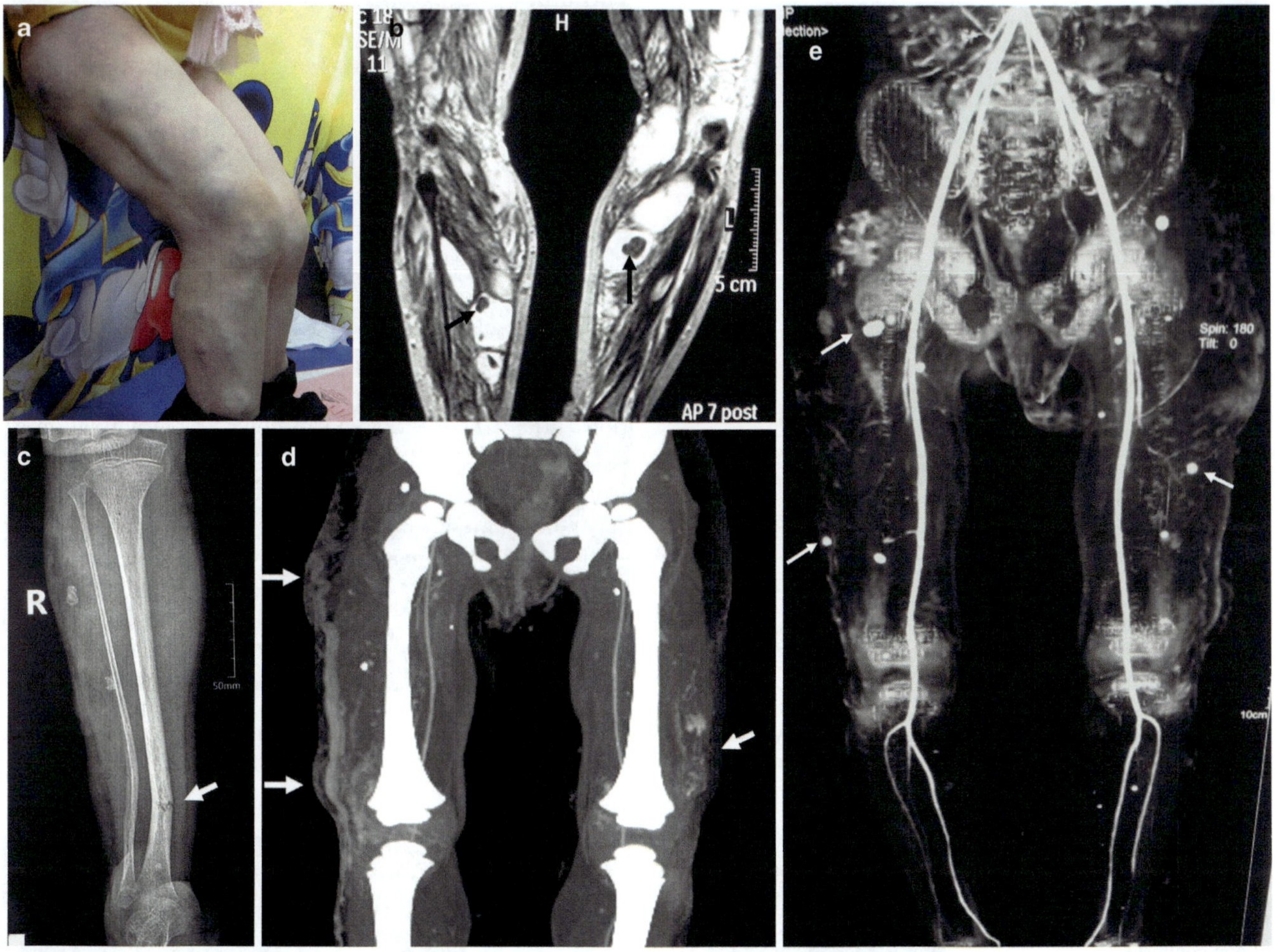

Fig. 14.4 Venous malformation of both lower limbs in a 5-year-old girl. (**a**) Clinical photograph. (**b**) Coronal T2-weighted MRI shows trans-spatial hyperintense lesions involving the muscles with phleboliths (arrows). (**c**) Plain X-ray of the right leg demonstrates overtubulation of the tibia and fibula with bowing and fracture (arrow). (**d**) Coronal contrast-enhanced CT in the venous phase shows delayed enhancement of the malformation (arrows). (**e**) Maximum intensity projection of contrast-enhanced CT in the arterial phase also demonstrates phleboliths (arrows)

Clinical Presentation

All VMs are present at birth; however, they may not be obvious except later in life especially when small or deep. VMs of the extremities vary in size and location, potentially affecting any region of the limb from proximal to distal up to fingers and toes (Fig. 14.5). VMs may be asymptomatic; however, functional impairment is often related to the lesion's size, weight, and anatomical location (Figs. 14.6 and 14.7) [1]. Pain and paresthesia are not uncommon with VMs, which may be explained by local inflammation around intralesional thrombi or nerve compression usually accompanying lesions located near joints such as elbows or knees (Fig. 14.8). Symptoms are usually aggravated following physical activity [4–6]. Extremity VMs involving synovial components are prone to spontaneous bleeding, hemarthrosis, and progressive hemosiderin-induced arthropathy (Fig. 14.9). Early prophylactic treatment with combined intralesional sclerotherapy and synovial resection may help prevent these complications [5, 6].

Occasionally, VMs occurring within and around the muscles of an extremity may be exceptionally painful progressing to contractures and deformity (Fig. 14.10). This presentation is now recognized as Fibroadipose Vascular Anomaly (FAVA) [5, 7]. Such lesions typically show poor response to conventional therapies and sclerotherapy, often requiring alternative treatment strategies. Oral sirolimus or alpelisib serves as an important therapeutic option for managing unresectable lesions with significant nerve involvement [7, 8].

Genuine diffuse phlebectasia of Bockenheimer is an eponym referring to extensive venous malformation affecting most of the length of an extremity (Fig. 14.11). Disuse skeletal atrophy and weakness has been described with this condition, which may lead to pathological fracture (Fig. 14.12) [1, 5]. The condition may be confused with Klippel-Traunanay syndrome; the latter is a different entity being a combined capillary veno-lymphatic malformation with tissue overgrowth (see Chap. 20).

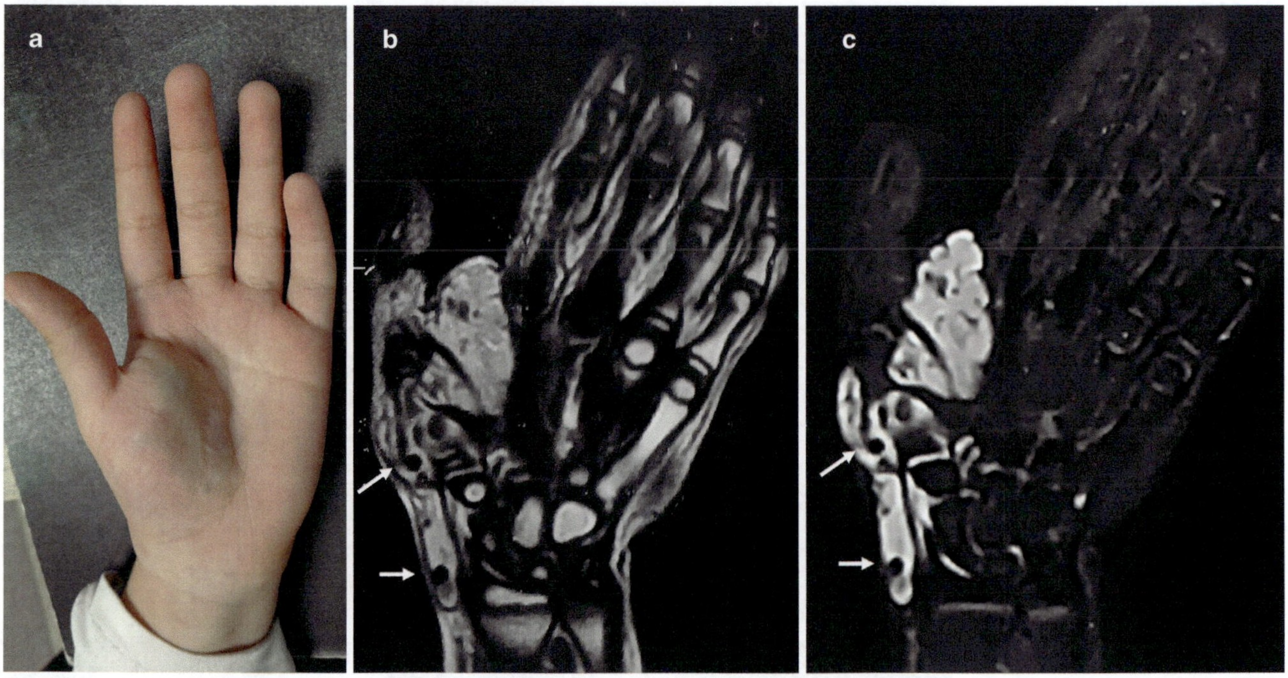

Fig. 14.5 (**a**) Venous malformation involving the hand (thenar eminence). (**b**) Axial MRI (T2-weighted image) showing the lesion with phleboliths (arrows). (**c**) MRI (T2-weighted fat-suppressed sequence) clearly demonstrating the lesion extension which appears hyperintense

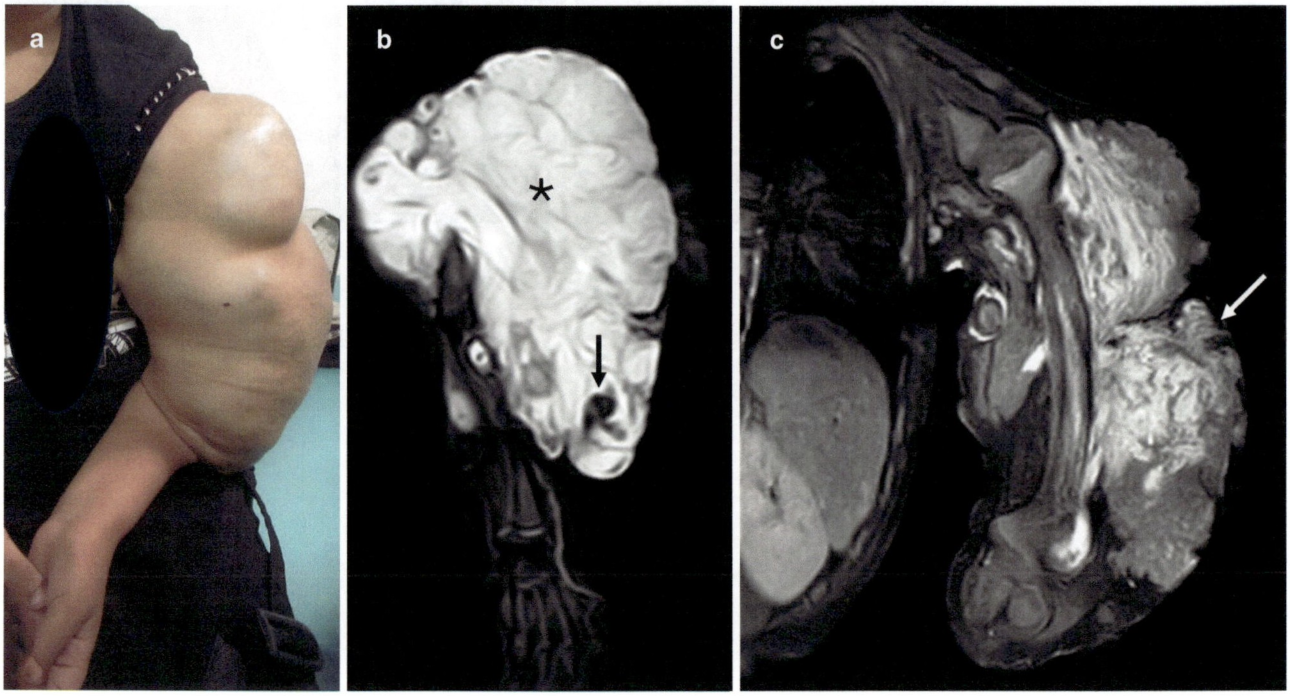

Fig. 14.6 (**a**) Extensive venous malformation involving the left arm of a 9-year-old boy. (**b**) Coronal STIR MRI showing an extensive hyperintense lesion (asterisk) with multiple phleboliths (black arrow). (**c**) Coronal contrast-enhanced T1-weighted MRI demonstrating the typical delayed, patchy enhancement pattern of the lesion (white arrow)

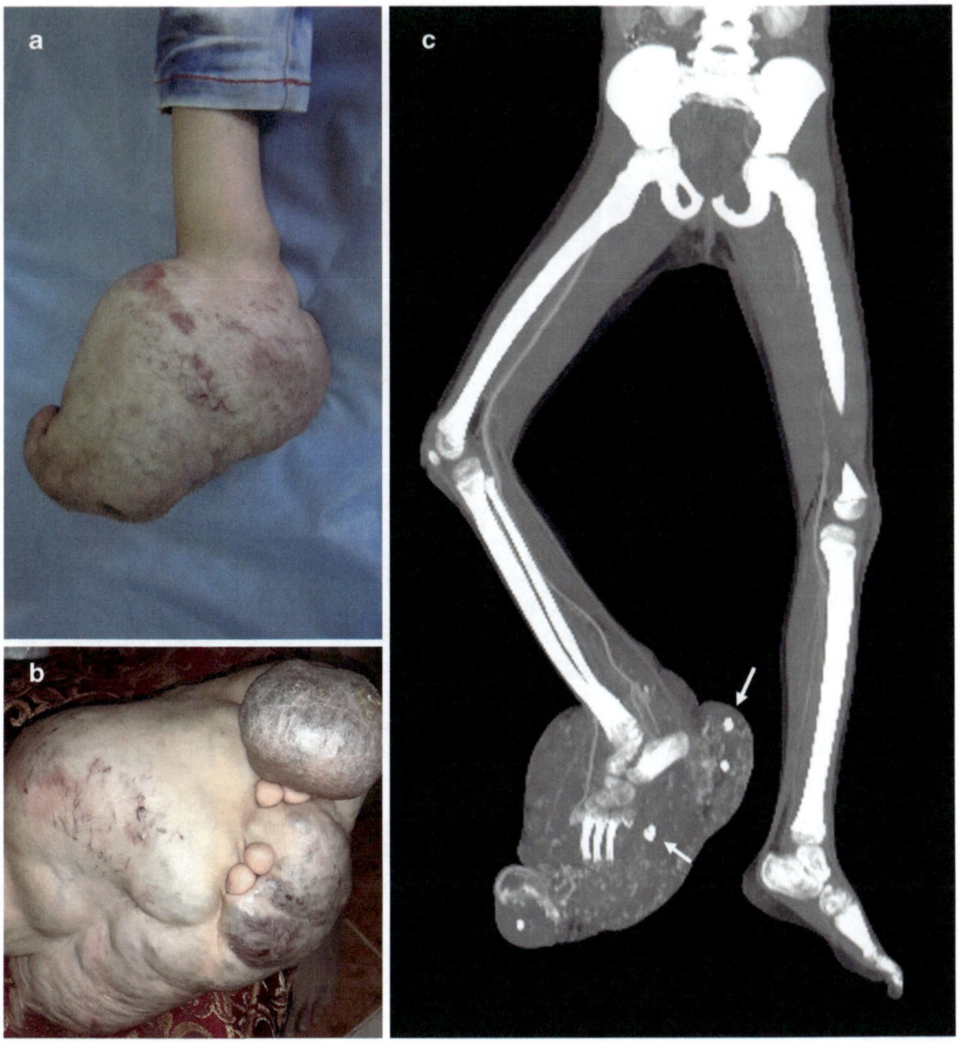

Fig. 14.7 (**a**, **b**) Extensive venous malformation of the foot in a 6-year-old boy. (**c**) Maximum intensity projection (MIP) CT of the lower extremities showing characteristic phleboliths within the lesion (arrows)

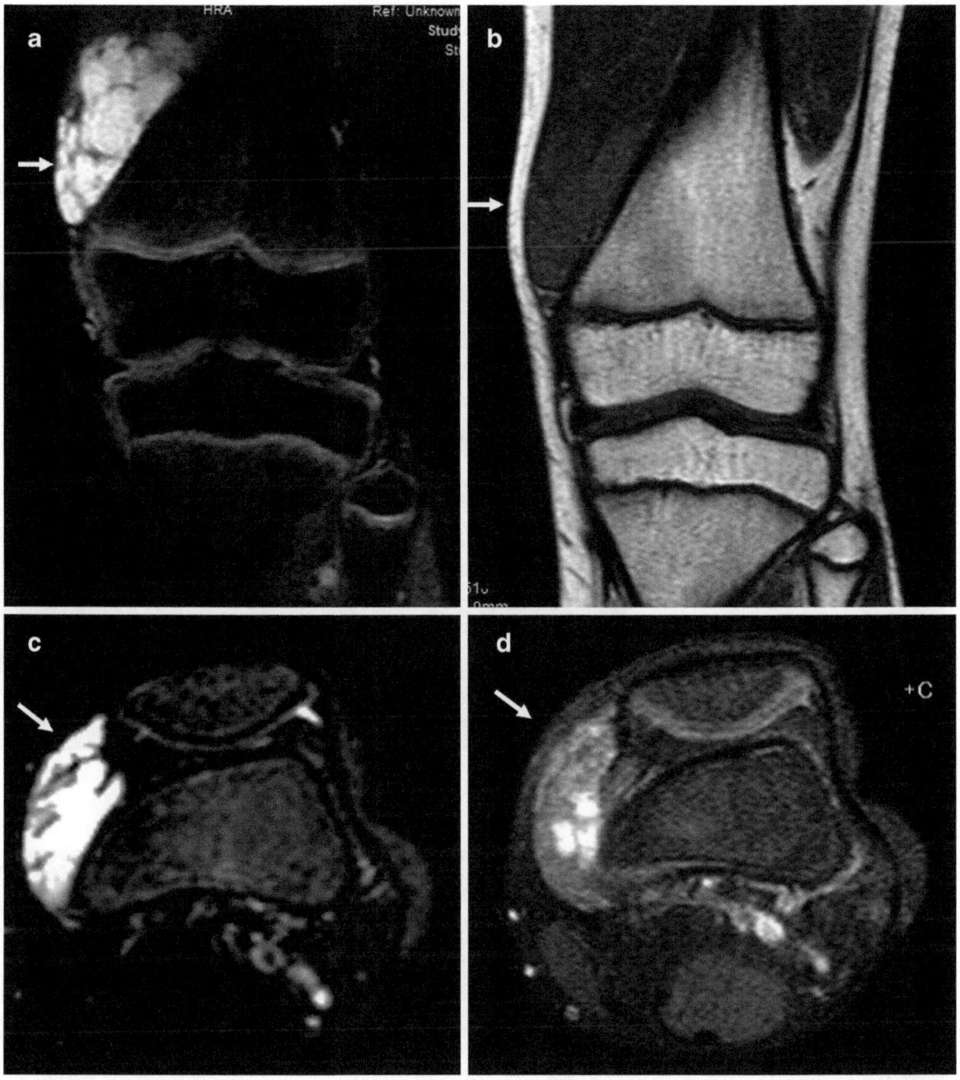

Fig. 14.8 MRI of venous malformation (arrow) adjacent to the knee joint without intra-articular extension. Coronal (**a**, **b**) and axial sections (**b**, **d**) demonstrate intramuscular venous malformation exhibiting hyperintense signal on STIR (**a**, **c**), intermediate signal on T1-WI (**b**), and with patchy contrast enhancement (**d**)

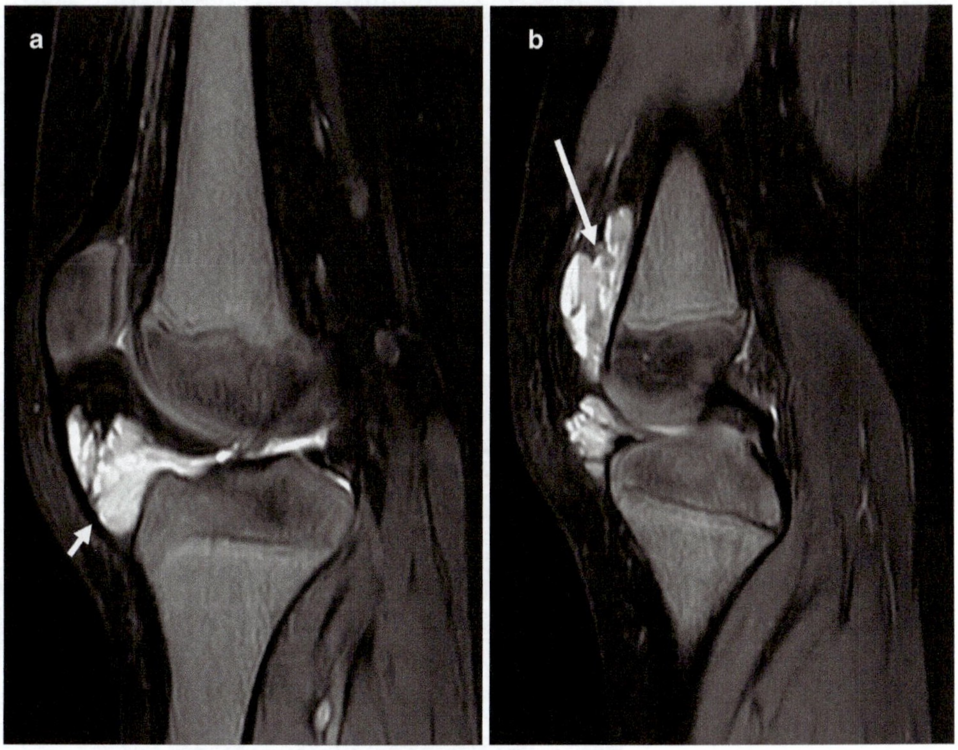

Fig. 14.9 MRI of intra-articular venous malformation in the knee joint. (**a**) Sagittal STIR MRI showing the intra-articular lesion (short arrow). (**b**) Sagittal STIR MRI demonstrating fluid–fluid levels within the lesion (long arrow)

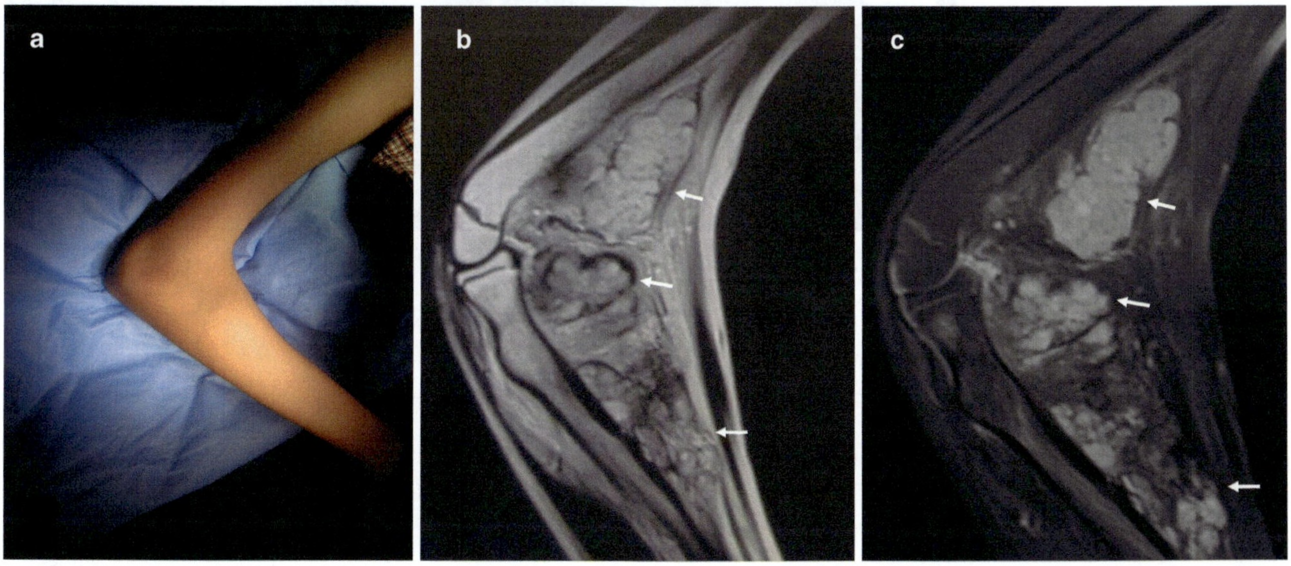

Fig. 14.10 Venous malformation at the right elbow of a 13-year-old girl, associated with contracture and disuse atrophy due to long-standing undiagnosed pain. (**a**) Clinical photograph. (**b**) Sagittal T2-weighted STIR MRI showing intramuscular venous malformation (arrows). (**c**) Sagittal contrast-enhanced fat-suppressed T1-weighted MRI demonstrating post-contrast enhancement of the lesions (arrows)

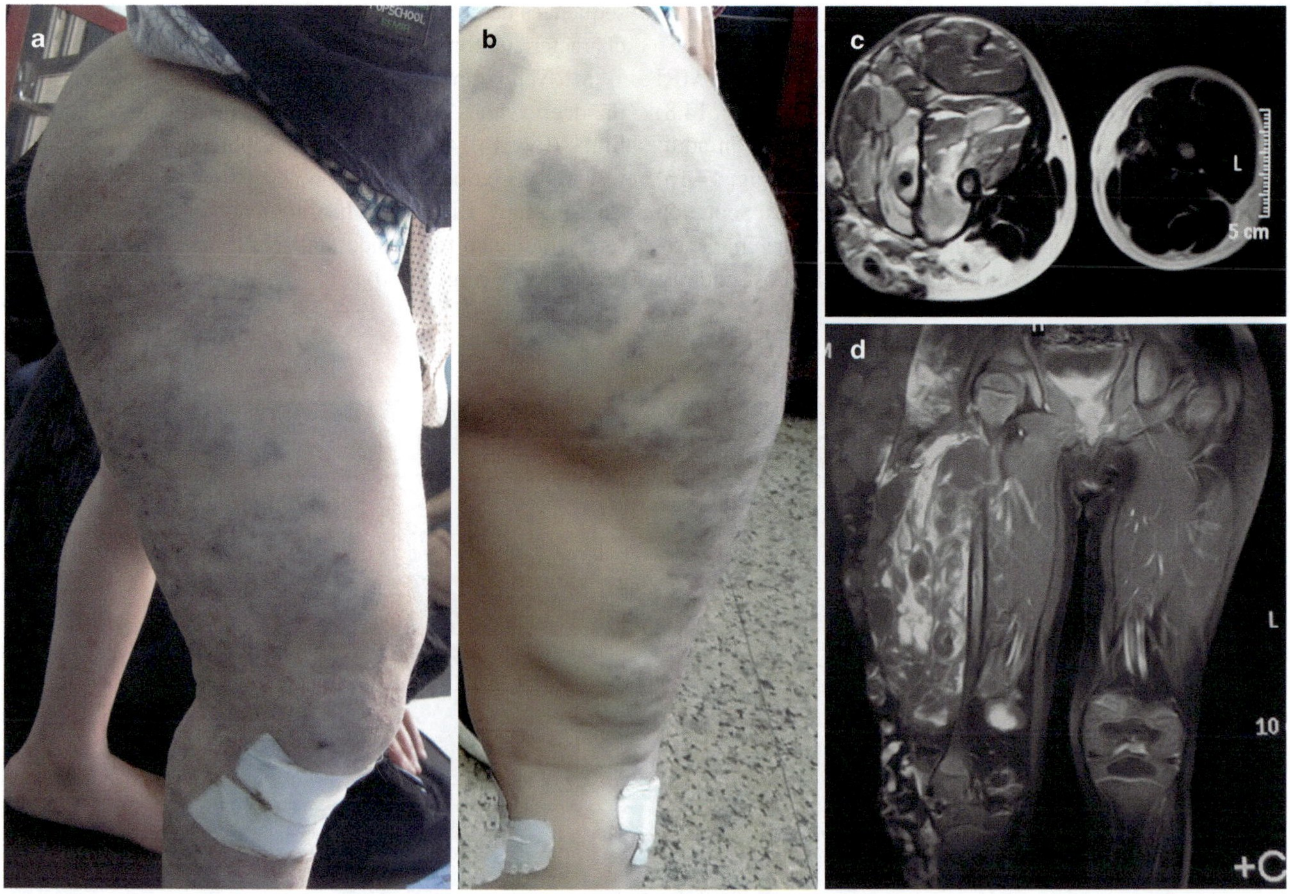

Fig. 14.11 Extensive venous malformation of the left lower limb. (**a**, **b**) Clinical photographs in lateral and posterior views, respectively. (**c**) Axial T2-weighted MRI demonstrates a trans-spatial lesion involving the skin, subcutaneous tissue, and muscles, showing fluid–fluid levels and phlebolith (arrow). (**d**) Coronal fat-suppressed contrast-enhanced T1-weighted MRI shows patchy enhancement

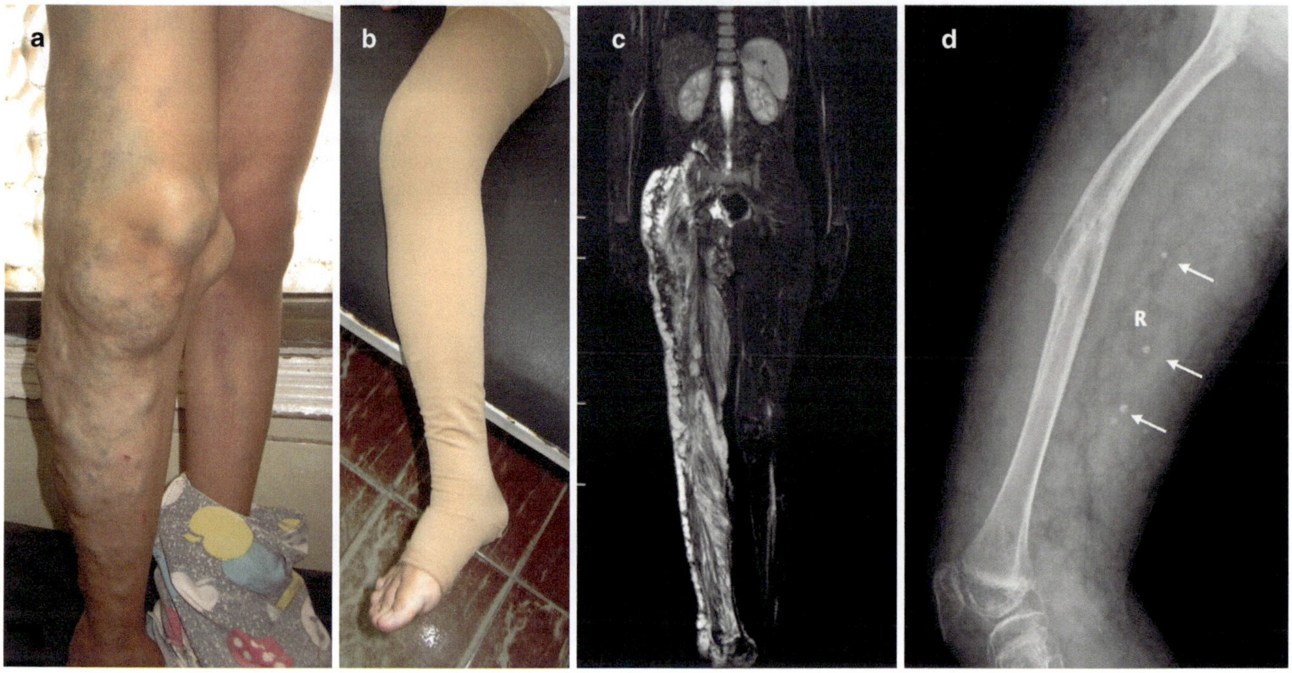

Fig. 14.12 (**a**) Extensive venous malformation (VM) of the right lower limb in a 9-year-old girl. (**b**) Ready-made compression garment used to control enlargement of VM. (**c**) Coronal STIR MRI demonstrating extensive involvement of the right lower extremity. (**d**) Healed pathological fracture of the femur in the affected limb, with characteristic calcifications/phleboliths visible (arrows)

Investigations

Ultrasound may be sufficient in small lesions; however, MRI is the gold standard for the diagnosis of most VMs (Fig. 14.8) [9, 10]. MRI can determine/confirm the diagnosis, in addition to delineation of the deep extent of lesions (Fig. 14.13) [1]. VMs appear isointense in T1-weighted images. Septation are evident in T2-weighted sequences besides the characteristic signal-voids of phleboliths (Fig. 14.4) [1]. Post-contrast sequences demonstrate gradual heterogeneous enhancement characteristic for VMS (Figs. 14.8 and 14.13) [9, 10].

MR venography is valuable for evaluating the integrity of the deep venous system in patients with diffuse VMs of the limbs (Fig. 14.14). Direct puncture phlebography is usually reserved to be performed at time of treatment by injection sclerotherapy. Biopsy and histological diagnosis of VMs are rarely indicated to exclude malignancy or when imaging in inconclusive (Fig. 14.10) [1].

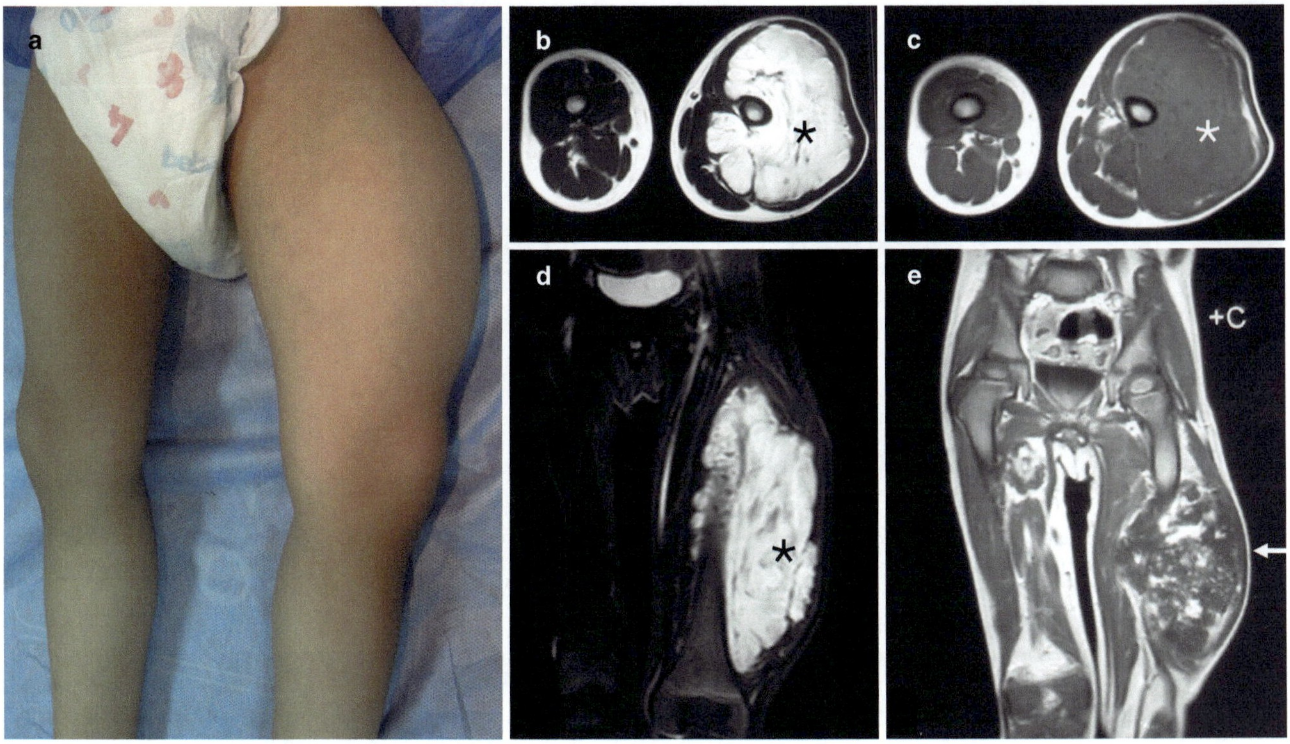

Fig. 14.13 Intramuscular venous malformation of the thigh in a 2-year-old boy. (**a**) Clinical photograph showing swelling of the left thigh. (**b, d**) Axial and coronal T2-weighted MRI demonstrating a hyperintense intramuscular lesion (asterisk). (**c**) Axial non-contrast T1-weighted MRI showing the lesion with intermediate signal intensity (asterisk). (**e**) Coronal contrast-enhanced T1-weighted MRI demonstrating patchy post-contrast enhancement (arrow)

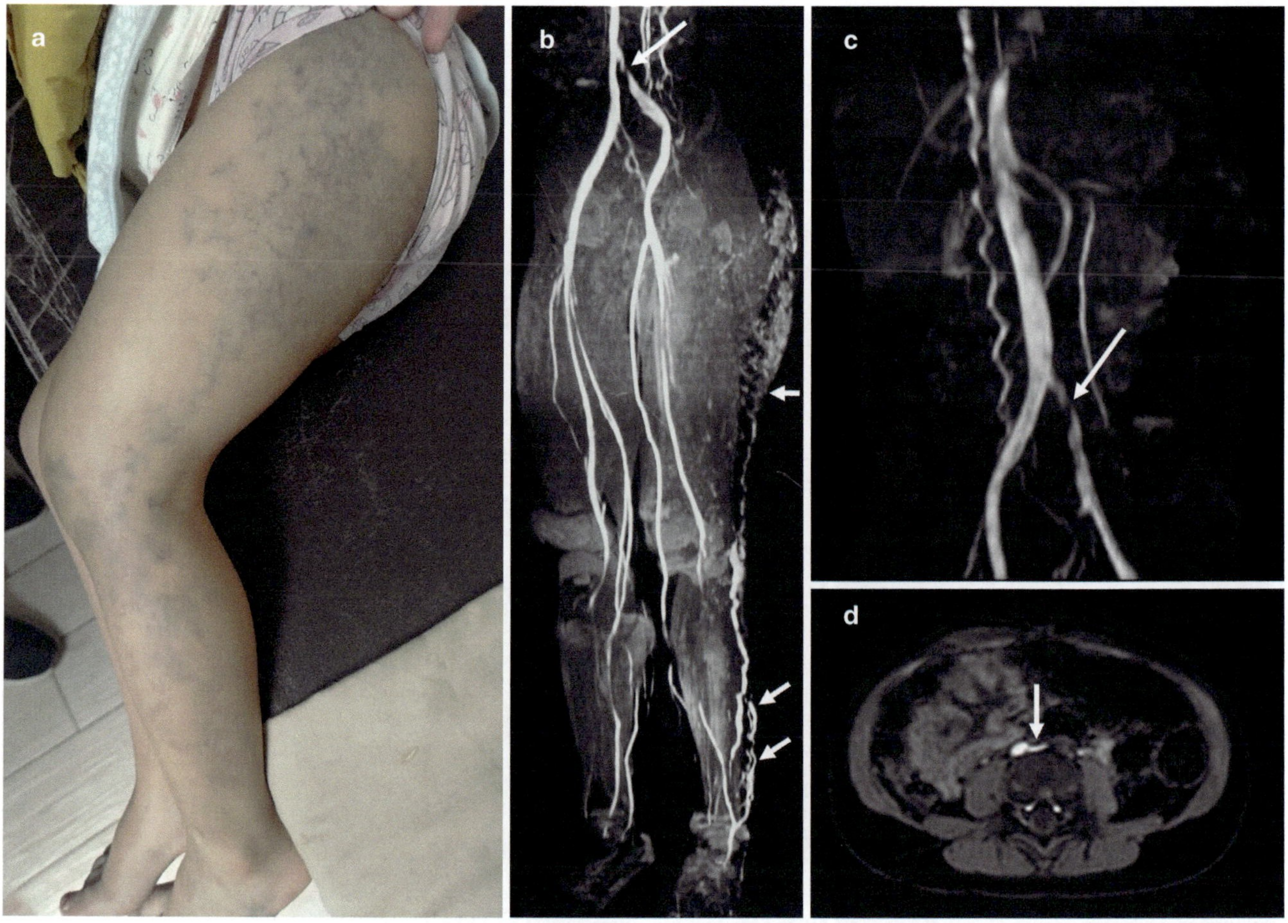

Fig. 14.14 Venous malformation of the left lower limb in a 3-year-old girl with May-Thurner syndrome. (**a**) Clinical photo showing cutaneous lesions. (**b**, **c**) MR venography of lower limb and abdomen showing narrowing of the left common iliac vein (long arrow) where it crosses under the right common iliac artery, plus abnormal veins in the lower limb (short arrows). (**d**) Axial non-contrast MR venography → again shows narrowing of left common iliac vein under right common iliac artery

Treatment

Conservative Management The initial management of all VMs is conservative. Carefully tailored compression garments help to control enlargement of VMs during and after exercise (Fig. 14.12). Daily low-dose aspirin helps to prevent thrombus formation. More definitive anticoagulation and invasive procedures like placement of inferior vena cava filter may be indicated in high-risk groups with large dilated redundant draining veins of the extremities [1]. In complicated and extensive cases, sirolimus (an m-TOR inhibitor) has shown promising symptom relief; however, its role in VMs management is still being actively studied [7, 8, 11].

Sclerotherapy Direct injection of sclerosing agents results in gradual shrinkage of VMs and is considered the primary treatment in most vascular anomaly centers. It has been recommended that patients with low baseline fibrinogen levels be treated with low-molecular weight heparin for 2 weeks prior to sclerotherapy [6]. Diffuse VMs require occlusion of venous outflow prior to sclerosant injection to prevent systemic leakage. Different sclerosing agents can be used. Absolute ethanol is the most potent but with the highest risk of both local and systemic complications. Therefore, ethanol should be used exclusively by skilled and experienced practitioners within a hospital setting equipped with appropriate supportive care facilities [12]. Sodium tetradecyl sulfate (surfactant sclerosant) is most popular for treating VMs, which is commonly injected as microfoam by mixing the sclerosant with air. Bleomycin is associated with least post injection swelling and is the preferred sclerosant for lesions in the hand. Generally, sclerotherapy is not preferred for those with multiple intralesional thromboses, neurologic impairment, and compressive symptoms and signs [6].

Surgery Surgery is indicated after failure of conservative measures and sclerotherapy to control symptoms. Surgery may be also requested for aesthetic reasons (contour deformity). It is important to discuss the risk of operative procedures that may include loss of function and a conspicuous scar. Excision of VMs of the extremities is a challenging task that should be performed by an experienced extremity surgeon. Every effort should be made to decrease blood loss at operation, which includes applying pneumatic tourniquet, hypotensive anesthesia, using cell saver and tissue sealants [1]. Localized subcutaneous lesions can be safely excised, offering a definitive cure and effectively simplifying management (Figs. 14.15, 14.16, and 14.17).

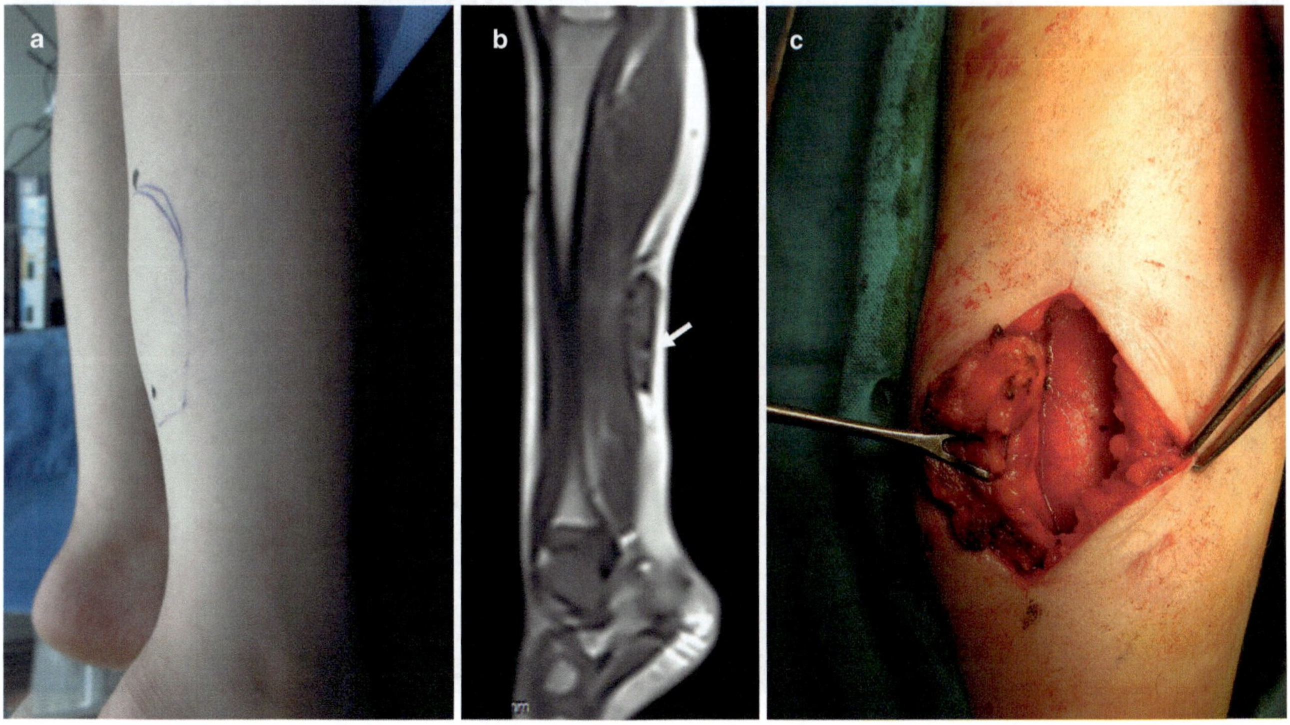

Fig. 14.15 Localized venous malformation at a subcutaneous site (back of leg), suitable for excision. (**a**) Clinical photograph showing the lesion. (**b**) Sagittal T1-weighted MRI showing subcutaneous lesion (arrow), with intermediate signal intensity. (**c**) Surgical excision

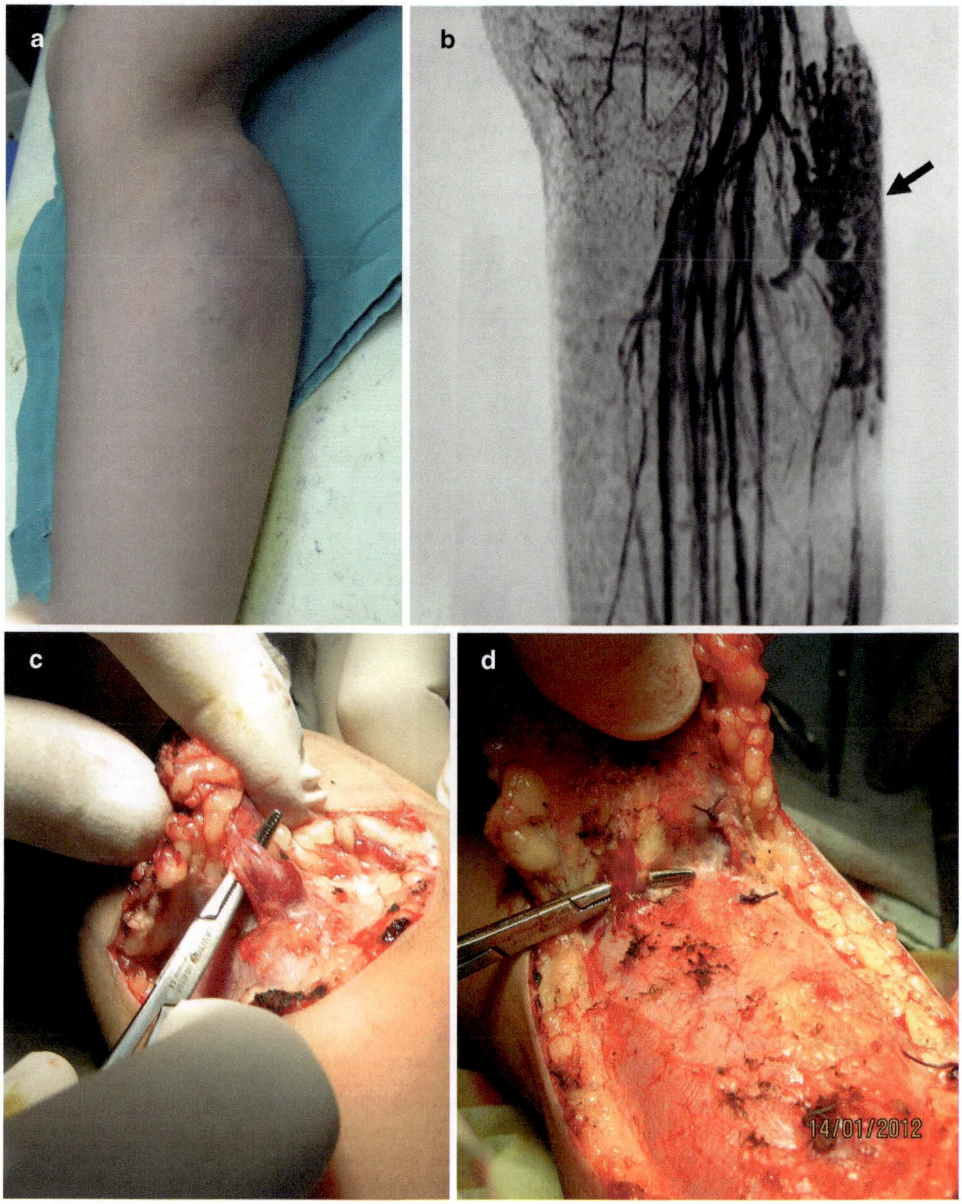

Fig. 14.16 Venous malformation of the leg. (**a**) Clinical photograph of the lesion. (**b**) MR venography showing multiple dilated venous channels (arrow). (**c**, **d**) Surgical excision: note isolation and ligation of communicating veins

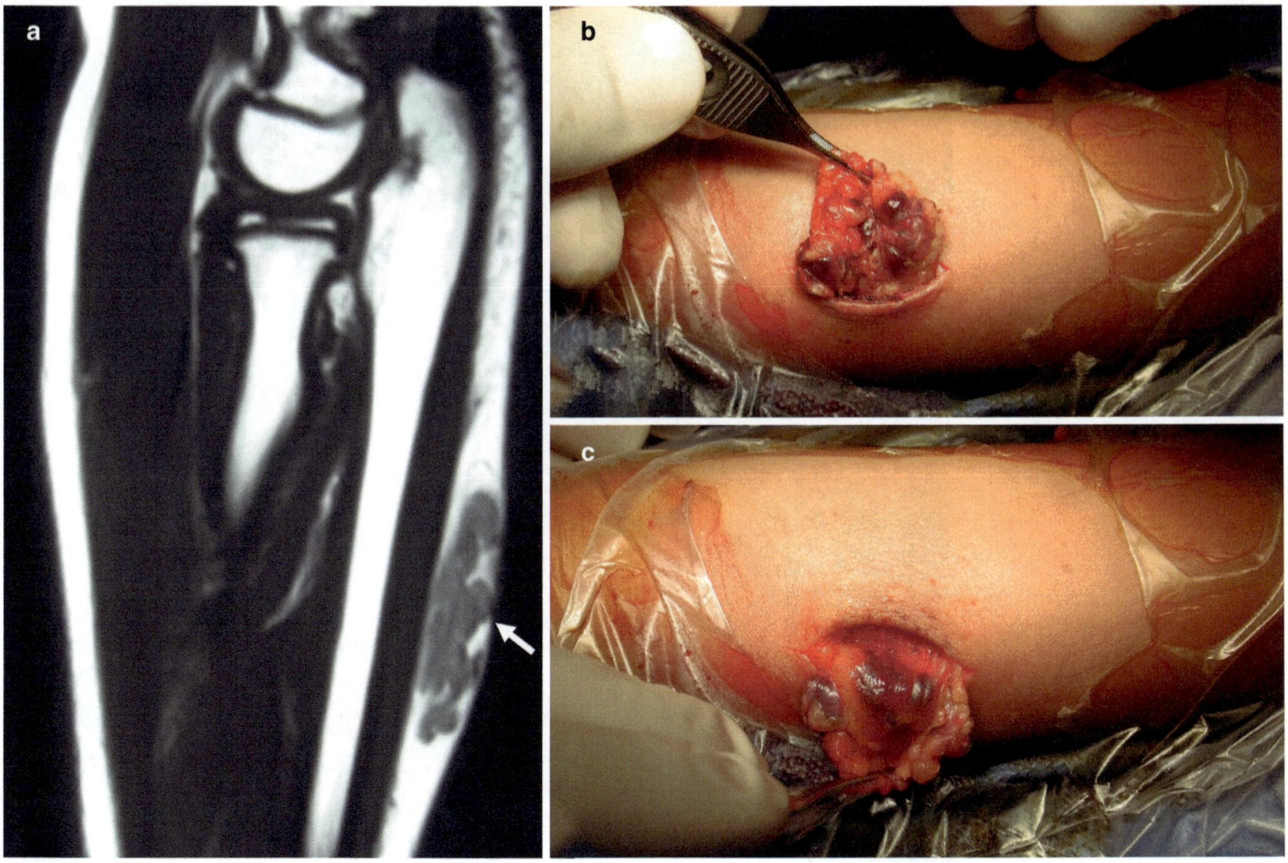

Fig. 14.17 Localized venous malformation at a subcutaneous site (forearm), suitable for excision. (**a**) MRI sagittal T1-WI shows a subcutaneous swelling (arrow) with intermediate signal intensity. (**b**, **c**) Surgical excision

References

1. Upton IIIJ. Vascular malformations of the extremities. In: Mulliken JB, Burrows PE, Fishman SJ, editors. Mulliken & Young's vascular anomalies: hemangiomas and malformations. Oxford University Press; 2013. p. 905–65.
2. Flors L, Hagspiel KD, Park AW, Norton PT, Leiva-Salinas C. Vascular malformations and tumors Part 2: low-flow lesions. Radiologia (English edition). 2019;61:124–33.
3. Gokani VJ, Sivakumar B, Kangesu L. Vascular anomalies. Surgery (Oxford). 2018;36:314–23.
4. Fishman SJ, Young AE. Clinical assessment of vascular malformations. In: Mulliken JB, Burrows PE, Fishman SJ, editors. Mulliken & Young's vascular anomalies: hemangiomas and malformations. Oxford University Press; 2013. p. 376–91.
5. Fishman SJ, Young AE. Slow-flow vascular malformations. In: Mulliken JB, Burrows PE, Fishman SJ, editors. Mulliken & Young's vascular anomalies: hemangiomas and malformations. Oxford University Press; 2013. p. 562–94.
6. Burrows PE. Percutaneous treatment of slow-flow vascular malformations. In: Mulliken JB, Burrows PE, Fishman SJ, editors. Mulliken & Young's vascular anomalies: hemangiomas and malformations. Oxford University Press; 2013. p. 661–709.
7. Wang H, Xie C, Lin W, et al. Fibro-adipose vascular anomaly (FAVA) – diagnosis, staging and management. Orphanet J Rare Dis. 2023;18:347. https://doi.org/10.1186/s13023-023-02961-6.
8. Adams DM. Practical genetic and biologic therapeutic considerations in vascular anomalies. Tech Vasc Interventional Rad. 2019;22:Article 100629.
9. Mamlouk MD, Nicholson AD, Cooke DL, Hess CP. Tips and tricks to optimize MRI protocols for cutaneous vascular anomalies. Clin Imaging. 2017;45:71–80.
10. Mohammad SA, AbouZeid AA, Fawzi AM, et al. Magnetic resonance imaging of head and neck vascular anomalies: pearls and pitfalls. Ann Pediatr Surg. 2017;13:116–24.
11. Abdelbaky MA, Ragab IA, AbouZeid AA, et al. Sirolimus: a rescue drug to control complications of extensive venous malformation. European J Pediatr Surg Rep. 2020;08(01):e90–4. https://doi.org/10.1055/s-0040-1716895.
12. Yakes WF, Haas DK, Parker SH, et al. Symptomatic vascular malformations: ethanol embolotherapy. Radiology. 1989;170:1059.

Truncal and Visceral Venous Malformations

15

Introduction

Venous malformations (VMs) may occur in the abdominal and chest walls, although these locations are less frequently involved compared to the head, neck, and extremities. VMs can also involve abdominal viscera, including solid organs such as the liver and intestines. The pelvis is another commonly affected site and is often associated with cutaneous VMs in the perineum. Visceral venous malformations are sometimes part of syndromic conditions. For instance, blue rubber bleb nevus syndrome (BRBNS) is characterized by multifocal venous malformations involving the skin, soft tissues, and gastrointestinal tract. Another example is Klippel-Trenaunay syndrome, a combined slow-flow vascular malformation primarily affecting the lower limbs, with frequent pelvic involvement (see Chap. 20).

Venous Malformations of the Trunk

Venous malformations (VMs) may involve various regions of the trunk, including the axilla, breast, back, abdominal wall, and chest wall (Fig. 15.1). Lesions are typically bluish and compressible [1–3]. MRI is the preferred imaging modality for confirming the diagnosis and assessing the deep extent of the lesions (Figs. 15.2, 15.3, and 15.4) [4, 5]. Localized VMs are often suitable for surgical excision or injection sclerotherapy. In contrast, more extensive lesions usually require a multimodal approach to manage symptoms, which may include pain or cosmetic concerns due to altered body contour. Treatment options may involve medical therapy (such as anticoagulants to reduce intralesional thrombosis), sclerotherapy, and debulking surgeries [6].

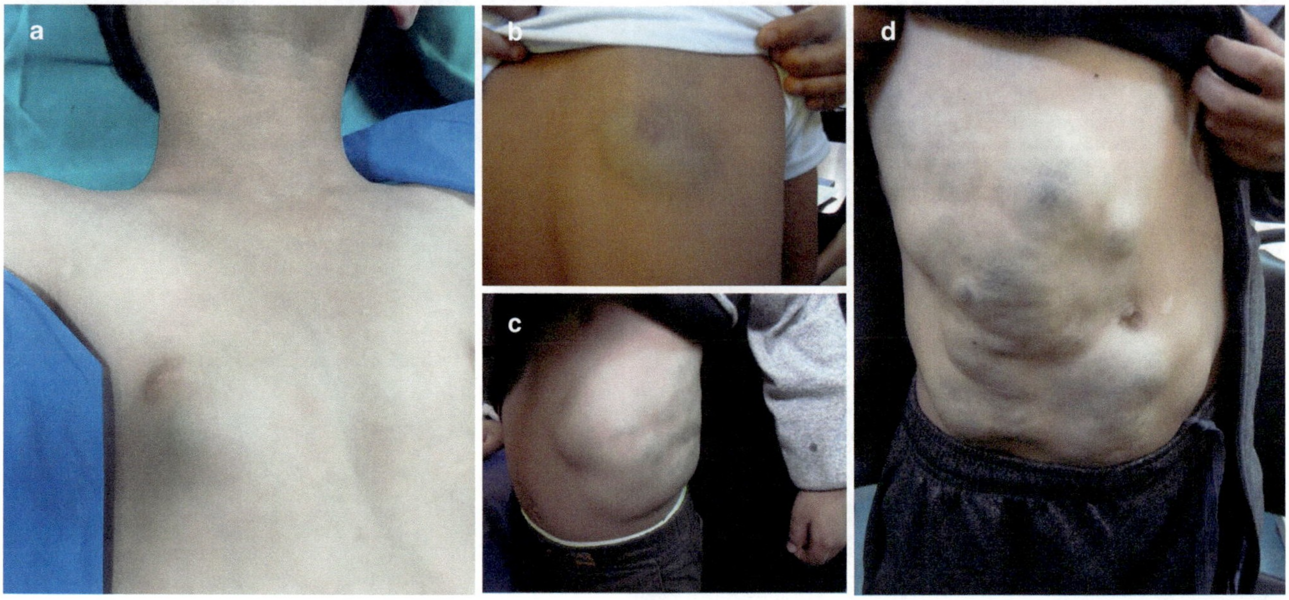

Fig. 15.1 Venous malformations located in different trunk regions: (**a**) breast, (**b**) back, (**c**) lateral chest wall, (**d**) diffuse lesion across both chest and abdominal walls

A. A. AbouZeid et al., *Atlas of Pediatric Vascular Anomalies*, https://doi.org/10.1007/978-3-032-30866-5_15

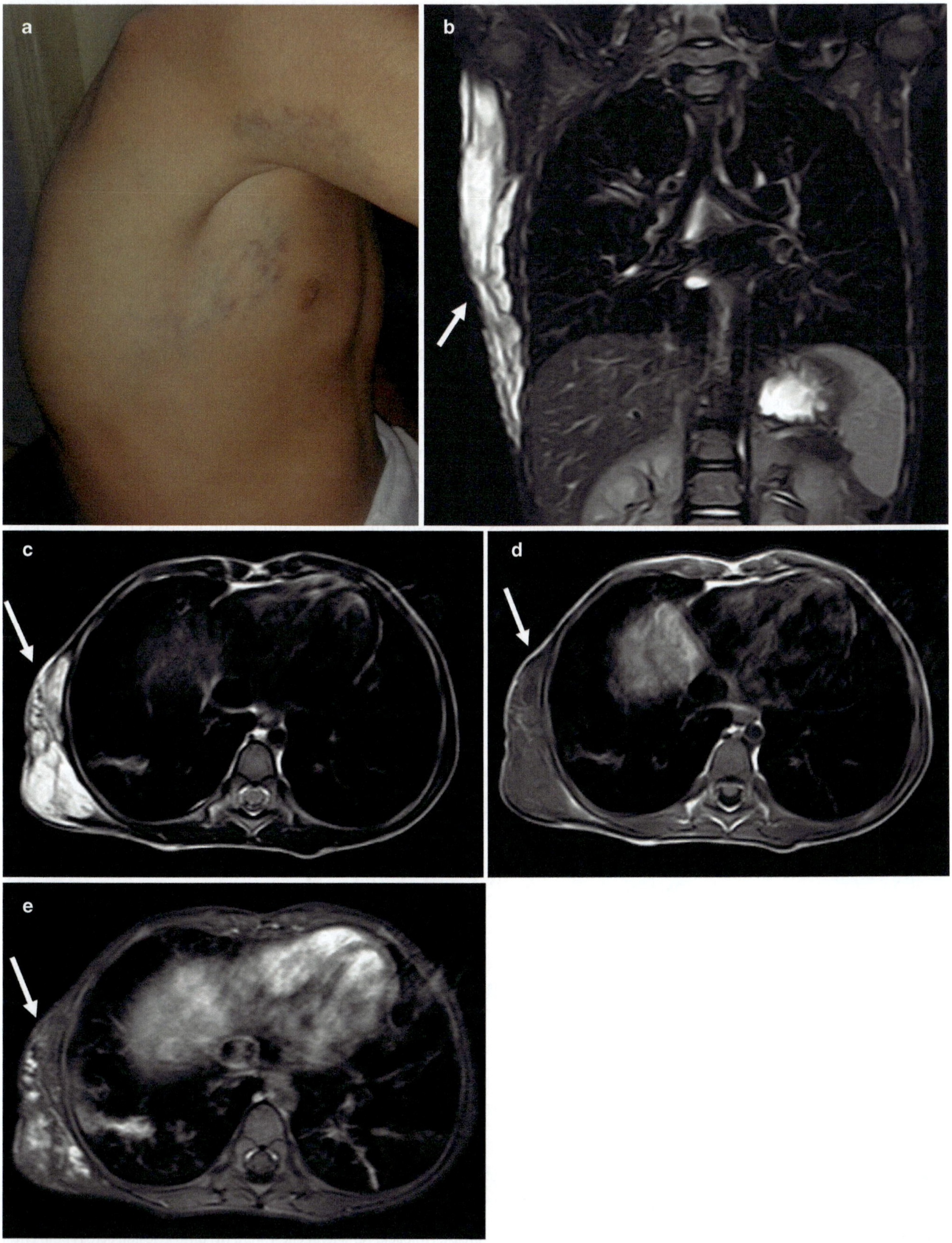

Fig. 15.2 Venous malformation in a 10-year-old girl. (**a**) Clinical photo shows bluish swelling of the arm and posterolateral chest wall. (**b–e**) MRI shows venous malformation (arrow): hyperintense signal on STIR (**b**) and T2-WI (**c**), intermediate signal on T1-WI (**d**), with typical patchy post-contrast enhancement (**e**)

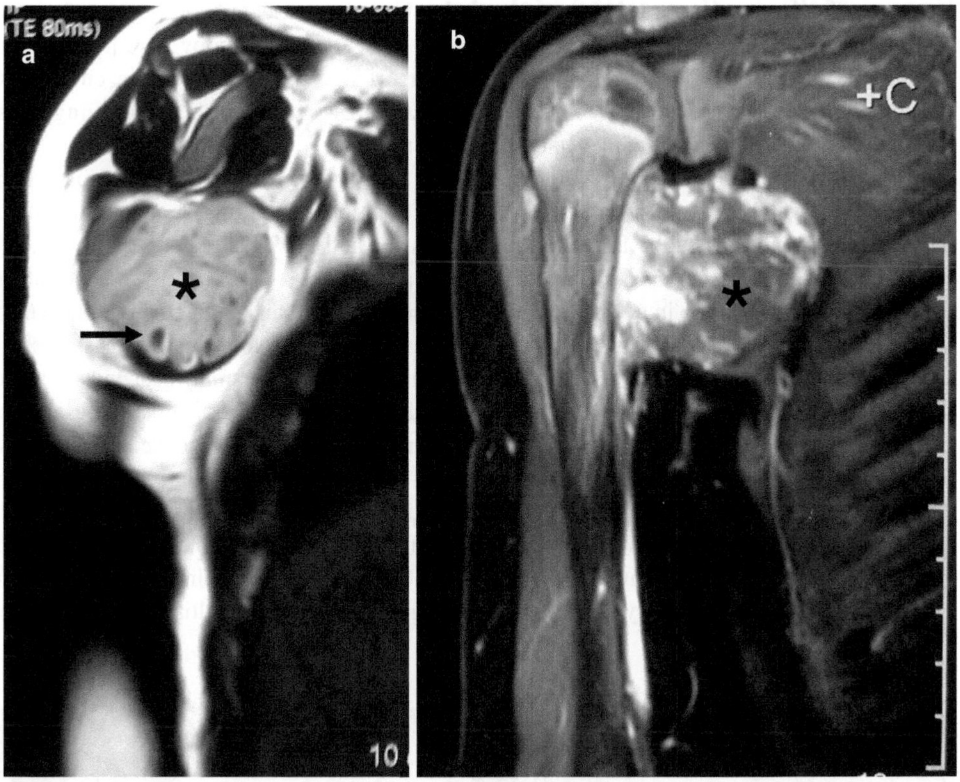

Fig. 15.3 MRI of venous malformation in the axilla. The lesion (asterisk) is hyperintense on T2-WI (**a**) with rounded phleboliths (arrow) and shows typical patchy post-contrast enhancement (**b**)

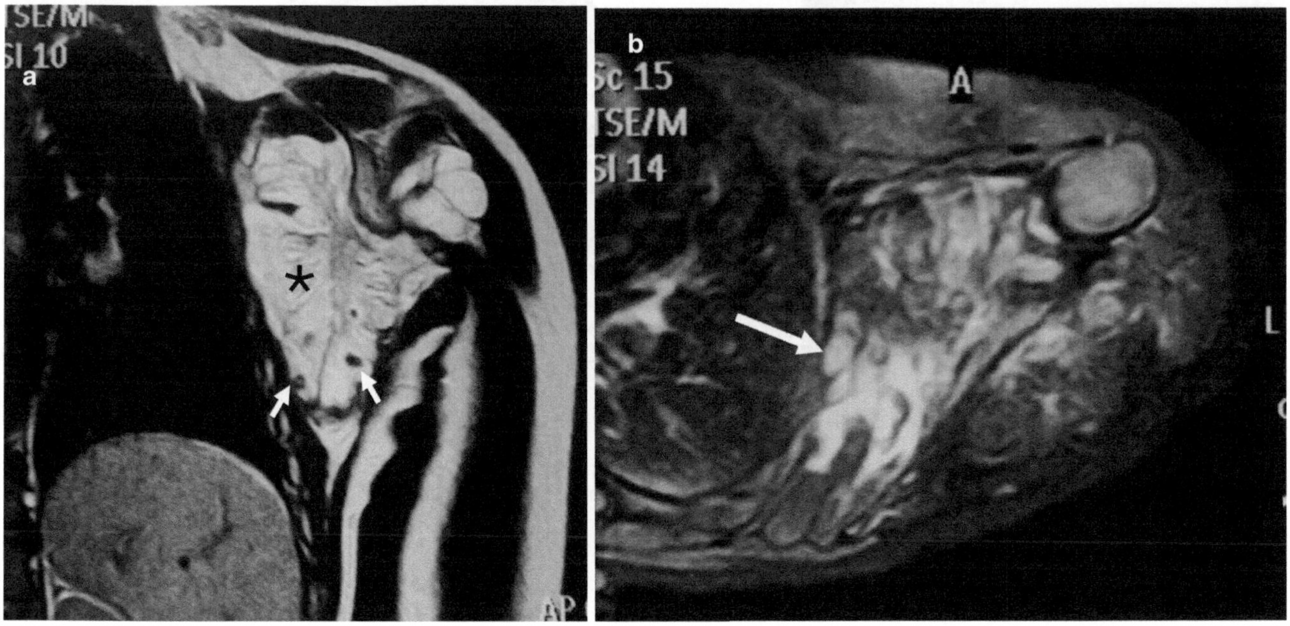

Fig. 15.4 Venous malformation of the left axilla. (**a**) Coronal T2-weighted MRI demonstrates a venous malformation (asterisk) exhibiting hyperintense signal with characteristic phleboliths (short arrows). (**b**) Axial fat-suppressed contrast-enhanced T1-weighted MRI shows patchy post-contrast enhancement (long arrow)

Venous Malformations (VMs) of the Intestine

Venous malformations (VMs) can involve any part of the intestine when they often present with recurrent gastrointestinal bleeding and/or iron-deficiency anemia [1, 2]. Intestinal VMs may occur as isolated lesions (Fig. 15.5), or as a part of the blue rubber bleb nevus syndrome (BRBNS), a condition characterized by multifocal VMs in the skin, soft tissue, and gastrointestinal tract (Fig. 15.6). Cutaneous lesions are typically small (1–2 cm), blue in color with "rubbery" sensation at palpation. In BRBNS, extensive soft tissue VMs carry increased risk of localized intravascular coagulopathy (LIC) leading to consumption of fibrinogen and platelets and thereby heightens the risk of bleeding from gastrointestinal lesions [2, 6].

The diagnostic approach is similar to that used for other causes of gastrointestinal bleeding and includes both upper and lower gastrointestinal endoscopy. Capsule endoscopy can be particularly useful in detecting lesions located in regions beyond the reach of conventional endoscopy [1, 2]. In patients with BRBNS, the presence of characteristic cutaneous lesions serves as a valuable clue to the underlying cause of gastrointestinal bleeding (Fig. 15.6). Triphasic CT scans, utilizing intravenous contrast (but not oral contrast), can aid in localizing bleeding venous malformations within the intestinal tract (Figs. 15.5 and 15.6) [1, 2].

Localized venous malformations (VMs) of the intestine can be effectively treated through surgical resection followed by intestinal re-anastomosis (Figs. 15.5 and 15.6). In cases with multifocal intestinal involvement, multiple resections may be necessary. Lesions that are accessible via endoscopy can be managed using endoscopic techniques such as banding or sclerotherapy (Fig. 15.7). Iron supplementation is essential to correct iron-deficiency anemia resulting from chronic blood loss. When surgical resection is not feasible, oral sirolimus has shown success in controlling bleeding from multiple intestinal lesions [2, 7].

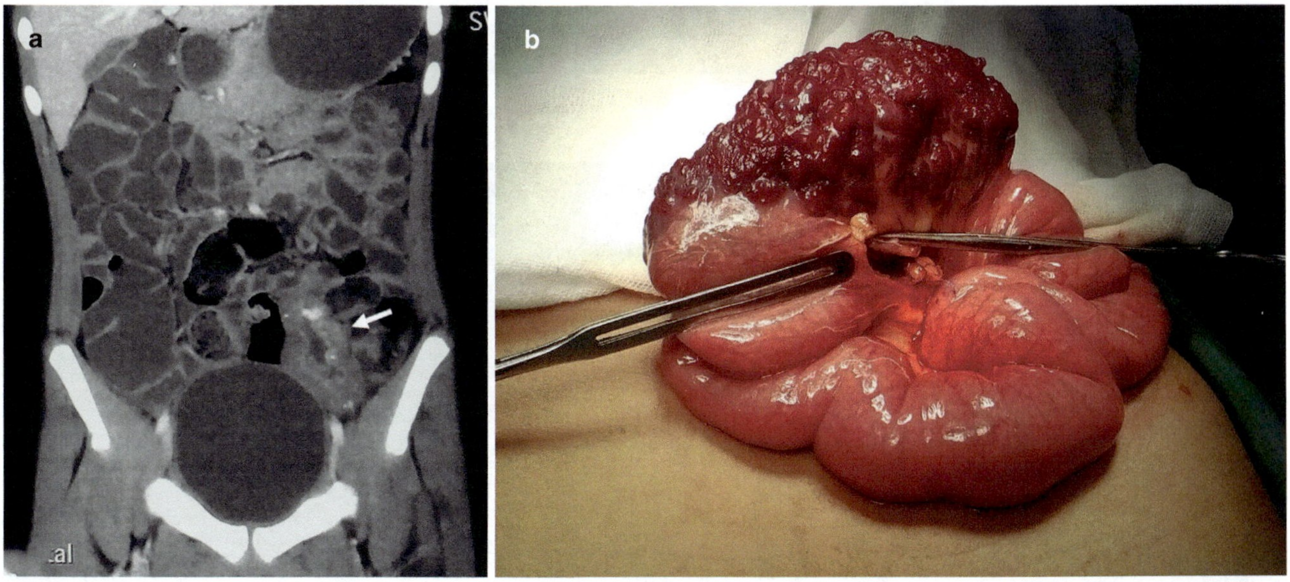

Fig. 15.5 Venous malformation of the small intestine in a 14-year-old boy presenting with rectal bleeding. (**a**) Coronal contrast-enhanced CT shows bowel wall thickening with patchy enhancement (arrow). (**b**) Intraoperative photo of the lesion before resection

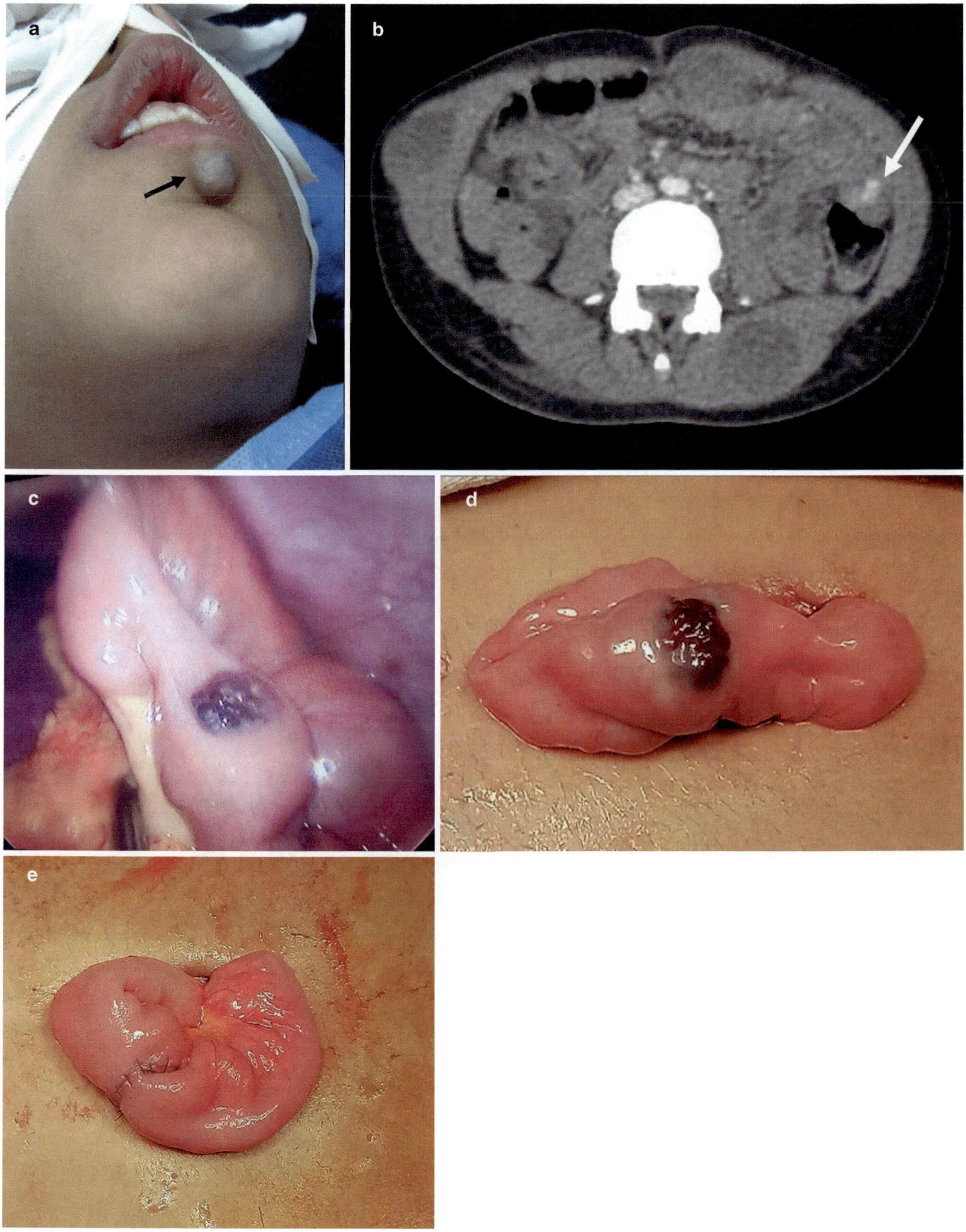

Fig. 15.6 An 11-year-old girl with blue rubber bleb nevus syndrome (multiple venous malformations) presented with a hemoglobin drop. (**a**) Clinical photo showing characteristic cutaneous lesion (black arrow). (**b**) Axial contrast-enhanced CT shows polypoidal enhancing venous malformation (white arrow) of the small intestine. (**c**) Laparoscopic view of the intestinal lesion. (**d**, **e**) Intestinal lesion exteriorized for resection and anastomosis

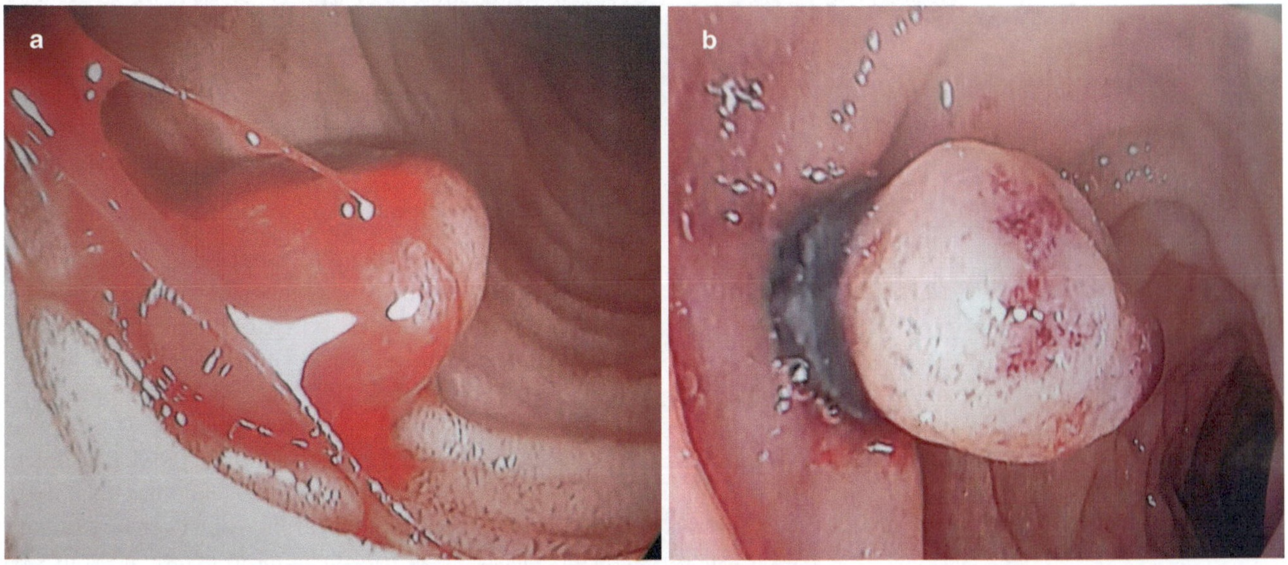

Fig. 15.7 Venous malformation in the duodenum presenting with gastrointestinal bleeding (**a**), managed by endoscopic banding (**b**)

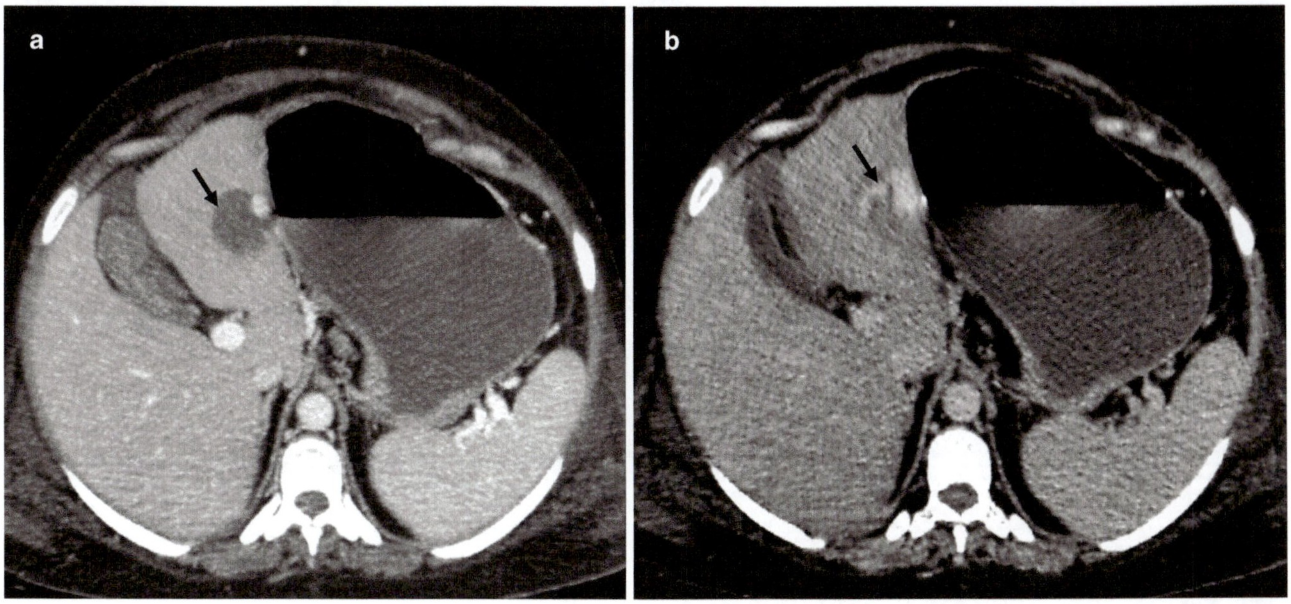

Fig. 15.8 A 53-year-old lady with intestinal obstruction. Axial contrast-enhanced CT shows an incidentally discovered venous malformation in the liver, commonly referred to as hepatic hemangioma (arrow). The lesion demonstrates early peripheral nodular hyperenhancement (**a**) and progressive filling in the delayed phase (**b**)

Venous Malformations (VMs) of the Liver

Hepatic venous malformations (VMs) are typically asymptomatic and are often discovered incidentally during routine imaging in adulthood (Fig. 15.8). They are frequently improperly diagnosed as cavernous hemangiomas. Hepatic VMs may also present in association with blue rubber bleb nevus syndrome (BRBNS) when they are often multiple in number but seldom lead to significant clinical problems (Fig. 15.9) [1, 2].

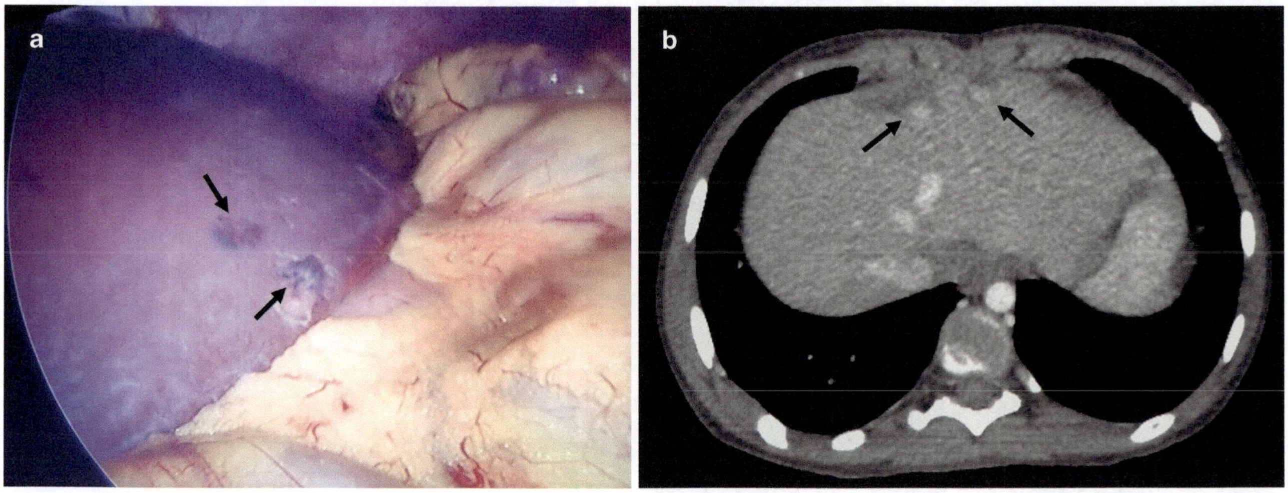

Fig. 15.9 Multiple venous malformations in an 11-year-old girl with blue rubber bleb nevus syndrome (same case as in Fig. 15.5). (**a**) Laparoscopic exploration showing multiple hepatic lesions (arrows). (**b**) Axial contrast-enhanced CT demonstrating patchy nodular enhancement corresponding to hepatic venous malformations (arrows)

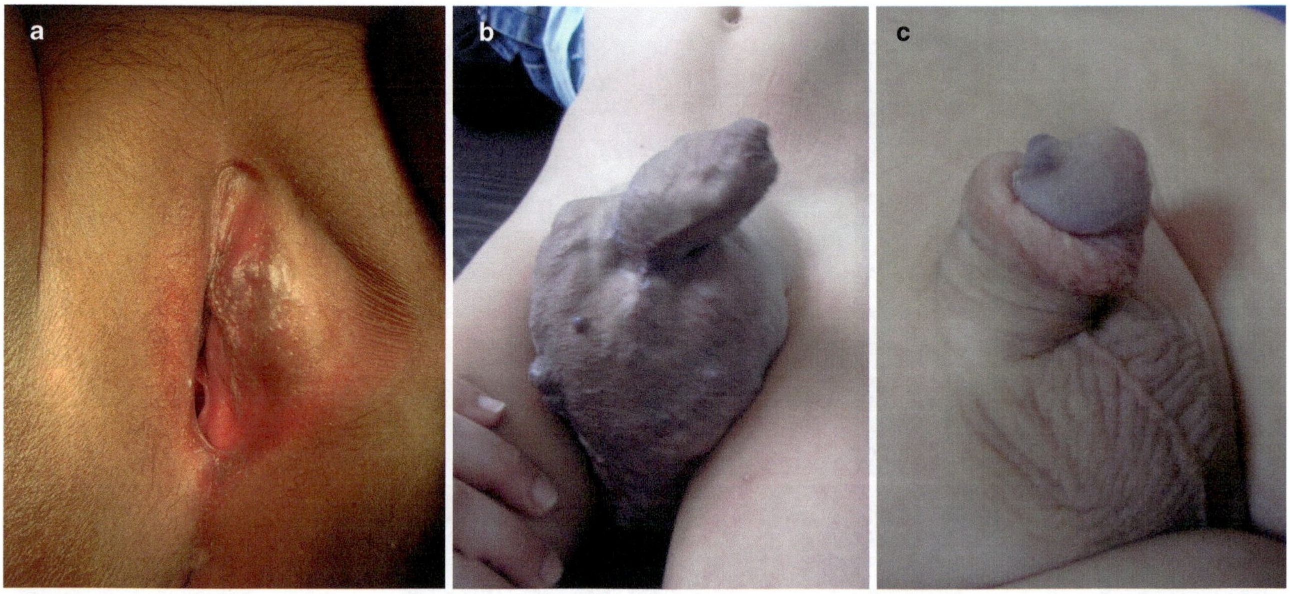

Fig. 15.10 Venous malformations (VMs) frequently affect the perineum and external genitalia, including the vulva (**a**), scrotum (**b**), and glans penis (**c**)

Venous Malformations (VMs) of the Pelvis and Perineum

Venous malformations (VMs) frequently affect the perineum and external genitalia, including the vulva, scrotum, and glans penis (Fig. 15.10). Similar to VMs in other regions, their size can vary significantly—from localized lesions (Fig. 15.11) to diffuse malformations (Fig. 15.12) that often extend deep into the pelvis and may envelop pelvic organs such as the rectum, vagina, and urinary bladder (Fig. 15.13). MRI plays a crucial role in identifying the deep pelvic extension of lesions (Figs. 15.14 and 15.15).

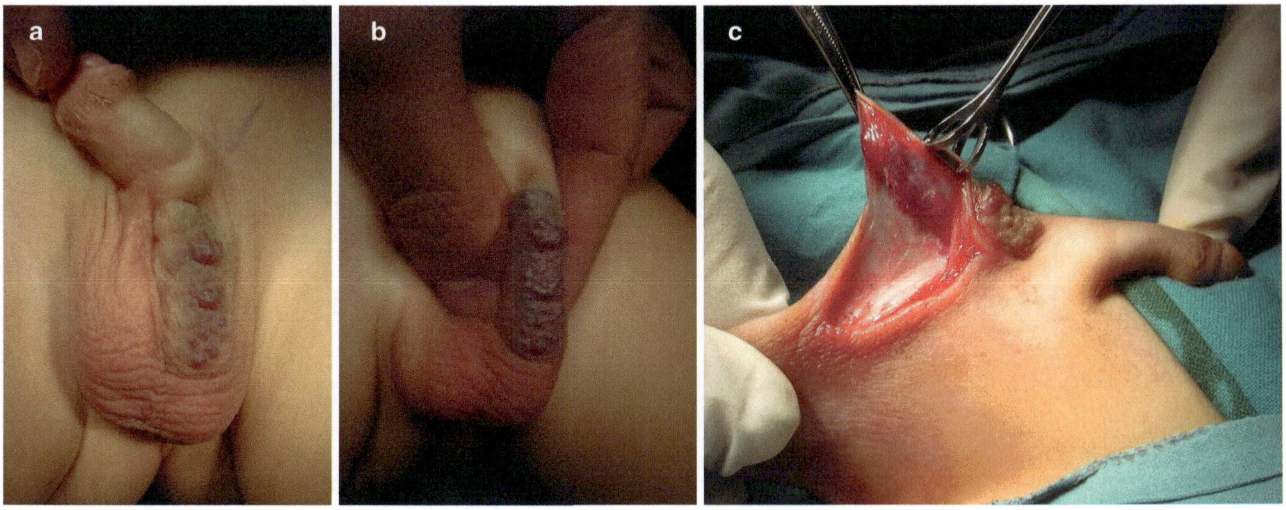

Fig. 15.11 Localized venous malformation of the left hemi-scrotum. (**a**, **b**) Clinical examination. (**c**) Surgical excision

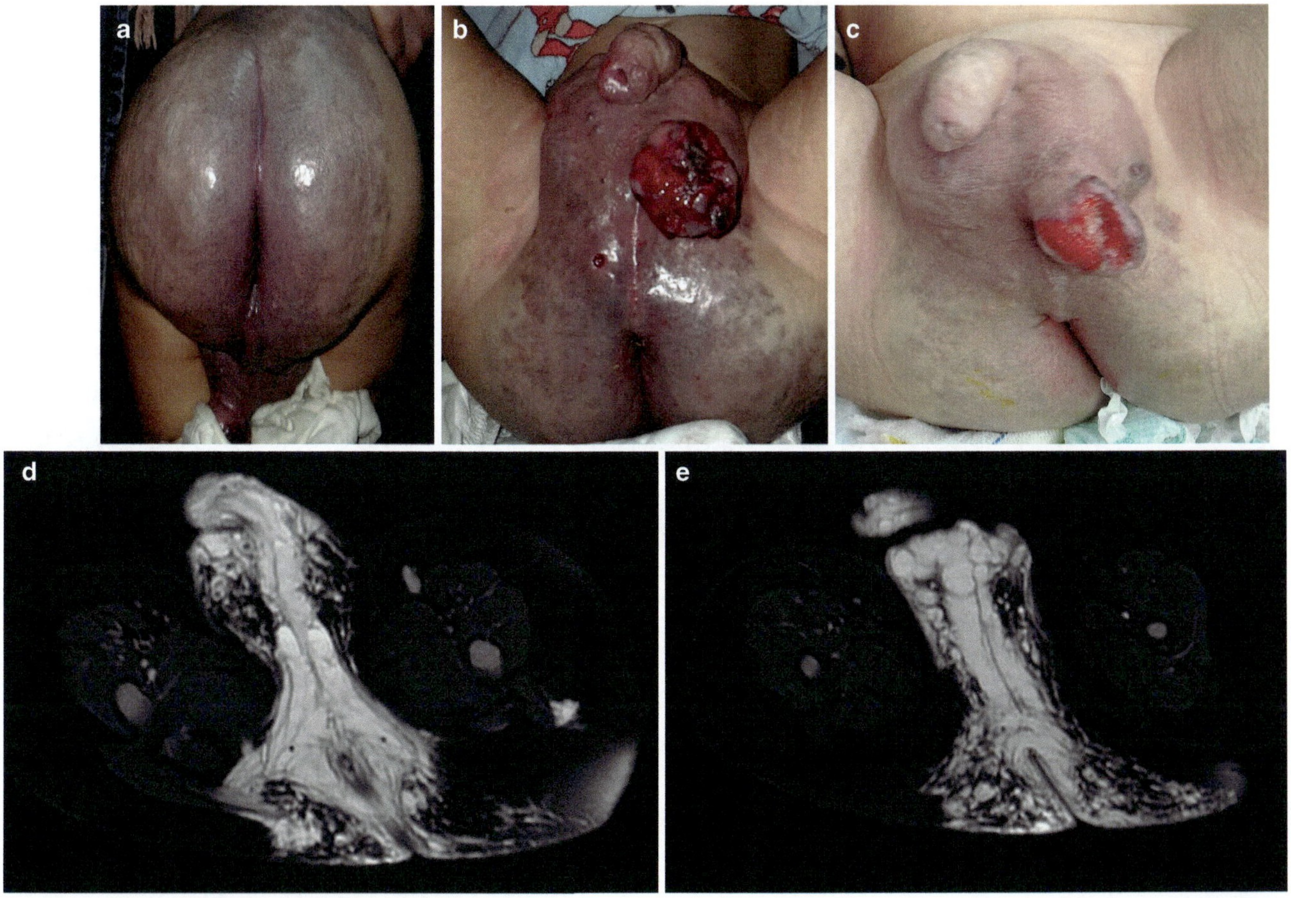

Fig. 15.12 Extensive venous malformation of the pelvis and perineum in a 2-year-old boy with fungating polyp at site of previous surgery. (**a**–**c**) Clinical photographs demonstrate the lesions before treatment (**a**, **b**) and after treatment with sirolimus (**c**). (**d**, **e**) Axial STIR MRI images reveal a trans-spatial lesion with hyperintense signal, extending through the skin, subcutaneous tissue, penile corpora, and scrotum

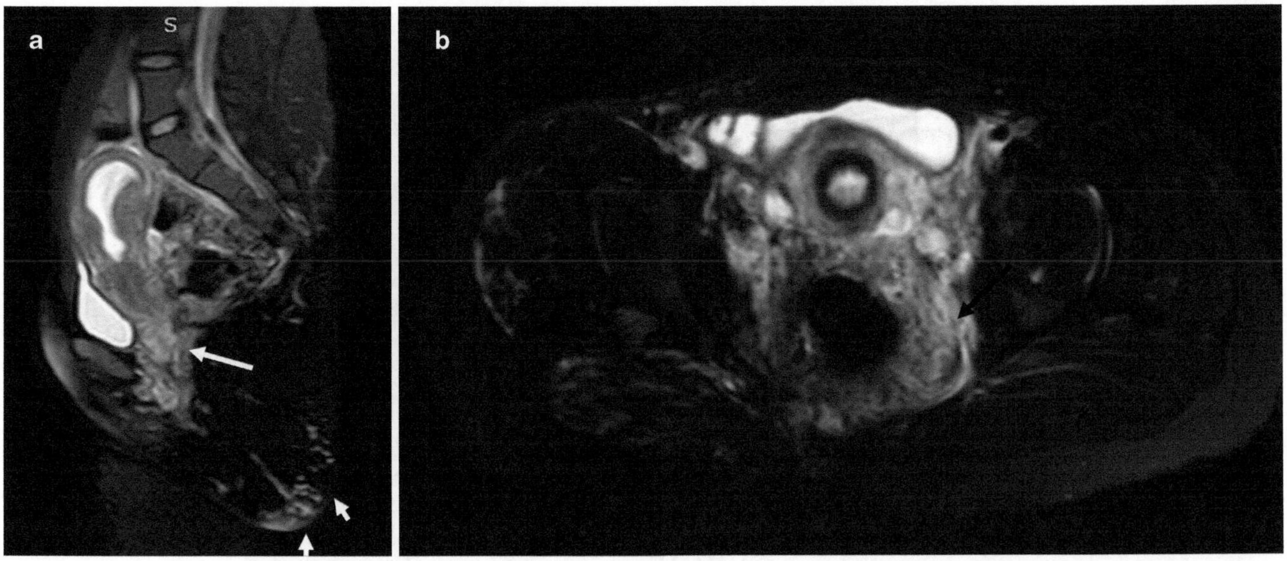

Fig. 15.13 Extensive venous malformation in the pelvis of an 18-year-old female presenting with menorrhagia and bleeding per rectum. (**a**) Sagittal and (**b**) axial STIR MRI demonstrate a trans-spatial hyperintense lesion involving the vagina (white arrow), rectal wall, and ischiorectal fossa (black arrow). Subcutaneous lesions are also noted (short arrows)

Extensive involvement of the rectum by VMs usually presents with dyschezia and fresh rectal bleeding (Fig. 15.16). Precise mapping of the lesion's extent is essential for appropriate planning and optimal management. A dilated (ectatic) inferior mesenteric vein has been reported in cases with extensive rectal VMs; this anomalous vein may divert blood flow from the portal vein down to the rectal malformations, thereby worsening venous congestion [1]. Therefore, all patients with extensive rectal VMs should be evaluated for this associated venous anomaly [1]. CT portal venography is the preferred diagnostic modality (Fig. 15.17). As with VMs elsewhere, management includes medical treatment (sirolimus), sclerotherapy, and surgical excision whenever feasible.

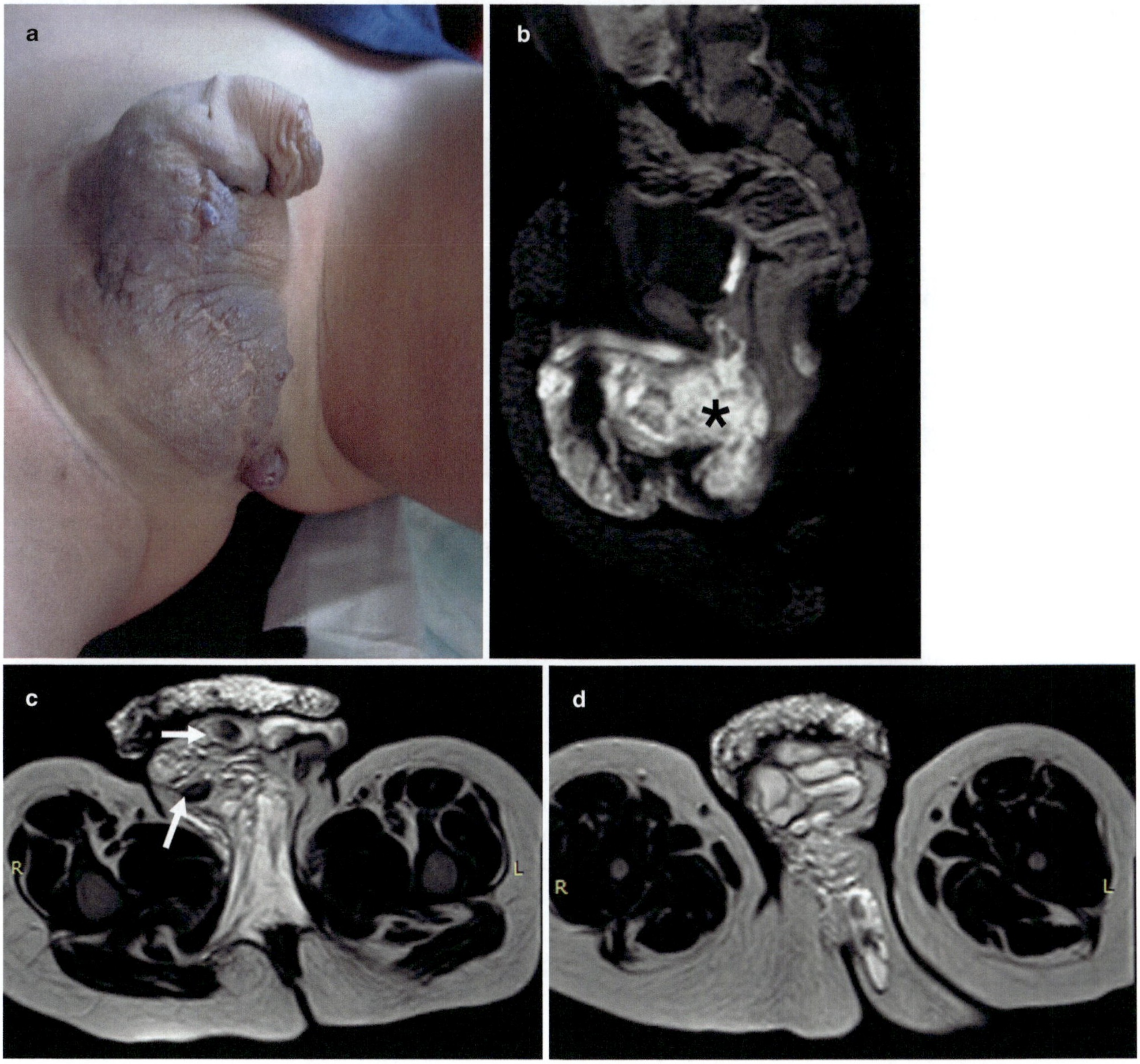

Fig. 15.14 Venous malformation of the scrotum in a 2-year-old boy. (**a**) Clinical photograph showing the midline scar from previous debulking surgery. (**b**) Sagittal post-contrast fat-suppressed MRI demonstrates the venous malformation (asterisk) with characteristic delayed contrast enhancement. (**c**, **d**) Axial T2-weighted MRI reveals a hyperintense lesion with extension and associated phleboliths (arrows)

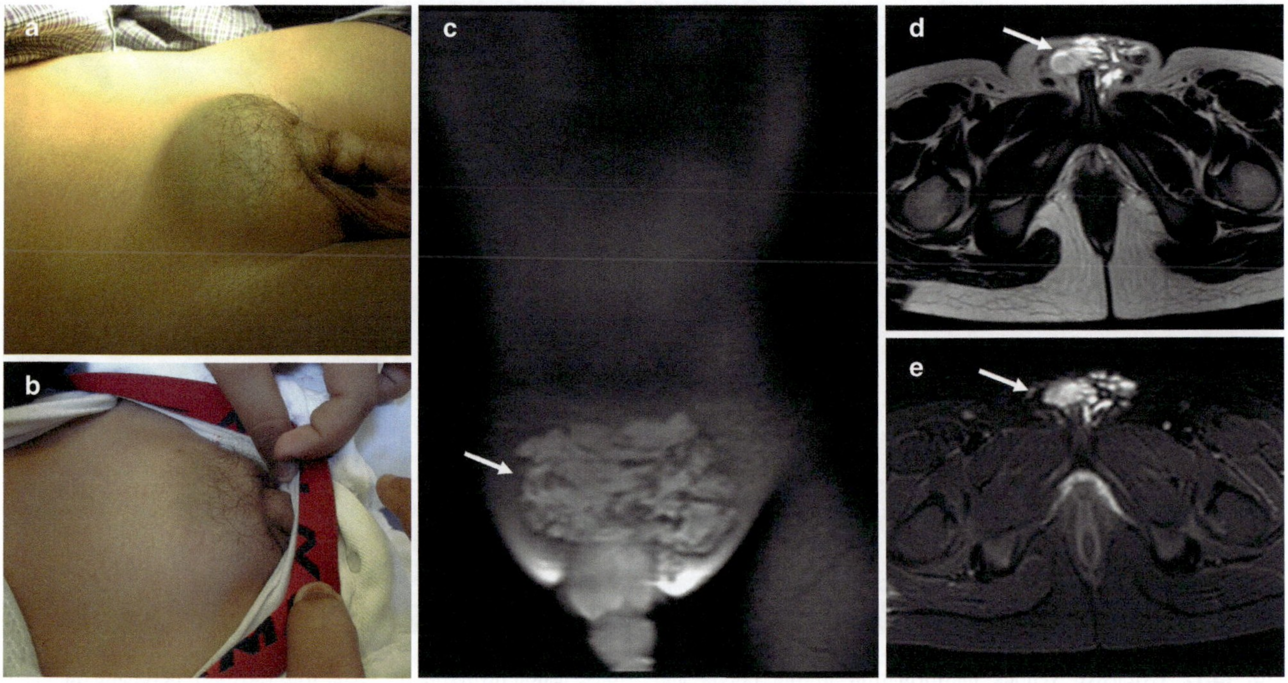

Fig. 15.15 Venous malformation of the suprapubic area in a 13-year-old boy. (**a**, **b**) Clinical photographs before and after injection sclerotherapy, respectively. (**c–e**) MRI demonstrates deep lesion extension appearing as a hyperintense lesion (arrow): (**c**) coronal T2-weighted image, (**d**) axial T2-weighted image, and (**e**) STIR sequence

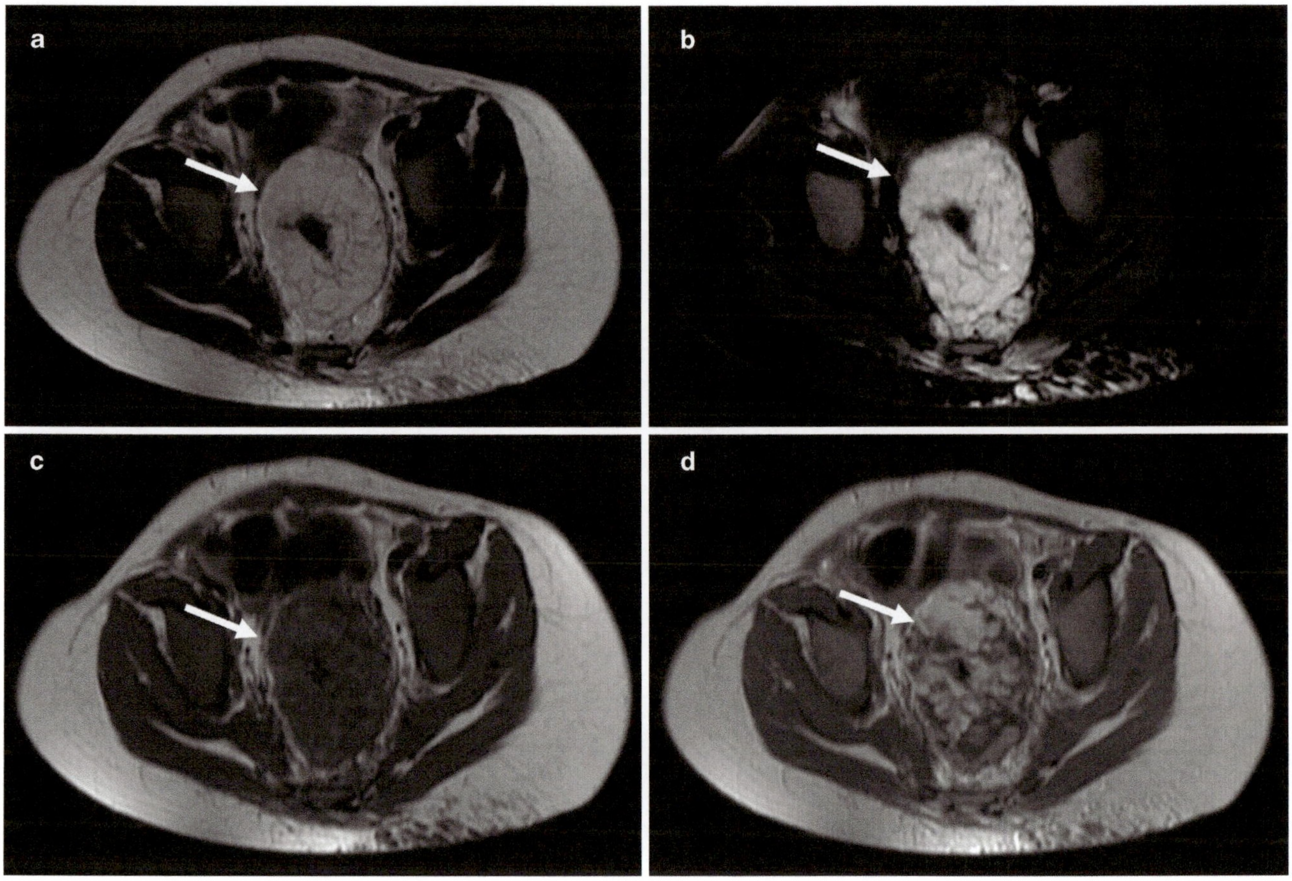

Fig. 15.16 Venous malformation of the rectal wall in a 2-year-old boy (same case as in Fig. 15.11). MRI demonstrates a venous malformation (arrow) with hyperintense signal on (**a**) T2-weighted image and (**b**) STIR, intermediate signal on (**c**) T1-weighted image, and patchy post-contrast enhancement on (**d**) contrast enhanced T1-weighted image

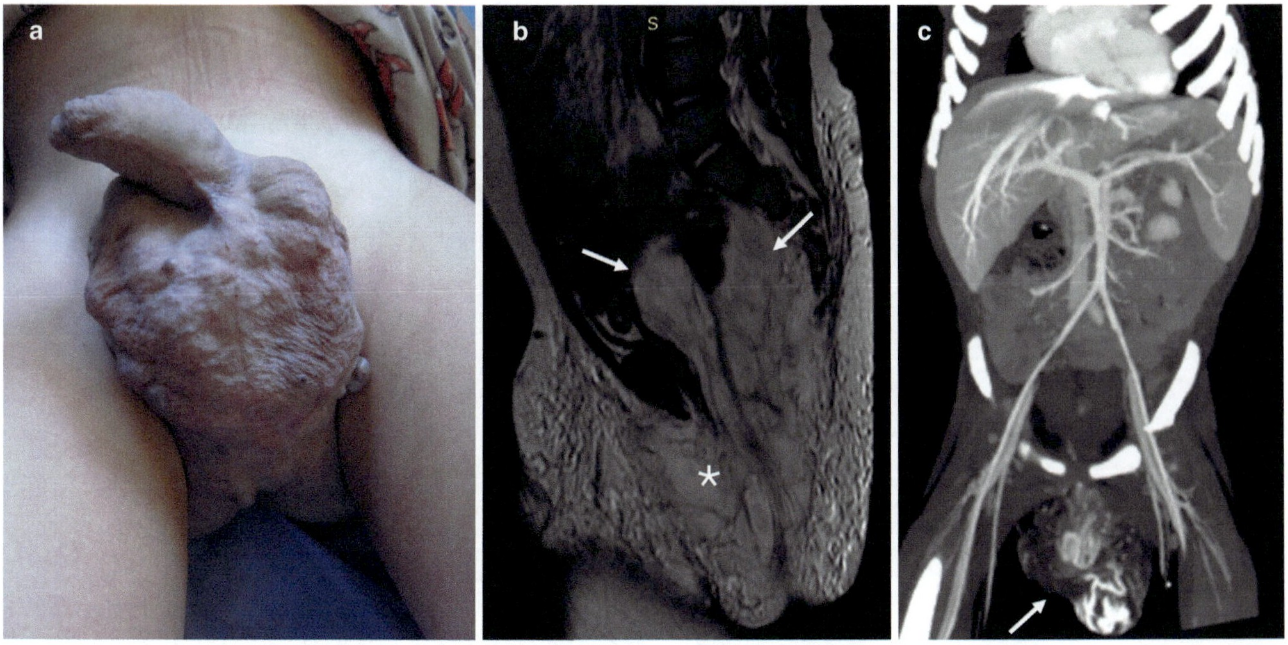

Fig. 15.17 Extensive venous malformation in the pelvis and perineum of a 2-year-old boy (same case as in Figs. 15.11 and 15.15). (**a**) Clinical photograph showing the scrotal lesion. (**b**) Sagittal T2-weighted image demonstrates a trans-spatial hyperintense lesion involving the rectal wall (arrows), perineum, and anal canal (asterisk). (**c**) CT portal venography reveals no associated venous anomalies; note the patchy contrast enhancement of the perineal lesions (arrow)

References

1. Fishman SJ. Truncal, visceral, and genital vascular malformations. In: Mulliken JB, Burrows PE, Fishman SJ, editors. Mulliken & Young's vascular anomalies: hemangiomas and malformations. Oxford University Press; 2013. p. 966–1016.
2. Ghaffarpour N. Vascular malformations in the viscera. In: Mattassi R, Loose D, Vaghi M, editors. Hemangiomas and vascular malformations. Milano: Springer; 2015. https://doi.org/10.1007/978-88-470-5673-2_46.
3. Flors L, Hagspiel KD, Park AW, Norton PT, Leiva-Salinas C. Vascular malformations and tumors Part 2: low-flow lesions. Radiologia (English edition). 2019;61:124–33.
4. Mamlouk MD, Nicholson AD, Cooke DL, Hess CP. Tips and tricks to optimize MRI protocols for cutaneous vascular anomalies. Clin Imaging. 2017;45:71–80.
5. Mohammad SA, AbouZeid AA, Fawzi AM, et al. Magnetic resonance imaging of head and neck vascular anomalies: pearls and pitfalls. Ann Pediatr Surg. 2017;13:116–24.
6. Fishman SJ, Young AE. Slow-flow vascular malformations. In: Mulliken JB, Burrows PE, Fishman SJ, editors. Mulliken & Young's vascular anomalies: hemangiomas and malformations. Oxford University Press; 2013. p. 562–94.
7. Abdelbaky MA, Ragab IA, AbouZeid AA, et al. Sirolimus: a rescue drug to control complications of extensive venous malformation. European J Pediatr Surg Rep. 2020;08(01):e90–4. https://doi.org/10.1055/s-0040-1716895.

Multifocal Venous Malformations

16

Introduction

Multifocal venous malformations are rare congenital vascular anomalies characterized by the presence of multiple, discrete venous malformations affecting different anatomical sites. They result from developmental errors in the venous system during embryogenesis and are classified under the spectrum of slow-flow vascular malformations. Multifocal venous malformations (VMs) may occur either sporadically or as inherited conditions.

First: Sporadic Multifocal Venous Malformations

Sporadic multifocal venous malformations encompass several syndromes, including blue rubber bleb nevus syndrome (BRBNS), Maffucci syndrome, and verrucous venous malformations (VVMs) [1].

Blue Rubber Bleb Nevus Syndrome

Although it remains a rare disorder, the most frequent sporadic multifocal venous malformation is Blue Rubber Bleb Nevus Syndrome (BRBNS); also known as Bean syndrome. It is characterized by multiple, widely distributed cutaneous and internal venous malformations (VMs) [2]. Patients may develop tens to hundreds of lesions, which often increase in both size and number with age [3]. The most commonly affected sites are the skin (93%) and gastrointestinal (GI) tract (76%), while other organs such as the central nervous system (13%), liver (11%), and muscles (9%) may also be involved [4].

Cutaneous lesions are usually small (less than 1–2 cm), bluish to purple in color (Fig. 16.1), compressible, and often hyperkeratotic. The term "rubber bleb" refers to cutaneous VMs that appear as small, nipple-like bluish nodules with a rubbery consistency (Fig. 16.1a). These can develop on any skin or mucosal surface and frequently cluster, particularly on

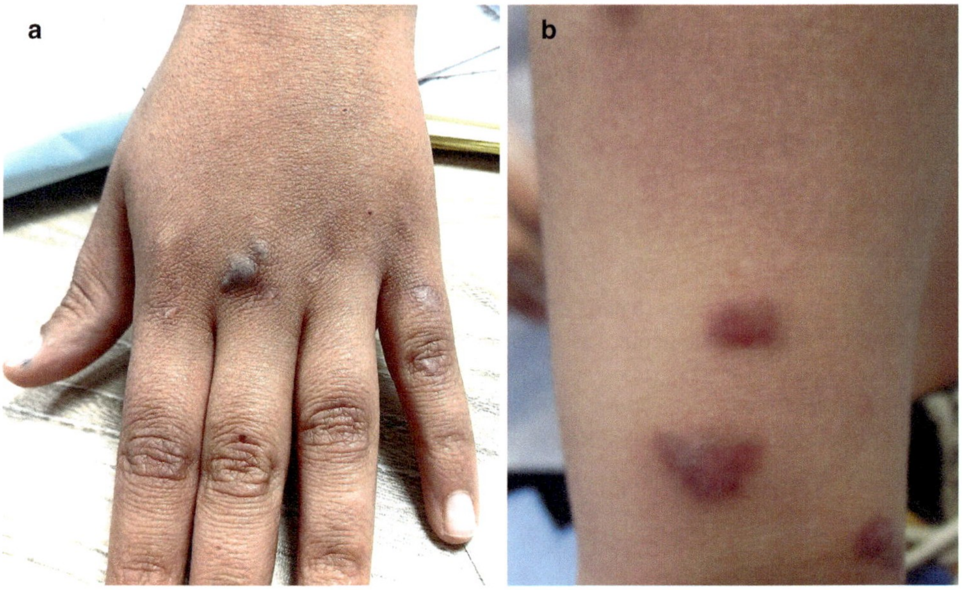

Fig. 16.1 Cutaneous manifestations of Blue Rubber Bleb Nevus Syndrome. (**a**) Characteristic small, bluish, nipple-like nodule on the dorsum of the hand. (**b**) Multiple purple cutaneous lesions on the leg of another patient

A. A. AbouZeid et al., *Atlas of Pediatric Vascular Anomalies*, https://doi.org/10.1007/978-3-032-30866-5_16

the palms and soles, where they often become hyperkeratotic (Fig. 16.2). In some patients, hundreds of cutaneous lesions may be present (Fig. 16.3) [5]. Gastrointestinal lesions, which are considered pathognomonic, are typically identified using endoscopy, or cross-sectional imaging (CT/MRI) (Fig. 16.4). They are most often located in the small intestine and may lead to complications such as hemorrhage (Fig. 16.5) or intussusception. The initial manifestation of BRBNS may be a large solitary venous malformation (VM), referred to as a "dominant VM." Such lesions typically display a central arborized or "fern-shaped" pattern (Fig. 16.6) [5].

BRBNS results from double somatic mutations (T1105N–T1106P) occurring on the same allele (cis) in the TEK/TIE2 gene [6]. Histologically, venous malformations (VMs) appear as large, thin-walled channels with little to no smooth muscle. In larger lesions, dysmorphic vascular channels may extend close to the epidermis, while intestinal lesions are predominantly located in the submucosa [7]. The major complications of BRBNS arise from gastrointestinal (GI) involvement, particularly GI bleeding. Lesions are most commonly found in the small intestine and may lead to recurrent hemorrhage, resulting in chronic anemia (Fig. 16.5). Affected patients often require repeated intravenous iron supplementation or blood transfusions. Additional GI complications, including volvulus and intussusception, may also occur.

Treatment of BRBNS is primarily supportive, focusing on managing recurrent blood loss. Surgical or endoscopic intervention may be required for lesions causing significant localized bleeding (Fig. 16.7), although these approaches are considered short-term solutions due to the high risk of recurrence [8]. Excision of cutaneous lesions, particularly those on pressure points such as the soles (Fig. 16.8), may be performed for symptomatic relief or cosmetic purposes. Medical therapy with sirolimus has shown benefit in reducing gastrointestinal bleeding, improving hemoglobin levels, and decreasing the need for transfusions and iron replacement in patients with BRBNS [9].

Maffucci Syndrome

It is a developmental disorder characterized by multiple enchondromas affecting the distal bones of the hands and feet, together with subcutaneous vascular malformations of the distal extremities. The subcutaneous vascular nodules typically appear later, most commonly on the fingers and toes. The condition carries a high risk of malignancy (approximately 40%), predominantly chondrosarcoma. The lesions are associated with mutations in the IDH1 or IDH2 genes [10].

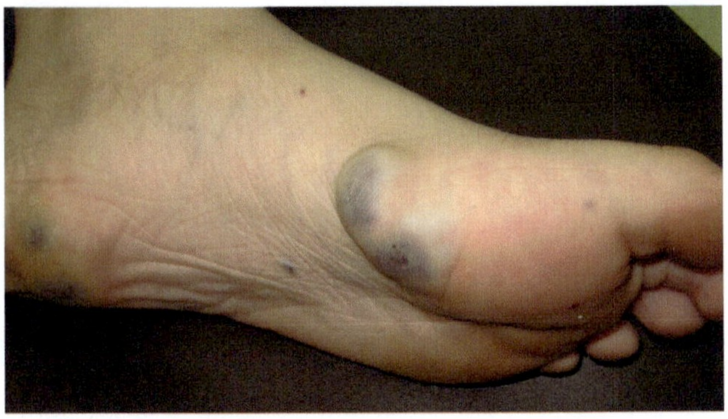

Fig. 16.2 Cutaneous lesions on the sole of the foot in a 14-year-old boy with Blue Rubber Bleb Nevus Syndrome

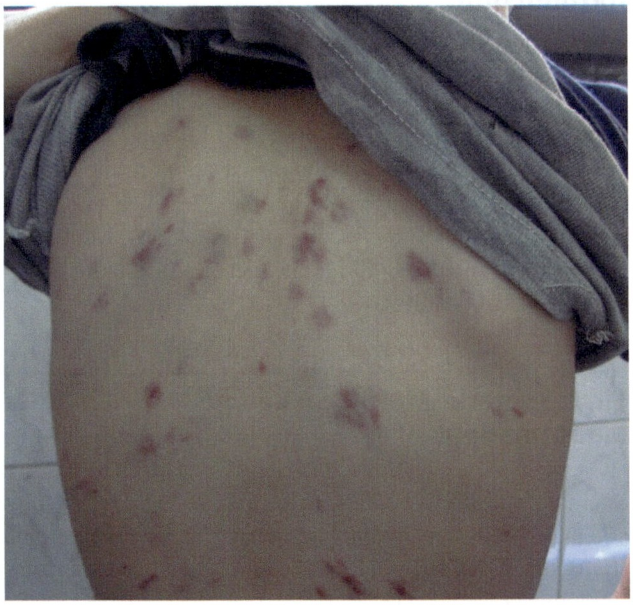

Fig. 16.3 Multiple cutaneous lesions on the back of a case with Multifocal Venous Malformations

Verrucous Venous Malformations

They are formed of a raised, purplish, hyperkeratotic papule, which could be multiple, with main distributions on extremities (Fig. 16.9). Histologically they are formed of venous-like channels with positive GLUT1 immunostaining. They often have a somatic *MAP 3 K3* mutation [11].

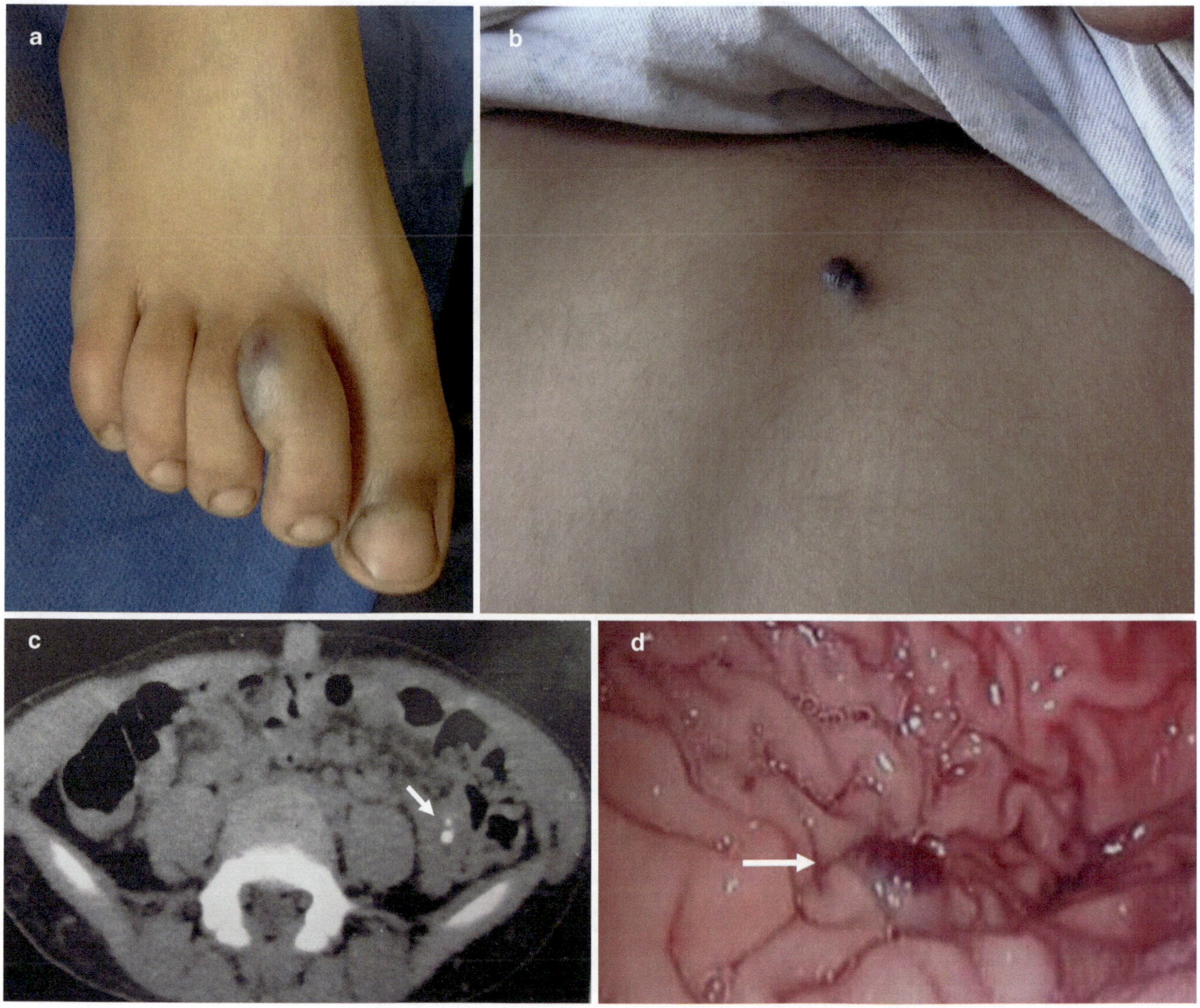

Fig. 16.4 A 12-year-old boy with Blue Rubber Bleb Nevus Syndrome. (**a**, **b**) Typical cutaneous lesions on the foot and back, respectively. (**c**) CT scan showing a phlebolith (arrow), indicative of an intestinal venous malformation. (**d**) Upper GI endoscopy revealing a venous malformation in the stomach (arrow)

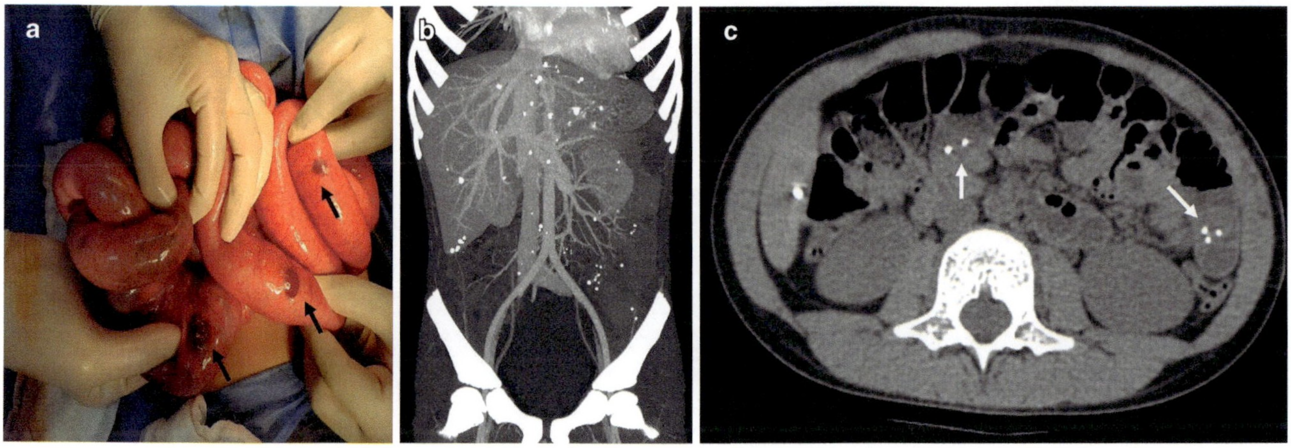

Fig. 16.5 A 9-year-old boy presenting with severe anemia and rectal bleeding. (**a**) Multiple small intestinal venous malformations (arrows) observed during surgical exploration. (**b**) Coronal maximum intensity projection CT showing multiple calcifications (phleboliths indicative of venous malformations) scattered throughout the intestine and liver. (**c**) Axial non-contrast CT demonstrating intestinal phleboliths (arrows)

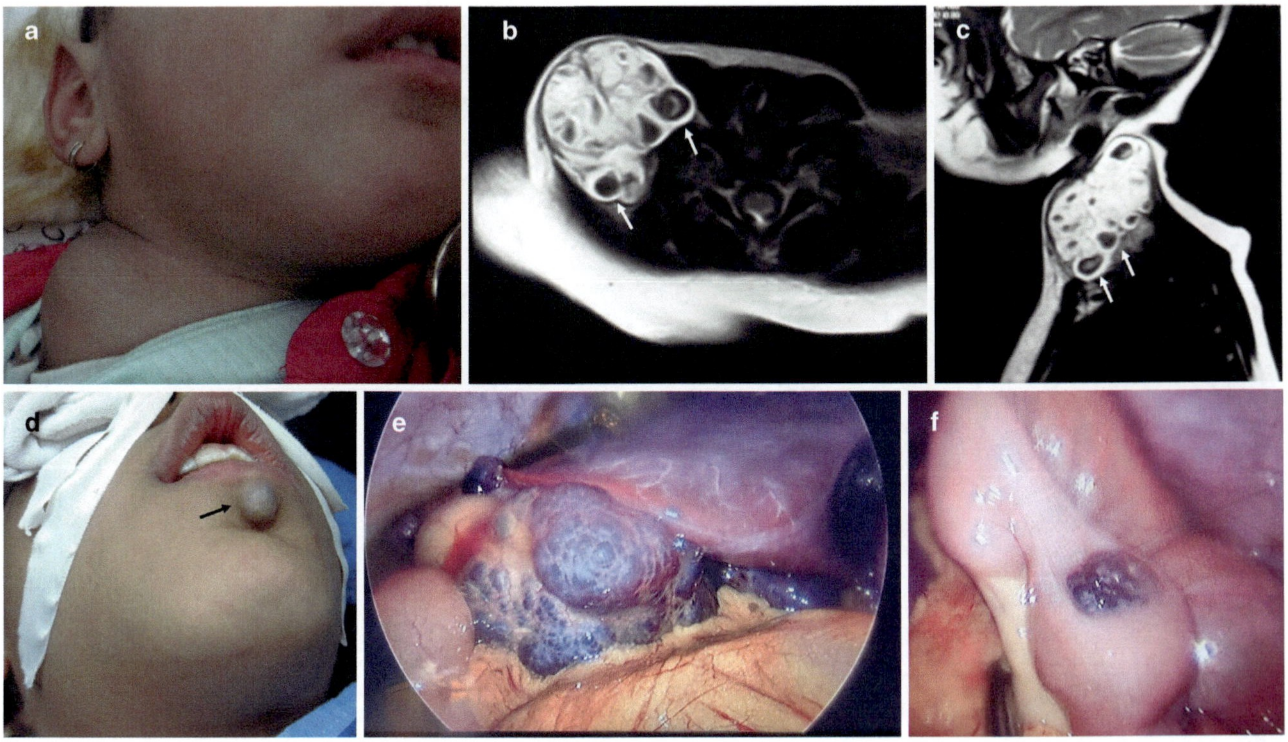

Fig. 16.6 (**a**) 18-month-old girl presenting initially with a solitary neck venous malformation. (**b**, **c**) MRI T2WI showing hyperintense lesion with phleboliths (arrows). (**d**) At 9 years, a new lower lip lesion (arrow) was excised. (**e**, **f**) Two years later, acute anemia and rectal bleeding led to laparoscopic exploration and detection of multiple venous malformations around and within the liver (**e**) and intestine (**f**)

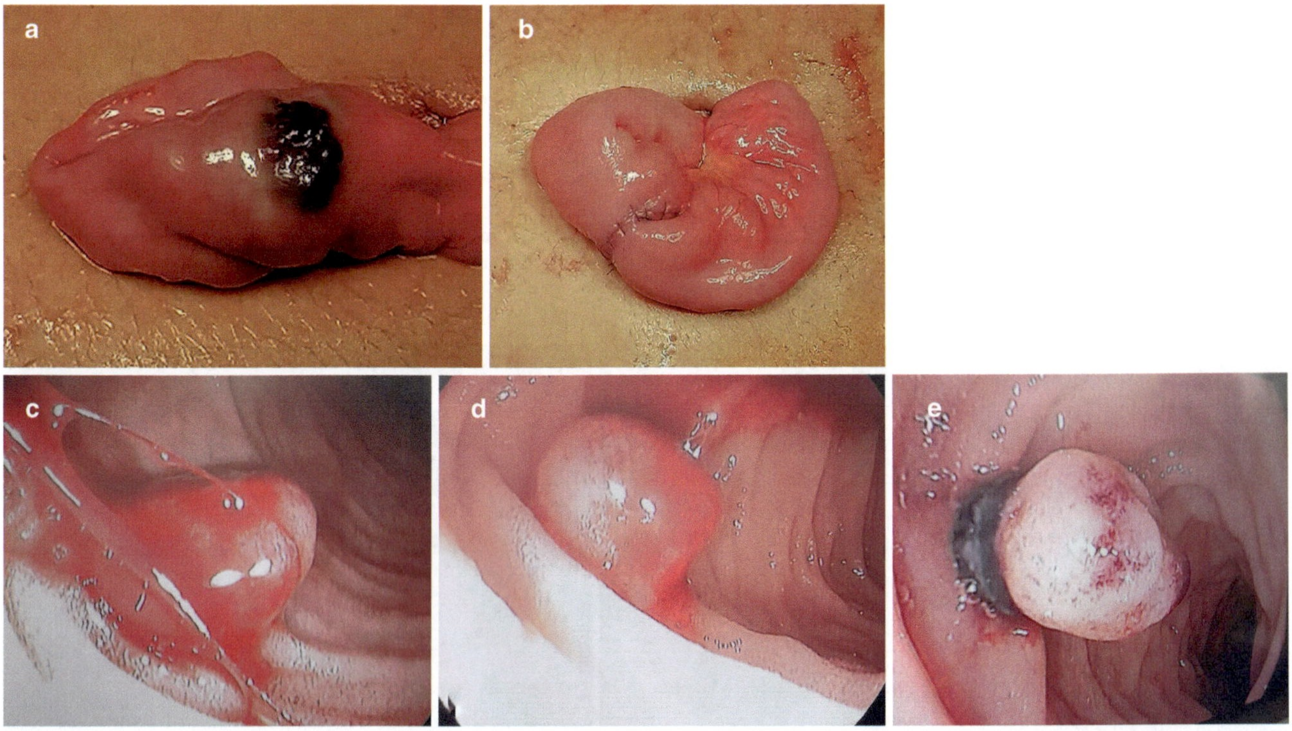

Fig. 16.7 (**a**, **b**) Surgical excision of venous malformation in the jejunum (same case as Fig. 16.6). (**c–e**) Bleeding venous malformation in the duodenum managed endoscopically by banding

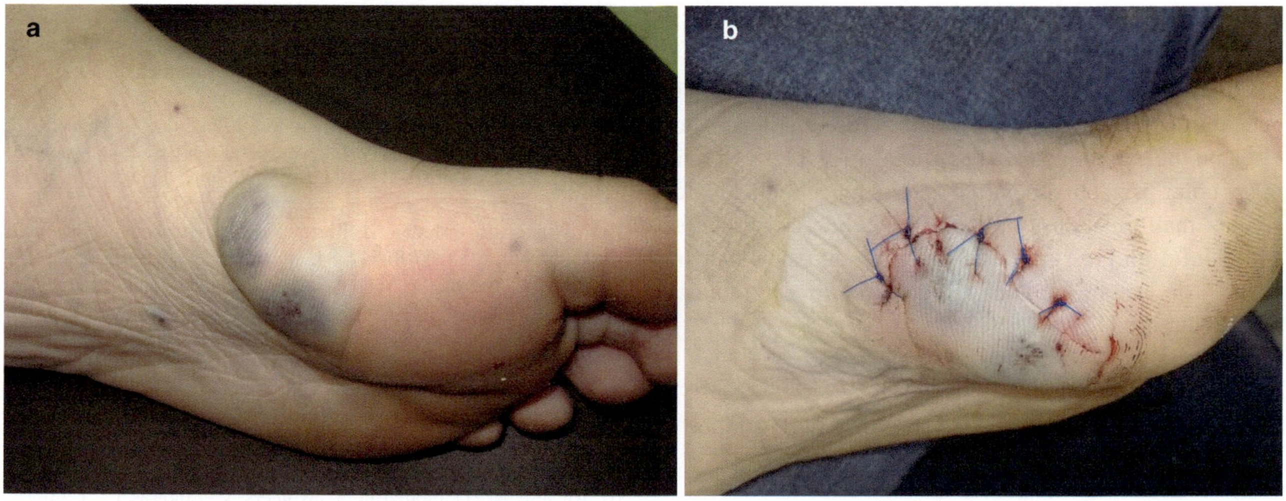

Fig. 16.8 Surgical excision of cutaneous lesion in a 14-year-old boy with Blue Rubber Bleb Nevus Syndrome. (**a**) before, and (**b**) after excision

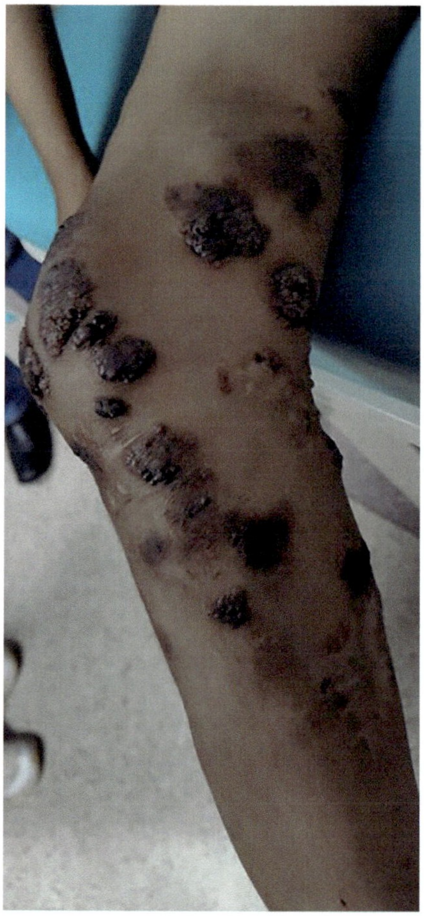

Fig. 16.9 Multifocal verrucous venous malformation affecting the lower extremity

Second: Familial Multifocal Venous Malformations

Familial multifocal venous malformations may result from inherited conditions such as cutaneo-mucosal venous malformations, glomuvenous malformations, and hyperkeratotic cutaneous capillary-venous malformations.

Familial Cutaneo-Mucosal Venous Malformation

The heritable form of multifocal venous malformations (VMs) is cutaneo-mucosal venous malformation (VMCM) [12]. VMCMs are usually small, multifocal lesions [13], composed of markedly dilated vascular spaces lined by a single continuous endothelial layer, with areas showing deficient mural cell support [14]. Familial VMCMs account for about 1–2% of all VMs and follow an autosomal dominant inheritance pattern. Clinically, the lesions are superficial, of small size, and rarely invade muscle [12]. The condition is caused by germline activating mutations in TEK/TIE2, leading to downstream activation of the PI3K/AKT pathway [12]. A common mutation involves a single amino acid substitution (R849W), but a second somatic hit in the same gene is typically required for lesion development.

Glomuvenous Malformations

These lesions are caused by mutations in the Glomulin gene (GLMN) [15]. They are usually present at birth, most often on the extremities, and appear as raised lesions ranging in color from pink to purple or dark blue. Unlike typical venous malformations, they are firm, non-compressible, and painful on pressure, involving skin and subcutaneous tissue. The lesions gradually increase in size and number throughout life [15].

Hyperkeratotic Cutaneous Capillary-Venous Malformations

They are caused by mutations of *KRIT1/CCM1* gene [15]. Lesions could be easily confused with verrucous venous malformations. Lesions are hyperkeratotic purple/blackish irregular plaques and located on the limbs.

References

1. Dompmartin A, Baselga E, Boon LM, Diociaiuti A, Dvorakova V, El Hachem M, et al. The VASCERN-VASCA working group diagnostic and management pathways for venous malformations. J Vasc Anom. 2023;4(2):e064.
2. Bean WB. Blue rubber-bleb nevi of the skin and gastrointestinal tract. In: Bean WB, editor. Vascular spiders and related lesions of the skin. Springfield: Thomas; 1958. p. 17–185.
3. Oranje AP. Blue rubber bleb nevus syndrome. Pediatr Dermatol. 1986;3(4):304–10.
4. Jin XL, Wang ZH, Xiao XB, Huang LS, Zhao XY. Blue rubber bleb nevus syndrome: a case report and literature review. World J Gastroenterol. 2014;20(45):17254–9.
5. Ivars M, Martin-Santiago A, Baselga E, Guibaud L, López-Gutiérrez JC. Fern-shaped patch as a hallmark of blue rubber bleb nevus syndrome in neonatal venous malformations. Eur J Pediatr. 2018;177(9):1395–8.
6. Soblet J, Kangas J, Nätynki M, Mendola A, Helaers R, Uebelhoer M, et al. Blue rubber bleb nevus (BRBN) syndrome is caused by somatic TEK (TIE2) mutations. J Invest Dermatol. 2017;137(1):207–16.
7. Mulliken JB, Fishman SJ, Burrows PE. Vascular anomalies. Curr Probl Surg. 2000;37(8):517–84.
8. Isoldi S, Belsha D, Yeop I, et al. Diagnosis and management of children with blue rubber bleb nevus syndrome: a multicenter case series. Dig Liver Dis. 2019;51(11):1537–46. https://doi.org/10.1016/j.dld.2019.04.020. Epub 2019 Jul 26. PMID: 31358484.
9. Wong XL, Phan K, Rodríguez Bandera AI, Sebaratnam DF. Sirolimus in blue rubber bleb naevus syndrome: a systematic review. J Paediatr Child Health. 2019;55(2):152–5.
10. Amyere M, Dompmartin A, Wouters V, Enjolras O, Kaitila I, Docquier PL, et al. Common somatic alterations identified in maffucci syndrome by molecular karyotyping. Mol Syndromol. 2014;5(6):259–67.
11. Couto JA, Vivero MP, Kozakewich HPW, Taghinia AH, Mulliken JB, Warman ML, et al. A somatic MAP3K3 mutation is associated with verrucous venous malformation. Am J Hum Genet. 2015;96(3):480–6.
12. Wouters V, Limaye N, Uebelhoer M, Irrthum A, Boon LM, Mulliken JB, et al. Hereditary cutaneomucosal venous malformations are caused by TIE2 mutations with widely variable hyperphosphorylating effects. Eur J Hum Genet. 2010;18(4):414–20.
13. Boon LM, Mulliken JB, Enjolras O, Vikkula M. Glomuvenous malformation (glomangioma) and venous malformation: distinct clinicopathologic and genetic entities. Arch Dermatol. 2004;140(8):971–6.
14. Calvert JT, Riney TJ, Kontos CD, Cha EH, Prieto VG, Shea CR, et al. Allelic and locus heterogeneity in inherited venous malformations. Hum Mol Genet. 1999;8(7):1279–89.
15. Brouillard P, Boon LM, Revencu N, Berg J, Dompmartin A, Dubois J, et al. Genotypes and phenotypes of 162 families with a glomulin mutation. Mol Syndromol. 2013;4(4):157–64.

Part V

Arteriovenous Malformations

Arteriovenous Malformations

17

Introduction

Arteriovenous malformations (AVMs) represent the rarest form of vascular malformations and the most difficult to treat. The presence of an arterial component is responsible for its classification as a fast-flow malformation. AVMs are composed of a tangled network of abnormal vascular channels that connect feeding arteries directly to draining veins, bypassing the normal intervening capillary bed. This central cluster is referred to as the "nidus" of the AVM. The absence of intervening capillary circulation in AVMs leads to direct arterial-to-venous shunting, resulting in significant hemodynamic consequences that vary based on the location and size of the AVM. Systemically, large proximal AVMs may cause a hyperdynamic circulatory state, potentially progressing to cardiac overload and heart failure. Locally, tissues may suffer ischemia due to the "steal phenomenon," where blood is diverted away from normal capillary beds. AVMs do not undergo spontaneous regression and typically exhibit a progressive course. Schobinger described their evolution through four clinical stages: an initial quiescent phase, followed by expansion, the onset of complications (such as ulceration or bleeding), and ultimately cardiac decompensation.

Clinical Picture

Arteriovenous malformations (AVMs) are congenital lesions, though they may remain clinically silent and undetected until later in life [1, 2]. Common anatomical sites include the head and neck region (Fig. 17.1), back (Fig. 17.2), and extremities (Fig. 17.3) [3, 4]. Intracranial AVMs fall outside the scope of this chapter and will not be addressed. Clinically, AVM often

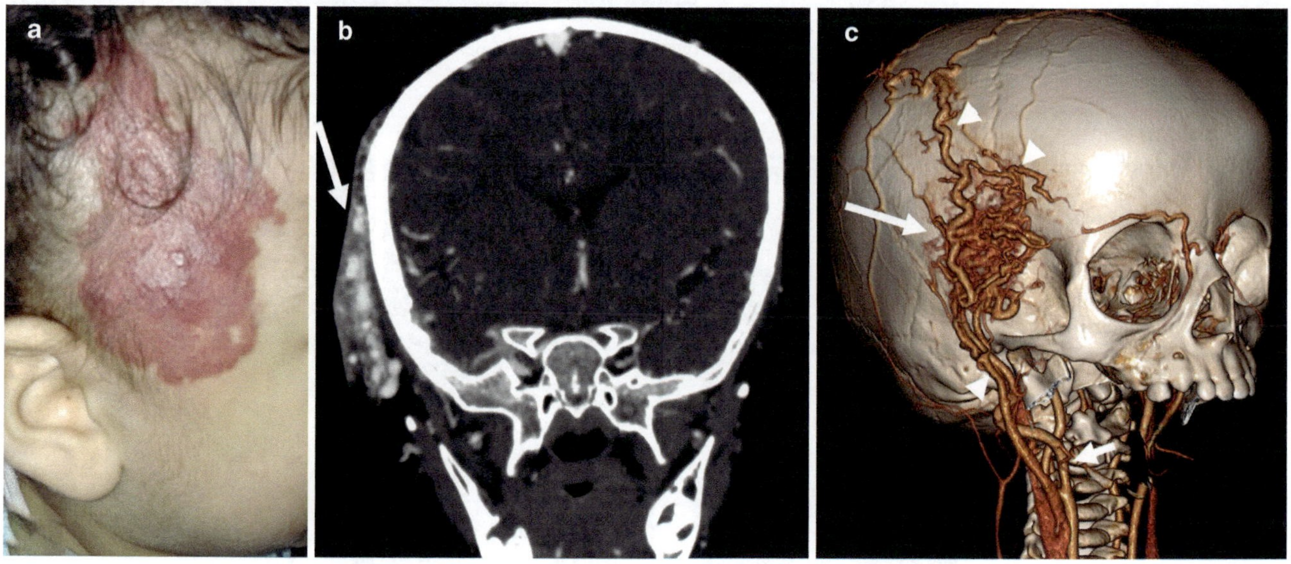

Fig. 17.1 Arteriovenous malformation (AVM) of the right temporal region in a one-year-old boy. (**a**) Clinical photograph of the lesion. (**b**) Coronal CT angiography demonstrates a vascular nidus (long arrow) in the right temporal region. (**c**) Three-dimensional reconstruction showing the nidus (long arrow) with a large feeding artery arising from the external carotid artery (short arrow) and multiple draining veins (arrowheads)

A. A. AbouZeid et al., *Atlas of Pediatric Vascular Anomalies*, https://doi.org/10.1007/978-3-032-30866-5_17

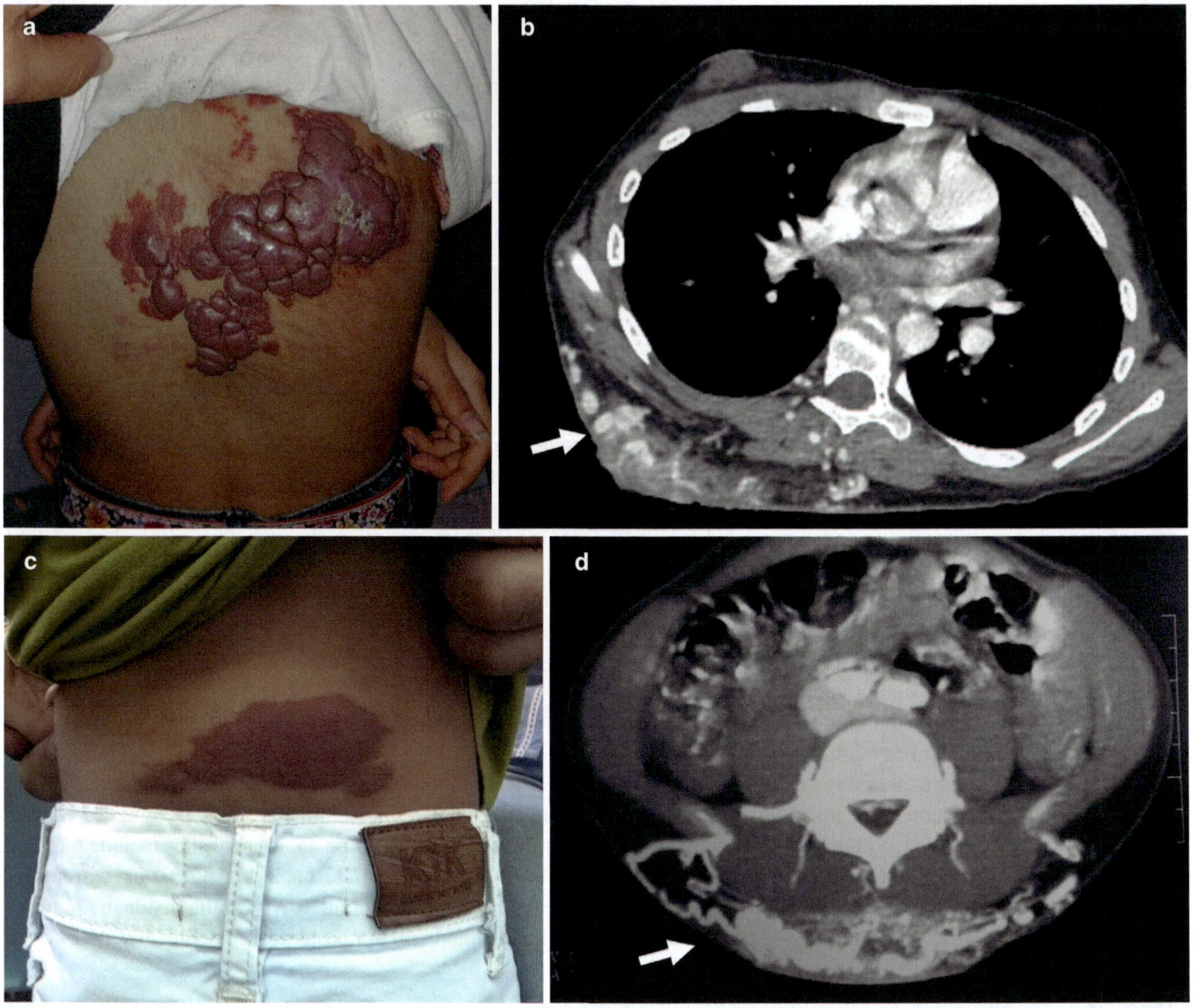

Fig. 17.2 Arteriovenous malformations (AVMs) of the back in two patients. (**a**, **c**) Clinical photographs showing lesions in the back. (**b**, **d**) Corresponding axial CT angiography images demonstrate enhancing vascular nidus (arrow)

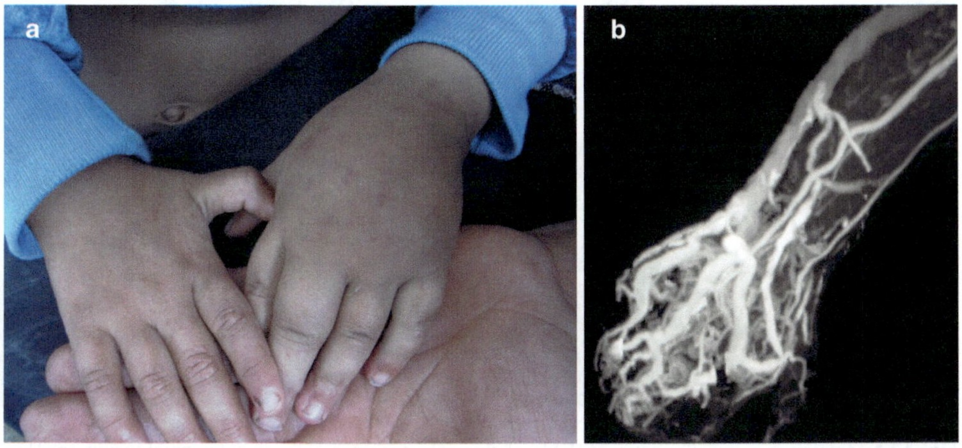

Fig. 17.3 Arteriovenous malformation (AVM) of the left hand in a 3-year-old girl. (**a**) Clinical photograph. (**b**) CT angiography demonstrates an infiltrative nidus with multiple draining veins

presents as a warm, pulsatile swelling with a palpable thrill [2]. They are frequently accompanied by a reddish discoloration of the overlying skin (Figs. 17.1 and 17.2) [4, 5]. Misdiagnosis as either congenital or infantile hemangiomas is not uncommon, which may lead to inappropriate treatment approaches (Fig. 17.4). Imaging is essential in distinguishing AVMs from vascular tumors such as hemangiomas, both of which are categorized as fast-flow lesions. However, unlike hemangiomas, AVMs typically lack a prominent soft tissue component and instead appear as a collection of dilated, tortuous vascular channels (Fig. 17.4) [6].

Pain is a frequent symptom in AVMs, particularly those affecting the extremities. It is often ischemic in origin, resulting from the steal phenomenon due to arterial-to-venous shunting, or may arise from compression of adjacent nerves. Additionally, elevated venous pressure in the draining veins—known as venous hypertension—can intensify the sensation of pain [3, 4]. As AVMs progress, other complications such as expansion, ulceration, and bleeding may also develop (Fig. 17.5) [7, 9].

Based on the extent of arteriovenous shunting and the stage of disease progression, patients may develop signs of a hyperdynamic circulatory state, including cardiomegaly, which can ultimately lead to heart failure (Fig. 17.6).

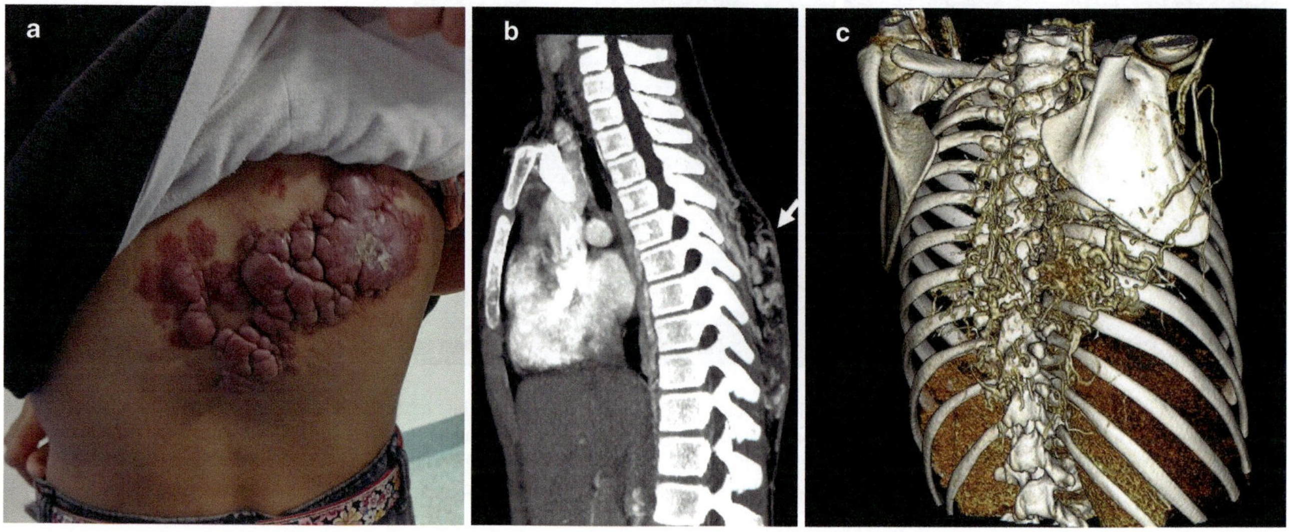

Fig. 17.4 Arteriovenous malformation (AVM) of the back in a 10-year-old girl. (**a**) Clinical photograph. (**b**) Sagittal CT angiography and (**c**) three-dimensional reconstruction show a tangle of enhancing vessels forming the nidus (arrow)

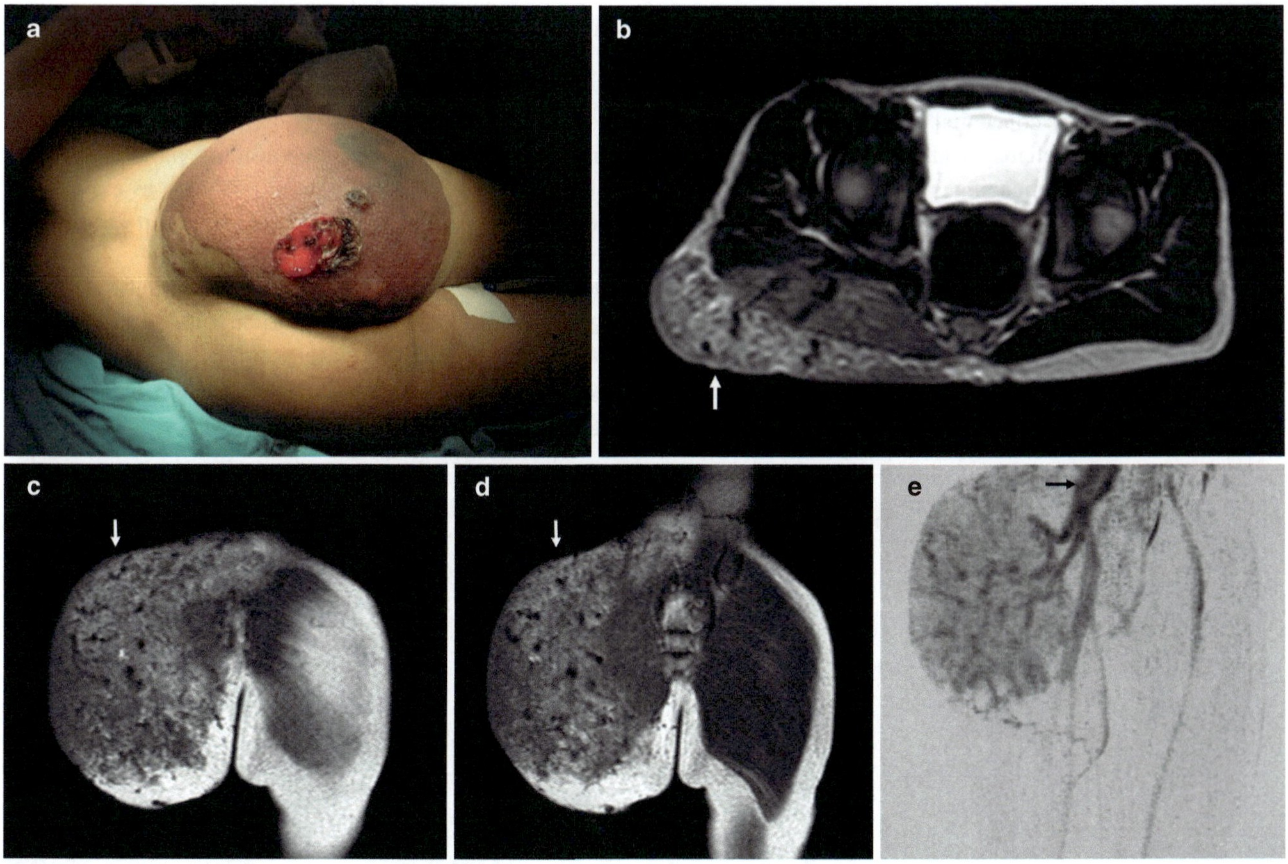

Fig. 17.5 Arteriovenous malformation (AVM) of the gluteal region in a 7-year-old boy. (**a**) Clinical photograph showing the lesion complicated by ulceration. (**b**) Axial T2-weighted image demonstrates the gluteal lesion with multiple flow voids (white arrow). (**c**, **d**) Coronal T1-weighted images show the lesion (white arrow) with associated soft tissue thickening due to fibrofatty matrix and muscle edema. (**e**) Arterial phase of dynamic contrast-enhanced MR angiography reveals a large enhancing lesion with early venous filling (black arrow), consistent with arteriovenous shunting

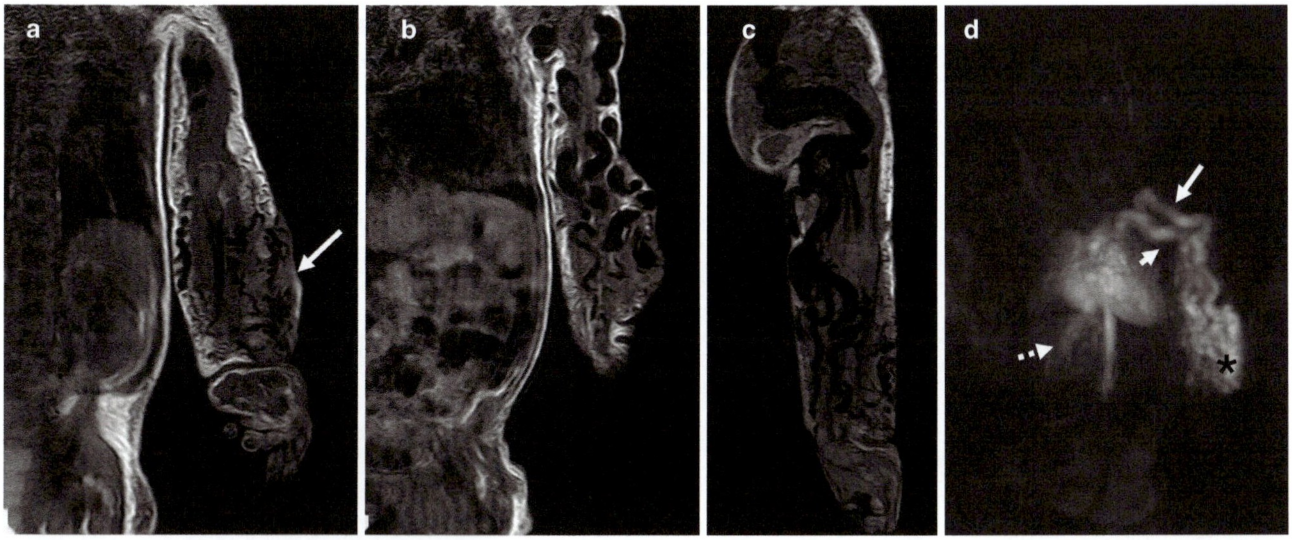

Fig. 17.6 Arteriovenous malformation (AVM) of the forearm in a 9-day-old girl. (**a**, **b**) Coronal T1-weighted images and (**c**) sagittal T1-weighted image show a large nidus (arrow) in the dorsum of the forearm. (**d**) Coronal maximum intensity projection of dynamic contrast-enhanced MR angiography demonstrates the nidus (asterisk), a dilated feeding artery (short arrow), and an early draining vein (long arrow), indicating arteriovenous shunting. Note the associated cardiomegaly and retrograde filling of the hepatic veins (dashed arrow), consistent with high-output cardiac failure

Investigations

Ultrasound is widely accessible and often employed as a first-line investigation (Fig. 17.7); nevertheless, more advanced imaging techniques are typically required for treatment planning. Magnetic resonance imaging (MRI) is a valuable tool for confirming the diagnosis of AVMs and assessing their full extent. The lesion primarily consists of dilated, tortuous abnormal vessels, which appear on MRI as characteristic flow voids (Fig. 17.6). A key distinguishing feature from vascular tumors is the absence of a significant soft tissue component in AVMs [8–10]. However, this distinction may be less clear when AVMs infiltrate muscle tissue or specific organs, such as the ear (Fig. 17.8) [6]. CT angiography has the advantage of producing "impressive" three-dimensional reconstruction images demonstrating the feeding arteries, draining veins, and involvement of surrounding organs or tissues (Figs. 17.9 and 17.10) [9, 10]. A hallmark feature of AVMs on post-contrast imaging is the early opacification of the efferent veins, reflecting the presence of arteriovenous shunting (Figs. 17.5e and 17.6d). Digital angiography remains the gold standard for evaluating AVMs when intervention is being planned (Fig. 17.11) [9]. It serves as the foundation for angiographic classification, which categorizes AVMs based on the configuration of their feeding arteries and draining veins [8].

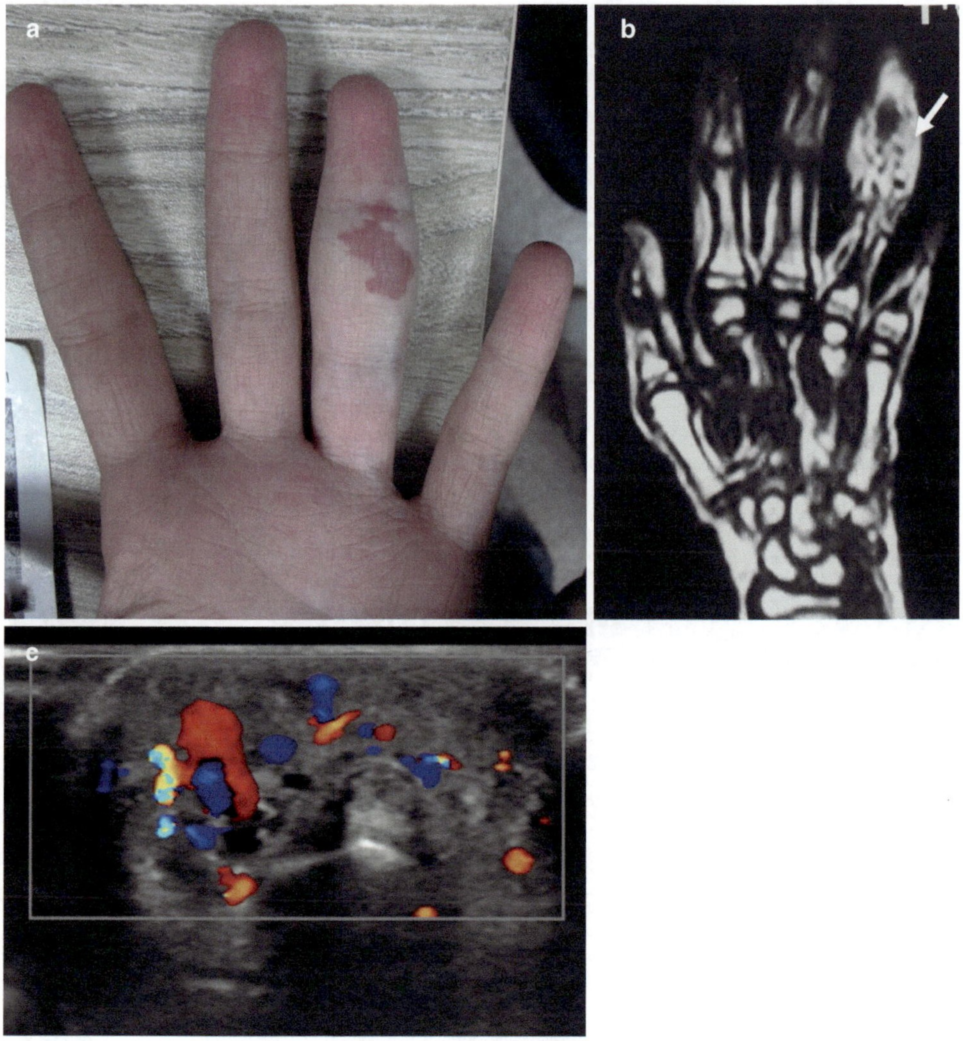

Fig. 17.7 Arteriovenous malformation (AVM) of the ring finger. (**a**) Clinical photograph. (**b**) Coronal T2-weighted image shows a hyperintense swelling (arrow) with multiple flow voids. (**c**) Color Doppler ultrasound demonstrates soft tissue thickening with increased vascularity

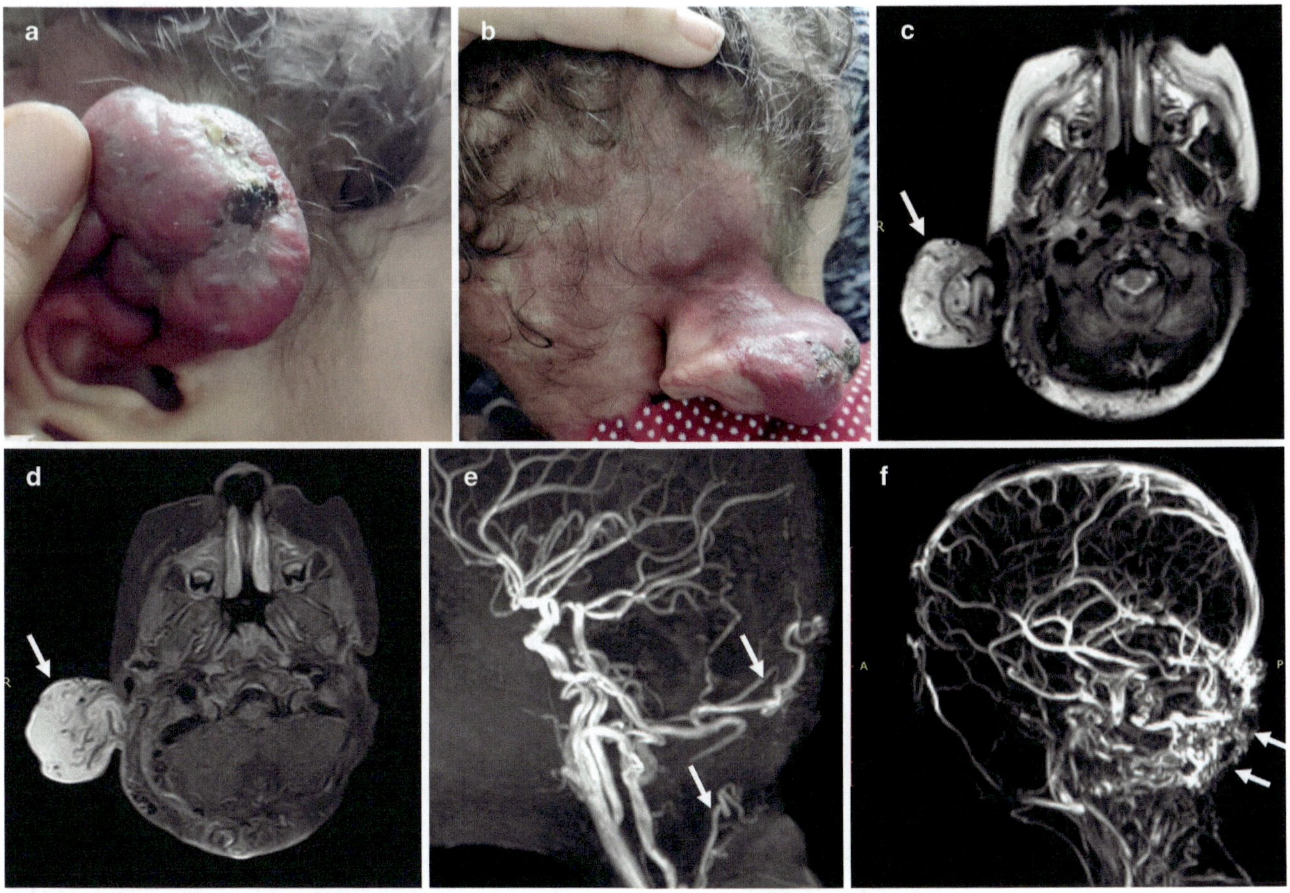

Fig. 17.8 Arteriovenous malformation (AVM) of the ear in a 1-year-old boy with atypical mass-like features. (**a**, **b**) Clinical photographs showing ulceration. (**c**) Axial T2-weighted image demonstrates a well-defined hyperintense mass (long arrow) with multiple flow voids. (**d**) Axial contrast-enhanced fat-suppressed T1-weighted image shows mass-like enhancement (arrow). (**e**) Sagittal non-contrast MR angiography depicts multiple arterial feeders (arrow) arising from the external carotid artery. (**f**) MR venography demonstrates multiple draining veins (arrows)

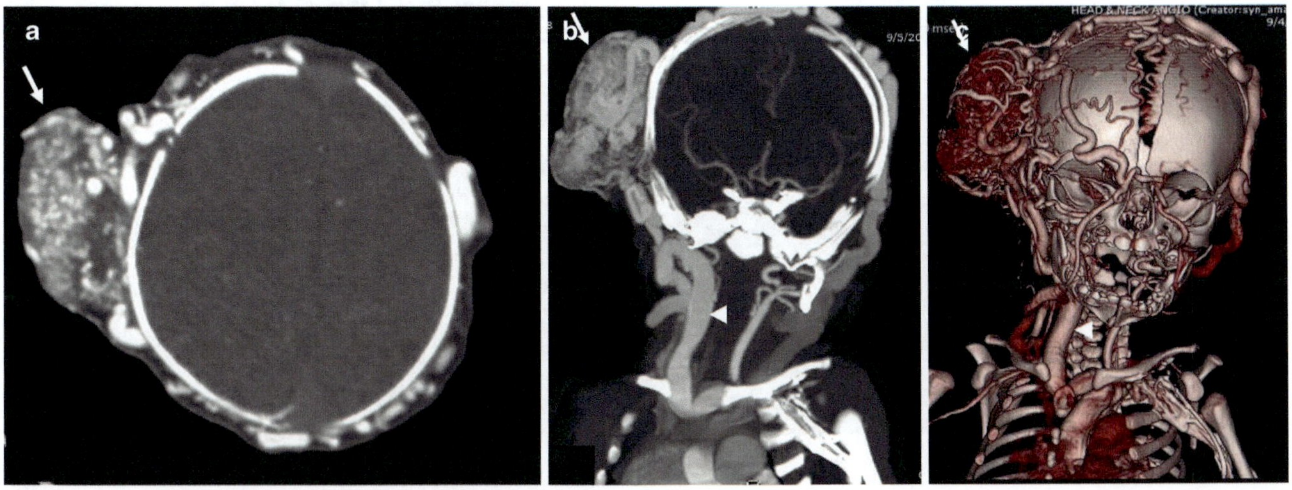

Fig. 17.9 Arteriovenous malformation (AVM) in a neonate. (**a**) Axial CT angiography, (**b**) coronal CT angiography, and (**c**) three-dimensional reconstruction demonstrate a large nidus (arrow) with multiple feeding arteries and draining veins. Note the congested internal jugular vein (arrowhead)

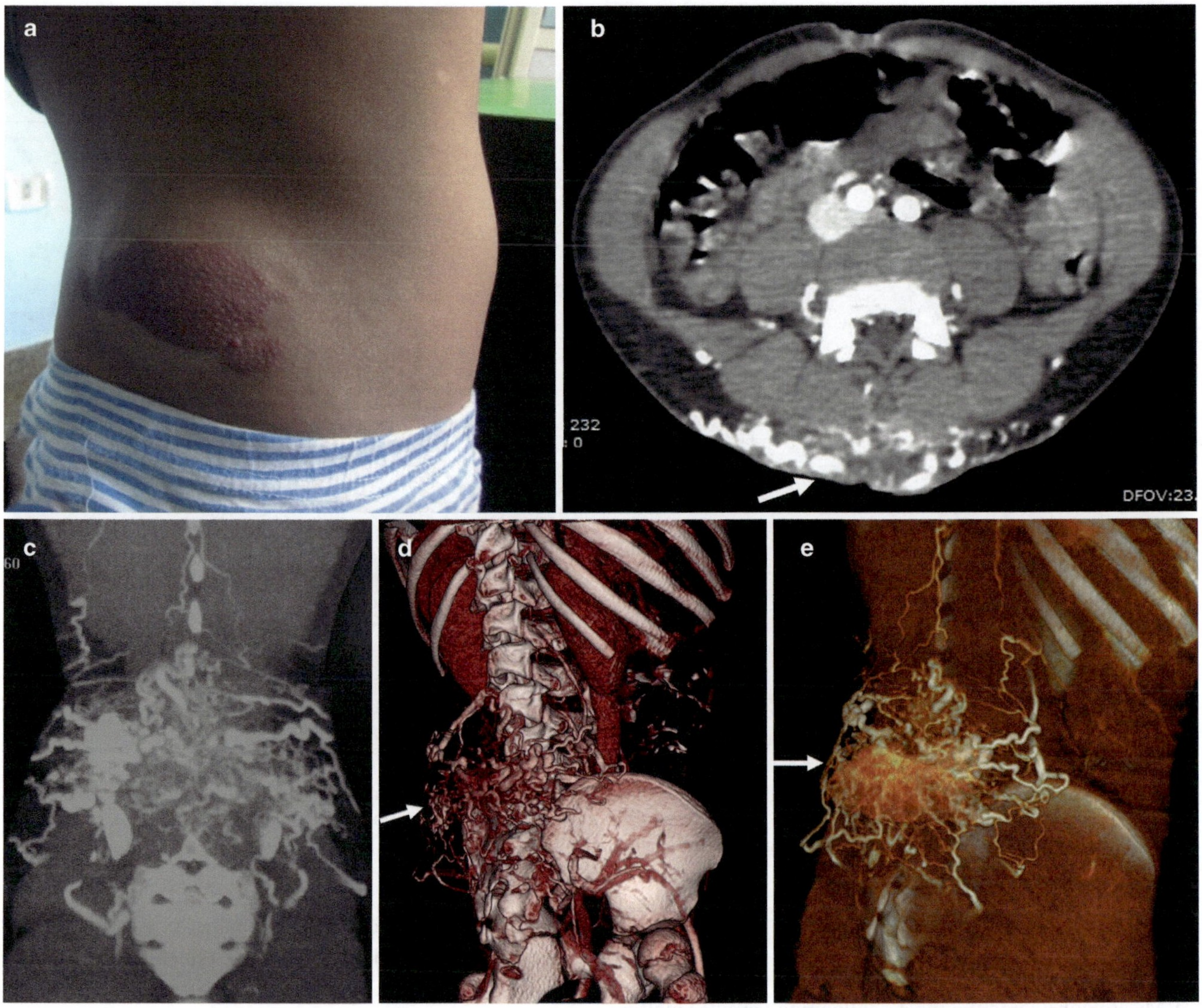

Fig. 17.10 Arteriovenous malformation (AVM) of the back in a 6-year-old boy. (**a**) Clinical photograph. (**b**) Axial CT angiography and (**c**) coronal CT angiography. (**d**, **e**) Three-dimensional reconstructions show an enhancing nidus (arrow) with multiple feeding vessels

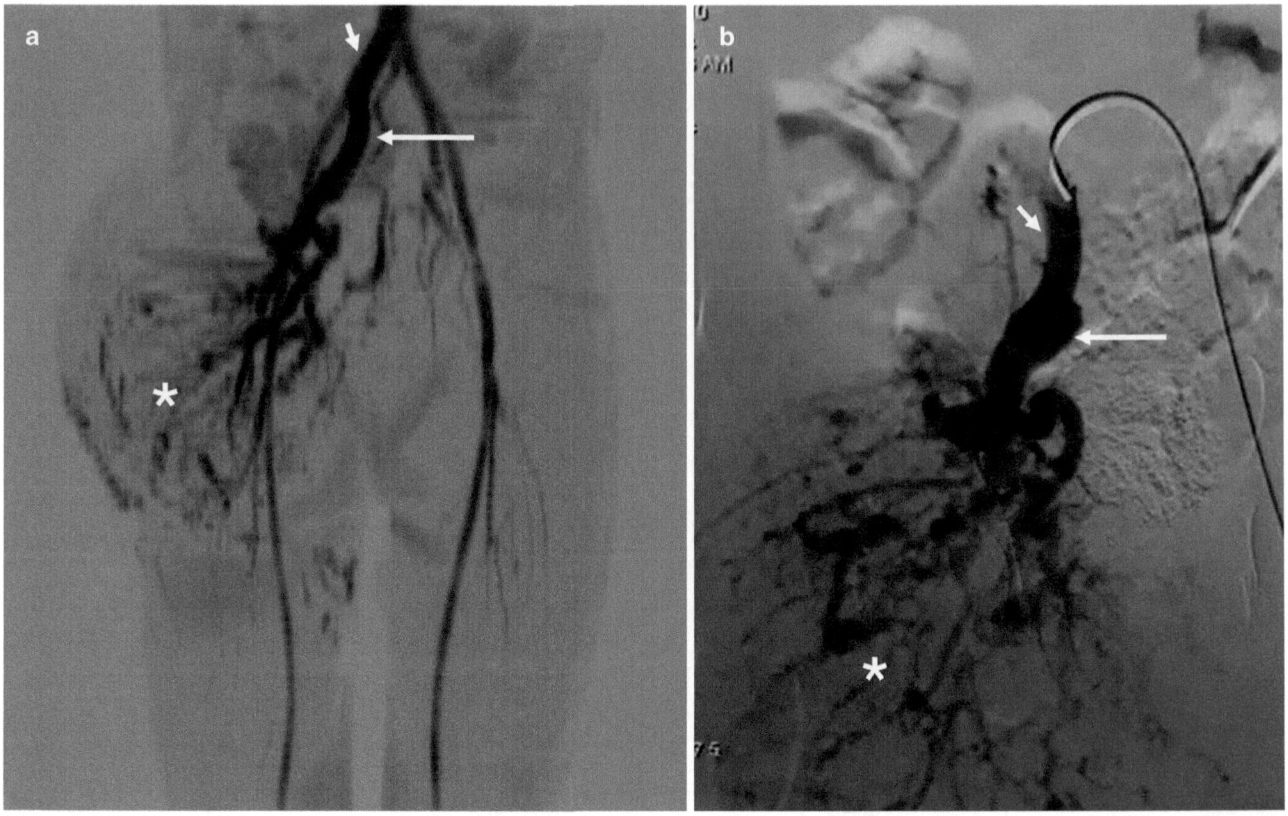

Fig. 17.11 Arteriovenous malformation (AVM) of the right gluteal region in a 7-year-old boy (same case as Fig. 17.5). (**a**) Non-contrast MR angiography and (**b**) digital subtraction angiography demonstrating a dilated common iliac artery (short arrow) giving rise to a dilated internal iliac artery (long arrow), which supplies a large nidus (asterisk)

Treatment

AVMs are considered the most challenging vascular malformations to manage. Inadequate treatment approaches—such as partial excision or mere occlusion of the feeding artery—can provoke a proliferative response within the lesion, often leading to rapid expansion and severe, uncontrollable complications [2, 7]. Recent advancements in endovascular therapy, utilizing various embolic and sclerosing agents either alone or in combination with surgical intervention, have emerged as an effective and widely accepted treatment strategy for AVMs [3–5, 8].

Embolization This technique is most frequently utilized to minimize blood loss during or after surgical resection and to provide symptomatic relief in patients with unresectable AVMs. However, AVMs tend to re-expand following embolization, especially if the central nidus and its feeding arteries are not completely obliterated [9, 10]. Several embolic agents are available for use, with N-butyl cyanoacrylate (NBCA) being one of the most commonly employed. NBCA is a clear, free-flowing adhesive liquid that rapidly polymerizes upon contact with ionic solutions such as blood. To control its polymerization rate and enhance visibility under imaging (adding radiopacity), it is typically mixed with ethiodized oil (Fig. 17.12) [3]. Angiography followed by super-selective embolization with NBCA is typically performed 24–72 h prior to surgical resection [11]. The embolized areas become readily visible and palpable, offering intraoperative landmarks to guide the surgeon during resection [9, 10].

Ethanol embolotherapy has been reported as potentially curative in the treatment of AVMs [8]. In other words, it can be sufficient to eliminate or improve symptoms of AVMs in a high percentage of patients, but with substantial risk of minor and major complications (see Chap. 13). Ethanol uniquely induces endothelial cell protein denaturation, leading to complete obliteration of the vessel lumen rather than simple obstruction. This mechanism prevents recanalization by irreversibly damaging the endothelium within the AVM nidus [3–5].

Surgery Surgical resection provides the most effective option for achieving long-term control of AVMs. However, incomplete (subtotal) resection is typically followed by recurrence, further lesion expansion, and occasionally, a more aggressive

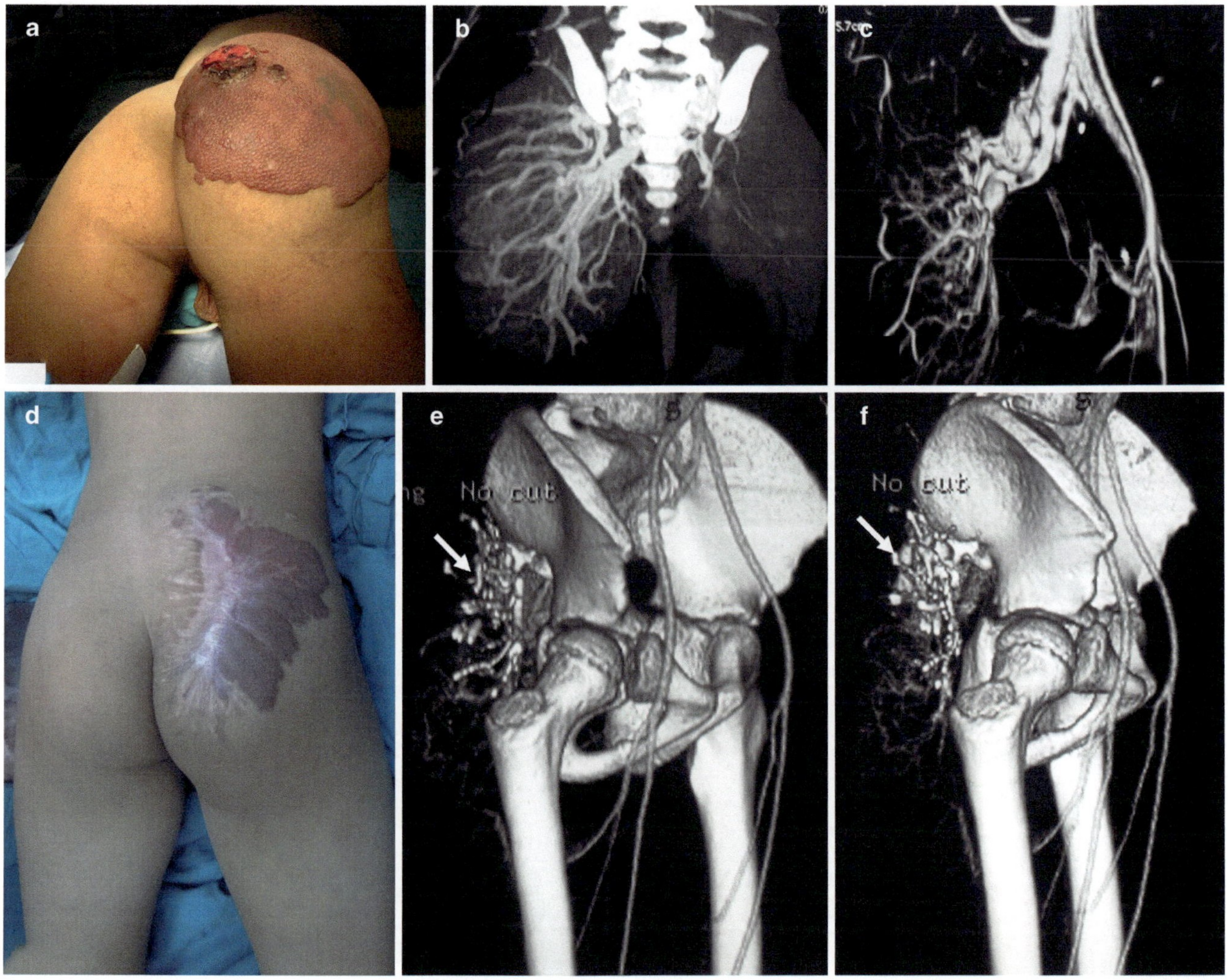

Fig. 17.12 Arteriovenous malformation (AVM) of the right gluteal region in a 7-year-old boy (same case as Figs. 17.5 and 17.11). Upper row (**a–c**), before surgical excision: (**a**) Clinical photograph. (**b**) Coronal CT angiography and (**c**) three-dimensional reconstruction demonstrate a large nidus with dilated common and internal iliac vessels. Lower row (**d–f**), after surgical excision: (**d**) Clinical photograph following excision. (**e, f**) Three-dimensional CT angiography reconstructions show hyperdense embolic material (arrow) within the AVM, applied preoperatively to reduce intraoperative bleeding

clinical course. Therefore, the primary objective—whenever feasible—is complete excision of the AVM nidus [7, 11]. Following resection of a small, well-localized AVM, linear closure may be possible. However, more frequently, alternative methods of primary closure—such as skin grafts or local/microvascular flaps—are required. Tissue expansion may also be considered as a preparatory step to facilitate skin closure after resection of AVMs [9, 10].

References

1. Gokani VJ, Sivakumar B, Kangesu L. Vascular anomalies. Surgery (Oxford). 2018;36:314–23.
2. Flors L, Park AW, Norton PT, Hagspiel KD, Leiva-Salinas C. Soft-tissue vascular malformations and tumors Part 1: classification, role of imaging and high-flow lesions. Radiologia (English edition). 2019;61:4–15.
3. Do YS, Park KB. Endovascular treatment of AVM: trunk and extremity. In: Kim YW, Lee BB, Yakes WF, Do YS, editors. Congenital vascular malformations. Berlin/Heidelberg: Springer-Verlag; 2017. p. 233–40.
4. Brassel F, Meila D, Schlunz-Hendann M. Interventional treatment in AVM. In: Mattassi R, Loose D, Vaghi M, editors. Hemangiomas and vascular malformations. Milano: Springer; 2015. p. 255–62.
5. Ritcher GT, Johnson AB. Arterioenous malformation. In: Perkins JA, Balakrishnan K, editors. Evidence-based management of head and neck vascular anomalies. Springer Nature Switzerland; 2018. p. 193–204.
6. Burrows PE, Paltiel HJ. Radiological imaging of hemangiomas and related vascular tumors. In: Mulliken JB, Burrows PE, Fishman SJ, editors. Mulliken & Young's vascular anomalies: hemangiomas and malformations. Oxford University Press; 2013. p. 111–60.
7. Uller W, Alomari AI, Richter GT. Arteriovenous malformations. Semin Pediatr Surg. 2014;23:203–7.

8. Yakes WF, Ivancev K, Vogelzang RL, Yakes AM. Endovascular treatment of AVMs: head and neck. In: Kim YW, Lee BB, Yakes WF, Do YS, editors. Congenital vascular malformations. Berlin/Heidelberg: Springer-Verlag; 2017. p. 223–32.
9. Mulliken JB. Vascular malformations of the head and neck. In: Mulliken JB, Burrows PE, Fishman SJ, editors. Mulliken & Young's vascular anomalies: hemangiomas and malformations. Oxford University Press; 2013. p. 839–904.
10. Upton IIIJ. Vascular malformations of the extremities. In: Mulliken JB, Burrows PE, Fishman SJ, editors. Mulliken & Young's vascular anomalies: hemangiomas and malformations. Oxford University Press; 2013. p. 905–65.
11. Johnson AB, Richter GT. Surgical considerations in vascular malformations. Tech Vasc Interv Radiol. 2019;22 https://doi.org/10.1016/j.tvir.2019.100635.

Part VI

Capillary Malformations

18 Capillary Malformations

Capillary Malformations

Capillary malformations (CMs), also known as port-wine birthmarks, are congenital slow-flow vascular malformations characterized by an increased number of dilated dermal capillaries. They affect approximately 0.1–2% of newborns [1], typically presenting at birth and grow proportionately with the individual. Clinically, they appear as light pink to red patches (Fig. 18.1) that may darken and thicken over time. In some cases, hyperkeratosis and soft tissue hypertrophy develop, particularly in facial lesions (Fig. 18.2) [2]. Additionally, eczematous dermatitis, known as the Meyerson phenomenon, can occur (Fig. 18.3) [2]. Beyond cosmetic concerns, CMs may significantly affect quality of life [3]—for example, lip hypertrophy can interfere with eating or dental function, while eyelid thickening may impair complete closure. On the face, capillary malformations (CMs) often follow a dermatomal distribution. In the early neonatal period, before the proliferative phase of infantile hemangioma (IH), it may be challenging to distinguish CMs from IH (see Chap. 3).

Nevus simplex, also known as a salmon patch, stork bite, or angel's kiss, is a special type of benign vascular birthmark present at birth and seen in up to 50% of newborns. It is caused by dilated capillaries within the papillary dermis and are likely due to a lack of local autonomic regulation in the affected skin area [4, 5]. It appears as a flat, pink to red patch, most often located on the glabella, eyelids, or nape of the neck (Fig. 18.4). The lesion becomes more noticeable when the infant cries, strains, or has a fever, but it remains flat, asymptomatic, and ill-defined. Unlike port-wine stains, nevus simplex is harmless and self-limiting, with most lesions fading spontaneously within the first one to two years of life, although those on the nape may persist into adulthood but are usually hidden by hair. Large, persistent facial Nevus simplex can be associated with underlying syndromes such as Beckwith–Wiedemann syndrome and macrocephaly-CM syndrome (M-CM) [5].

Diagnosis of CMs is essentially a clinical diagnosis while imaging is ordered to exclude the presence of associated anomalies (Fig. 18.5). Histopathological examination is rarely performed in CMs. Most of the involved vessels are located in the papillary and reticular dermis with decreasing number of abnormal vessels in deeper areas [6]. They are caused by a sporadic somatic mosaic activating mutation in *GNAQ or GNA11* with defective expression of smooth muscle actin (SMA) in the pericytes [7].

Although isolated cutaneous capillary malformations (CMs) are not life-threatening and are primarily a cosmetic concern, their location may signal underlying pathology. For example, facial CMs, particularly those involving the upper face and forehead, may be associated with Sturge–Weber syndrome (Fig. 18.6) [8], while midline back lesions can indicate underlying spinal anomalies [9]. Of particular importance is the association of CMs with other vascular anomalies and tissue growth abnormalities (overgrowth or undergrowth), which may occur as part of syndromes such as Klippel–Trenaunay syndrome (Fig. 18.7) or other PIK3CA-related overgrowth spectrum (PROS) disorders (Fig. 18.8). In addition, certain special subtypes of CMs are linked to internal organ arteriovenous malformations, with notable concern for involvement of the central nervous system (CNS).

A. A. AbouZeid et al., *Atlas of Pediatric Vascular Anomalies*, https://doi.org/10.1007/978-3-032-30866-5_18

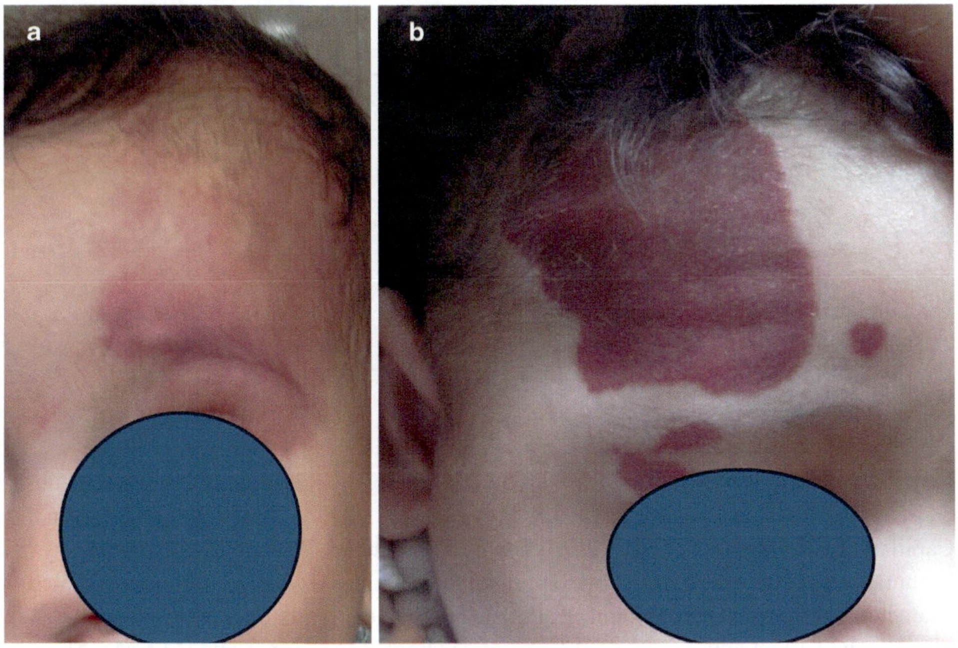

Fig. 18.1 Capillary malformations typically presenting as flat skin lesions ranging in color from light pink (**a**) to red (**b**)

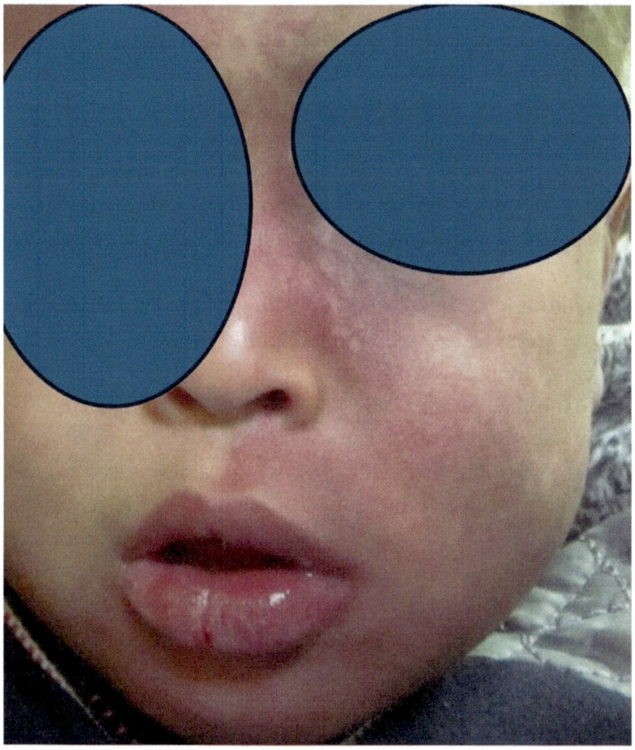

Fig. 18.2 Soft tissue hypertrophy associated with capillary malformations, demonstrated in this case by hypertrophy of the left cheek and lips

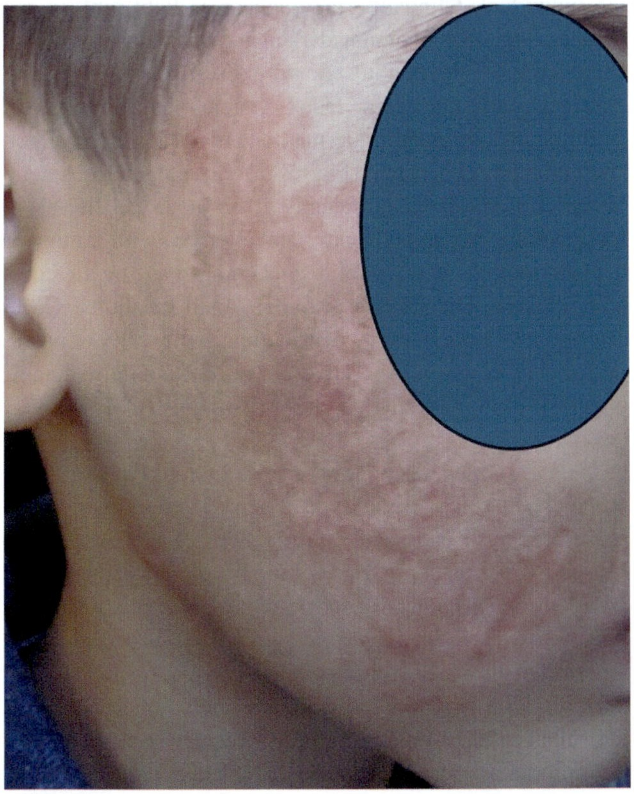

Fig. 18.3 Eczematous dermatitis arising within a capillary malformation

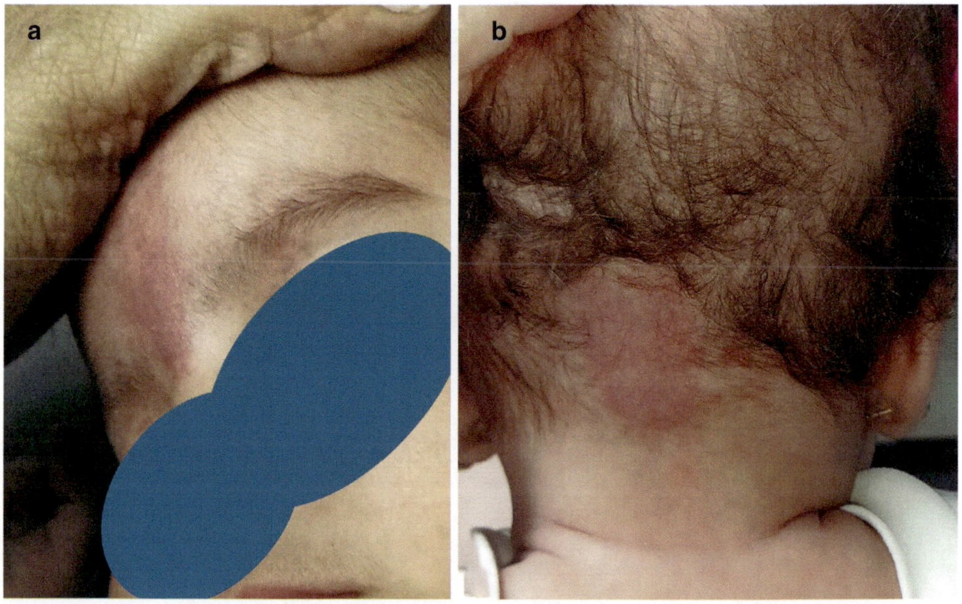

Fig. 18.4 Common sites of nevus simplex involving the glabella (**a**) and the nape of the neck (**b**)

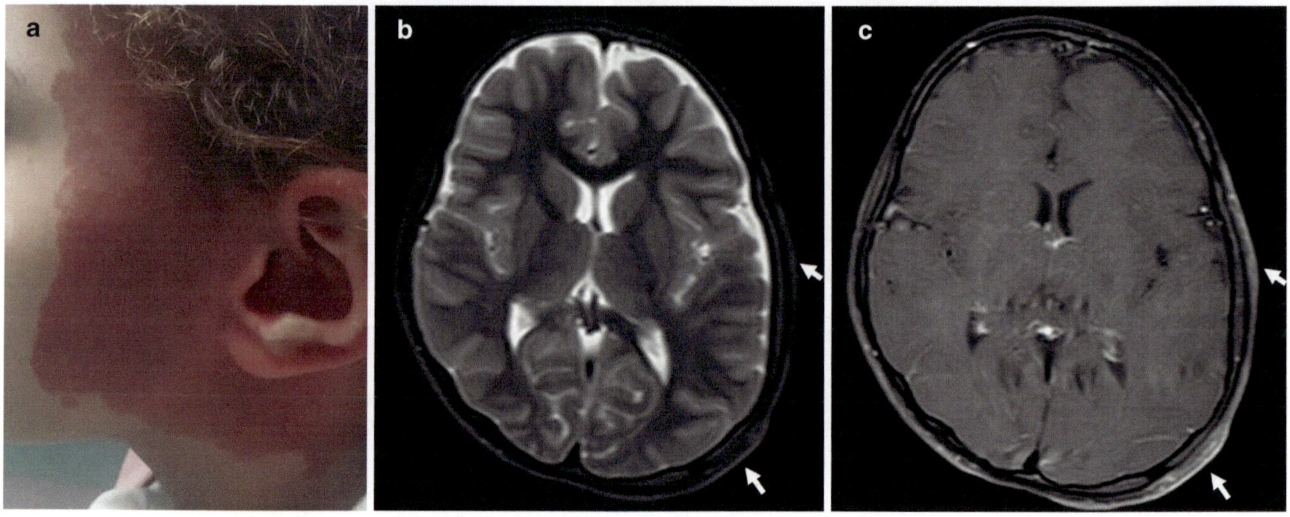

Fig. 18.5 (**a**) Capillary malformation in a 9-year-old girl. (**b**) Axial T2-weighted MRI and (**c**) axial contrast-enhanced fat-suppressed T1-weighted MRI demonstrate cutaneous thickening (arrows) appearing hyperintense with evident contrast enhancement

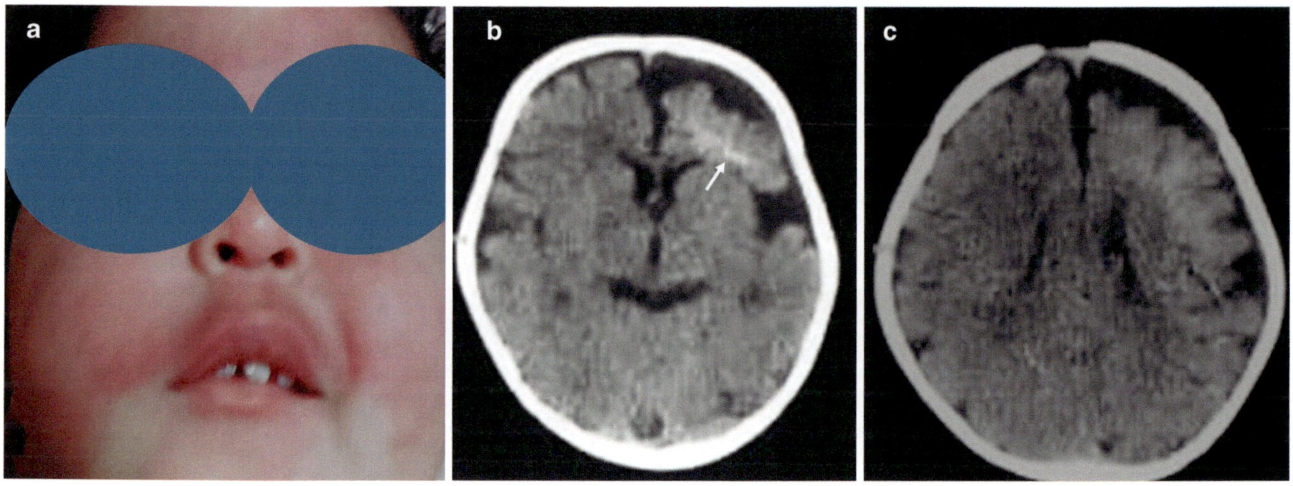

Fig. 18.6 Sturge–Weber syndrome. (**a**) Capillary malformation following a frontonasal distribution. (**b**, **c**) Axial non-contrast CT show left cerebral hemiatrophy and subcortical calcification (arrow)

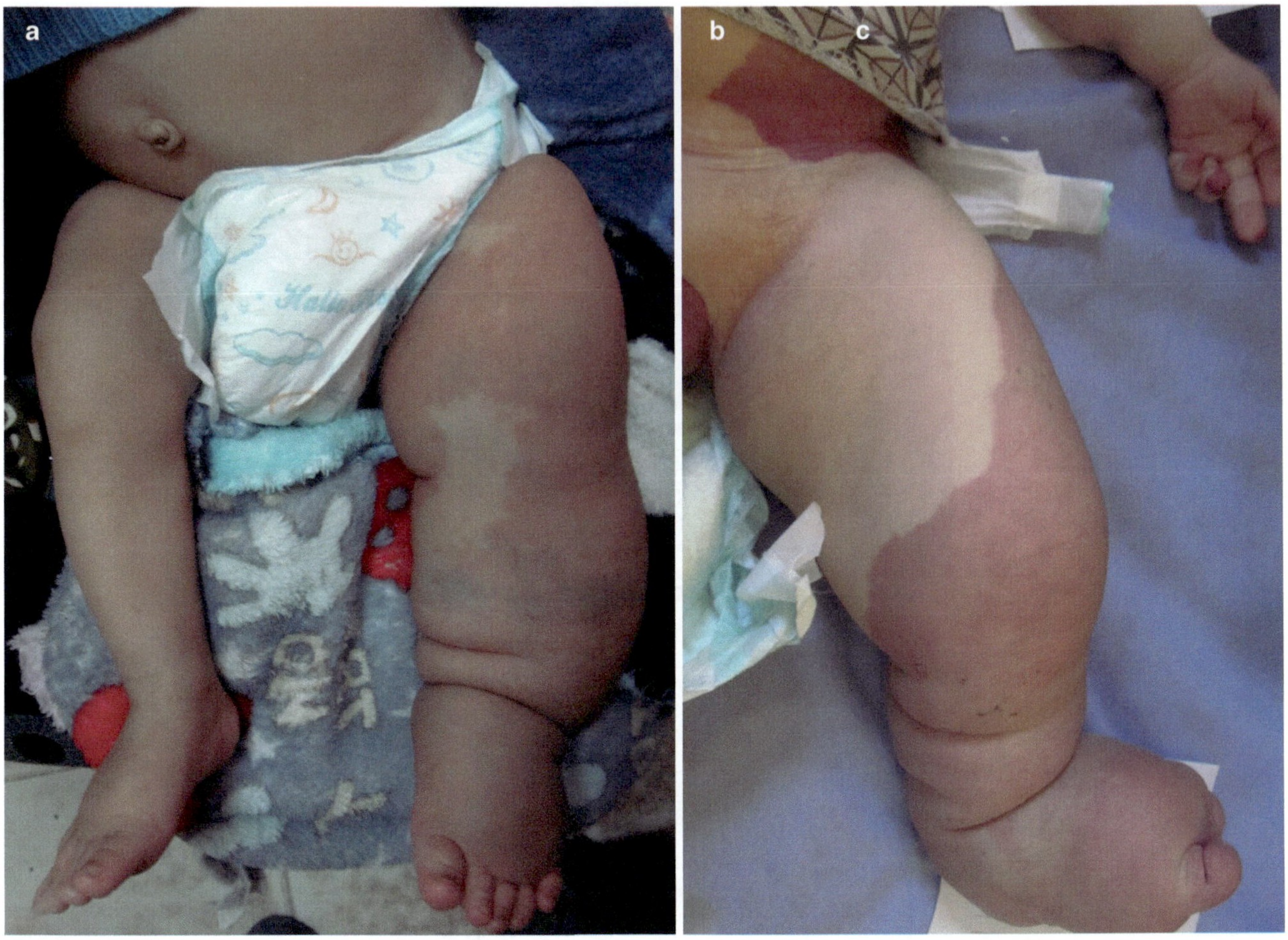

Fig. 18.7 Capillary malformations of the lower extremities in Klippel–Trénaunay syndrome in two different cases

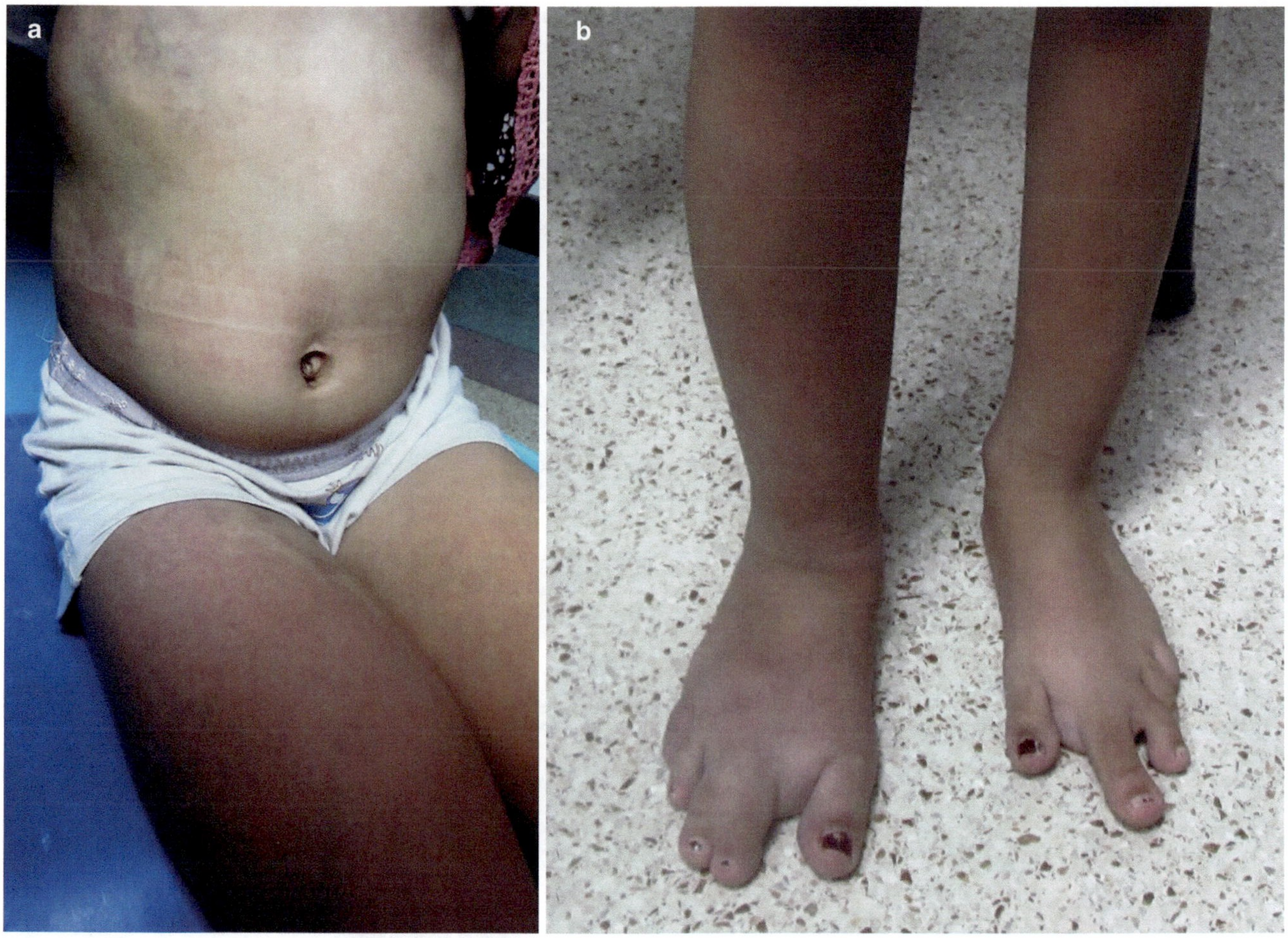

Fig. 18.8 Capillary malformation (CM) associating PIK3CA-related overgrowth spectrum (PROS) in a 7-year-old girl. (**a**) CM involves the right lower limb and extending up to lower lateral trunk. (**b**) The feet show sandal gap deformity (wide first interdigital gap), syndactyly, and toe hypertrophy

Syndromes Associated with Capillary Malformations

- *Sturge Weber Syndrome (SWS)*: SWS is a rare, sporadic neurocutaneous disorder with an estimated incidence of 1 in 50,000 live births. It is classically defined by a triad consisting of facial capillary malformations (CMs), ipsilateral leptomeningeal angiomatosis, and ocular abnormalities, which may be accompanied by bone and/or soft tissue involvement [10]. The facial CM typically follows a frontonasal distribution in most patients. When the lesion is multi-dermatomal or bilaterally distributed, the risk of SWS is significantly increased (Fig. 18.6) [11]. Ocular manifestations of Sturge–Weber Syndrome most commonly present as glaucoma or elevated intraocular pressure. Additional findings may include choroidal vascular lesions, characterized by intraocular capillary proliferation, which can increase the risk of retinal detachment. Neurological involvement typically results from capillary–venous malformations of the leptomeninges. On contrast-enhanced MRI, these appear as leptomeningeal enhancement, ranging from localized areas to extensive hemispheric involvement. Frequently associated radiological features include cortical atrophy and intracranial calcifications (Fig. 18.9) [12]. Clinically, neurological symptoms often include seizures, headaches, stroke or stroke-like episodes, developmental delay, cognitive impairment, and attention difficulties.
- *Microcephaly-Capillary Malformation (MIC-CAP)*: MIC-CAP is a rare disorder defined by congenital microcephaly, global developmental delay, seizures, optic atrophy, poor somatic growth, and the presence of small cutaneous capillary malformations (CMs) [13]. The condition results from homozygous or compound heterozygous mutations in the STAM-binding protein (STAMBP) gene, leading to aberrant activation of the RAS-MAPK and PI3K-AKT-mTOR signaling pathways [14].
- *Megalencephaly-Capillary Malformation-Polymicrogyria (MCAP)*: Patients with MCAP typically present with congenital or early postnatal megalencephaly, segmental

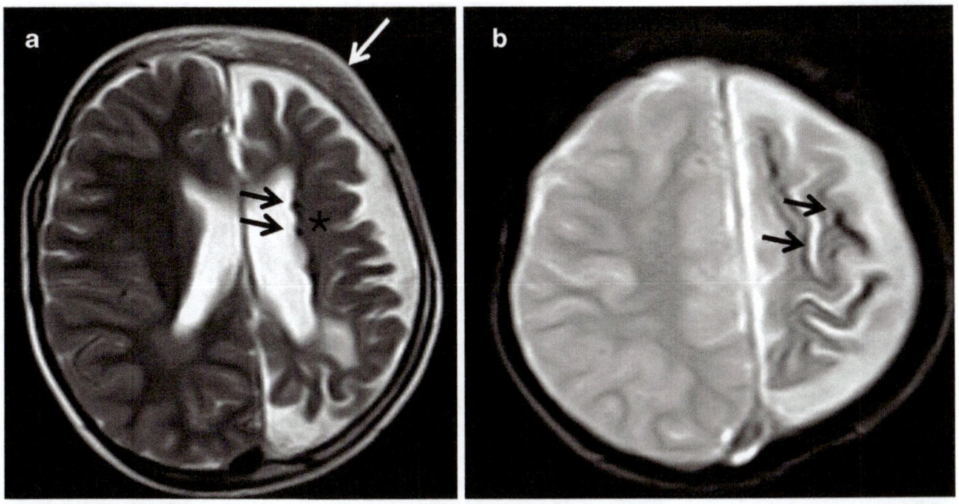

Fig. 18.9 Five-year-old boy with facial capillary malformation and Sturge–Weber syndrome. (**a**) Axial T2-weighted MRI showing left cerebral hemiatrophy (*) and dilated deep veins (double arrows) and cortical expansion of the left frontal bone (single arrow) exhibiting bright signal. (**b**) T2* sequence demonstrating gyral low-signal intensity consistent with gyral calcifications (arrows)

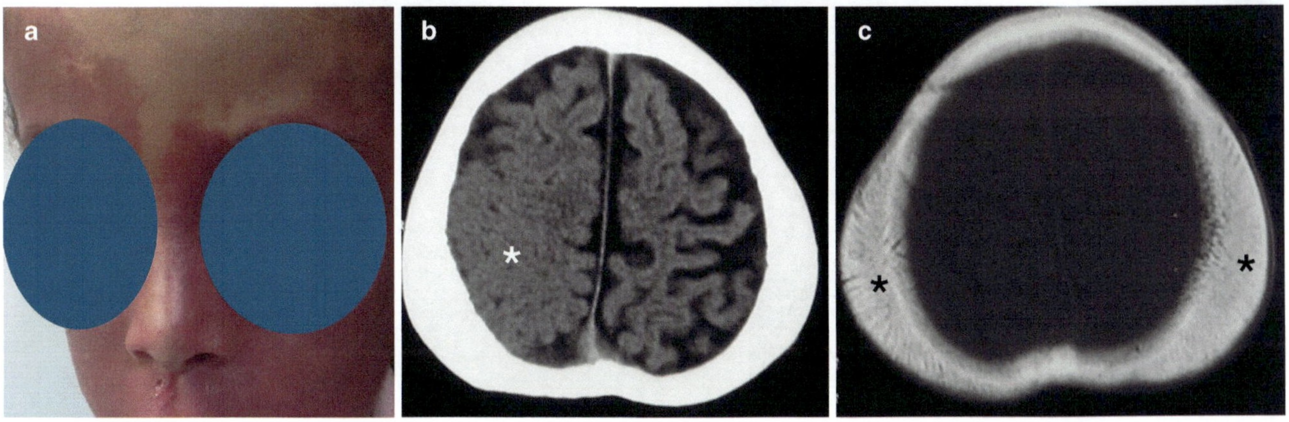

Fig. 18.10 Megalencephaly-capillary malformation–polymicrogyria syndrome. (**a**) Midline facial capillary malformation. (**b, c**) Axial CT of the cranium in soft tissue window (**b**) and bone window (**c**) shows polymicrogyria (white asterisk) in the right cerebral hemisphere, with left cerebral atrophy. There is associated osseous expansion (black asterisk) of the parietal eminence on both sides

overgrowth, capillary malformations (CMs), and polymicrogyria [15]. A characteristic feature is a midline facial CM (Fig. 18.10), often associated with overgrowth and digital anomalies such as polydactyly or syndactyly [13]. Neurological abnormalities may include ventriculomegaly, cerebellar tonsillar ectopia, developmental delay, and seizures [13]. MCAP is caused by activating somatic mutations in the PIK3CA gene [15].

- *Cutis Marmorata Telangiectatica Congenita (CMTC)*: CMTC is characterized by a persistent reticulated, marbled erythema that blanches with pressure and does not resolve with warming (Fig. 18.11) [16]. Affected areas may show cutaneous atrophy or ulceration and can be associated with body asymmetry. The condition has also been linked to anomalies such as congenital glaucoma, limb asymmetry (Fig. 18.12), and central nervous system involvement [17]. In some cases, CMTC co-occurs with Mongolian spots ("blue spots" or dermal melanocytosis, Fig. 18.13), a presentation described as phacomatosis pigmento-vascularis type V [18]. Kienast et al. proposed diagnostic criteria for CMTC, in which the presence of three major and two minor features is considered diagnostic. Major criteria are congenital reticulate (marmorated) erythema, absence of venectasia within the affected area by 1 year of age, and lack of improvement with warming. Minor criteria are fading of erythema within 2 years, telangiectasia within the CMTC-affected area, port-wine stain outside the CMTC region, ulceration, and cutaneous atrophy [16]. Less commonly, CMTC may be associated with multiple anomalies, including body asymmetry (hypertrophy or hypotrophy), neurological abnormalities (such as seizures and developmental delay), congenital glaucoma, cardiovascular malformations, Mongolian spots, as well as genitourinary and endocrine defects [19]. Currently, no standardized treatment exists; however, laser therapy, sympathectomy, and vasodilator treatment have been employed in some cases [20, 21].

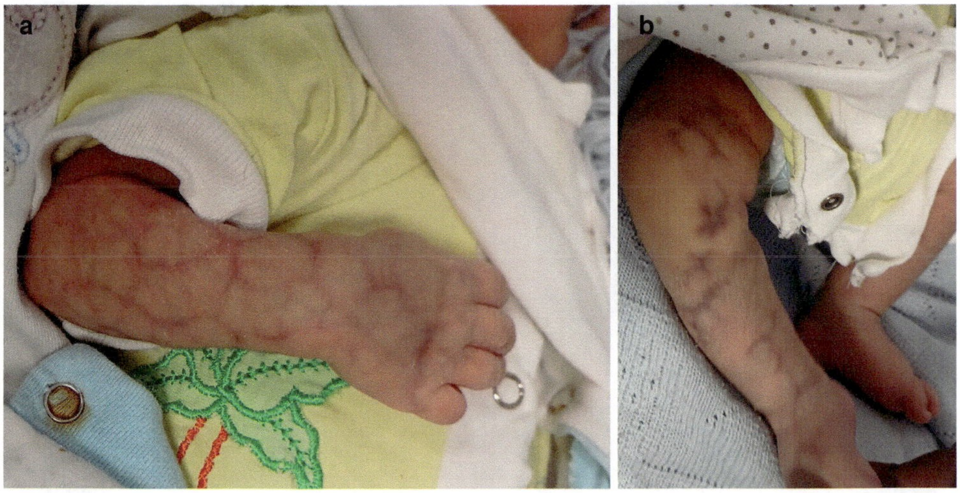

Fig. 18.11 Cutis marmorata telangiectatica congenita: reticulated, marbled erythema affecting upper (**a**) and lower extremities (**b**)

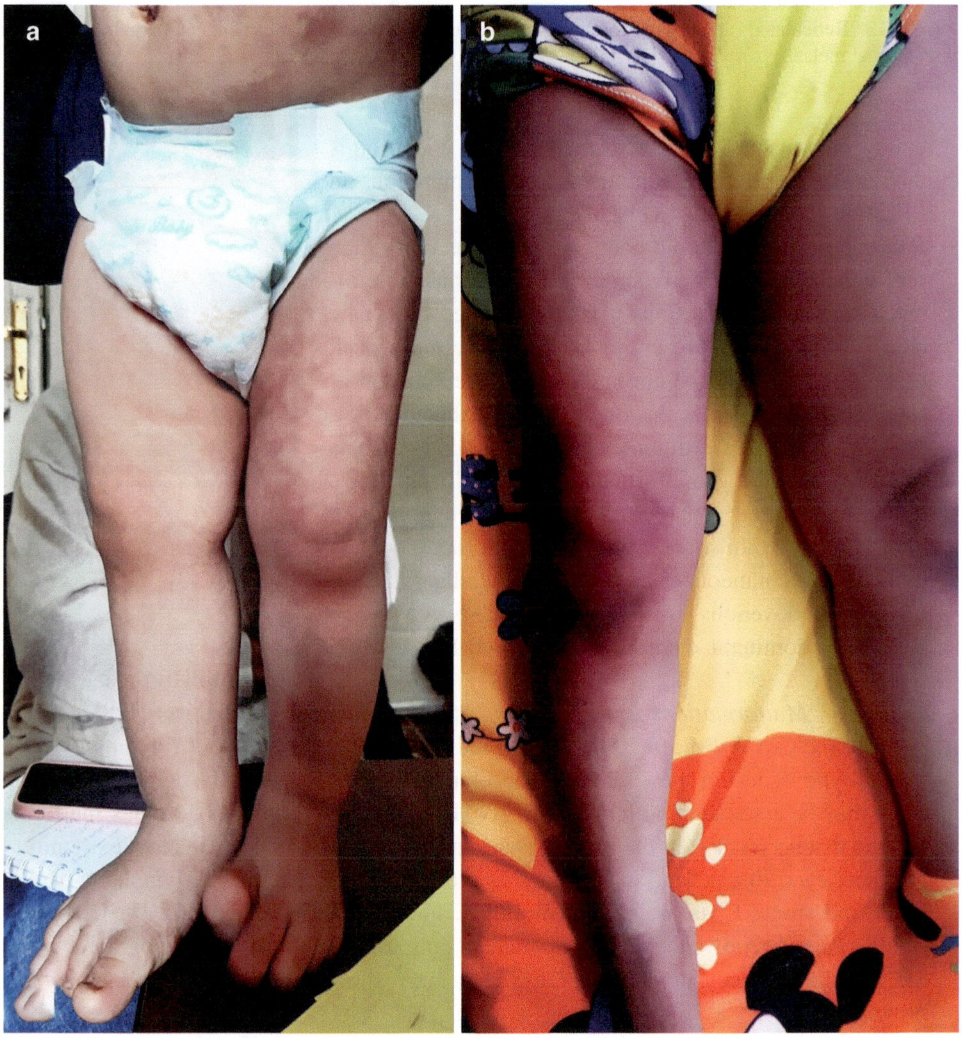

Fig. 18.12 Cutis marmorata telangiectatica congenita (CMTC). (**a**) Involvement of the left lower limb with normal limb size. (**b**) Involvement of the right lower limb with reduced limb size

- *Diffuse Capillary Malformations with Overgrowth (DCMO)*: DCMO is defined by extensive capillary malformations (CMs) associated with overgrowth of soft tissue or bone in an extremity [22]. The CMs are typically pale, and diffuse, often involving contiguous body regions [23]. Patients with DCMO may exhibit prominent subcutaneous veins and varicosities, but lymphatic anomalies are not a feature [4]. Overgrowth may occur either ipsilat-

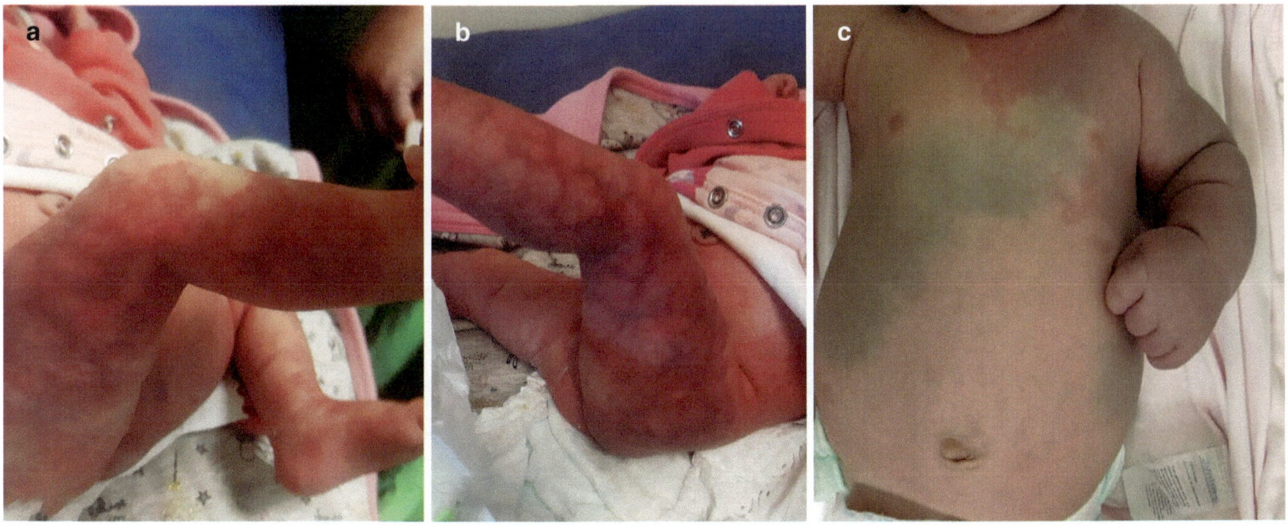

Fig. 18.13 Reticulated capillary malformation (cutis marmorata telangiectatica congenita). (**a**, **b**) Involvement of both lower limbs. (**c**) Association with dermal melanocytosis

eral or contralateral to the affected CM. The condition is thought to result from somatic activating mutations in PIK3CA, GNAQ, or GNA11 [24].

- *Rhodoid naevus*: Rhodoid naevi are lighter in color than port-wine stains, typically small, and appear as disseminated round or oval lesions often surrounded by a pale halo [25]. Most are present at birth and are multifocal, measuring less than 1–3 cm in diameter. They present as round or oval pink macules or patches distributed across the face, trunk, and extremities, although solitary lesions and larger capillary malformations (up to 15 cm) have also been reported. Doppler ultrasound may demonstrate arterial flow within some lesions. Multiple rhodoid naevi represent the cutaneous manifestation of capillary malformation–arteriovenous malformation (CM-AVM), an autosomal dominant disorder caused by RASA1 mutations [26].
- *Capillary Malformations-Arteriovenous Malformation (CM-AVM)*: CM-AVM affects 1/100,000 individuals [6]. In this type of lesion, new CM may develop over time. They may be associated with high-flow AVMs or arteriovenous fistulas (AVFs) in the skin, muscles, and bones of the face, ears, thorax, and extremities, as well as in the brain and spine. CMs are usually multiple, multifocal, small (ranging from 1 to 3 cm in diameter), pink to dull red annular macules or papules [26]. They may show brownish hue, a perilesional whitish halo of vasoconstriction, and hypotrichosis. These pink macules are considered cutaneous micro-AVMs [27]. Magnetic resonance angiography (MRA) screening for high-flow brain or spinal AVMs is recommended [13]. CM-AVM is an autosomal dominant disorder caused by germline heterozygous inactivating mutations in the RASA1 gene or the EPHB4 gene causing CM-AVM1 and CM-AVM2 respectively [28].

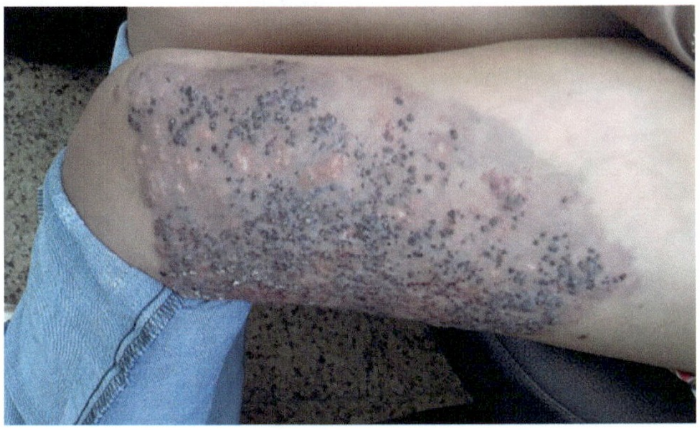

Fig. 18.14 Sharply circumscribed, geographic violaceous capillary malformations with visible nodules (lymphatic blebs) in Klippel–Trénaunay syndrome (KTS)

- *Klippel Trenaunay–Weber Syndrome (KTS)*: KTS is classically defined by the triad of capillary malformations (CMs), venous malformations, and limb hypertrophy of the affected extremity [13]. Additional features may include lymphatic or veno-lymphatic malformations (see Chap. 20). The CMs in KTS are typically sharply circumscribed, geographic violaceous plaques that may contain visible nodules (lymphatic blebs). These lesions tend to thicken with age and are prone to significant bleeding (Fig. 18.14). In some cases, non-geographic CMs may also occur, presenting as scattered pink lesions over the affected limb [17].
- *Congenital Lipomatous Overgrowth, Vascular Malformations, Epidermal Nevis, Spinal/Skeletal Anomalies/Scoliosis Syndrome (CLOVES)*: CLOVES

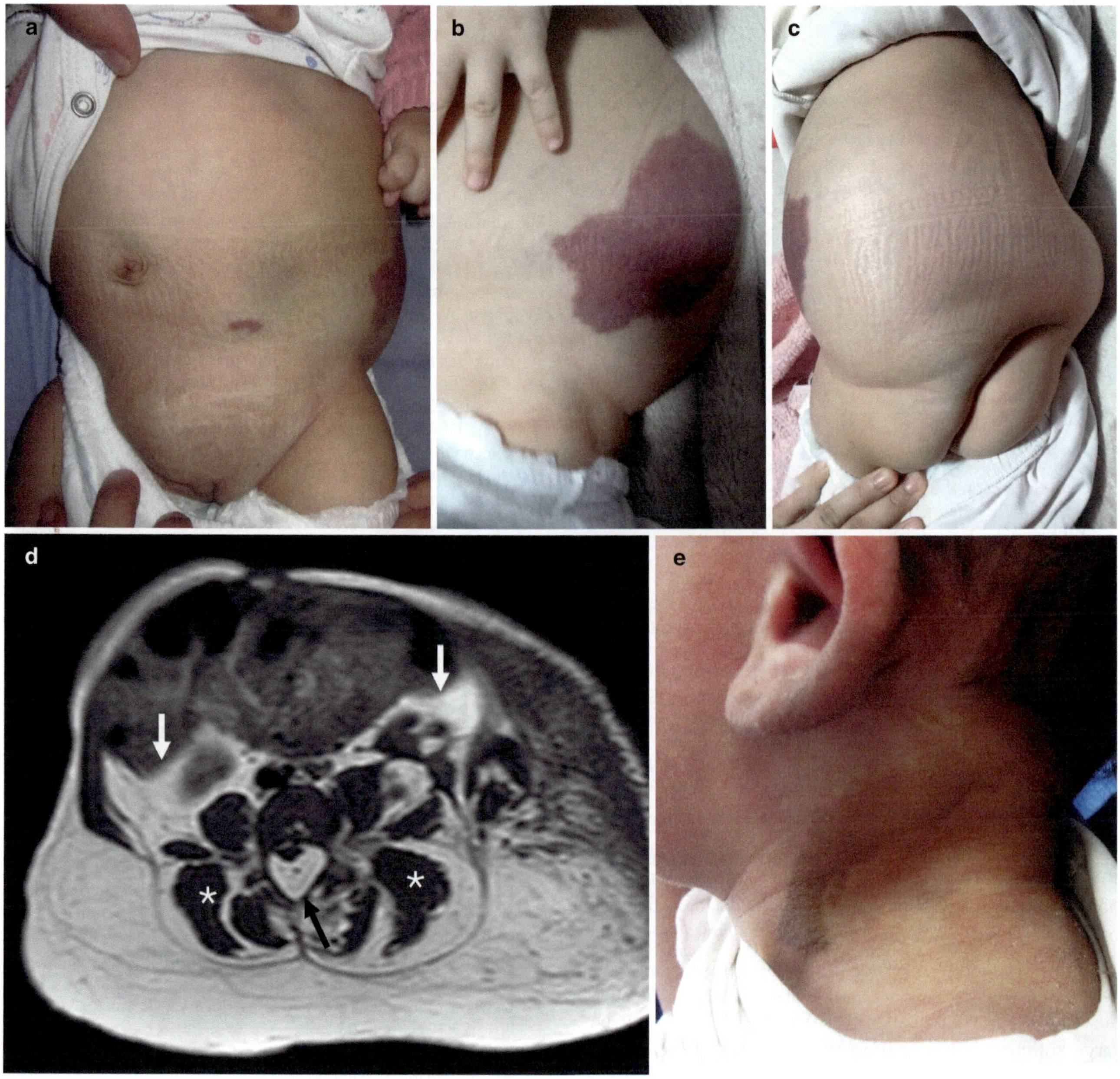

Fig. 18.15 A 4-month-old girl with CLOVES syndrome. (**a–c**) Anterior, lateral, and posterior views showing truncal lipomatous overgrowth with overlying capillary malformation. (**d**) Axial T1WI MRI revealing deep extension of lipomatous overgrowth into back muscles (asterisk), spinal canal (black arrow), and retroperitoneum (white arrows). (**e**) Linear epidermal nevus on the neck of the same patient

syndrome is classified as a PIK3CA-related overgrowth disorder [13]. The associated capillary malformations typically have a deep purple coloration and are most often geographic in pattern and lateralized in distribution (Fig. 18.15) [29].

- *Capillary Vascular Malformation of the Lower Lip, Lymphatic Malformations of the Head and Neck, Asymmetry, and Partial or Generalized Overgrowth Syndrome (CLAPO)*: CLAPO syndrome is thought to occur sporadically due to somatic activating mutations in the PIK3CA gene [30]. It is characterized by midline lower-lip capillary malformations (CMs), often associated with facial or cervical lymphatic malformations (LMs), and in some cases accompanied by asymmetric overgrowth [31].
- *Proteus Syndrome*: Proteus syndrome results from a somatic activating mutation in the AKT gene [13]. It is characterized by asymmetric overgrowth, connective tissue and epidermal nevi, cranial hyperostosis, visceral hamartomas, and various vascular anomalies, including capillary malformations. The most distinctive clinical feature is the presence of plantar cerebriform connective tissue nevi [8].

References

1. Jacobs AH, Walton RG. The incidence of birthmarks in the neonate. Pediatrics. 1976;58(2):218–22.
2. Escobar K, Pandher K, Jahnke MN. Capillary malformations. Dermatol Clin. 2022;40(4):425–33.
3. Nguyen HL, Bonadurer GF, Tollefson MM. Vascular malformations and health-related quality of life: a systematic review and meta-analysis. JAMA Dermatol. 2018;154(6):661–9.
4. Rozas-Muñoz E, Frieden IJ, Roé E, Puig L, Baselga E. Vascular stains: proposal for a clinical classification to improve diagnosis and management. Pediatr Dermatol. 2016;33(6):570–84.
5. Maguiness SM, Liang MG. Management of capillary malformations. Clin Plast Surg. 2011;38(1):65–73.
6. Garzon MC, Huang JT, Enjolras O, Frieden IJ. Vascular malformations: part I. J Am Acad Dermatol. 2007;56(3):353–70; quiz 371–4.
7. Valdivielso-Ramos M, Torrelo A, Martin-Santiago A, Hernández-Nuñez A, Azaña JM, Campos M, et al. Histopathological hallmarks of cutaneous lesions of capillary malformation-arteriovenous malformation syndrome. J Eur Acad Dermatol Venereol. 2020;34(10):2428–35.
8. Waelchli R, Aylett SE, Robinson K, Chong WK, Martinez AE, Kinsler VA. New vascular classification of port-wine stains: improving prediction of Sturge-Weber risk. Br J Dermatol. 2014;171(4):861–7.
9. Ben-Amitai D, Davidson S, Schwartz M, Prais D, Shamir R, Metzker A, et al. Sacral nevus flammeus simplex: the role of imaging. Pediatr Dermatol. 2000;17(6):469–71.
10. Martinez-Lopez A, Salvador-Rodriguez L, Montero-Vilchez T, Molina-Leyva A, Tercedor-Sanchez J, Arias-Santiago S. Vascular malformations syndromes: an update. Curr Opin Pediatr. 2019;31(6):747–53.
11. Tallman B, Tan OT, Morelli JG, Piepenbrink J, Stafford TJ, Trainor S, et al. Location of port-wine stains and the likelihood of ophthalmic and/or central nervous system complications. Pediatrics. 1991;87(3):323–7.
12. Yeom S, Comi AM. Updates on Sturge-Weber Syndrome. Stroke. 2022;53(12):3769–79.
13. McCuaig CC. Update on classification and diagnosis of vascular malformations. Curr Opin Pediatr. 2017;29(4):448–54.
14. McDonell LM, Mirzaa GM, Alcantara D, Schwartzentruber J, Carter MT, Lee LJ, et al. Mutations in STAMBP, encoding a deubiquitinating enzyme, cause microcephaly-capillary malformation syndrome. Nat Genet. 2013;45(5):556–62.
15. Ustaszewski A, Janowska-Głowacka J, Wołyńska K, Pietrzak A, Badura-Stronka M. Genetic syndromes with vascular malformations – update on molecular background and diagnostics. Arch Med Sci. 2021;17(4):965–91.
16. Kienast AK, Hoeger PH. Cutis marmorata telangiectatica congenita: a prospective study of 27 cases and review of the literature with proposal of diagnostic criteria. Clin Exp Dermatol. 2009;34(3):319–23.
17. Garzon MC, Huang JT, Enjolras O, Frieden IJ. Vascular malformations. Part II: associated syndromes. J Am Acad Dermatol. 2007;56(4):541–64.
18. Torrelo A, Zambrano A, Happle R. Cutis marmorata telangiectatica congenita and extensive mongolian spots: type 5 phacomatosis pigmentovascularis. Br J Dermatol. 2003;148(2):342–5.
19. Bui TNPT, Corap A, Bygum A. Cutis marmorata telangiectatica congenita: a literature review. Orphanet J Rare Dis. 2019;14(1):283.
20. Kumar A, Zastrow DB, Kravets EJ, Beleford D, Ruzhnikov MRZ, Grove ME, et al. Extracutaneous manifestations in phacomatosis cesioflammea and cesiomarmorata: case series and literature review. Am J Med Genet A. 2019;179(6):966–77.
21. Sahin A, Celebi N, Doğan R, Canbay O, Uzümcügil F, Aypar U. Lumbar sympathetic blockade in a patient with cutis marmorata telangiectatica congenita. Paediatr Anaesth. 2006;16(12):1292–3.
22. Goss JA, Konczyk DJ, Smits P, Sudduth CL, Bischoff J, Liang MG, et al. Diffuse capillary malformation with overgrowth contains somatic PIK3CA variants. Clin Genet. 2020;97(5):736–40.
23. Hughes M, Hao M, Luu M. PIK3CA vascular overgrowth syndromes: an update. Curr Opin Pediatr. 2020;32(4):539–46.
24. Couto JA, Huang L, Vivero MP, Kamitaki N, Maclellan RA, Mulliken JB, et al. Endothelial cells from capillary malformations are enriched for somatic GNAQ mutations. Plast Reconstr Surg. 2016;137(1):77e–82e.
25. Revencu N, Boon LM, Mendola A, Cordisco MR, Dubois J, Clapuyt P, et al. RASA1 mutations and associated phenotypes in 68 families with capillary malformation-arteriovenous malformation. Hum Mutat. 2013;34(12):1632–41.
26. Orme CM, Boyden LM, Choate KA, Antaya RJ, King BA. Capillary malformation–arteriovenous malformation syndrome: review of the literature, proposed diagnostic criteria, and recommendations for management. Pediatr Dermatol. 2013;30(4):409–15.
27. Valdivielso-Ramos M, Martin-Santiago A, Azaña JM, Hernández-Nuñez A, Vera A, Perez B, et al. Capillary malformation-arteriovenous malformation syndrome: a multicentre study. Clin Exp Dermatol. 2021;46(2):300–5.
28. Eerola I, Boon LM, Mulliken JB, Burrows PE, Dompmartin A, Watanabe S, et al. Capillary malformation-arteriovenous malformation, a new clinical and genetic disorder caused by RASA1 mutations. Am J Hum Genet. 2003;73(6):1240–9.
29. Happle R. Capillary malformations: a classification using specific names for specific skin disorders. J Eur Acad Dermatol Venereol. 2015;29(12):2295–305.
30. Rodriguez-Laguna L, Ibañez K, Gordo G, Garcia-Minaur S, Santos-Simarro F, Agra N, et al. CLAPO syndrome: identification of somatic activating PIK3CA mutations and delineation of the natural history and phenotype. Genet Med. 2018;20(8):882–9.
31. Ivars M, Boixeda P, Triana P, Martinez-Glez V, Rodríguez-Laguna L, Agra N, et al. Clinical overlap between CLAPO syndrome and macrocephaly-capillary malformation syndrome. J Dtsch Dermatol Ges. 2020;18(5):479–82.

Part VII

Cerebrovascular Malformations

Cerebral Vascular Malformations

19

Introduction

Cerebral vascular malformations (CVMs) represent a heterogeneous group with a wide range of clinical presentations. While some CVMs, such as developmental venous anomalies, may be asymptomatic and discovered incidentally, others like arteriovenous malformations are associated with significant morbidity and mortality [1]. These malformations can be classified based on several criteria, including the type of vessels involved, the presence of abnormal vessels within the brain parenchyma, the morphology of the nidus, and the existence of early draining veins [1, 2]. Various classification schemes exist for CVMs, one of which is based on the presence or absence of arteriovenous shunting. From a radiological perspective, CVMs can also be categorized according to whether abnormal parenchymal vessels are present. Those involving intraparenchymal vessels are further divided into two types: lesions with a compact and well-defined nidus and those with a diffuse nidus [1, 2] (Fig. 19.1).

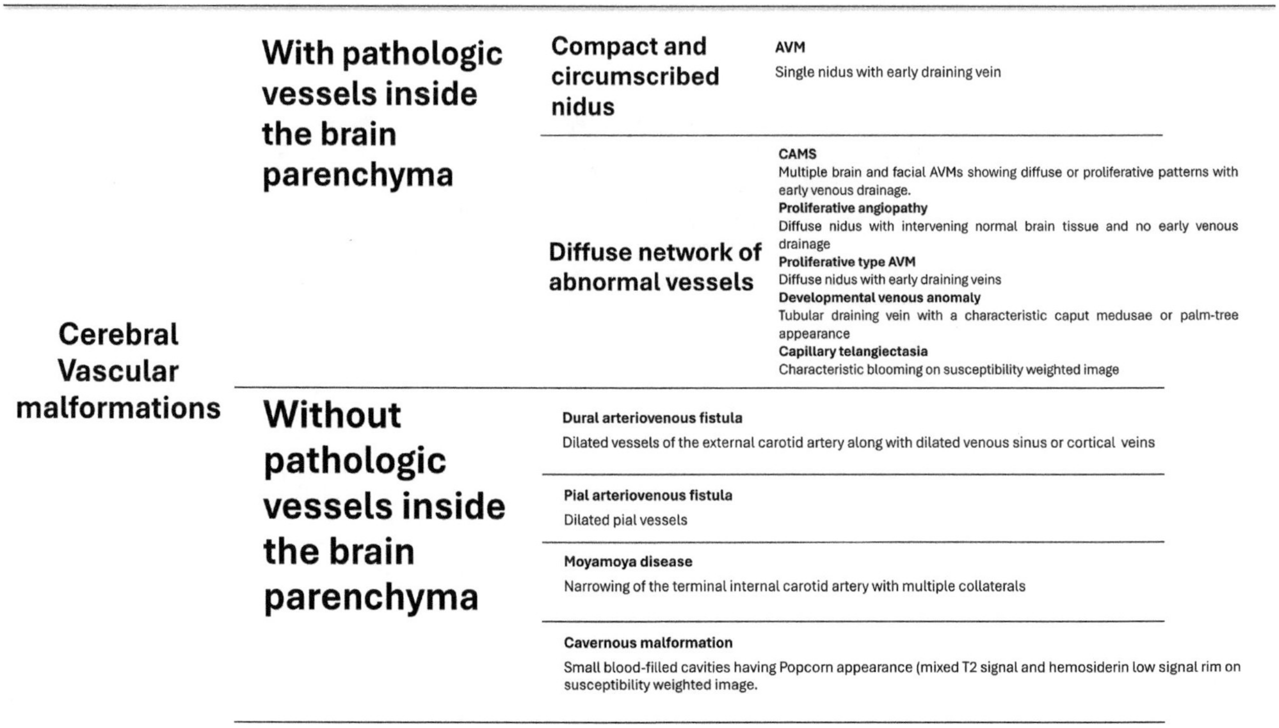

Fig. 19.1 Schematic representation of cerebral vascular malformations. AVM arteriovenous malformation, CAMS Cerebrofacial arteriovenous metameric syndrome

A. A. AbouZeid et al., *Atlas of Pediatric Vascular Anomalies*, https://doi.org/10.1007/978-3-032-30866-5_19

Cerebrovascular Malformation with Pathologic Vessels Inside the Brain Parenchyma

Arteriovenous Malformation

Arteriovenous malformation (AVM) involves direct abnormal connections between arteries and veins, bypassing the normal capillary network. Approximately 25% of AVM cases manifest during early adolescence, often by the age of 15. Hemorrhage is the most common initial presentation, occurring in about 50% of cases. Other possible clinical manifestations include headaches, seizures, or varying degrees of neurological deficits, depending on the size and location of the malformation [1, 2].

Imaging of arteriovenous malformations (AVMs) reveals characteristic features across different modalities (Figs. 19.2, 19.3, and 19.4). On CT scans, AVMs appear as hyperdense, serpentine vascular structures and may show associated calcifications. MRI demonstrates flow voids on T2-weighted images with surrounding gliosis (most clearly visualized on FLAIR sequences). Hemorrhage at the time of diagnosis is not uncommon, frequently accompanied by perilesional edema and mass effect (Figs. 19.2, 19.3, and 19.4). Vascular imaging, including CTA and MRA, typically shows a nidus composed of tangled vessels, along with dilated feeding arteries and draining veins. The Spetzler-Martin grading system is used to assess surgical risk, based on three criteria: lesion size (small <3 cm = 1 point; medium 3–6 cm = 2 points; large >6 cm = 3 points), location (0 points for non-eloquent areas; 1 point for eloquent regions), and venous drainage (0 for superficial only; 1 for deep venous drainage). Eloquent brain areas include critical functional zones such as the primary motor cortex, somatosensory cortex, visual and auditory cortices, as well as Broca's and Wernicke's areas [3]. It is essential to differentiate arteriovenous malformations (AVMs) from other intraparenchymal high-flow shunt-related vascular anomalies. While AVMs are defined by a compact nidus, proliferative angiopathy presents with a diffuse nidus, within which normal brain parenchyma is interspersed (Fig. 19.5). This distinction is important for both diagnosis and management planning [1].

Treatment options for arteriovenous malformations (AVMs) include endovascular embolization, stereotactic radiosurgery, and microsurgical resection, often selected based on the size, location, and accessibility of the lesion. Importantly, the risk of life-threatening hemorrhage associated with AVMs tends to increase with advancing age, underscoring the need for timely intervention when appropriate [4].

Proliferative Angiopathy

Proliferative angiopathy is a rare vascular anomaly, accounting for approximately 2–4% of all cerebral arteriovenous malformations (AVMs). It is marked by ongoing angiogenesis and vascular proliferation and was previously referred to

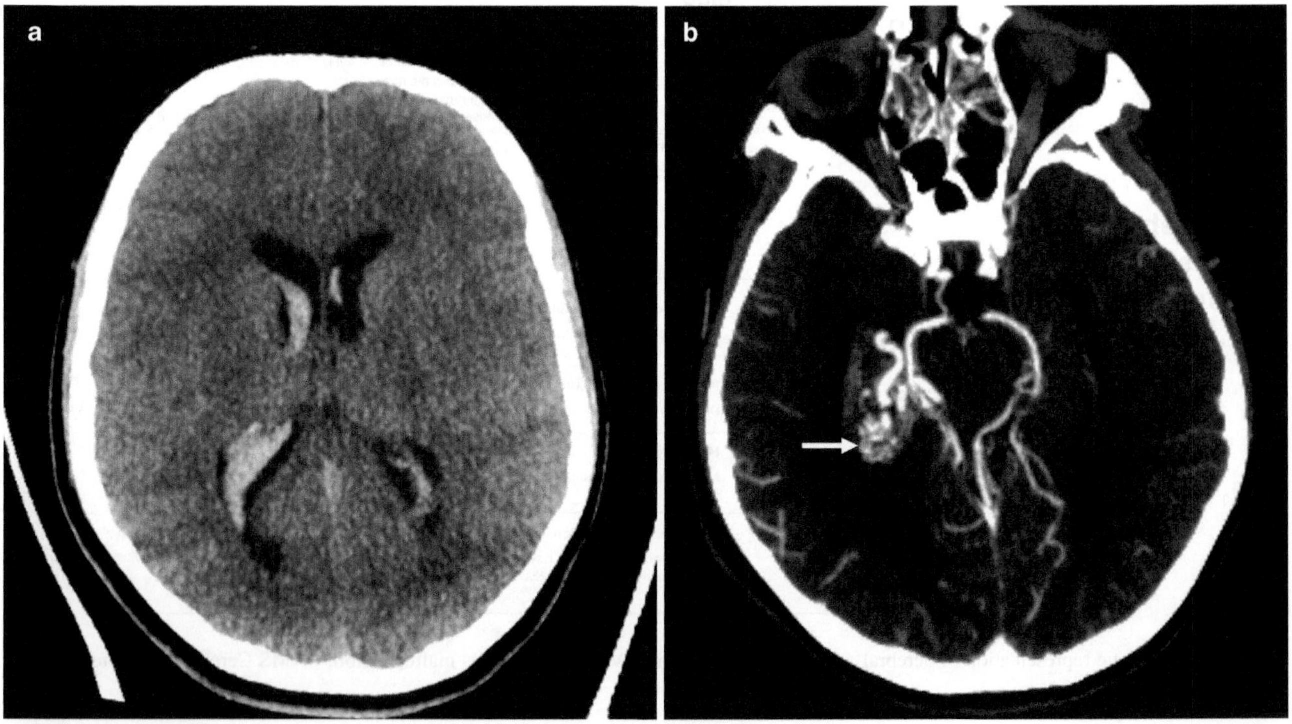

Fig. 19.2 A 13-year-old boy presents with sudden onset of impaired consciousness. (**a**) Axial non-contrast CT reveals intraventricular hemorrhage. (**b**) CT angiography demonstrates the arteriovenous malformation nidus (arrow) located in the right hippocampal region

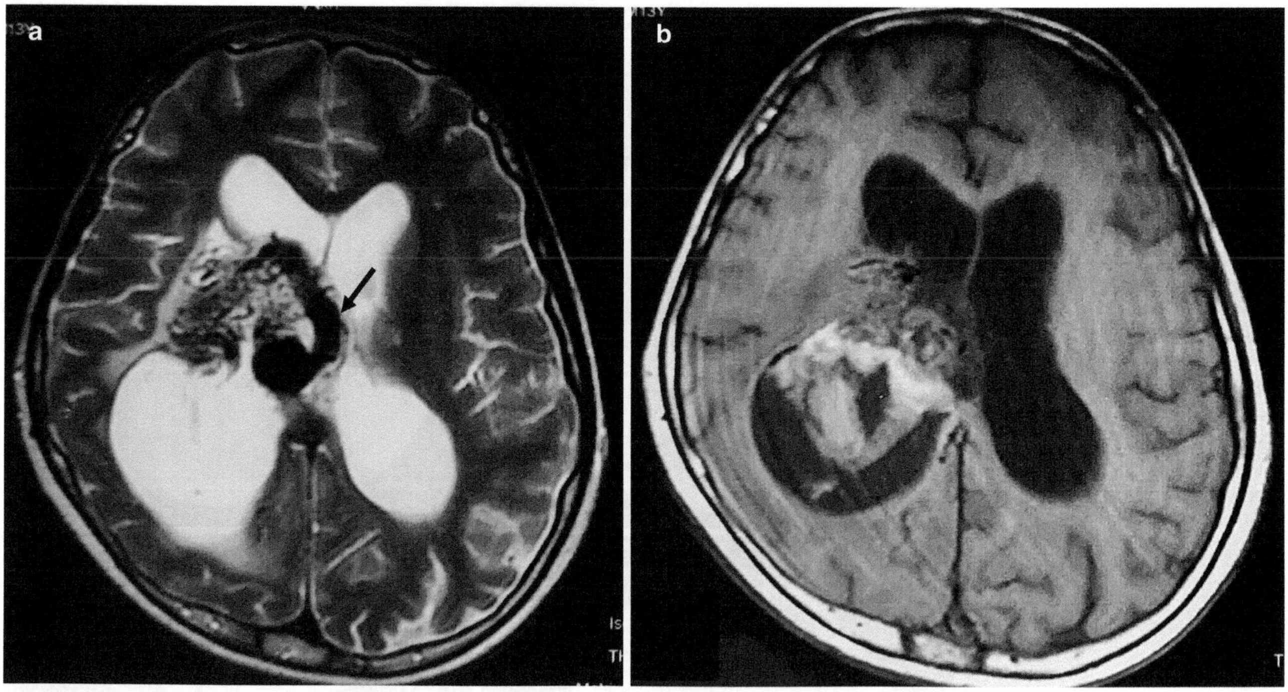

Fig. 19.3 A 13-year-old boy with arteriovenous malformation. (**a**) Axial T2-weighted MRI reveals the arteriovenous malformation nidus with a prominent draining vein (arrow). Bilateral ventricular dilatation is evident. (**b**) Axial T1-weighted image shows high signal intensity within the right ventricle indicating intraventricular hemorrhage

as diffuse nidus AVM due to its non-compact architecture. Proliferative angiopathy typically affects young female patients who may present with progressive neurological deficits, transient ischemic attacks, seizures, or headaches. Unlike classic AVMs, these lesions rarely present with hemorrhage or sudden-onset neurological deficits [1].

On contrast-enhanced CT and MRI, the nidus appears diffuse with abnormal vessels interspersed with normal brain parenchyma, often involving an entire lobe or even a cerebral hemisphere. MR angiography demonstrates similar pattern (Fig. 19.5). T2-weighted MRI typically shows flow voids coursing through the parenchyma. Digital subtraction angiography reveals normal or mildly enlarged arterial feeders without early venous drainage, a key distinguishing feature. Proximal arterial stenosis may be observed, along with possible flow-related aneurysms. Additionally, there is often transdural arterial supply from branches of the external carotid artery [1, 5].

Management of proliferative angiopathy is primarily symptomatic, with medical therapy aimed at controlling associated symptoms such as seizures. In selected cases, burr-hole therapy may be considered, particularly in patients with disabling symptoms like severe headaches or intractable seizures, especially when transdural arterial supply is limited. Additionally, endovascular intervention may be indicated for the treatment of associated flow-related aneurysms [5].

Developmental Venous Anomaly

Developmental venous anomaly (DVA), also referred to as a venous angioma, is regarded as a variation of normal venous drainage in the brain. DVAs are the most frequently encountered type of cerebral vascular anomaly. It can occur alone or in conjunction with a cavernous malformation, forming what is known as a mixed vascular malformation. DVAs are most often identified incidentally during neuroimaging. However, the presence of thrombosis or an associated cavernous malformation can elevate the risk of intracranial hemorrhage. DVAs typically do not require any medical or surgical intervention [6, 7].

On imaging, DVAs are most located in the frontoparietal region or the cerebellar hemispheres. CT may appear normal, but if associated with a cavernous malformation, calcification may be seen. Hemorrhagic features may be evident if thrombosis has occurred. MRI may also appear normal or may reveal a signal void, branching tubular structure often described as resembling a "Medusa head." There may be a surrounding bright signal on T2 or FLAIR which may represent edema or gliosis. DVA are best visualized using susceptibility-weighted imaging, post-contrast T1-weighted imaging, and MR venography. MRI may show multiple small veins draining into a single collector vein, which subsequently empties into an ependymal vein or a dural venous sinus (Figs. 19.6 and 19.7). Magnetic resonance angiography

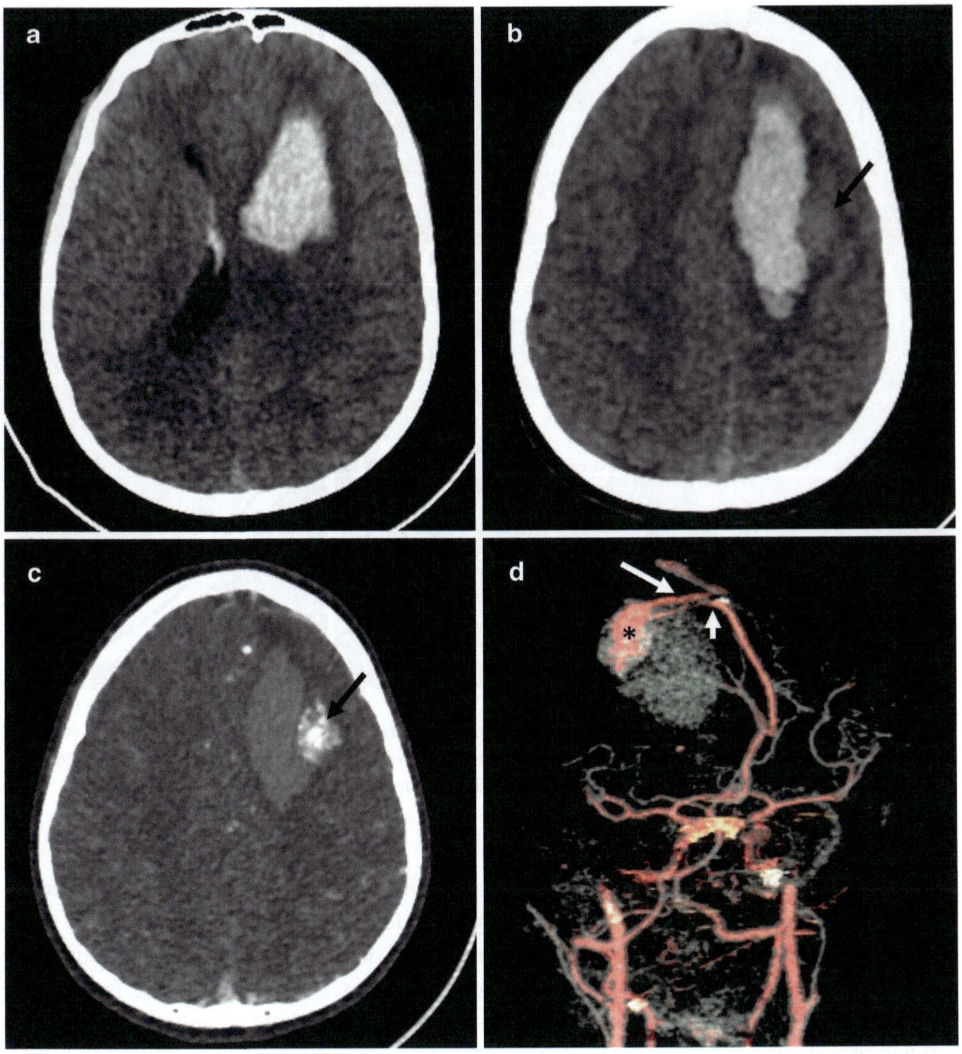

Fig. 19.4 A 12-year-old boy with arteriovenous malformation. (**a**, **b**) Axial non-contrast CT shows parenchymal and intraventricular hemorrhage. Note the nearby nidus appear as relatively hyperdense lesion (arrow). (**c**) Contrast-enhanced CT reveals enhancement of the nidus (arrow). (**d**) Three-dimensional reconstruction of CT cerebral angiography shows enhancing nidus (asterisk), feeding artery (short arrow) arising from the anterior cerebral artery, and a superficial venous drainage (long arrow)

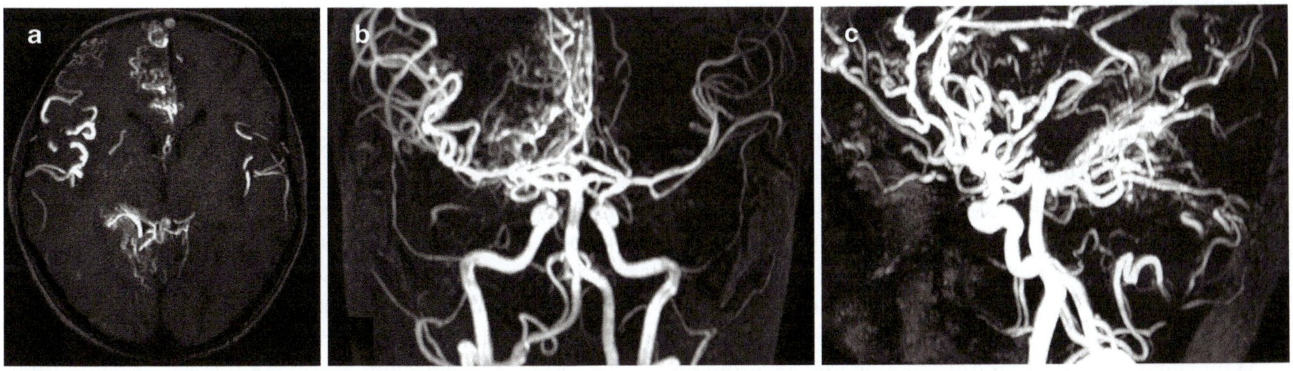

Fig. 19.5 A 9-year-old boy with proliferative angiopathy. (**a**) Axial time-of-flight MR angiography shows multiple dilated vessels with intervening normal brain parenchyma. (**b**, **c**) Coronal and sagittal maximum intensity projection of MR angiography shows multiple serpiginous vessels arising from the anterior, middle, and posterior cerebral arteries without identifiable nidus

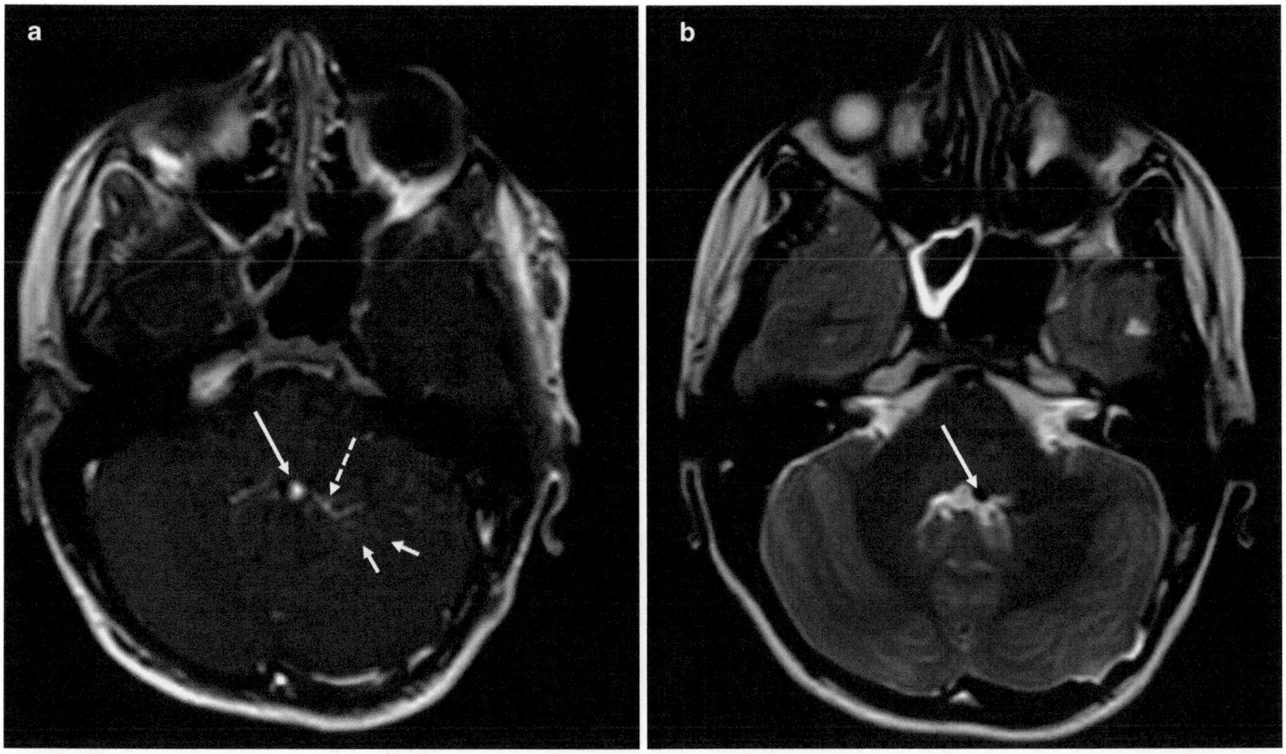

Fig. 19.6 A 10-year-old boy with developmental venous anomaly. (**a**, **b**) Contrast-enhanced T1-weighted MRI (**a**) and axial T2-weighted image (**b**) show the developmental venous anomaly as branching venous tributaries (short arrows) draining into a collector vein (dashed arrow) that drains into an enlarged ependymal vein (long arrow)

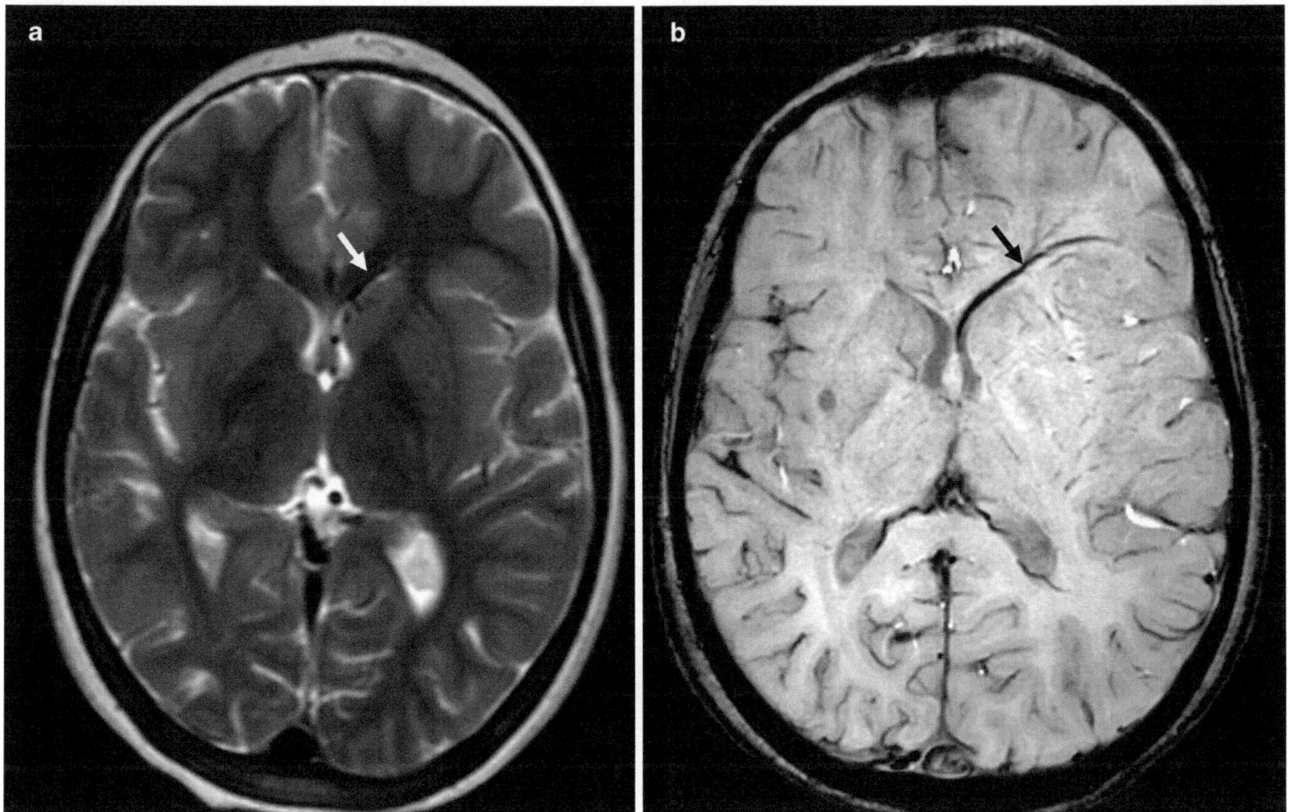

Fig. 19.7 A 9-year-old girl with capillary malformation (note the soft tissue thickening on the forehead). (**a**, **b**) Axial T2-weighted image (**a**) and axial susceptibility weighted image (**b**) demonstrate developmental venous anomaly showing branching venous tributaries draining into a collector vein (arrow). Note that developmental venous anomaly is more appreciated on the susceptibility weighted image (**b**)

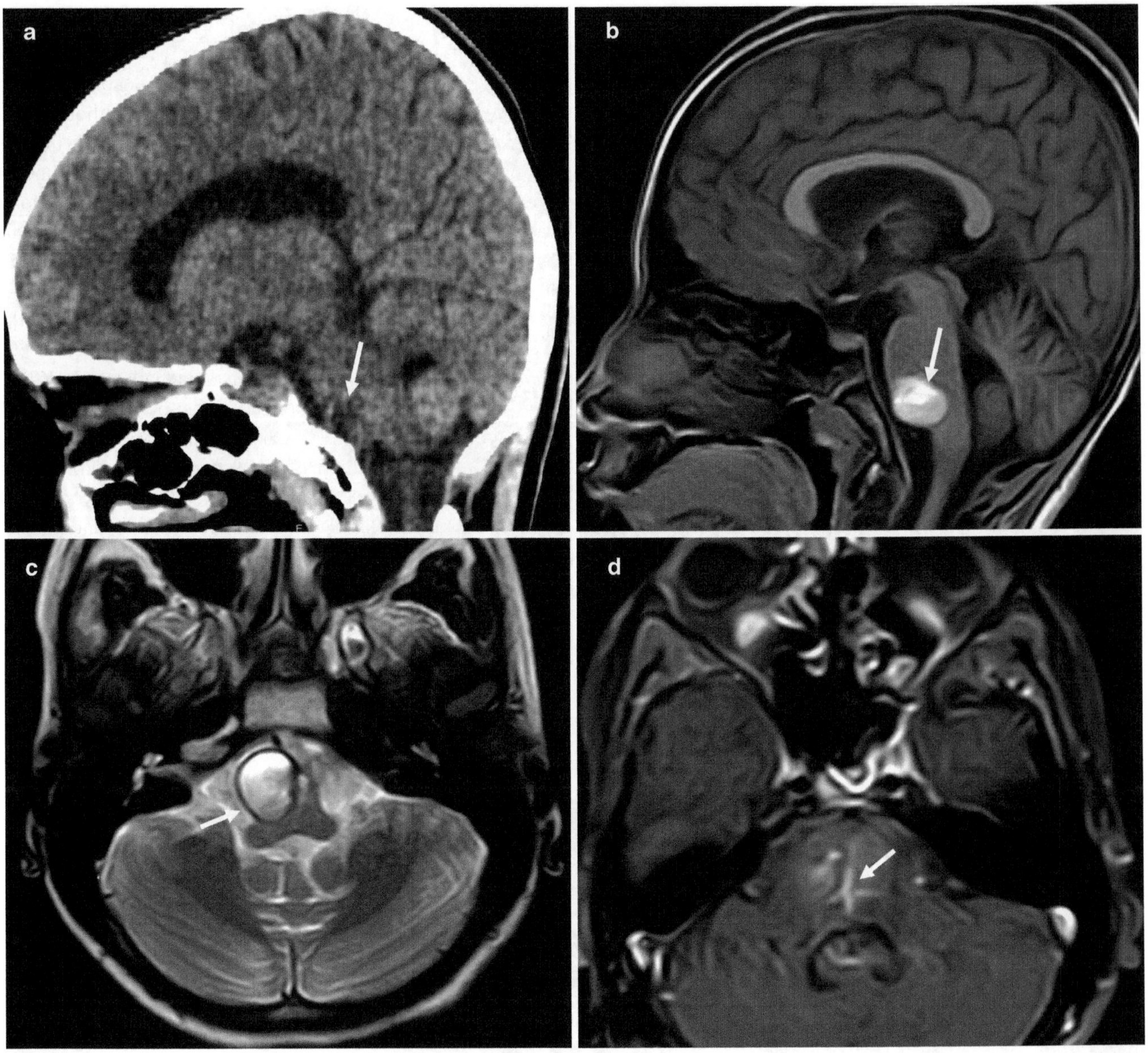

Fig. 19.8 A 13-year-ol girl with cavernous malformation (Zabramski type 1) associated with developmental venous anomaly. (**a**) Sagittal reconstruction of non-contrast CT reveals iso- to hypodense lesion in the pons (arrow). (**b**) Sagittal T1-weighted MRI demonstrates a well-defined rounded lesion exhibiting hyperintense signal. (**c**) Axial T2-weighted image reveals a hyperintense lesion with hypointense hemosiderin rim (arrow). (**d**) Axial contrast-enhanced T1-weighted imaging shows enhancing branching vessels characteristic of developmental venous anomaly

of the cerebral arteries generally appears normal. In some cases, DVAs may be accompanied by a cavernoma (Fig. 19.8) or signs of hemorrhage [6, 7].

Capillary Telangiectasia

Capillary telangiectasia consists of a network of small, dilated capillaries dispersed within the brain parenchyma. It displays characteristic hypointense signal on susceptibility weighted image (Fig. 19.9) with brush-like faint contrast enhancement [2].

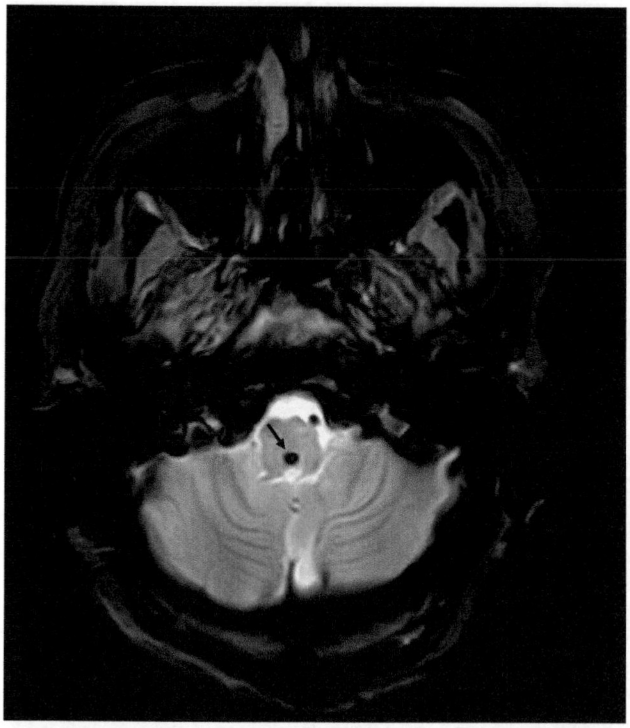

Fig. 19.9 Capillary telangiectasia. Axial T2* weighted imaging at the level of the medulla oblongata demonstrates capillary telangiectasia (arrow) with its characteristic hypointense signal

Cerebrovascular Malformation Without Pathologic Vessels Inside the Brain Parenchyma

Dural Arteriovenous Fistula

Dural arteriovenous fistulas (DAVFs) are characterized by abnormal direct connections between dural arteries and either dural venous sinuses or cortical veins, without an intervening nidus. Though relatively rare, DAVFs account for approximately 10–15% of all intracranial vascular malformations. DAVFs typically manifest during mid to late adulthood, although they can occasionally be congenital, idiopathic, or secondary to head trauma or thrombosis of a dural venous sinus. Carotid-cavernous fistulas are a distinct subtype of DAVFs characterized by an abnormal communication between the internal or external carotid artery and the cavernous sinus (Fig. 19.10). These lesions may develop spontaneously, often following the rupture of an intracavernous aneurysm, or may occur secondary to head trauma [1, 8].

In pediatric patients, DAVFs can be further classified into three types: dural sinus malformations, infantile-type DAVFs, and adult-type DAVFs, each with distinct clinical and radiological features. Dural sinus malformations are congenital lesions, typically identified prenatally or in early infancy. When associated with arteriovenous shunting, the clinical course tends to be more complicated (Fig. 19.11). Infantile or juvenile-type DAVFs typically present in older infants and young children. They are characterized by multiple high-flow arteriovenous shunts draining into an enlarged dural venous sinus. In contrast, adult-type DAVFs appear in older children and closely resemble the angiographic and clinical features seen in adults (Fig. 19.12) [9].

DAVFs may present early in life with signs such as hydrocephalus or high-output cardiac failure. Patients may present with intracranial hemorrhage or non-hemorrhagic neurological deficits (NHND), both of which are often attributed to cortical venous hypertension (Fig. 19.12). Additionally, symptoms such as pulsatile tinnitus and ophthalmologic findings (such as proptosis, visual disturbances, and chemosis) may occur due to increased venous sinus drainage [8, 9].

On CT, DAVFs may be associated with intracranial hemorrhage or vasogenic edema, which can appear distant from the actual fistula site. Chronic venous congestion may lead to white matter calcifications due to long-standing perfusion deficits. MRI typically shows flow voids on T2-weighted images, reflecting dilated arterialized veins, and may reveal white matter edema on both T2 and FLAIR sequences (Fig. 19.12). Susceptibility-weighted imaging can detect microhemorrhages and white matter calcification. On MR angiography, serpiginous dilated vessels adjacent to a dural sinus are suggestive of DAVF. Phase-contrast angiography with low-velocity settings may reveal the fistula and flow reversal in draining veins. Time-resolved dynamic contrast-enhanced angiography provides high-resolution visualization of the fistula. MR venography is useful for identifying associated venous sinus thrombosis (Fig. 19.12) [8, 9].

Digital subtraction angiography remains the most sensitive modality for evaluating DAVFs. It allows precise visualization of the fistulous point, arterial feeders, and venous drainage patterns. The Borden-Shucart classification system is commonly used to categorize DAVFs based on their venous outflow. Type I lesions drain into a dural venous sinus with normal antegrade flow and no cortical venous involvement. Type II DAVFs exhibit both antegrade sinus drainage and retrograde flow into cortical veins. Type III lesions have direct retrograde cortical venous drainage, with or without venous ectasia. Types II and III are considered high-grade fistulas due to the presence of cortical venous drainage, which significantly increases the risk of hemorrhagic or neurological complications [8].

Management of DAVFs may involve endovascular or surgical intervention, depending on the lesion's characteristics. Prognosis is closely tied to the lesion's location and venous drainage pattern. Type I DAVFs, which lack cortical venous drainage, typically follow a benign course and rarely result in intracranial hemorrhage or NHND. However, these lesions may progress to a higher grade over time. In contrast, higher-

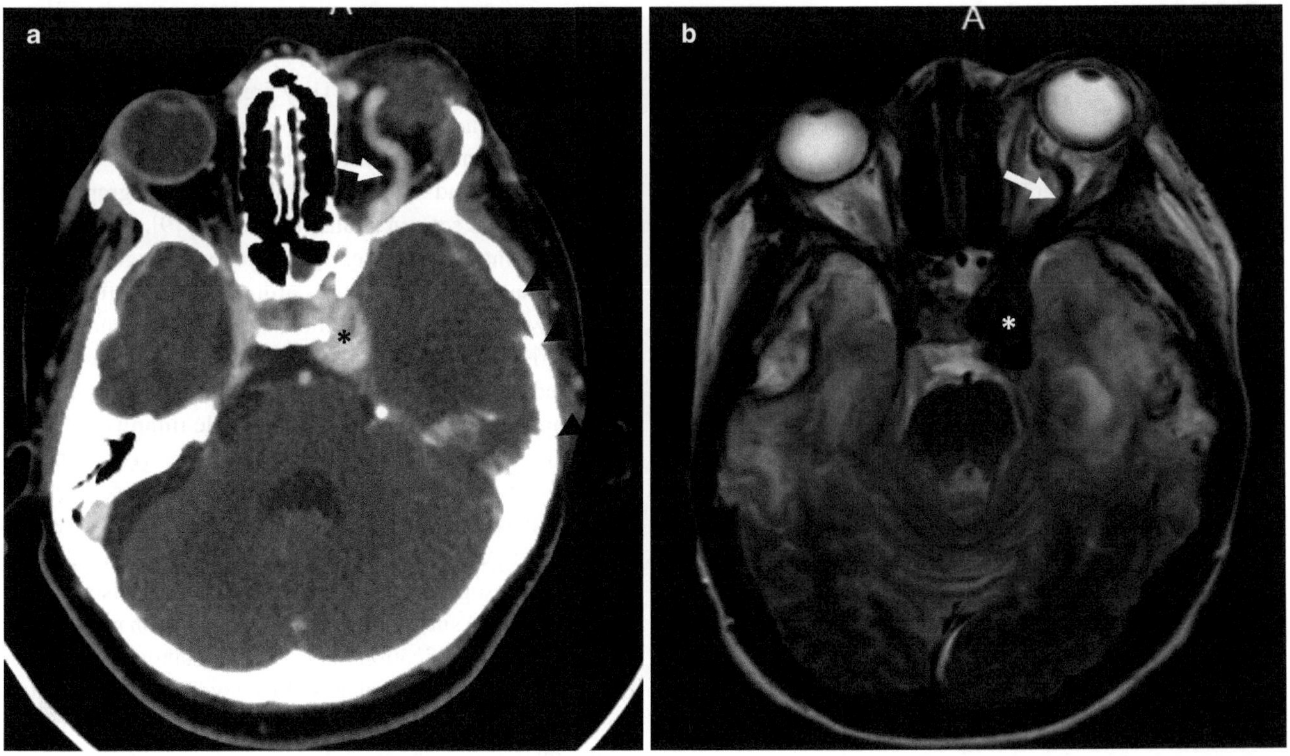

Fig. 19.10 Post-traumatic carotid-cavernous fistula. (**a, b**) Axial contrast-enhanced CT (**a**) and axial T2-weighted image (**b**) show congested cavernous sinus (asterisk) and dilated superior ophthalmic vein (arrow). Note left eye proptosis, skull fractures (arrowheads), and brain contusions

grade DAVFs carry a significantly increased risk of intracranial hemorrhage or NHND, with an estimated annual mortality rate of 3.8% [8].

Pial Arteriovenous Fistula

Pial arteriovenous fistulas (PAVFs) are vascular anomalies characterized by a direct connection between a pial artery and a vein, without an intervening nidus which increases the risk of rupture. PAVFs are more commonly observed in children and may be associated with underlying conditions such as hereditary hemorrhagic telangiectasia or Klippel-Trenaunay syndrome. PAVFs have a variable clinical presentation. Patients may present with symptoms such as headache, seizures, or intracranial hemorrhage [1, 2].

On cross-sectional imaging, pial arteriovenous fistulas (PAVFs) appear as dilated vessels along the brain surface. CT and MR angiography typically demonstrate an enlarged pial feeding artery, which may arise from cortical branches or vessels at the level of the circle of Willis—commonly the anterior, middle, or posterior cerebral arteries. These arterial dilations are often accompanied by prominent venous pouches visible at the brain surface (Fig. 19.13) [1, 2].

Management of PAVFs involves either surgical intervention or endovascular embolization. If left untreated, PAVFs carry a high risk of complications, with reported mortality rates reaching up to 63% [1, 2].

Vein of Galen Aneurysmal Malformation

Vein of Galen aneurysmal malformation (VGAM) is a misnomer, as it does not involve the true vein of Galen. Instead, it represents a congenital arteriovenous fistula between the median prosencephalic vein (MPV), the embryologic precursor of the vein of Galen, and the choroidal arteries, typically forming between the 6th and 11th weeks of gestation. The MPV normally drains into the straight sinus, although in approximately 50% of VGAM cases, the straight sinus may be absent, and drainage instead occurs via a persistent falcine sinus. Clinically, VGAM often presents during antenatal ultrasound screening in the third trimester or postnatally with signs of high-output cardiac failure due to the significant arteriovenous shunting. It may also be associated with hydrocephalus, which can result either from venous hypertension or from aqueductal stenosis caused by the mass effect of the dilated venous structure [10–12].

Imaging plays a critical role in the diagnosis and classification of VGAM. On prenatal or neonatal cranial ultrasound, VGAM typically appears as an anechoic midline

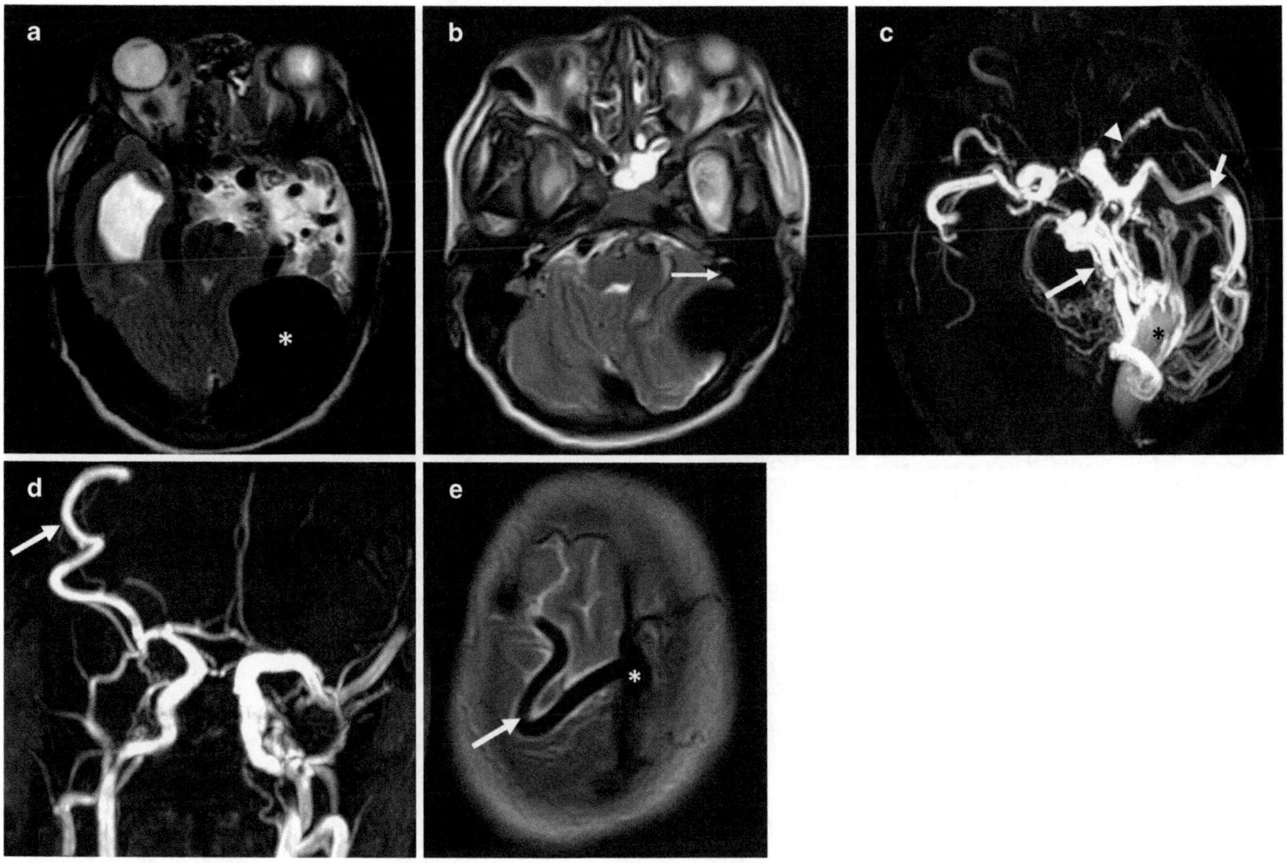

Fig. 19.11 Dural sinus malformation with associated dural and pial arteriovenous fistula. (**a**) Axial T2-weighted MRI shows evident dilatation of the transverse venous sinuses with a large venous lake (asterisk). (**b**) Axial T2-weighted image demonstrate hypoplasia of the internal jugular bulb on the left side (arrow). (**c**) Three-dimensional reconstruction of MR angiography shows multiple dilated vessels arising from the middle cerebral artery (short arrow), posterior cerebral artery (long arrow) and external carotid artery (arrowhead) supplying pial and dural arteriovenous fistulas with dilated venous sinus (asterisk). (**d**, **e**) Coronal maximum intensity projection of time-of-flight angiography (**d**) and axial T2-weighted MRI (**e**) shows a large arterial branch (arrow) arising from the right middle cerebral artery and ending at the superior sagittal sinus (asterisk)

lesion with detectable color Doppler flow, often accompanied by hydrocephalus. On CT imaging, it presents as a hyperdense midline venous pouch, while MRI, particularly T2-weighted imaging, shows multiple serpiginous signal void vessels consistent with high-flow vascular channels. Mural calcifications may be observed, and post-contrast studies reveal prominent enhancing arterial feeders and draining veins (Fig. 19.14). Associated findings may include hydrocephalus and dystrophic parenchymal calcifications. Angiography remains the gold standard for detailed vascular mapping and treatment planning. VGAM is classified based on the pattern of arterial supply, with the choroidal type representing the more complex form, characterized by numerous arterial feeders arising from the choroidal, callosal, and thalamoperforating arteries. In contrast, the mural type is simpler, characterized by fewer arterial feeders, typically from the posterior choroidal or collicular arteries. It is important to distinguish VGAM from vein of Galen aneurysmal dilatation, which refers to an AVM located in the subpial space that drains into one of the tributaries of the vein of Galen, resulting in secondary dilatation of the vein (Fig. 19.13) [10–12].

Initial management in the neonatal period focuses on medical stabilization of high-output cardiac failure. In cases where medical therapy fails, early neurointervention is considered. The primary treatment modality is transcatheter embolization using coils or liquid acrylic agents to occlude the abnormal arteriovenous shunt. Management of hydrocephalus remains controversial; ventricular shunting may be considered only in patients with refractory hydrocephalus after all feasible embolization attempts have been exhausted. Without treatment, VGAM carries a dismal prognosis, with a nearly 100% mortality rate [10–12].

Moyamoya Disease

Moyamoya disease (MMD) is an idiopathic, progressive narrowing of the distal internal carotid arteries (ICA), leading to the formation of a network of fragile collateral ves-

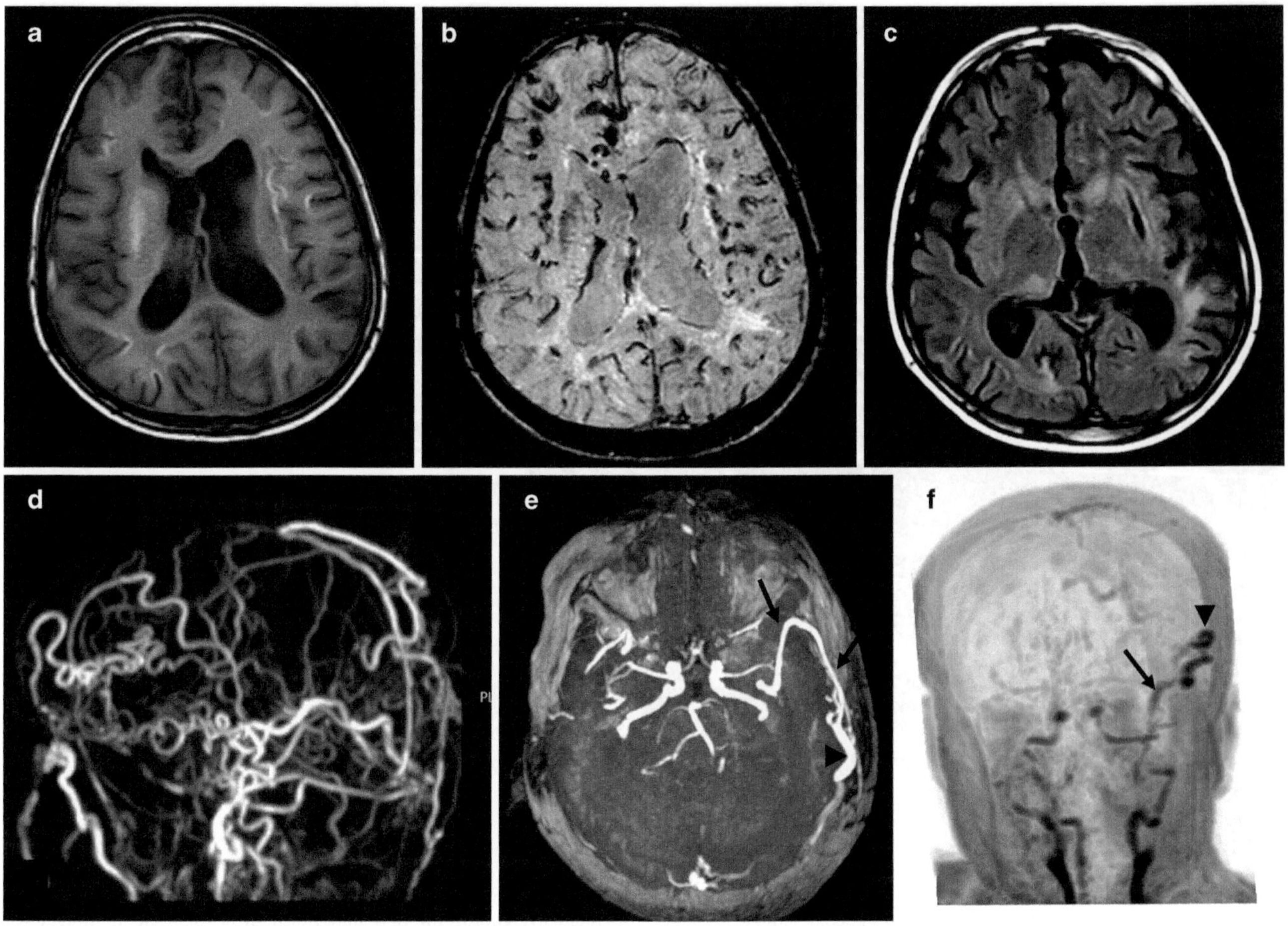

Fig. 19.12 A 13-year-old boy with dural arteriovenous fistula and venous sinus thrombosis. (**a**, **b**) Axial T1-weighted image (**a**) and susceptibility weighted image (**b**) show subcortical and basal ganglia abnormal signal being bright on T1-weighted image (**a**) and dark on T2*-weighted image (**b**) consistent with calcifications. (**c**) Axial FLAIR shows white matter abnormal signal with encephalomalacia in the left basal ganglia. (**d**) Three-dimensional reconstruction of the MR phase-contrast venography reveals thrombosis of the cerebral sinuses with multiple dilated superficial veins. (**e**, **f**) Axial maximum intensity projection of time-of-flight angiography (TOF) (**e**) and coronal maximum intensity projection of time-resolved MR angiography (**f**) show dilated middle meningeal artery (arrow) anastomosing with a superficial vein (arrowhead) which shows early venous filling (**f**)

sels, characteristically described as a "moyamoya pattern." This vascular alteration results in chronic cerebral ischemia and recurrent strokes. Children with MMD typically present with recurrent transient ischemic attacks and ischemic strokes. When similar vascular changes occur in association with an underlying condition (such as neurofibromatosis type 1, prior cranial radiotherapy, or sickle cell anemia) the condition is referred to as Moyamoya syndrome (Fig. 19.15) [13].

Imaging plays a crucial role in the diagnosis and staging of Moyamoya disease. On contrast-enhanced CT- and T2-weighted MRI, the presence of multiple basal ganglia collaterals may appear as bright dots and signal voids, respectively. The characteristic "leptomeningeal Ivy sign" can be seen on FLAIR images as a bright signal smearing the subarachnoid space (Figs. 19.15 and 19.16). CT angiography and MR angiography reveal stenosis in the terminal internal carotid arteries along with the formation of numerous moyamoya collaterals [13].

Disease severity is often graded using the Suzuki classification: Stage I involves narrowing of the terminal ICA or its proximal branches without visible collaterals; Stage II marks the initiation of moyamoya collateral formation; Stage III shows intensified moyamoya collaterals with progressive ICA stenosis; Stage IV includes the development of external carotid artery (ECA) collaterals (Fig. 19.16); Stage V is characterized by the disappearance of major cerebral arteries with decreasing moyamoya collaterals and more ECA contribution (Fig. 19.17); and Stage VI indicates complete occlusion of major cerebral arteries and moyamoya vessels, with cerebral perfusion relying solely on ECA-derived supply [14].

Revascularization is the mainstay of treatment for Moyamoya disease and has been shown to improve cognitive

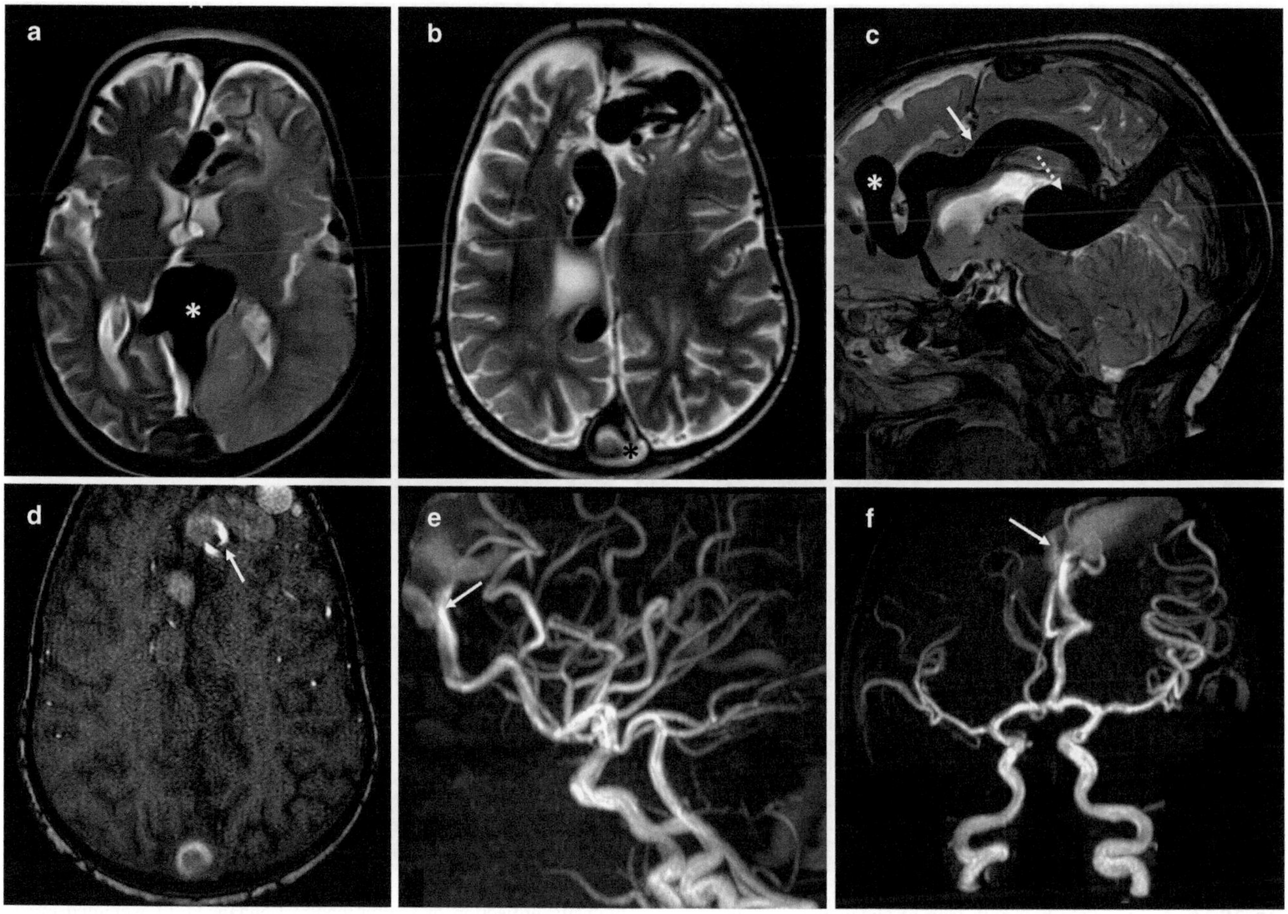

Fig. 19.13 A 4-year-old boy with pial arteriovenous fistula. (**a, b**) Axial T2-weighted image shows serpentine vessels in the subarachnoid space with dilated superior sagittal sinus (black asterisk) which shows flow-related artifacts associated with aneurysmal dilatation of the vein of Galen (white asterisk). (**c**) Minimal intensity projection of sagittal T2-weighted image show a saccular venous dilatation (venous pouch) (asterisk) draining into the congested inferior sagittal sinus (arrow). Note the dilated vein of Galen (dashed arrow). (**d**) Axial time-of-flight MR angiography shows the feeding pial artery (arrow) arising from the anterior cerebral artery. (**e, f**) Sagittal and coronal maximum intensity projection of MR angiography reveals the pial arteriovenous fistula (arrow). The abrupt change in caliber and signal intensity between the feeding artery and draining vein demarcate the site of the fistula

function, particularly when performed before irreversible brain damage occurs. Surgical approaches include direct and indirect revascularization. Direct revascularization involves creating an anastomosis between branches of the external carotid artery (such as the superficial temporal artery) and the internal carotid artery or the middle cerebral artery. Indirect revascularization techniques, on the other hand, aim to stimulate angiogenesis by placing a vascularized flap from the external carotid system onto the brain surface [14].

Cavernous Malformation

Cavernous malformation is the third most common cerebral vascular anomaly, following developmental venous anomaly and capillary telangiectasia. It is classified as a slow-flow vascular malformation by the International Society for the Study of Vascular Anomalies (ISSVA). It consists of tightly packed, immature vascular channels lacking intervening neural tissue. This malformation may occur in isolation or be associated with a DVA. In approximately 40% of cases, it is discovered incidentally during imaging studies. However, it may also develop as a late complication of cerebral radiation. Clinically, it can present with intracerebral hemorrhage, seizures, or focal neurological deficits. In the context of familial cerebral cavernous malformation syndrome, linked to a founder mutation in the KRIT1 gene, multiple lesions may be present (Fig. 19.18). Asymptomatic lesions typically do not require treatment; however, if the lesion becomes symptomatic, surgical resection is considered curative [14].

On imaging, cerebral cavernous malformations may show variable appearances. CT scans may be normal or reveal a slightly hyperdense, non-enhancing lesion, occasionally with calcifications or signs of hemorrhage. MRI provides more detailed characterization, with the Zabramski classification being widely used. Type 1 lesions, representing acute

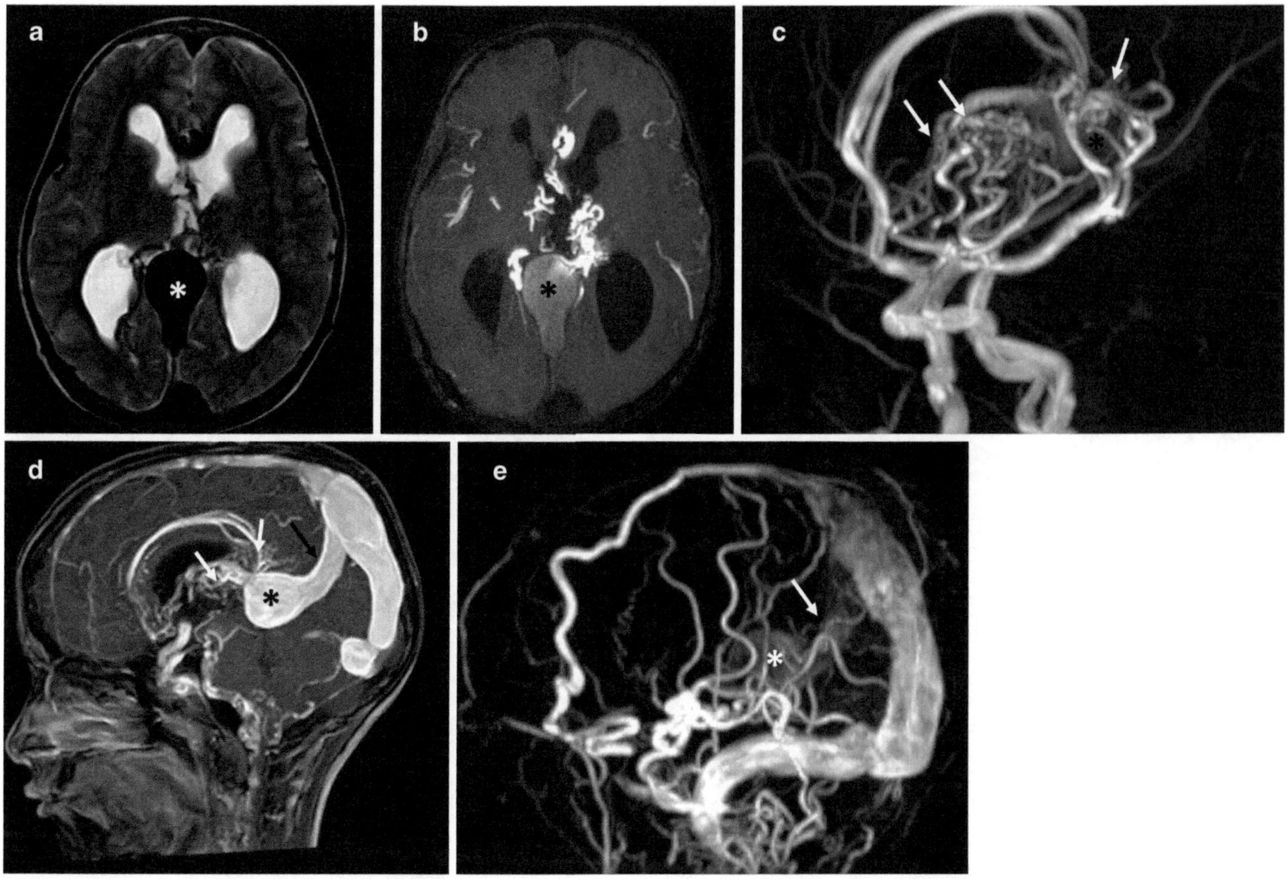

Fig. 19.14 A 7-year-old boy with vein of Galen aneurysmal malformation. (**a**) Axial T2-weighted image demonstrates multiple serpentine signal void vessels draining into the median prosencephalic vein (asterisk). (**b**, **c**) Axial (**b**) and sagittal (**c**) maximum intensity projection of time-of-flight MR angiography demonstrate multiple vessels (arrows) draining into the median prosencephalic vein (asterisk). (**d**) Maximum intensity projection of sagittal contrast-enhanced T1-weighted image shows multiple vessels (white arrows) draining into the dilated median prosencephalic vein (asterisk) which drains into persistent falcine sinus (black arrow). (**e**) Maximum intensity projection of the MR phase-contrast venography shows dilated median prosencephalic vein (asterisk), persistent falcine sinus (arrow), and other venous sinuses

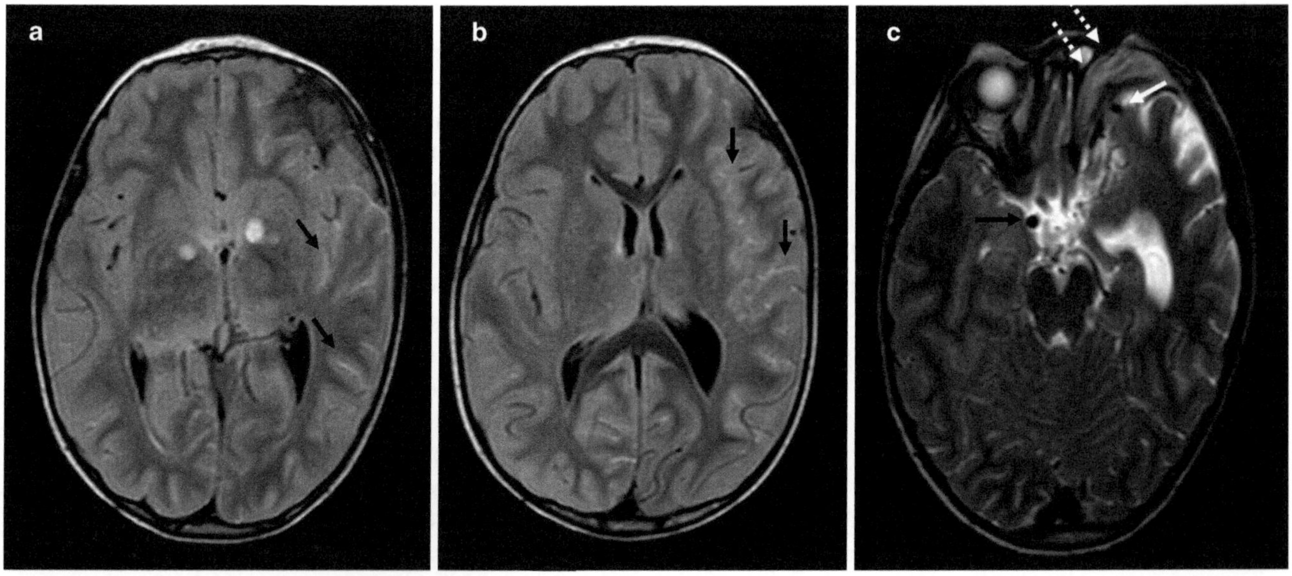

Fig. 19.15 An 8-year-old boy with neurofibromatosis and moyamoya syndrome. (**a**, **b**) Axial FLAIR shows abnormal signal in the basal ganglia corresponds to unidentified bright objects characteristic of neurofibromatosis. Note is made to the bright signal in the subarachnoid space corresponds to ivy sign (arrows). (**c**) Axial T2-weighted image demonstrates sphenoid wing dysplasia (dashed arrows) on the left side and nonvisualized left internal carotid artery compared to the right (black arrow) and dilated left middle meningeal artery (white arrow)

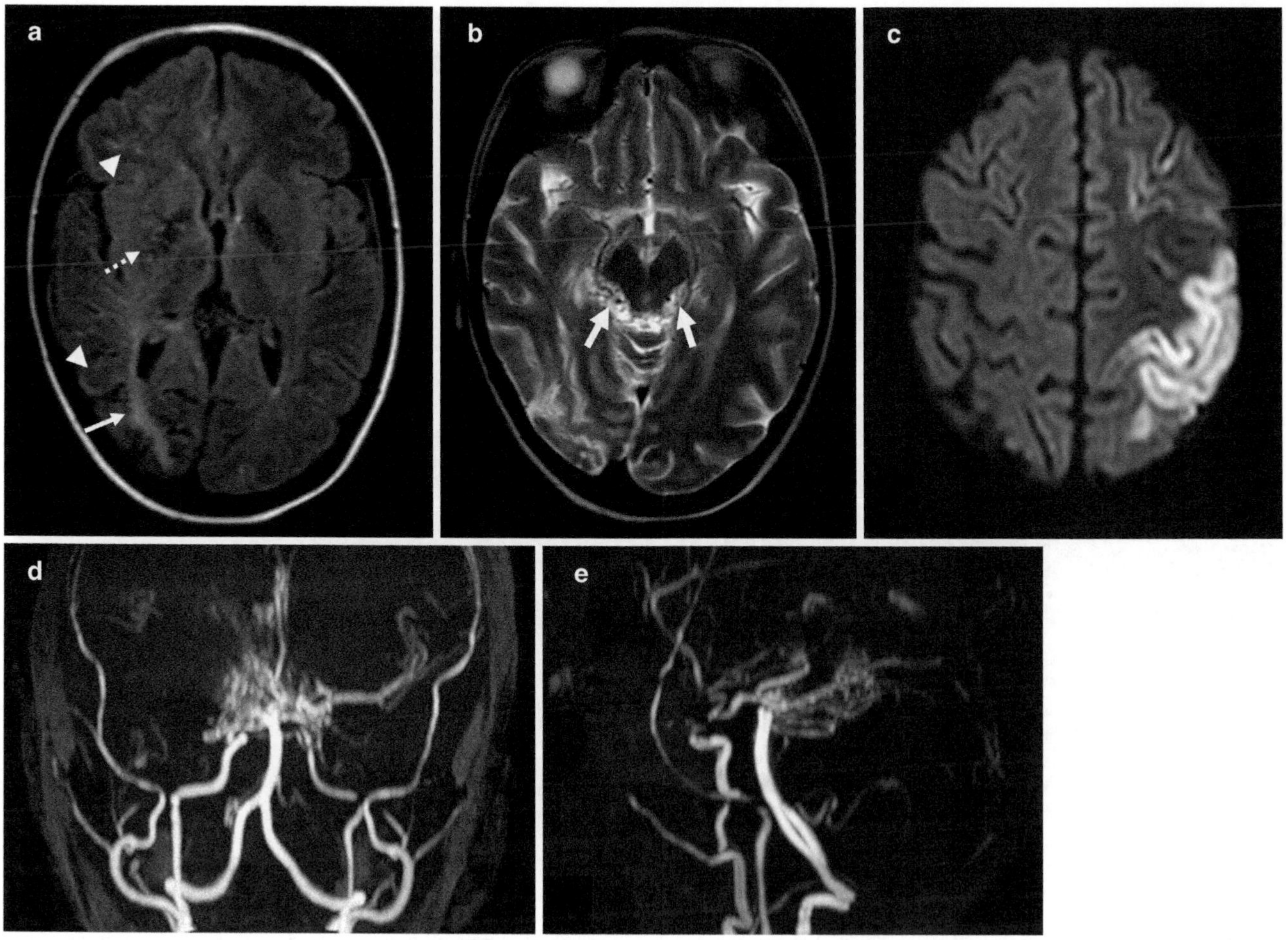

Fig. 19.16 A 10-year-old girl with beta thalassemia and moyamoya syndrome presented with acute neurologic deficit. (**a**) Axial FLAIR shows asymmetric brain atrophy more appreciated on the right cerebral hemisphere associated with white matter signal abnormality (arrow) representing gliotic changes. Note is made to bright dots (dashed arrow) in the basal ganglia representing lenticulostriate vessels and bright signal in the subarachnoid space (ivy sign) (arrowheads). (**b**) Axial T2-weighted image shows moyamoya collaterals in the subarachnoid space (ambient and quadrigeminal cistern) (arrows). (**c**) Axial diffusion-weighted image demonstrates restricted diffusion in the left parietal lobe in keeping with acute infarct. (**d, e**) Coronal and sagittal maximum intensity projection of time-of-flight MR angiography reveal multiple moyamoya collaterals, stenosis of the middle cerebral artery with presence of external carotid artery collaterals (Suzuki stage IV)

or subacute hemorrhage, appear as a hyperintense core on T1-weighted images and may be hypo- or hyperintense on T2, surrounded by a low-signal hemosiderin ring (Fig. 19.8). Type 2, the classic "popcorn-like" lesion, shows a mixed-signal, reticulated core on both T1 and T2, also encased by a hemosiderin ring (Figs. 19.18 and 19.19). Type 3 lesions, which indicate chronic hemorrhage, appear hypointense on both T1- and T2-weighted images. Type 4 lesions are not visible on conventional MRI sequences but can be detected using susceptibility-weighted imaging (SWI) or T2*-weighted sequence [15]. Cavernous malformations can be difficult to diagnose and must be differentiated from other hemorrhagic lesions (Figs. 19.20 and 19.21). Hemorrhagic neoplasms may not exhibit the classic low-signal hemosiderin rim and often present with heterogeneous or irregular enhancement [1] (Fig. 19.21). The persistence of edema, enhancement, and Zabramski type 1 cavernous malformation features should raise the concern of hemorrhagic neoplasm [16, 17]. Moreover, perilesional hyperintense signal on T1-weighted image was found to be highly specific and predictive of cavernous malformation (Fig. 19.18). The high T1 signal could result from the extravascular leakage of red blood cells and plasma outside, possibly related to active bleeding within the cavernous malformation [17].

Sinus Pericranii

Sinus pericranii (SP) is an uncommon venous malformation characterized by an abnormal connection between extracranial veins and the dural venous sinuses within the cranium. Clinically, it typically presents as a soft, non-tender, and fluctuant scalp mass that becomes more prominent with dependency or valsalva maneuver and decreases in size when

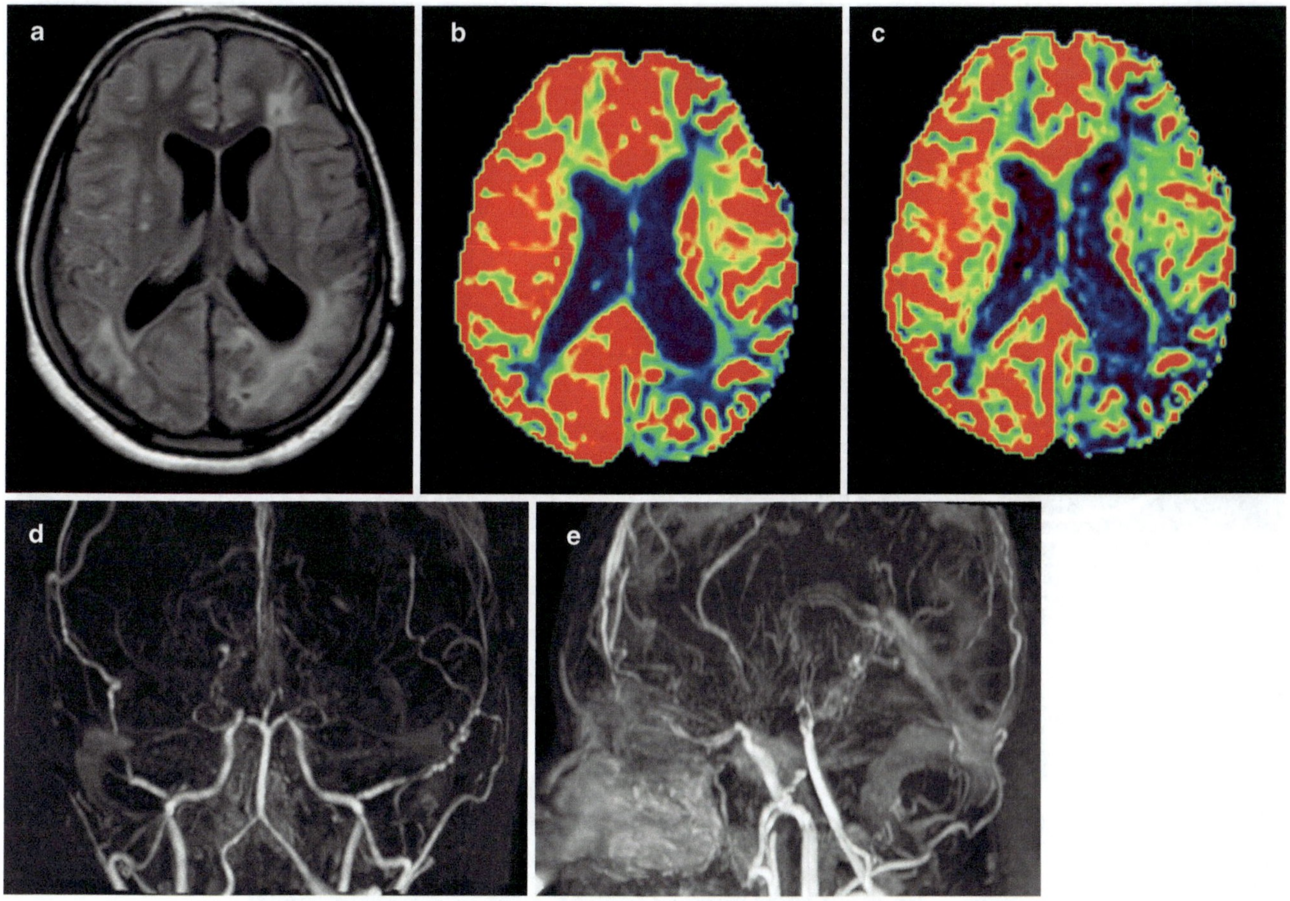

Fig. 19.17 A 12-year-old boy with moyamoya disease. (**a**) Axial FLAIR shows abnormal white matter signal denoting ischemic leukoencephalopathy and gliotic changes due to old infarct. (**b**, **c**) Color map of cerebral blood flow (CBF) (**c**) and cerebral blood volume (CBV) (**d**) show more reduction of CBF and CBV in the left hemisphere compared to the right. (**d**, **e**) Coronal and sagittal maximum intensity projection of MR angiography demonstrates few moyamoya collaterals, absent anterior cerebral, middle cerebral and posterior cerebral arteries with external carotid artery collaterals (Suzuki stage V)

the patient is in an upright position (Fig. 19.22). These lesions are most commonly found in the midline or paramidline regions of the scalp [18].

Imaging plays a key role in the diagnosis of SP. On ultrasound, SP appears as an anechoic vessel exhibiting a venous waveform pattern, traversing the hyperechoic skull bone. CT typically reveals a well-defined bony defect in the skull, and contrast-enhanced CT or CT venography demonstrates the presence of a vein connecting the extracranial venous system with the dural venous sinus (Fig. 19.22). MRI further characterizes SP, where the lesion appears iso- to hypointense on T1-weighted images and hyperintense on T2-weighted images, although it may show as a signal void if a rapidly flowing varix is present. Post-contrast T1-weighted images and MR venography effectively delineate all the venous structures involved in the SP [18]. Sinus pericranii should be distinguished from other scalp or calvarial masses in children, such as vascular anomalies, cephaloceles, and lesions like Langerhans cell histiocytosis, neuroblastoma metastases, or epidermoid cysts [19] (Figs. 19.23, 19.24, 19.25, and 19.26).

Management of SP includes surgical excision or endovascular/percutaneous embolization, often utilizing hydrocoils or ethylene vinyl alcohol copolymer. With the advent of advanced endovascular techniques, most cases of SP are effectively treated, and the overall prognosis is favorable [20].

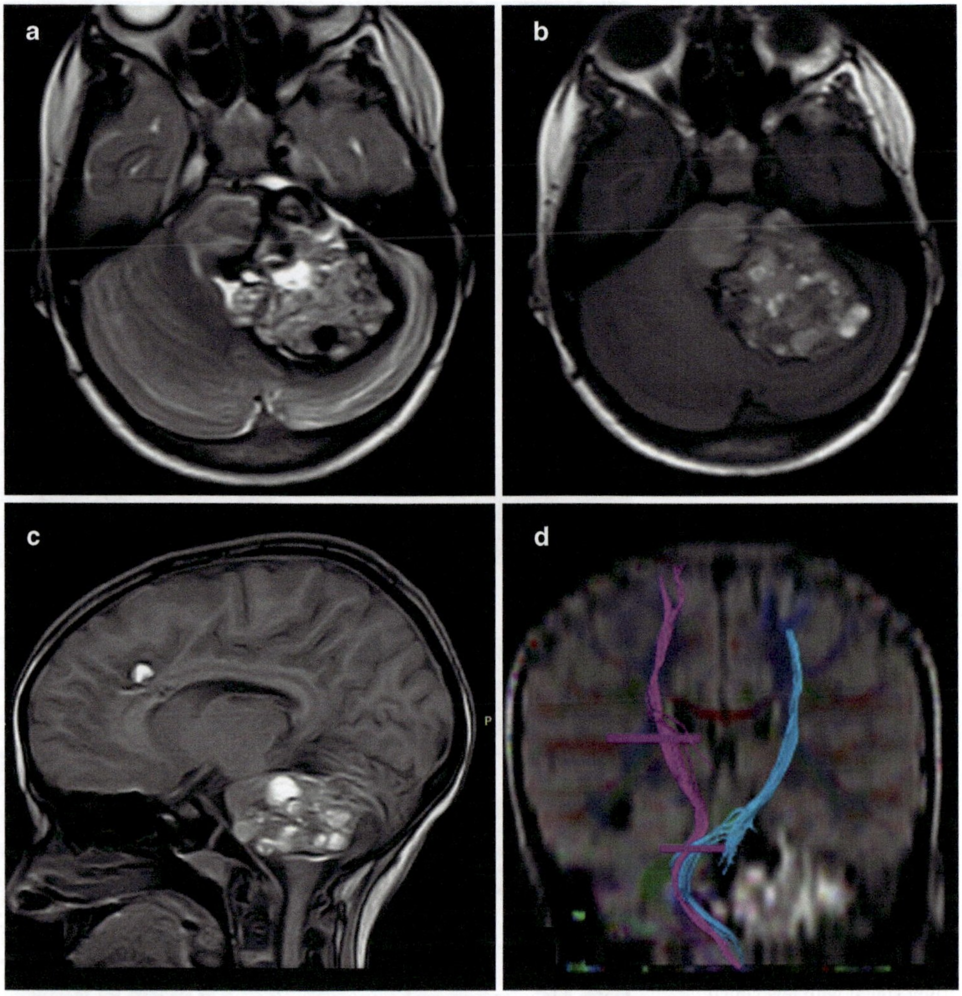

Fig. 19.18 An 8-year-old girl with multiple cavernous malformations. (**a–c**) Axial T2-weighted image (**a**), axial T1-weighted image, (**b**) and sagittal T1-weighted image (**c**) show a large cavernoma with its typical popcorn appearance and characteristic hypointense hemosiderin rim. Associated perilesional abnormal signals appear bright on T2-weighted image (**a**) and T1-weighted image (**b**). (**d**) Coronal FLAIR with diffusion tensor tractography shows displacement of both pyramidal tracts by the large cavernous malformation

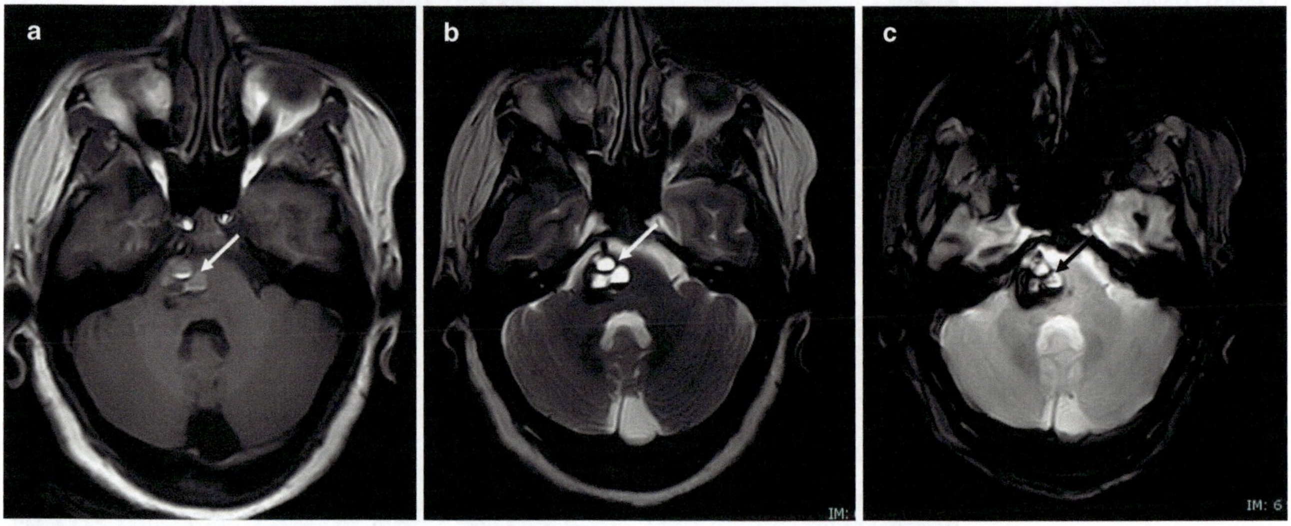

Fig. 19.19 Pontine cavernous malformation. (**a–c**) Axial T1-weighted (**a**), Axial T2 weighted (**b**), axial T2* (**c**) shows cavernous malformation (arrow) with its characteristic mixed signal (popcorn appearance) and hemosiderin low signal rim and blooming on T2*-weighted image (**c**)

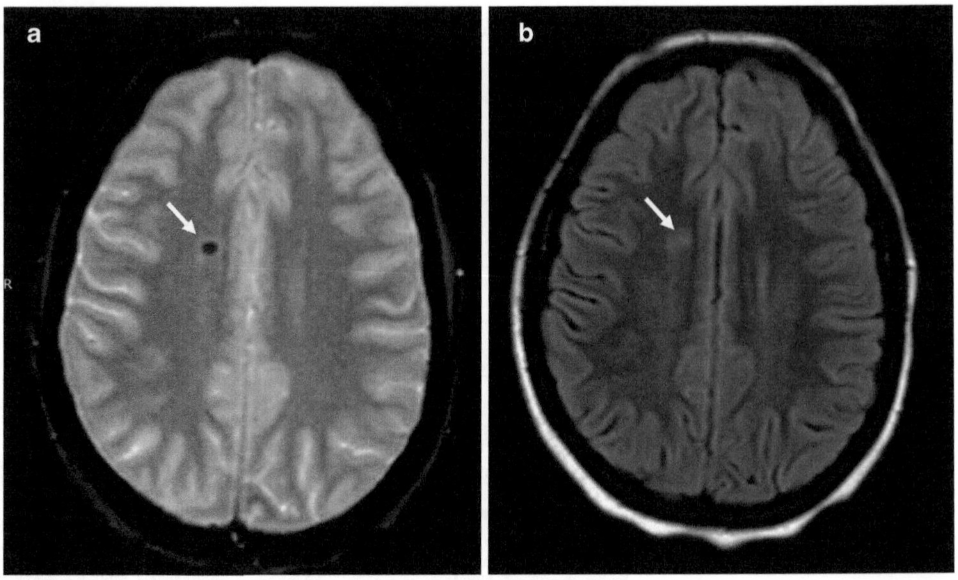

Fig. 19.20 A 10-year-old boy with acute lymphoblastic leukemia developed brain parenchymal hemorrhage (arrow). Brain MRI shows characteristic hypointense signal on T2*-weighted image (**a**) and bright signal on FLAIR (**b**). Correlation with patient's history is mandatory

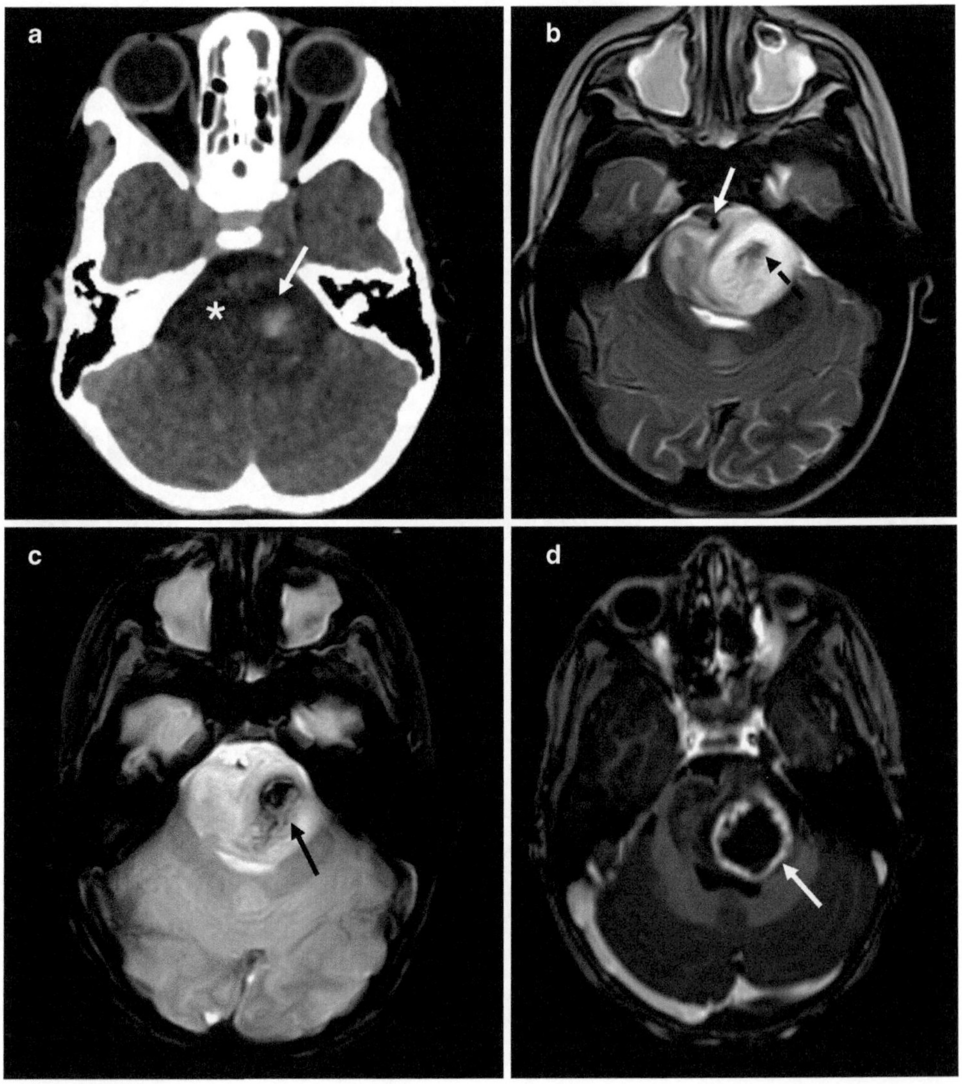

Fig. 19.21 A 3-year-old girl with high-grade pontine glioma presented with acute disturbance of conscious level. (**a**) Non-contrast CT demonstrate enlarged hypodense pons (asterisk) with hyperdense hemorrhagic area (arrow). (**b**) Axial T2-weighted MRI shows enlarged pons engulfing the basilar artery (arrow). The pons is enlarged exhibiting bright signal with low signal intensity hemorrhage (dashed arrow). (**c**) Axial T2*-weighted imaging confirms intralesional hemorrhage (arrow). (**d**) Axial contrast-enhanced T1-weighted image shows a large area of irregular marginal enhancement

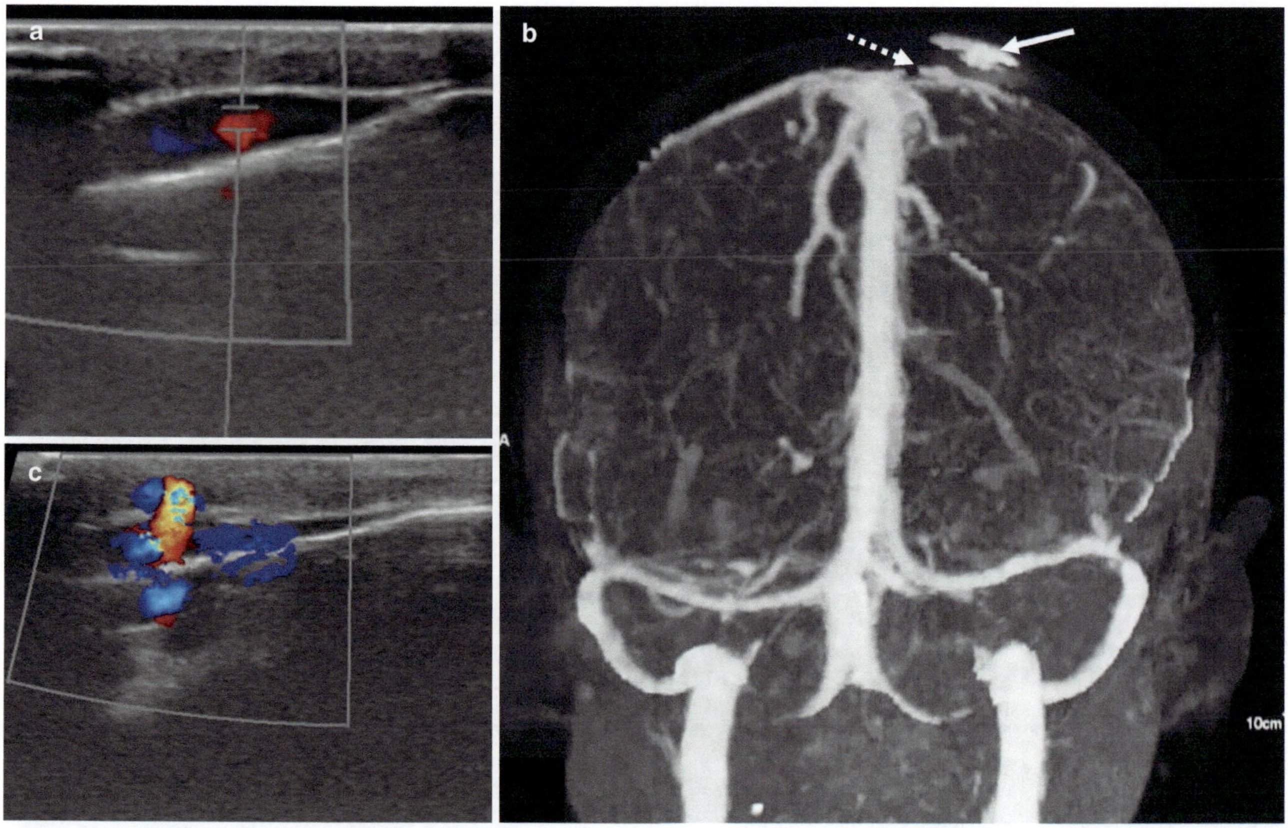

Fig. 19.22 A 9-year-old boy with sinus pericranii presented with a soft compressible scalp swelling. (**a**, **b**) Color Doppler ultrasound shows more flow at dependent position (**b**) compared to upright position (**a**). (**c**) Maximum intensity projection of CT venography demonstrates the dilated superficial veins (arrow). There is a vein crossing the calvarium (dashed arrow)

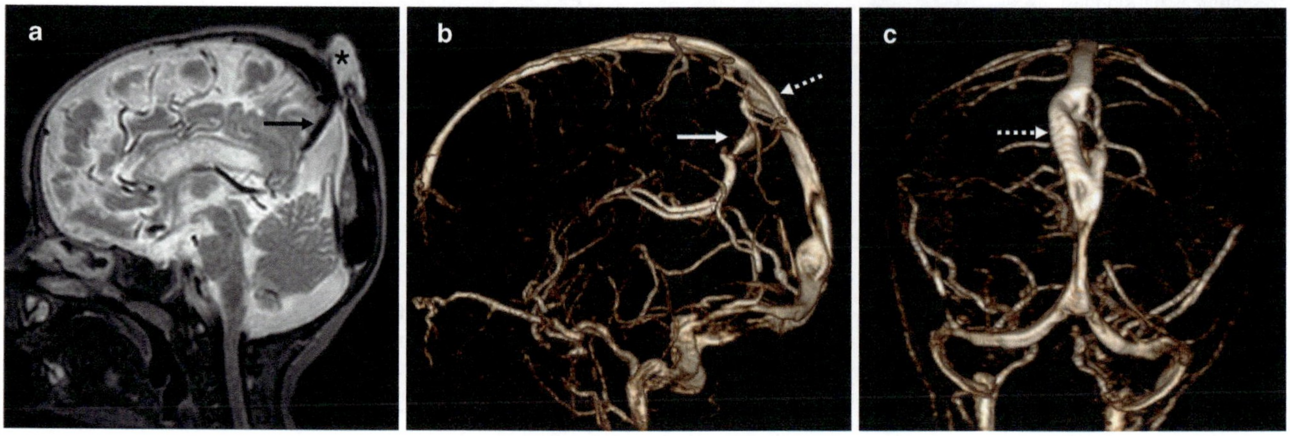

Fig. 19.23 A 3-month-old boy with atretic parietal cephalocele. (**a–c**) Sagittal T2-weighted image (**a**) and three-dimensional reconstruction of MR venography (**b**, **c**) show cystic scalp swelling (asterisk) associated with vertically oriented falcine sinus (arrow) draining into the superior sagittal sinus (dashed arrow). The superior sagittal sinus (dashed arrow) is bifid at the site of the cephalocele

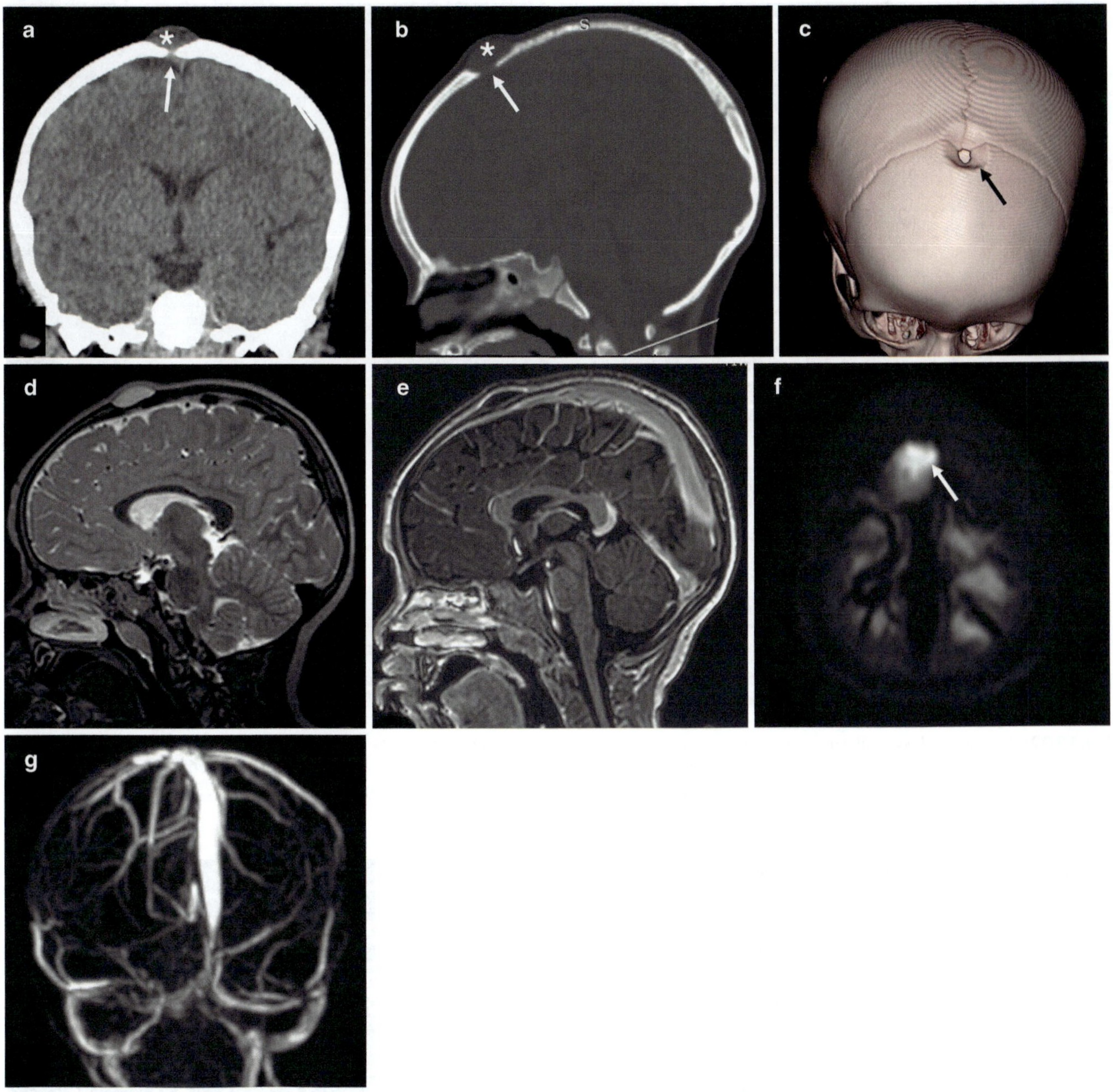

Fig. 19.24 A 2-year-old boy with scalp epidermoid. (**a**, **b**) Coronal and sagittal CT of the skull show cystic swelling (asterisk) with underlying osseous defect (arrow). (**c**) Three-dimensional reconstruction of the skull demonstrates the skull defect (arrow). (**d**, **e**) Sagittal T2-weighted image (**d**) and sagittal contrast-enhanced T1-weighted image (**e**) show that the lesion is hyperintense (**d**) with no contrast enhancement (**e**). (**f**) Axial diffusion-weighted image demonstrates the characteristic diffusion restriction (arrow). (**g**) Phase-contrast MR venography confirms absent communication with the lesion

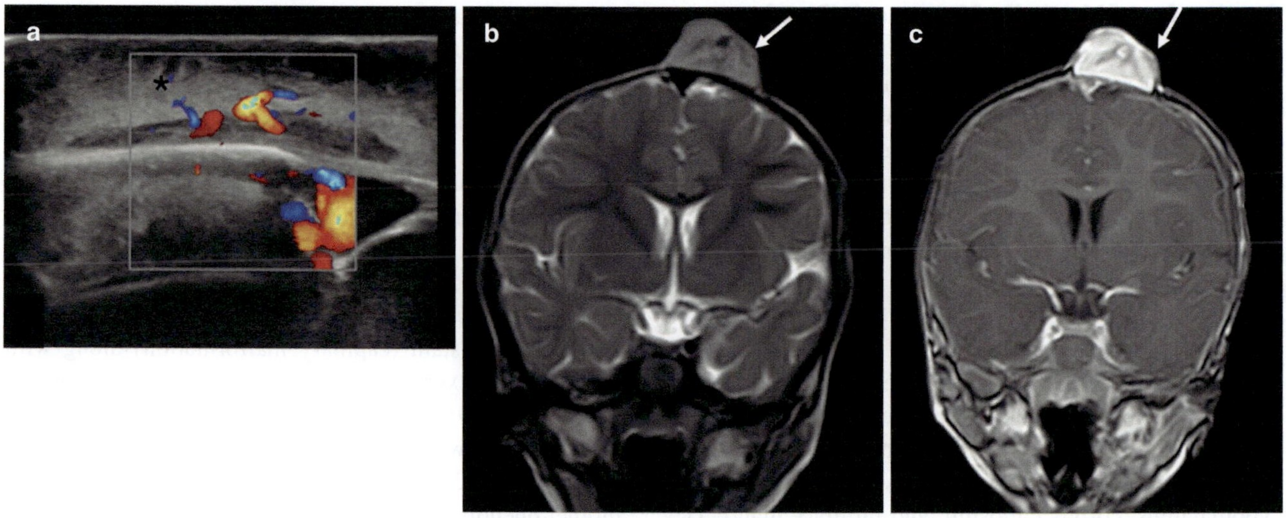

Fig. 19.25 A 1-year-old girl with scalp infantile hemangioma. (**a**) Color Doppler ultrasound shows soft tissue mass (asterisk) with internal color flow. No crossing veins identified through the skull bones. (**b, c**) Coronal T2-weighted image (**b**), Coronal contrast enhanced T1-weighted image (**c**) shows soft tissue mass (arrow) with bright signal on T2-weighted image, showing internal signal voids (**b**) and remarkable contrast enhancement (**c**)

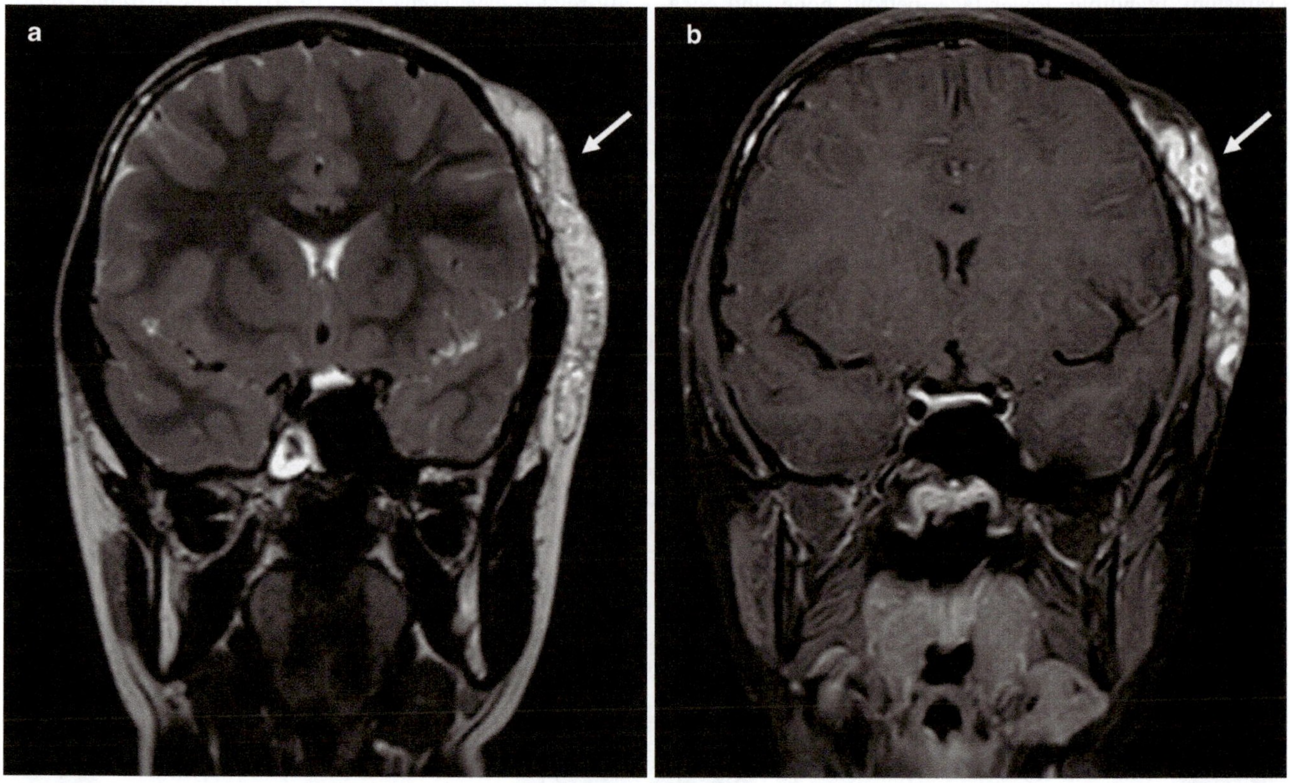

Fig. 19.26 A 12-year-old girl with scalp venous malformation (arrow). (**a**) Coronal T2-weighted image and (**b**) contrast-enhanced T1-weighted image. The venous malformation exhibits bright signal on T2-weighted image (**a**) with appreciable contrast enhancement (**b**), with no evidence of veins crossing the calvarium

Cerebrofacial Vascular Metameric Syndrome

The brain and spinal cord develop from a series of 34 metameres or somites (3 dedicated to the brain and 31 to the spinal segments). Each metamere contains distinct structural elements derived from the neural tube, neural crest, mesoderm, musculature, and skin. Cerebrofacial vascular metameric syndrome refers to a group of complex congenital disorders characterized by vascular anomalies, primarily affecting arteries or veins, in regions corresponding to specific embryological metamere [21].

The condition is divided into three types based on the specific metameres affected during embryologic development. Type 1, known as the medial prosencephalic group, involves midline structures such as the forehead, nose, hypothalamus, corpus callosum, and pituitary gland. Type 2, or the lateral prosencephalic (optic) group, includes the optic apparatus, retina, thalamus, temporo-parietal-occipital lobes, eye, cheek, and maxilla. Type 3, referred to as the rhombencephalic (Otic) group, affects the cerebellum, brainstem, mandible, lower face, petrous bone, and occasionally the maxilla [21, 22].

Cerebrofacial arteriovenous metameric syndrome (CAMS) involves multiple AVMs located in both the brain and facial regions. These lesions often feature a diffuse, proliferative nidus and are associated with multiple small arterial feeders and early venous drainage, making them particularly challenging to manage [22] (Fig. 19.27).

Cerebrofacial venous metameric syndrome (CVMS) encompasses a range of slow-flow vascular malformations that may affect the skin, soft tissues, dura mater, brain, orbit, and eye. Sturge-Weber syndrome is the most common phenotypic variant of CVMS in which there is cutaneous port wine stain (capillary malformation) along with leptomeningeal venous malformation and ispsilateral hemispheric atrophy and gyral calcification (Figs. 19.28 and 19.29). CVMS with developmental venous anomaly associating head and neck venous vascular malformation is another phenotypic variant (Fig. 19.30). Most developmental venous anomalies are supratentorial, ipsilateral to the side of facial vascular malformation, and have large venous radicles draining into tortuous deep venous system. Patients with CVMS also may have developmental venous anomaly-related cavernoma (Fig. 19.30). In the extreme end of the spectrum, patients with head and neck venous malformation may have developmental venous anomaly associating cavernous sinus hemangioma [21].

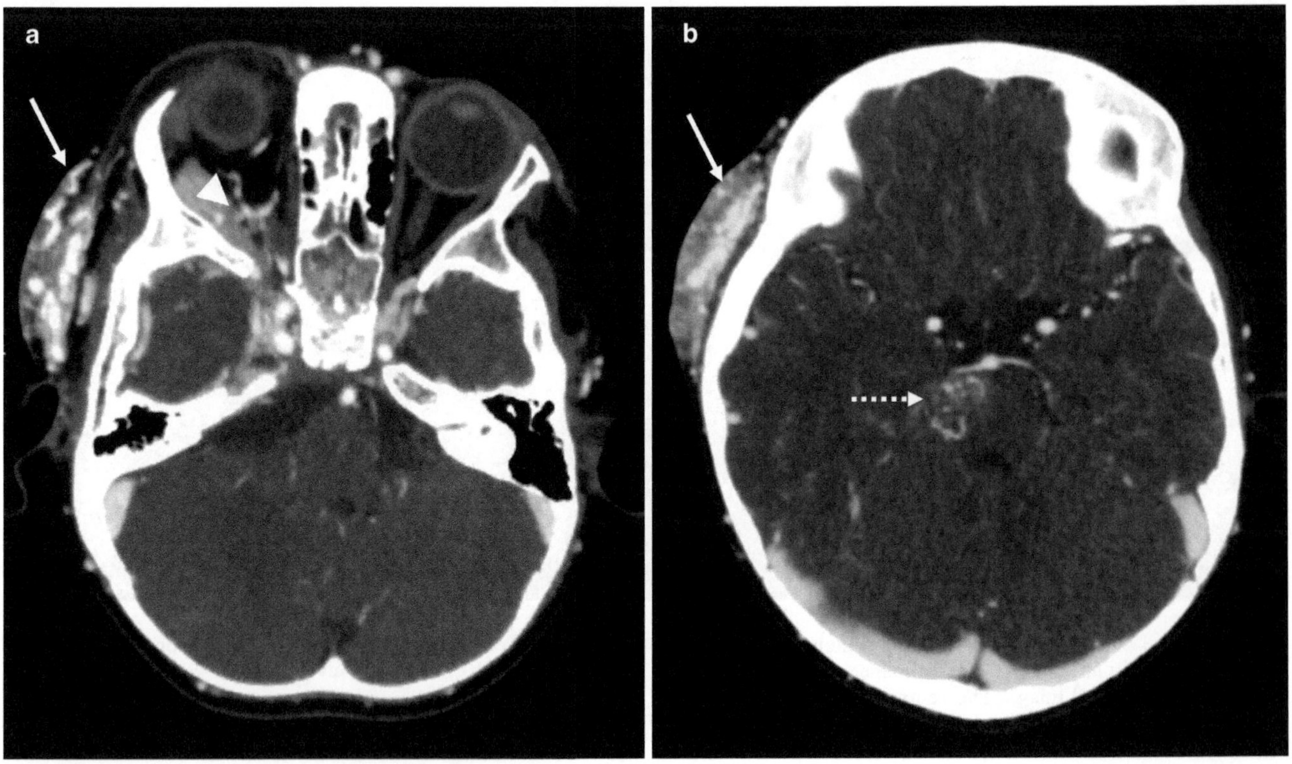

Fig. 19.27 A two-year-old boy with cerebrofacial arteriovenous metameric syndrome. (**a**, **b**) Axial contrast-enhanced CT cerebral angiography shows arteriovenous malformation at the right temporal region (arrow), right orbit (arrowhead), and in the pons (dashed arrow)

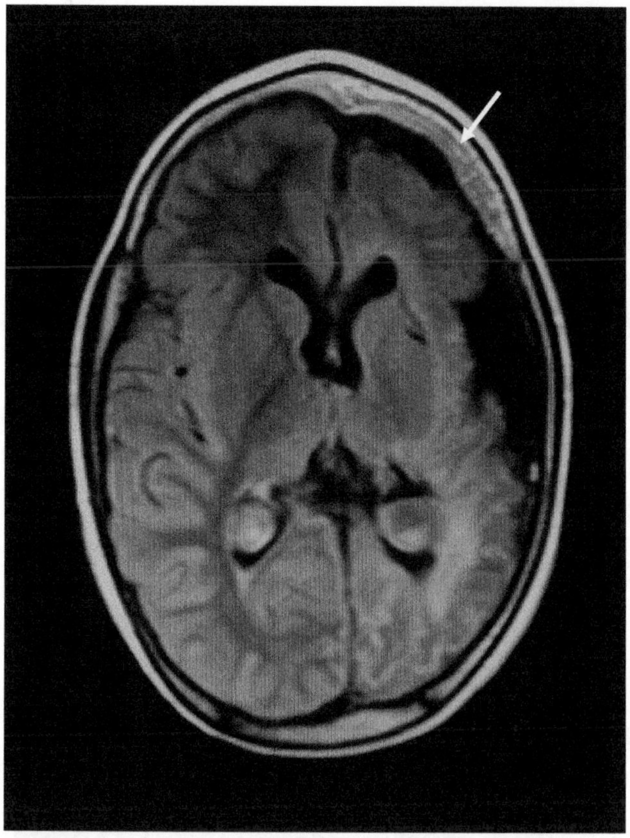

Fig. 19.28 Sturge-Weber syndrome. Axial FLAIR shows left cerebral hemiatrophy, bright signal in the sulci of the left cerebral hemisphere due to leptomeningeal angiomatosis associated with osseous expansion of the left frontal bone (arrow)

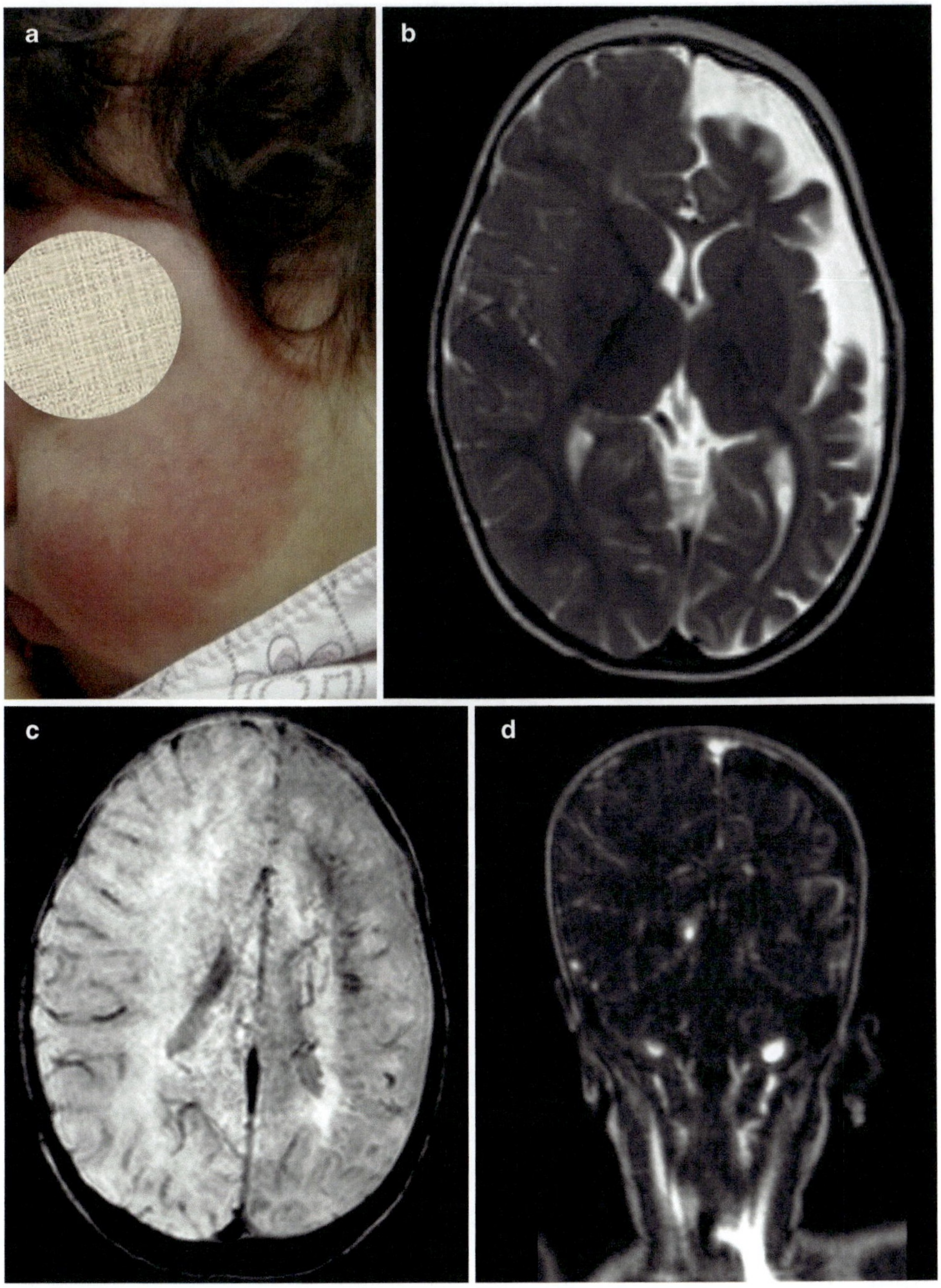

Fig. 19.29 A one-year-old girl with Sturge–Weber syndrome. (**a**) Clinical photograph shows port wine stain representing capillary malformation. (**b**) Axial T2-weighted MRI shows left cerebral hemiatrophy. (**c**) Axial T2* shows subcortical low signal intensity representing calcification associated with multiple linear signal voids representing congested medullary veins. (**d**) Coronal contrast-enhanced dynamic MR angiography at the venous phase shows leptomeningeal enhancement representing leptomeningeal angiomatosis

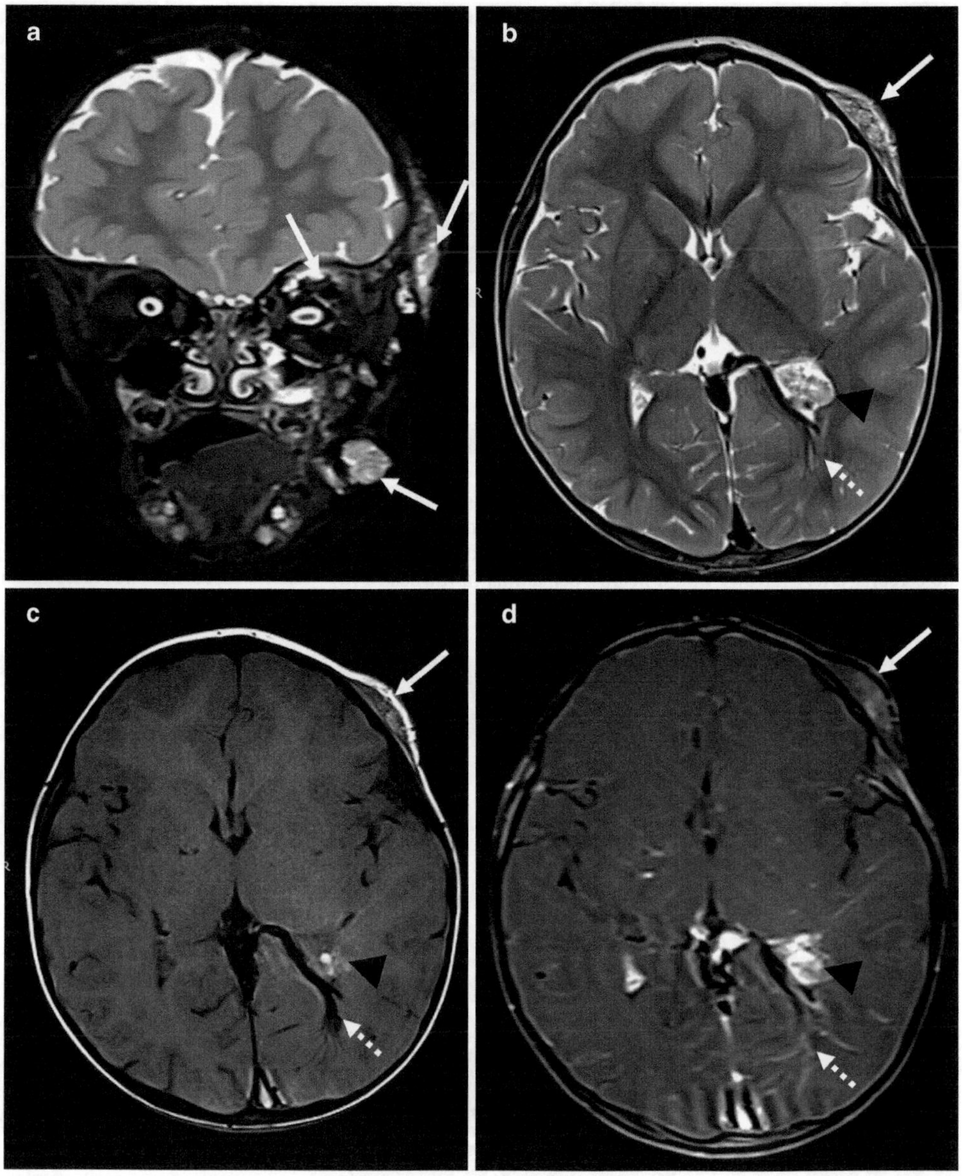

Fig. 19.30 A one-year-old boy with cerebrofacial venous metameric syndrome. (**a**) Coronal T2-fat saturated image shows left hemifacial venous malformation (arrows). (**b–d**) Axial T2-weighted image (**b**), T1-weighted image (**c**), and contrast-enhanced T1-weighted image (**d**) demonstrate the cutaneous venous malformation (arrow), developmental venous anomaly (dashed arrow), and choroid plexus angioma (arrowhead)

Intracranial Arterial Aneurysms in Pediatric Population

Intracranial arterial aneurysms (IAA), though uncommon, are responsible for 10–15% of hemorrhagic strokes occurring during the first two decades of life. While the majority are idiopathic, some cases may be associated with trauma, arteriopathies, or infections. In young children, most of the aneurysms develop distal to the circle of Willis (Fig. 19.31). Excessive hemodynamic stress in school-aged children and adolescents can lead to the development of IAA. These stresses may result from flow overload, as seen in arteriovenous malformations (AVMs); vibrational stress, such as that associated with aortic coarctation (Fig. 19.32); or pressure overload, observed in juvenile hypertension [23].

Intracranial aneurysms most commonly manifest as subarachnoid hemorrhage, a critical medical emergency associated with approximately 50% mortality and considerable long-term morbidity in survivors, despite advancements in treatment strategies. Non-contrast CT is typically the first imaging modality of choice, as the pattern of bleeding can often indicate the location of the ruptured aneurysm. It is also effective in identifying intraventricular hemorrhage and assessing the severity of associated hydrocephalus (Figs. 19.31 and 19.32). However, its sensitivity for detecting subarachnoid hemorrhage decreases significantly after 6 h. CT angiography using multidetector CT, with its ability to produce multiplanar and 3D reconstructions, can visualize aneurysms as small as 4 mm (Figs. 19.31 and 19.32). Digital subtraction angiography is considered the standard of care in

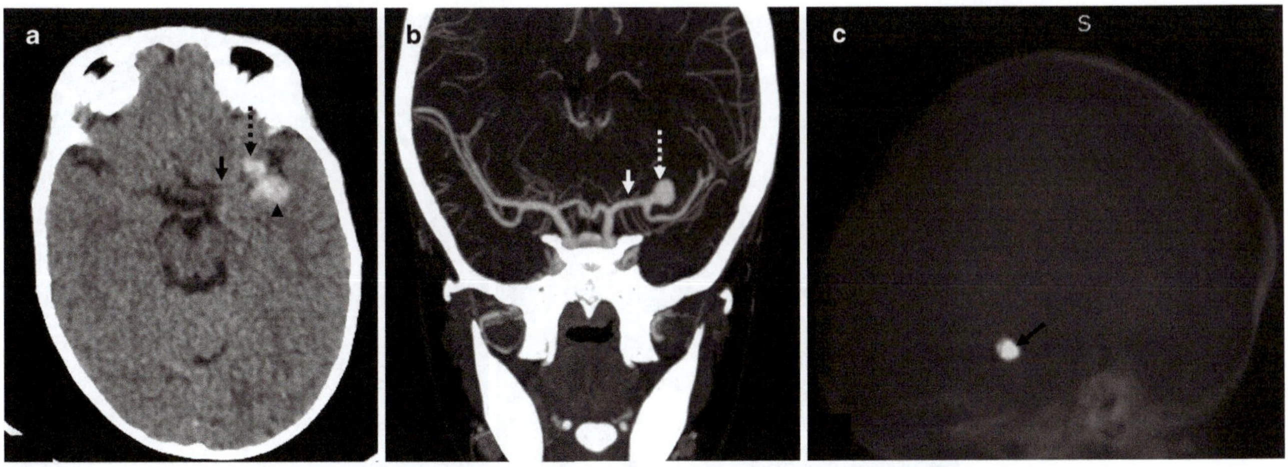

Fig. 19.31 A one-year-old girl with aneurysm of the left middle cerebral artery underwent endovascular coiling. (**a**) Axial non-contrast CT shows hyperdense aneurysm (dashed arrow) arising from the left middle cerebral artery (arrow) with a nearby hematoma (arrowhead). (**b**) Coronal maximum intensity projection of CT angiography shows saccular aneurysm (dashed arrow) arising from the left middle cerebral artery (arrow). (**c**) Sagittal average intensity projection of head CT shows successful endovascular coiling (arrow)

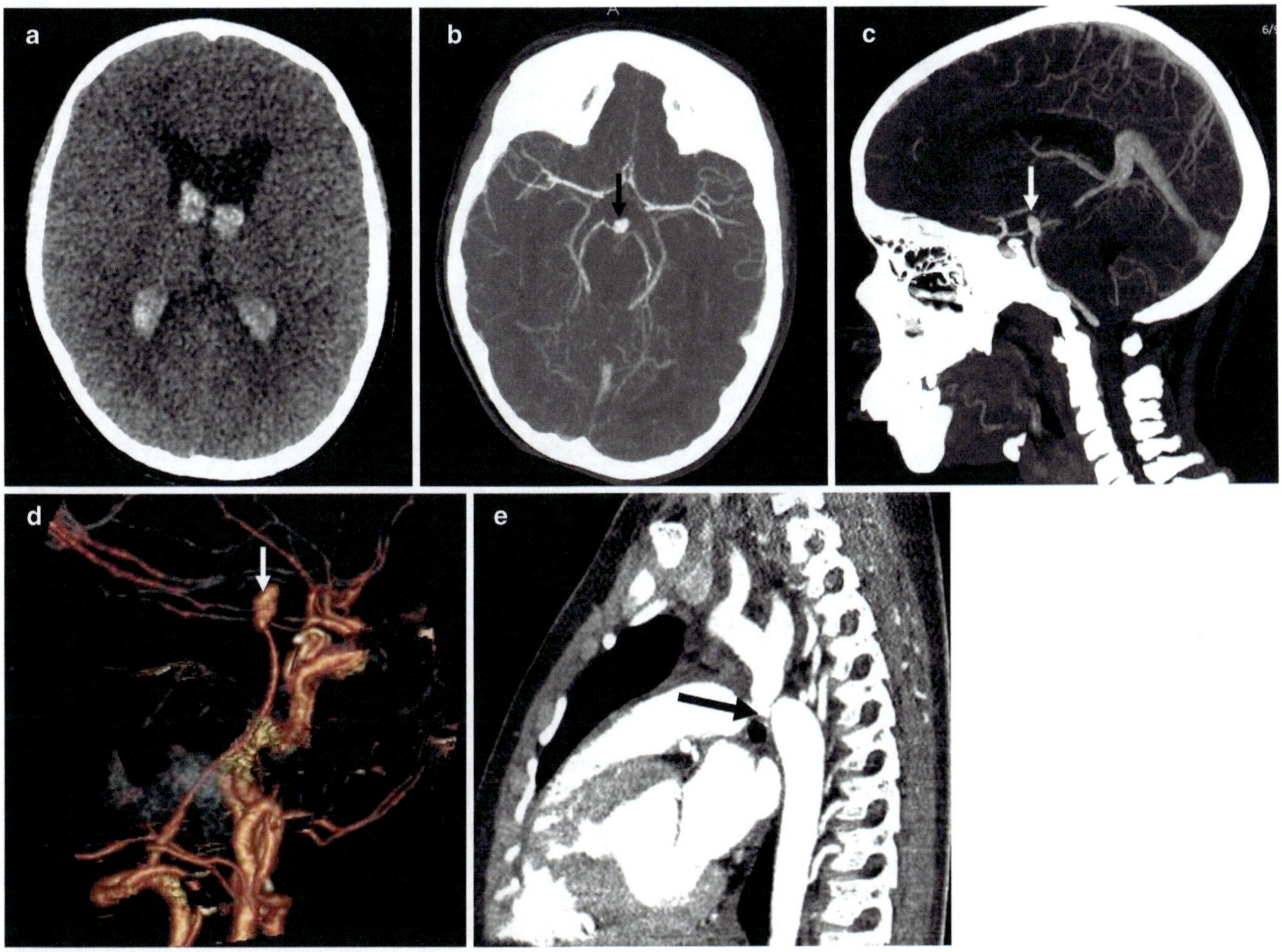

Fig. 19.32 A 12-year-old boy with coarctation of the aorta and basilar tip aneurysm presented with intraventricular hemorrhage. (**a**) Non-contrast CT at presentation shows intraventricular hemorrhage and ventricular dilatation. (**b–d**) Axial (**b**), sagittal (**c**) maximum intensity projection and three-dimensional reconstruction (**d**) demonstrate an oval shaped aneurysm (arrow) at the tip of the basilar artery. (**e**) Sagittal reconstruction of CT aortography demonstrates coarctation of the aorta (arrow)

diagnosing cerebral aneurysms. Moreover, three-dimensional rotational angiography has higher sensitivity in detecting aneurysms less than 3 mm. Cerebral aneurysms may be managed successfully by endovascular intervention [24] (Fig. 19.31).

Spinal Vascular Anomalies

Spinal vascular anomalies are group of complex and critical conditions often presenting with acute neurological manifestations that result in significant morbidity. The diagnosis of spinal vascular anomalies may be more challenging compared to cerebral vascular anomalies due to its smaller size and spinal angiography is technically more difficult than cerebral angiography. In addition, their angiographic features are variable according to the spinal cord level and the type of the anomaly.

There are different classifications of spinal vascular anomalies according to their location and type of shunt. Spetzler and Takai are the most widely used classifications. Spetzler classified vascular anomalies according to their anatomical location, pathophysiology, neuroimaging findings, and intraoperative observations into four groups (arteriovenous malformation, arteriovenous fistula, neoplastic vascular lesions, and spinal aneurysms). On the other hand, Takai classified spinal vascular anomalies according to their angioarchitecture into five types (type I: dural AVF; type II: intradural intramedullary glomus AVM; type III: intradural intramedullary juvenile AVM; type IV: perimedullary AVF; type V: extradural AVF) [25].

Digital subtraction angiography remains the gold standard for accurately identifying the specific type of spinal vascular malformation and for precisely determining the location of the arteriovenous fistula. Nevertheless, MRI is typically the first imaging modality used when evaluating spinal cord pathology in patients presenting with neurological symptoms [26].

In cases of dural arteriovenous fistula, MRI often reveals intramedullary hyperintensity consistent with spinal cord edema caused by venous hypertension along with segmental enhancement of the spinal cord that indicates disruption of the blood–spinal cord barrier. Multiple dilated perimedullary vessels representing enlarged pial veins are also observed (Fig. 19.33) [26]. Dilated vessels appear as serpiginous flow void that should be differentiated from cerebrospinal fluid (CSF)-flow-related artifact especially in fast spin echo MRI sequence. A common location of this artifact is in the dorsal spine (Fig. 19.34). This artifact arises from a combination of pulsatile cerebrospinal fluid flow driven by both respiratory and cardiac cycles, overlaid on

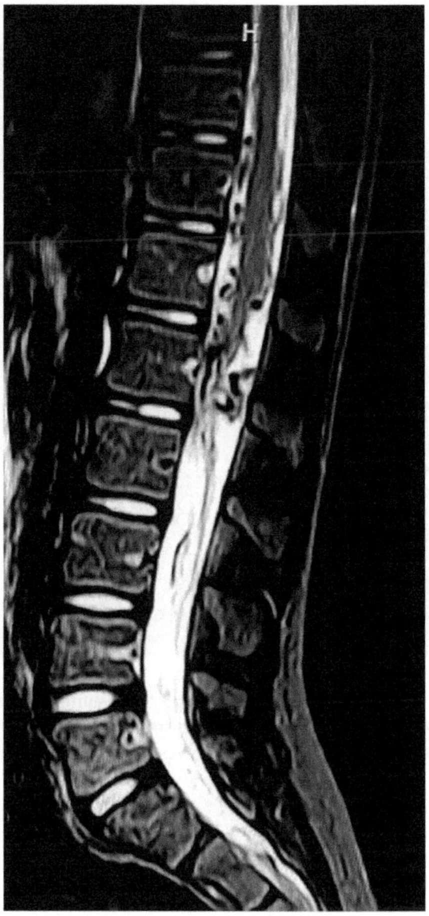

Fig. 19.33 An 11-year-old girl with spinal arteriovenous fistula (AVF). Sagittal T2-MRI shows multiple serpentine flow voids representing dilated veins. Spinal dural AVF and epidural arteriovenous fistula with perimedullary venous drainage has similar MR findings. Final diagnosis should be assessed by digital subtraction angiography

the overall cranially directed CSF movement. Additionally, turbulence generated as CSF shifts from the ventral to the dorsal subarachnoid space contributes to the disturbance. The resulting complex CSF dynamics cause phase incoherence, which manifests as signal loss on imaging [27]. Flow voids of spinal dural artiovenous fistula tend to be more hypointense and sharply defined. If doubt remains, gadolinium enhanced sequence may be necessary to exclude true pathology (Fig. 19.34) [28].

For spinal arteriovenous malformations, MRI demonstrates a classic nidus located either intramedullary or at the intra-perimedullary region. Spinal cavernomas appear as well-defined intramedullary lesions with mixed signal intensity on T1- and T2-weighted images and a surrounding hypointense rim, creating the characteristic "popcorn" appearance with minimal or absent contrast enhancement [26].

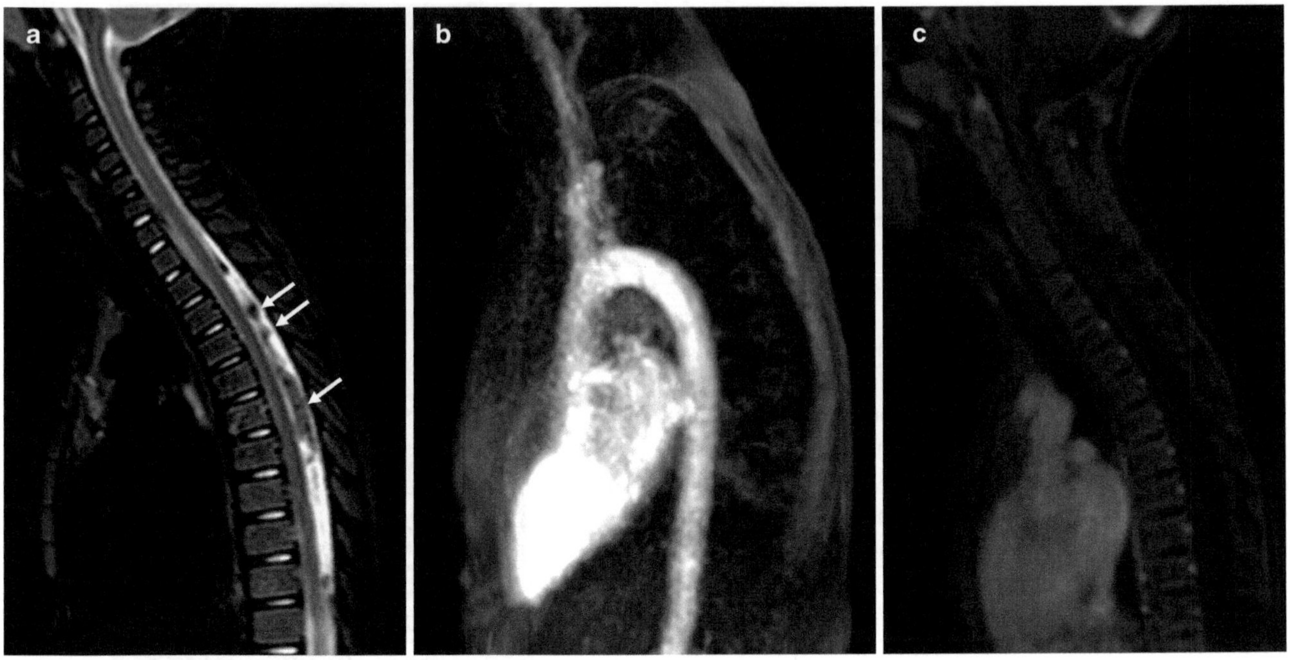

Fig. 19.34 A 5-year-old boy referred for dynamic study due to suspected spinal vascular malformation. (**a**) Sagittal T2-weighted image shows globular signal loss (arrows) in the dorsal subarachnoid space resulting from CSF flow turbulence. (**b**, **c**) Maximum intensity projection of time-resolved MR angiography at the arterial phase (**b**) and contrast-enhanced fat-saturated T1-weighted image at the venous phase shows no evidence of vascular malformation

References

1. Geibprasert S, Pongpech S, Jiarakongmun P, Shroff MM, Armstrong DC, Krings T. Radiologic assessment of brain arteriovenous malformations: what clinicians need to know. Radiographics. 2010;30(2):483–501. https://doi.org/10.1148/rg.302095728. Erratum in: Radiographics. 2011 May–Jun;31(3):904. PMID: 20228330.
2. Vollherbst DF, Bendszus M, Möhlenbruch MA. Vascular malformations of the brain and its coverings. J Neuroendovasc Ther. 2020;14(8):285–94. https://doi.org/10.5797/jnet.ra.2020-0020. Epub 2020 May 28. PMID: 37502170; PMCID: PMC10370599.
3. Assker MM, Youssef AM, Mohammed SA, Akar NM, Hashim MA, Kadhim N, Al-Saadi N, Algabri MH, Shukur MJ, Ismail M, Muthana A. Cerebral arteriovenous malformations classification systems in comparison with Spetzler-Martin: a comparative review. Surg Neurol Int. 2025;16:173.
4. Plasencia AR, Santillan A. Embolization and radiosurgery for arteriovenous malformations. Surg Neurol Int. 2012;3(Suppl 2):S90.
5. Brown NJ, Lien BV, Ehresman J, Rahmani R, Catapano JS, Lawton MT. Proliferative angiopathy: a systematic review. Stroke Vasc Interv Neurol. 2024;4(3):e001186.
6. Cogswell PM, Pillai JJ, Lanzino G, Flemming KD. Prevalence of developmental venous anomalies in association with sporadic cavernous malformations on 7T MRI. Am J Neuroradiol. 2024;45(1):72–5.
7. Aoki R, Srivatanakul K. Developmental venous anomaly: benign or not benign. Neurol Med Chir (Tokyo). 2016;56(9):534–43. https://doi.org/10.2176/nmc.ra.2016-0030. Epub 2016 Jun 1. PMID: 27250700; PMCID: PMC5027236.
8. Reynolds MR, Lanzino G, Zipfel GJ. Intracranial dural arteriovenous fistulae. Stroke. 2017;48(5):1424–31.
9. Smajda SJ, Söderman M, Dorfmüller G, Dorison N, Nghe MC, Rodesch GL. Paediatric intracranial dural arteriovenous shunts: types, clinical presentation and therapeutic management. Brain Commun. 2022;4(2):fcac043.
10. Jones BV, Ball WS, Tomsick TA, Millard J, Crone KR. Vein of Galen aneurysmal malformation: diagnosis and treatment of 13 children with extended clinical follow-up. AJNR Am J Neuroradiol. 2002;23(10):1717–24. PMID: 12427630; PMCID: PMC8185849.
11. Alvarez H, Garcia Monaco R, Rodesch G, Sachet M, Krings T, Lasjaunias P. Vein of galen aneurysmal malformations. Neuroimaging Clin N Am. 2007;17(2):189–206. https://doi.org/10.1016/j.nic.2007.02.005. Erratum in: Neuroimaging Clin N Am. 2007 Nov;17(4):xi. PMID: 17645970.
12. Shigematsu T, Bazil MJ, Fifi JT, Berenstein A. Fine, vascular network formation in patients with vein of galen aneurysmal malformation. AJNR Am J Neuroradiol. 2022;43(10):1481–7. https://doi.org/10.3174/ajnr.A7649. Epub 2022 Sep 22. PMID: 36137661; PMCID: PMC9575532.
13. Suzuki J, Takaku A. Cerebrovascular "moyamoya" disease. Disease showing abnormal net-like vessels in base of brain. Arch Neurol. 1969;20(3):288–99. https://doi.org/10.1001/archneur.1969.00480090076012. PMID: 5775283.
14. Houkin K, Nakayama N, Kuroda S, Nonaka T, Shonai T, Yoshimoto T. Novel magnetic resonance angiography stage grading for moyamoya disease. Cerebrovasc Dis. 2005;20(5):347–54. https://doi.org/10.1159/000087935. Epub 2005 Aug 30. PMID: 16131804.
15. Zabramski JM, Wascher TM, Spetzler RF, Johnson B, Golfinos J, Drayer BP, Brown B, Rigamonti D, Brown G. The natural history of familial cavernous malformations: results of an ongoing study. J Neurosurg. 1994;80(3):422–32.
16. Kumar S, Brinjikji W, Lanzino G, Flemming KD. Distinguishing mimics from true hemorrhagic cavernous malformations. J Clin Neurosci. 2020;74:11–7.

17. Yun TJ, Na DG, Kwon BJ, Rho HG, Park SH, Suh YL, Chang KH. A T1 hyperintense perilesional signal aids in the differentiation of a cavernous angioma from other hemorrhagic masses. Am J Neuroradiol. 2008;29(3):494–500.
18. Manjila S, Bazil T, Thomas M, Mani S, Kay M, Udayasankar U. A review of extraaxial developmental venous anomalies of the brain involving dural venous flow or sinuses: persistent embryonic sinuses, sinus pericranii, venous varices or aneurysmal malformations, and enlarged emissary veins. Neurosurg Focus. 2018;45(1):E9. https://doi.org/10.3171/2018.5.FOCUS18107. PMID: 29961384.
19. Choudhary G, Udayasankar U, Saade C, Winegar B, Maroun G, Chokr J. A systematic approach in the diagnosis of paediatric skull lesions: what radiologists need to know. Pol J Radiol. 2019;84:92–111.
20. Zamora C, Castillo M. Sinus Pericranii. In: Agrawal A, Britz G, editors. Pediatric vascular neurosurgery. Cham: Springer; 2016. https://doi.org/10.1007/978-3-319-43636-4_13.
21. Brinjikji W, Nicholson P, Hilditch CA, Krings T, Pereira V, Agid R. Cerebrofacial venous metameric syndrome—spectrum of imaging findings. Neuroradiology. 2020;62:417–25.
22. O'Loughlin L, Groves ML, Miller NR, Pearl MS. Cerebrofacial arteriovenous metameric syndrome (CAMS): a spectrum disorder of craniofacial vascular malformations. Childs Nerv Syst. 2017;33:513–6.
23. Aeron G, Abruzzo TA, Jones BV. Clinical and imaging features of intracranial arterial aneurysms in the pediatric population. Radiographics. 2012;32(3):667–81.
24. Yoon NK, McNally S, Taussky P, Park MS. Imaging of cerebral aneurysms: a clinical perspective. Neurovasc Imaging. 2016;2(1):6.
25. TaKai K. Spinal arteriovenous shunts: angioarchitecture and historical changes in classification. Neurol Med Chir. 2017;57(7):356–65.
26. Vargas MI, Bing F, Gariani J, Dietemann JL. Spinal vascular imaging: technique. In: Saba L, Raz E, editors. Neurovascular imaging. New York: Springer; 2016. https://doi.org/10.1007/978-1-4614-9029-6_13.
27. Lisanti C, Carlin C, Banks KP, Wang D. Normal MRI appearance and motion-related phenomena of CSF. Am J Roentgenol. 2007;188(3):716–25.
28. Larsen DW, Teitelbaum GP, Norman D. Cerebrospinal fluid flow artifact a possible pitfall on fast-spin-echo MR imaging of the spine simulating intradural pathology. Clin Imaging. 1996;20(2):140–2.

Part VIII

Combined Vascular Malformations and Overgrowth Syndromes

20 Klippel-Trenaunay Syndrome

Introduction

Klippel Traunanay Syndrome (KTS) has been described as "the prototype of complex overgrowth syndromes associated with vascular anomalies" [1]. The syndrome is classically defined by a triad of capillary malformation (commonly port-wine stain), soft tissue and/or bony overgrowth, and a combination of venous and lymphatic malformations (Fig. 20.1) [2, 3]. KTS most often affects the lower extremities (Fig. 20.2), which may be involved unilaterally, bilaterally, or along with other regions such as the lower trunk, abdomen, pelvis, and occasionally the upper extremities (Fig. 20.3). In some cases, however, lesions may appear in the trunk or upper limbs while the lower limbs are spared (Fig. 20.4) [2]. The condition, first described in 1900 by two French physicians—Klippel and Trenaunay—has an uncertain incidence, though it is estimated to affect about 1 in 100,000 births [4]. Multiple gene mutations have been identified in individual cases of KTS. Recent advances in understanding somatic mosaicism have significantly contributed to uncovering the underlying cause of the condition. The majority of KTS cases are now attributed to somatic activating mutations in the PIK3CA gene, a key component of the mTOR signaling pathway [5].

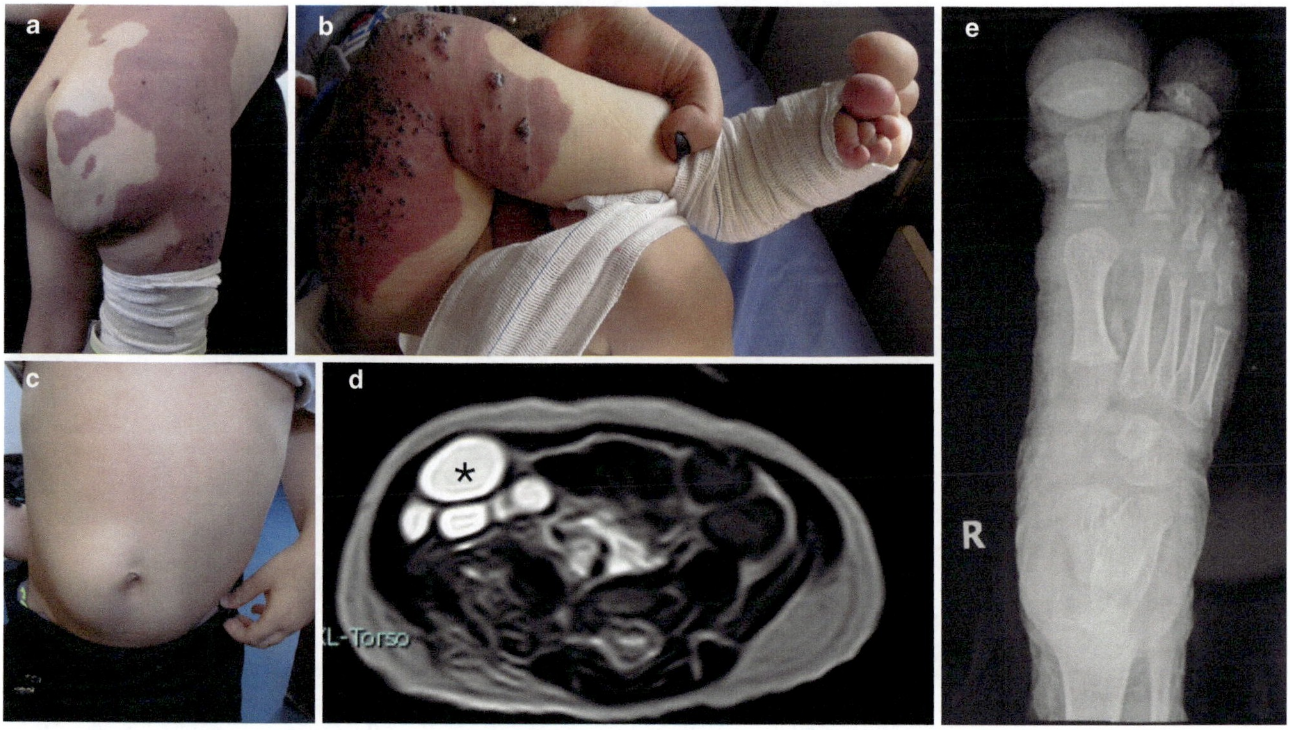

Fig. 20.1 A two-year-old boy diagnosed with Klippel–Trénaunay Syndrome. (**a**, **b**) Distribution of characteristic skin lesions (capillary malformations) along the right lower extremity and lower trunk, associated with soft tissue hypertrophy and bony deformity (notably toe hypertrophy). The child is wearing a compression bandage to reduce edema. (**c**, **d**) Right lower abdominal swelling, confirmed by imaging to represent a macrocystic lymphatic malformation (asterisk). (**e**) Plain X-ray of the foot showing bone and soft tissue hypertrophy

A. A. AbouZeid et al., *Atlas of Pediatric Vascular Anomalies*, https://doi.org/10.1007/978-3-032-30866-5_20

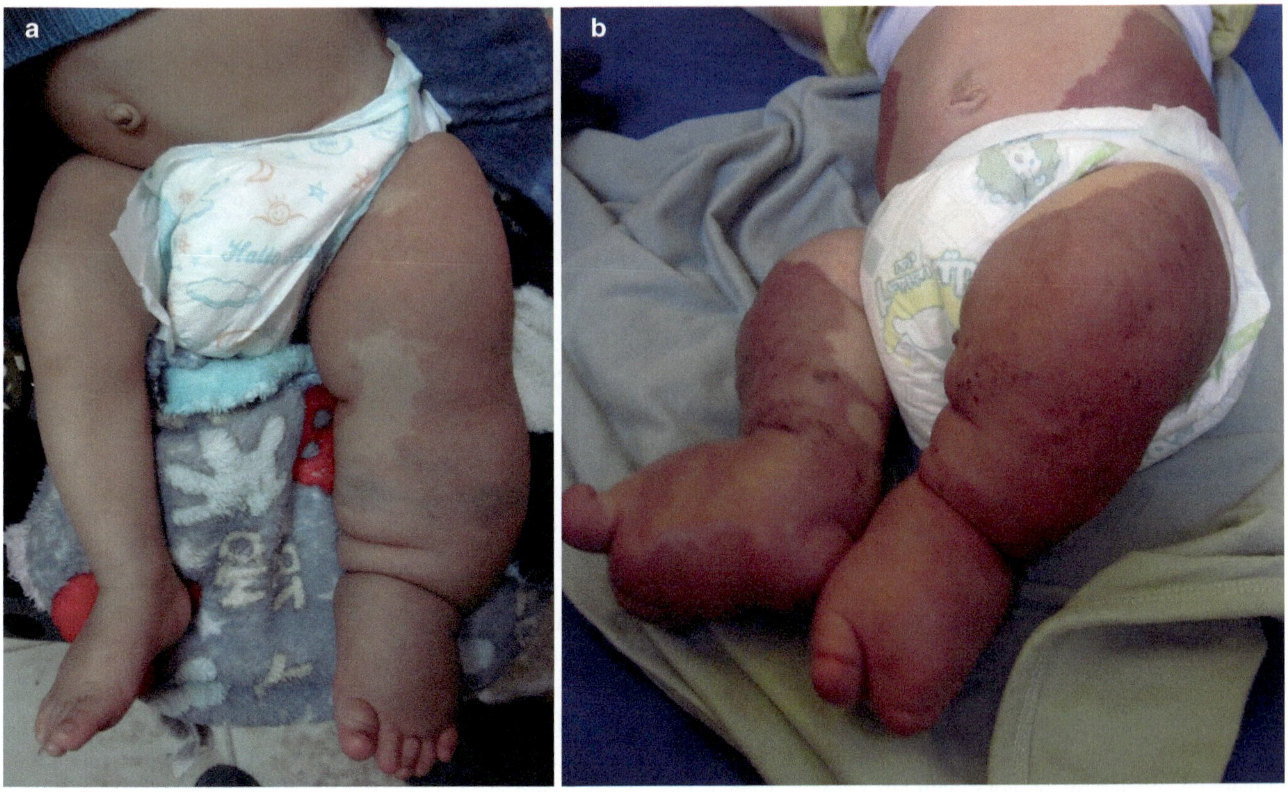

Fig. 20.2 Klippel–Trénaunay Syndrome most often affects the lower extremities, which may be unilateral (**a**) or bilateral (**b**)

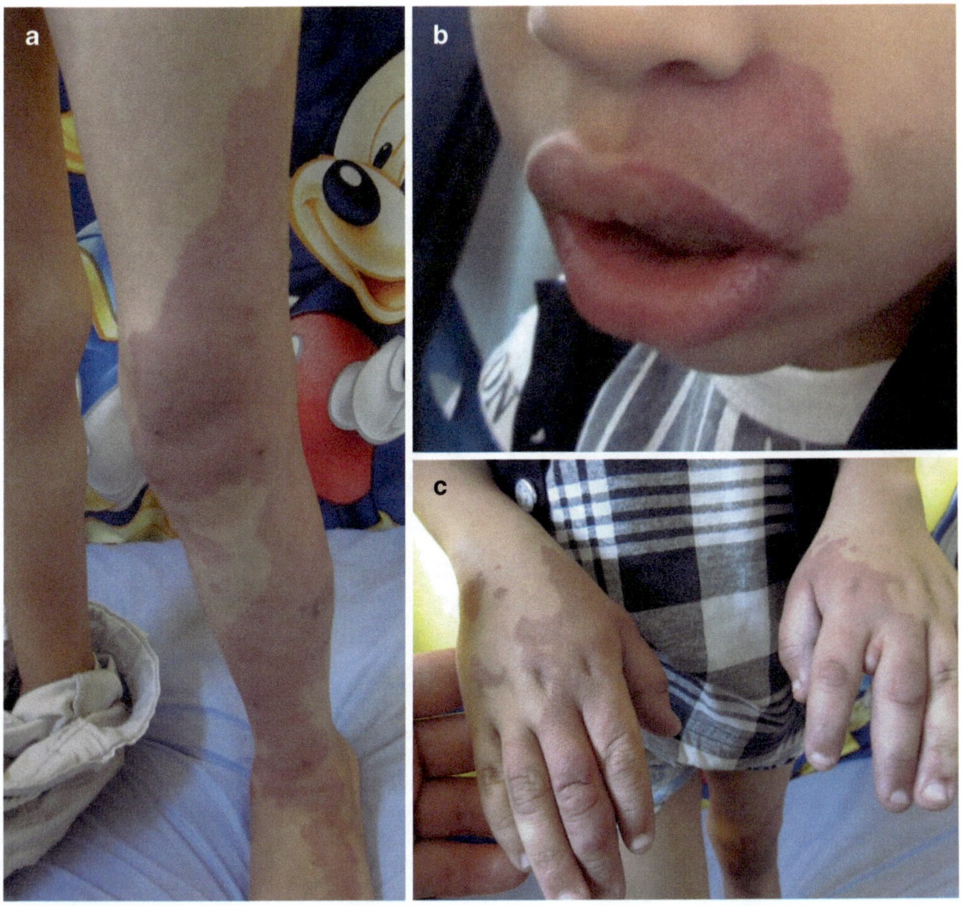

Fig. 20.3 A 7-year-old boy diagnosed with Klippel–Trénaunay Syndrome showing involvement of multiple regions: (**a**) lower extremities; (**b**) face; (**c**) upper extremities

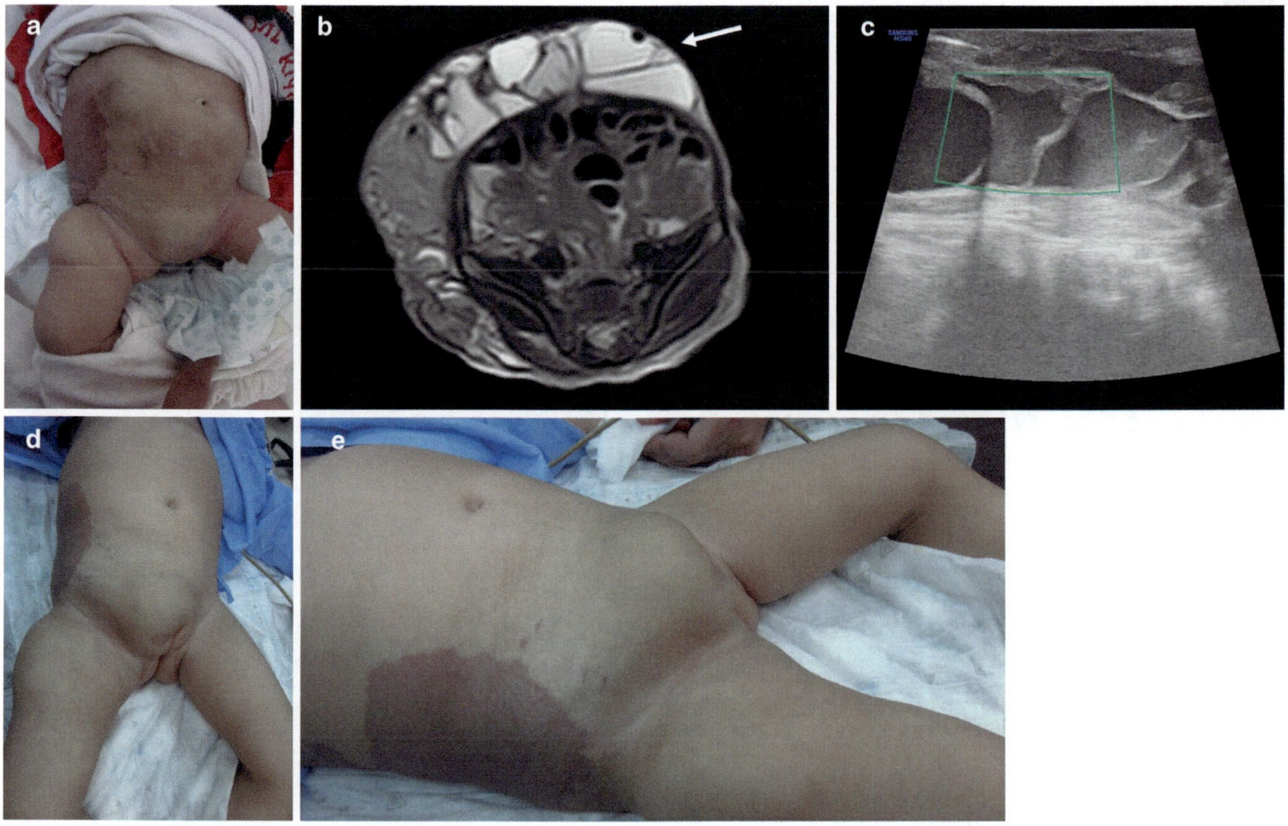

Fig. 20.4 Two-month-old girl with combined vascular malformation of the abdominal wall. (**a**) Clinical photo at presentation shows swelling with overlying capillary malformation. (**b**) Axial T2-WI demonstrates multilocular cystic lesion with hyperintense signal (arrow). (**c**) Ultrasound reveals multilocular cystic lesion with internal echoes, no color flow. (**d**, **e**) One-year follow-up after sclerotherapy shows reduced swelling

Clinical Presentation

Capillary Malformations Capillary malformations are cutaneous lesions and an almost constant finding in KTS (about 98% of cases), demonstrating wide variation in size, shape, and color [2]. CMs vary from light pink to deep red/purple in color. CMs may cover wide areas with irregular geographic distribution, often on the lateral aspect of the limb, or may be small or blotchy (Fig. 20.5). CMs in KTS may thicken over time and become raised over the skin surface with vascular blebs. The latter indicates the presence of associated lymphatic components. These blebs may be fragile and liable for spontaneous bleeding or after minor trauma. Occasionally, there is a localized fungating lesion caused by excessive hyperkeratosis associating the vascular skin lesion, which is referred to as "angiokeratoma circumscriptum" [6].

Lymphatic Malformations (LMs) Early accounts of KTS did not identify lymphatic anomalies as part of the condition. In 1988, Young expanded the definition to include lymphatic malformations, classifying KTS as a combined capillary-lymphatic-venous malformation. More recently, the International Society for the Study of Vascular Anomalies (ISSVA) has defined KTS as the presence of a capillary malformation and venous malformation, with or without lymphatic malformation, accompanied by limb overgrowth [7]. Lymphedema of the affected lower limb in KTS is common. Microcystic LMs may be associated with capillary malformations and appear as raised cutaneous blebs. The gluteal region is a common site for lymphatic malformations in KTS (Fig. 20.6). Macrocystic LMs are often located in the abdomen, pelvis, and retroperitoneum (Figs. 20.1 and 20.7) [2, 5].

Venous Malformations (VMs) VMs are a hallmark in KTS, often presenting as dilated tortuous veins; persistence of the embryonic marginal vein (so-called vein of Servelle) on the lateral aspect of the thigh is characteristic (Fig. 20.8) [2]. Abnormalities of the deep venous system can also occur in KTS (hypoplasia, aplasia, duplication) (Figs. 20.9 and 20.10) [8, 9]. In the affected limb, chronic venous insufficiency may present as significant edema and a dull, aching pain that worsens throughout the day. Although congenital, venous varicosities are not always visible at birth and often become more apparent as the child grows. In KTS, venous malformations can extend into the pelvis, involving the genitourinary

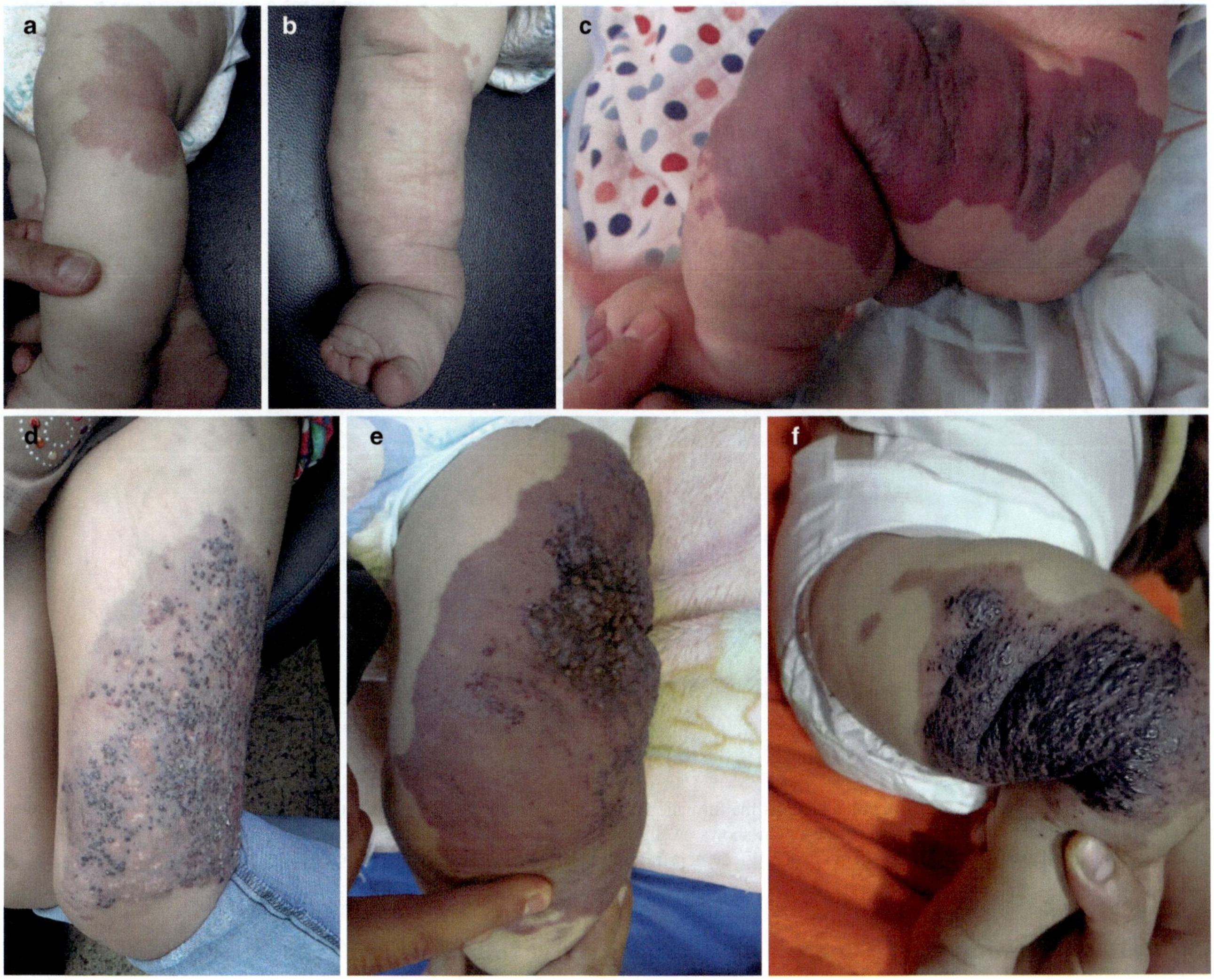

Fig. 20.5 Variable forms of skin manifestations in Klippel–Trenaunay Syndrome (KTS), including: (**a**, **b**): Typical port-wine stains, mostly on the lateral aspect of the lower limb. (**c**): Darker (purple) capillary malformation. (**d**–**f**): Raised capillary malformations with vascular blebs

or lower gastrointestinal tract, potentially leading to hematuria or rectal bleeding (Fig. 20.11) [2, 5].

Because of the dilated and incompetent superficial veins, patients with KTS are prone to developing thrombophlebitis [1–3]. Patients with large, dilated, tortuous veins that communicate directly with the central circulation may have an increased risk of pulmonary embolism (Fig. 20.12). This may necessitate obliteration of these abnormal veins or implementation of other specific prophylactic measures—such as initiating anticoagulation therapy or placing an inferior vena cava filter—to prevent this potentially fatal complication. Those with extensive venous malformations are also prone to developing localized intravascular coagulopathy, characterized by elevated D-dimer levels and reduced fibrinogen concentrations [2, 5].

Soft Tissue and/or Bony Overgrowth Tissue overgrowth is a defining feature of KTS. The extent and pattern of soft tissue enlargement vary, but it is typically fatty in nature and mainly situated in the extrafascial subcutaneous compartment (Fig. 20.13) [1]. This overgrowth can cause a bulky appearance, altered body contour, and increased circumference of the affected limb. In contrast, bony overgrowth may result in limb length discrepancies. Additional skeletal abnormalities, such as toe hypertrophy and/or fusion, may also be observed [2, 5].

With few exceptions, the phenotype at birth defines the appearance of the child and young children. Exceptions may include the change in color of CMs, lymphatic vesicle eruptions, and increase in limb length discrepancy. Parents should be reassured that the unaffected extremities and organs will not become involved in the future [2].

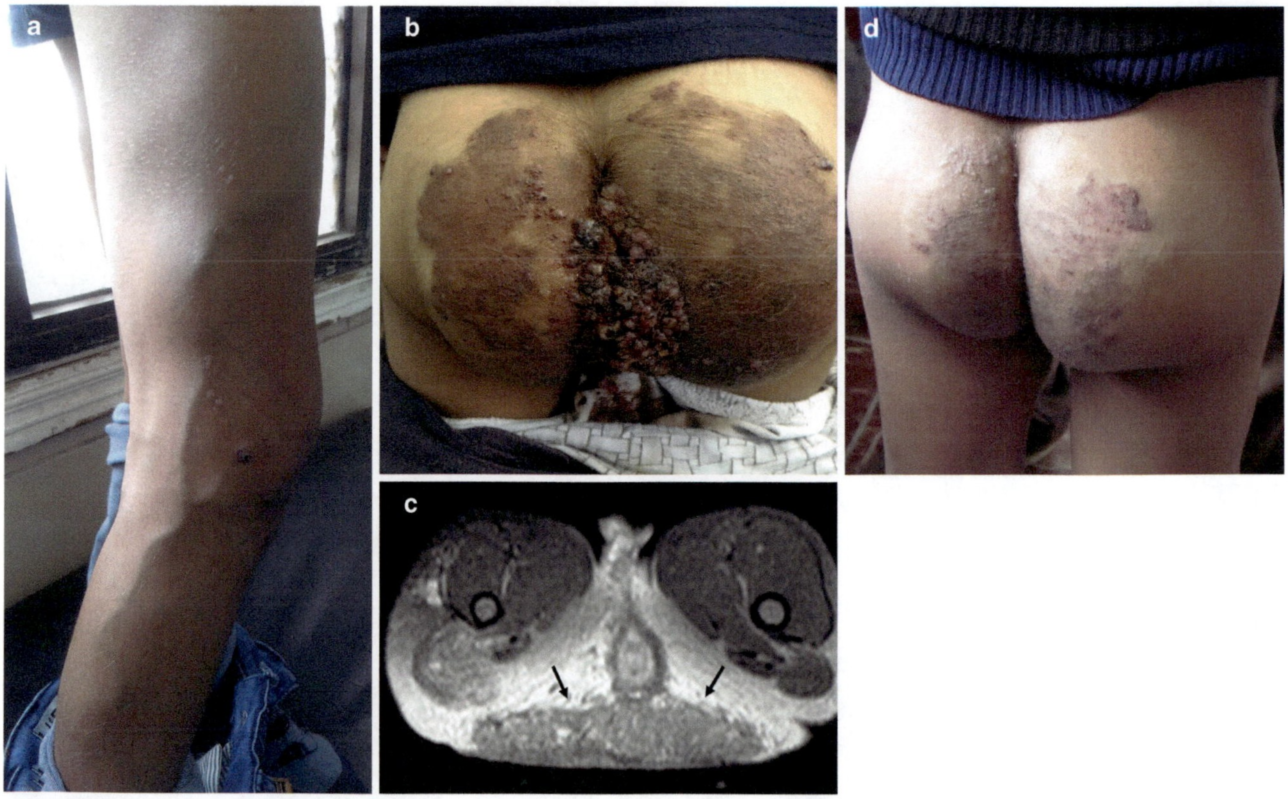

Fig. 20.6 Nine-year-old boy with Klippel-Trénaunay syndrome. (**a**) Dilated marginal vein of the lower extremity (typical finding). (**b**) Associated gluteal skin lesions presenting with recurrent bleeding. (**c**) Marked clinical improvement after 6 months of oral sirolimus therapy. (**d**) Axial MRI demonstrating deep extension of the cutaneous lesions (arrows)

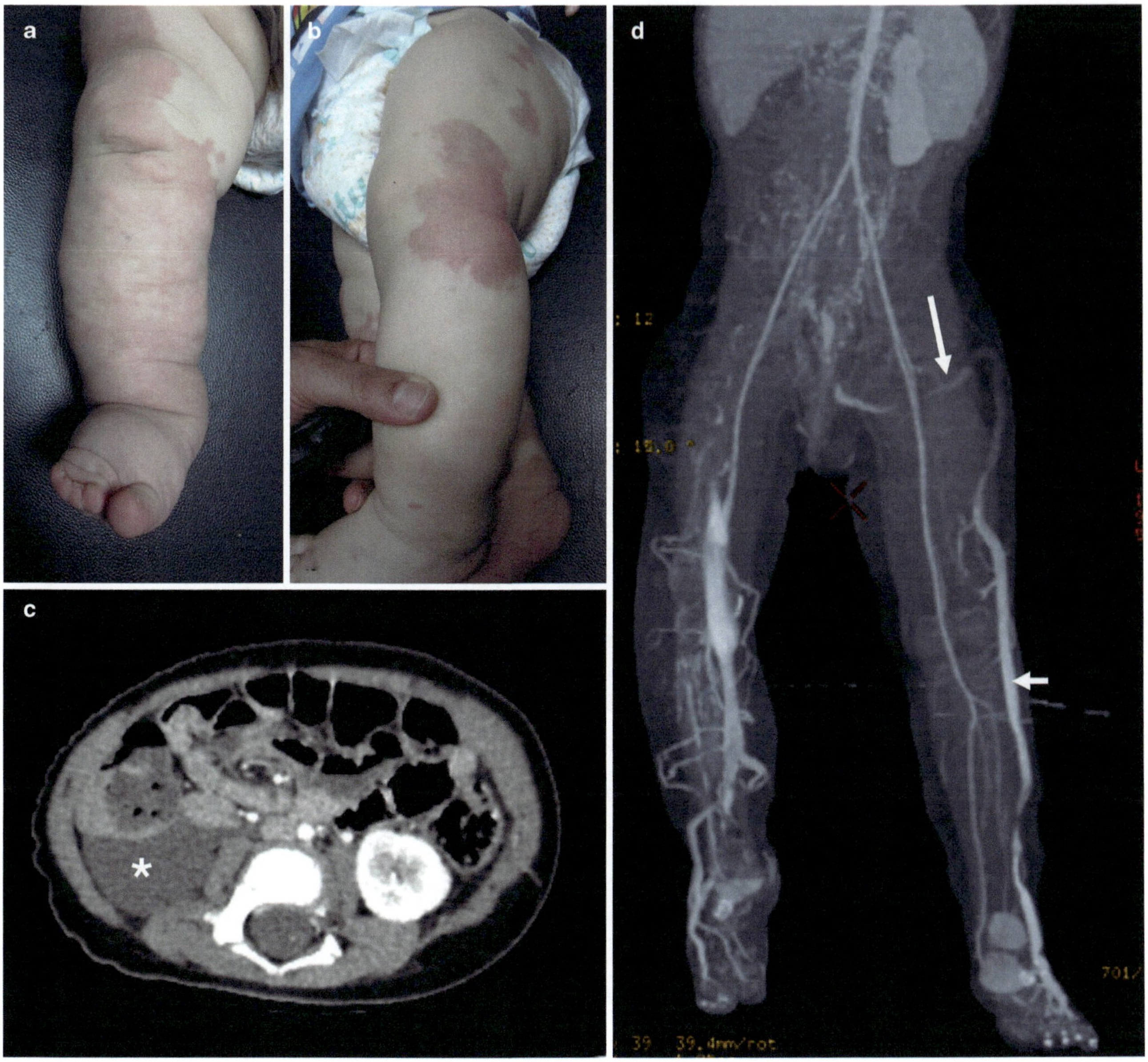

Fig. 20.7 Eight-month-old boy with Klippel-Trénaunay syndrome. (**a**, **b**) Clinical photographs showing bilateral lower limb involvement. (**c**) Contrast-enhanced CT demonstrating a retroperitoneal lymphatic malformation, appearing as a non-enhancing cystic lesion (asterisk). (**d**) Coronal CT venography showing limb length discrepancy with anomalous veins bilaterally. On the left side, the lateral marginal vein of Servelle (short arrow) extends from the foot to the thigh, where it continues as the sciatic vein (long arrow)

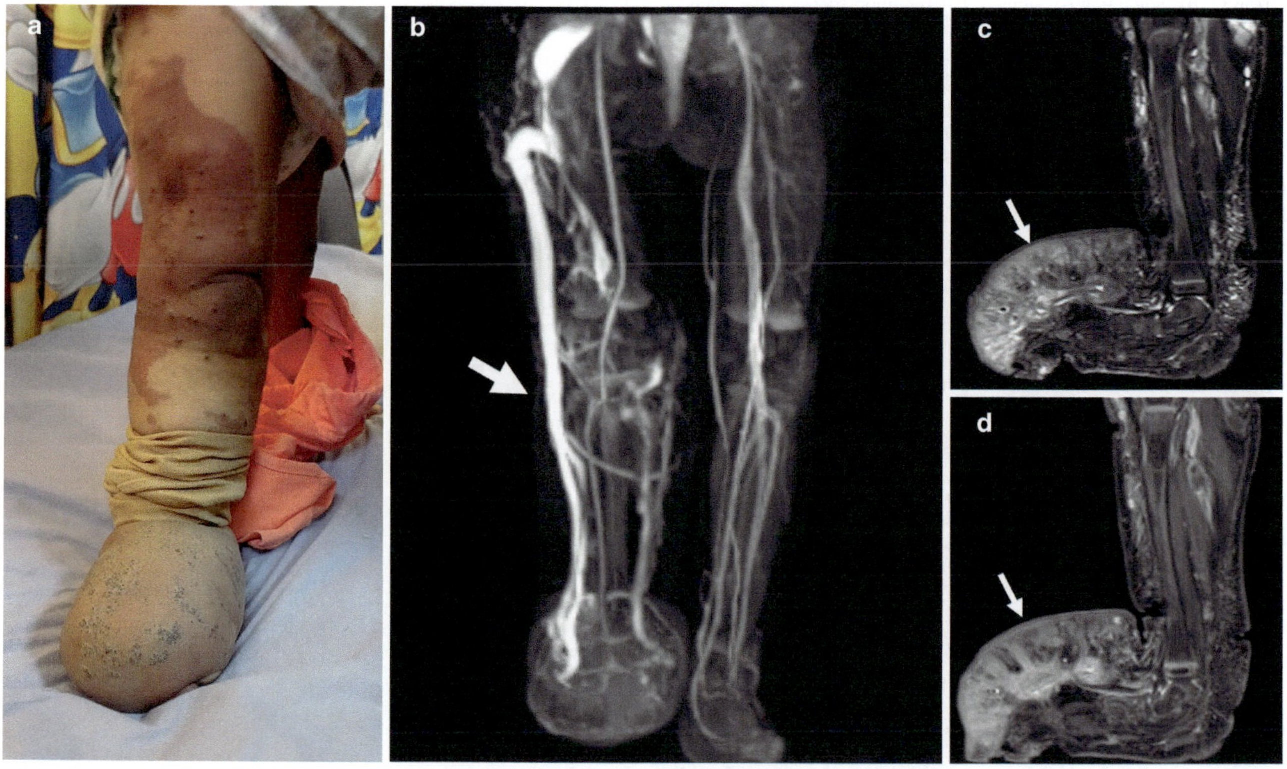

Fig. 20.8 One-year-old girl with Klippel-Trénaunay syndrome. (**a**) Clinical photograph. (**b**) MR venography showing the lateral marginal vein of Servelle (arrow) with a hypoplastic deep venous system. (**c**, **d**) Sagittal STIR and contrast-enhanced fat-suppressed T1-weighted images demonstrating soft tissue thickening involving multiple tissue planes, with bright signal intensity and contrast enhancement most pronounced at the dorsum of the foot (arrow)

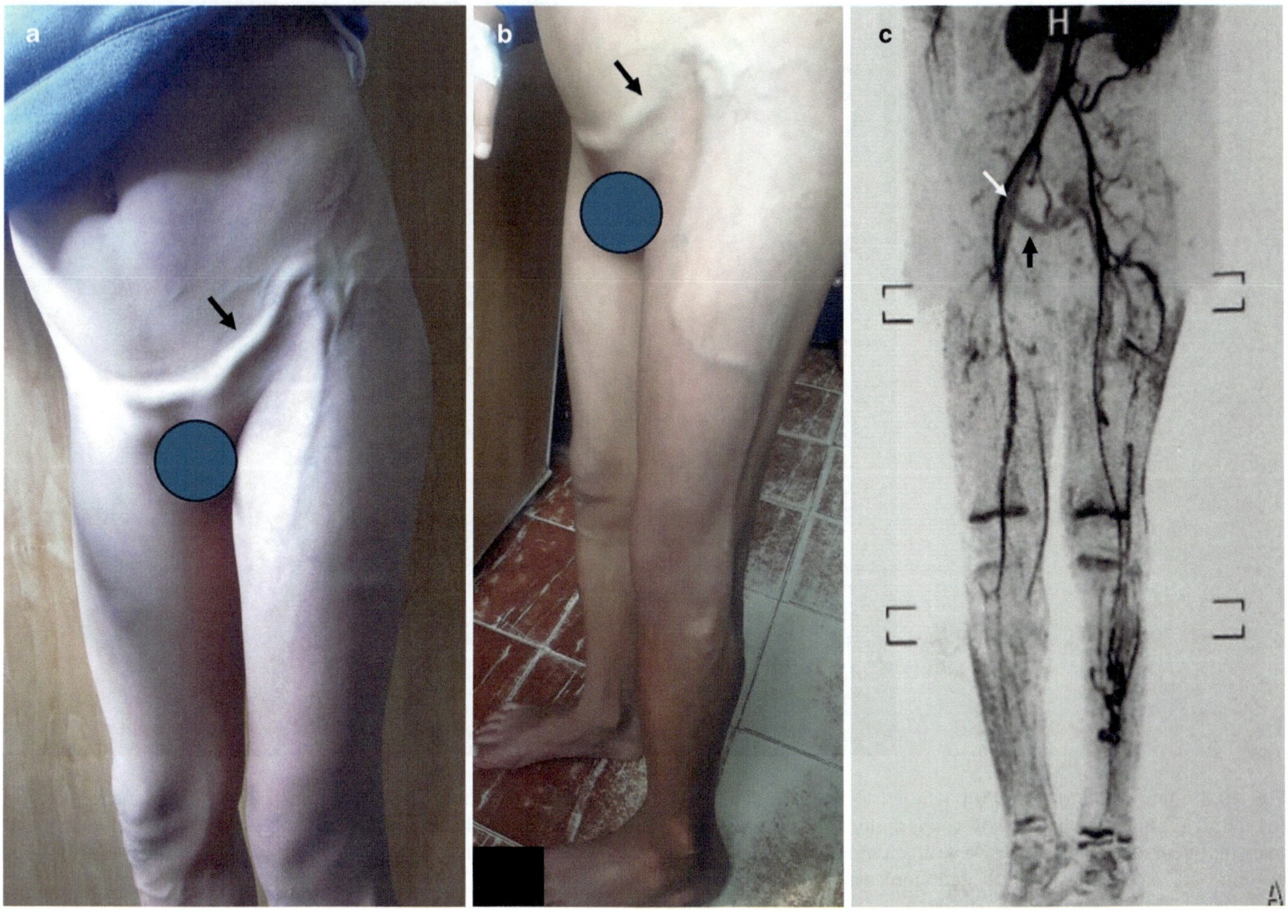

Fig. 20.9 Nine-year-old boy diagnosed as Klippel Trenaunay Syndrome. (**a**, **b**) Clinical appearance: overgrowth of the left lower extremity with varicose veins and port wine stain. Note the abnormal dilated subcutaneous trans-pubic vein (black arrow) denoting obstructed deep venous system on the left side (hypoplastic/atretic). (**c**) MRI angiography demonstrating aplasia/hypoplasia of left external iliac vein with abnormal dilated trans-pubic vein (black arrow) draining into contralateral (right) iliac vein (white arrow)

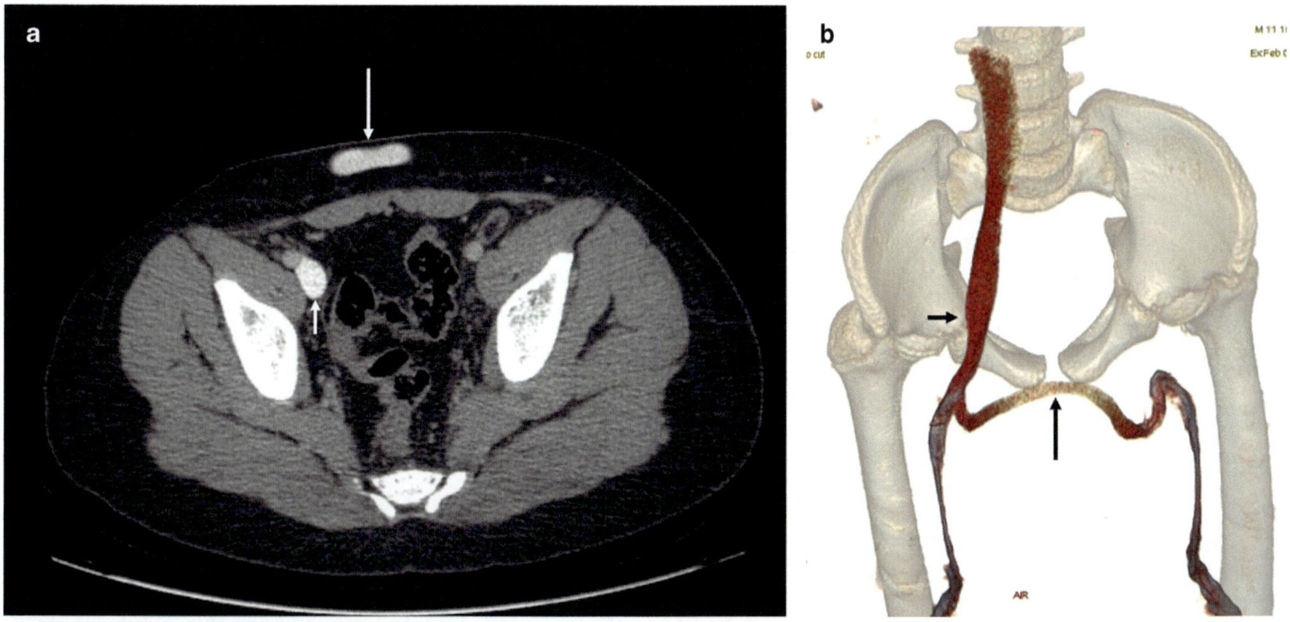

Fig. 20.10 Agenesis of the left iliac veins in an 11-year-old boy. CT venography of both lower limbs using direct injection at the dorsum of both feet (**a**), and 3D volume rendering (**b**), demonstrating non visualized left iliac veins with crossing subcutaneous vein (long arrow), draining the veins of the left lower limb to the contralateral right side (short arrow)

Fig. 20.11 Nine-year-old boy with Klippel-Trénaunay syndrome. Coronal STIR MRI demonstrating abnormal signal diffusely involving the entire muscular compartments of the thigh and upper leg (long arrows), extending into the pelvis and perineum (short arrows)

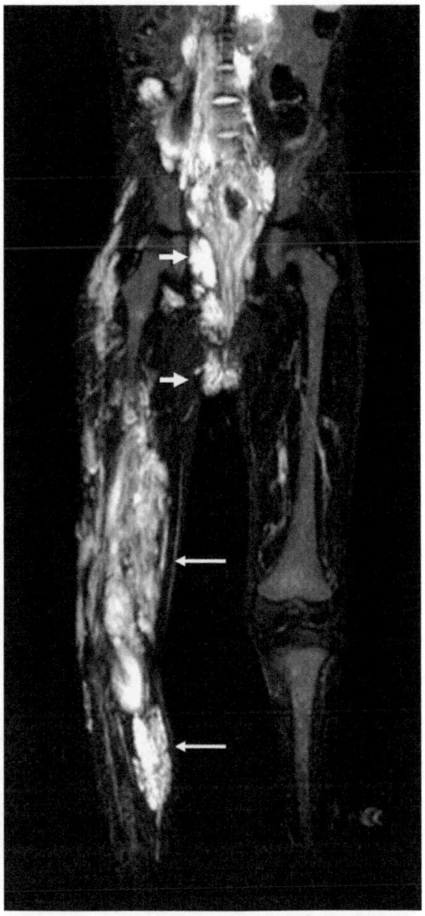

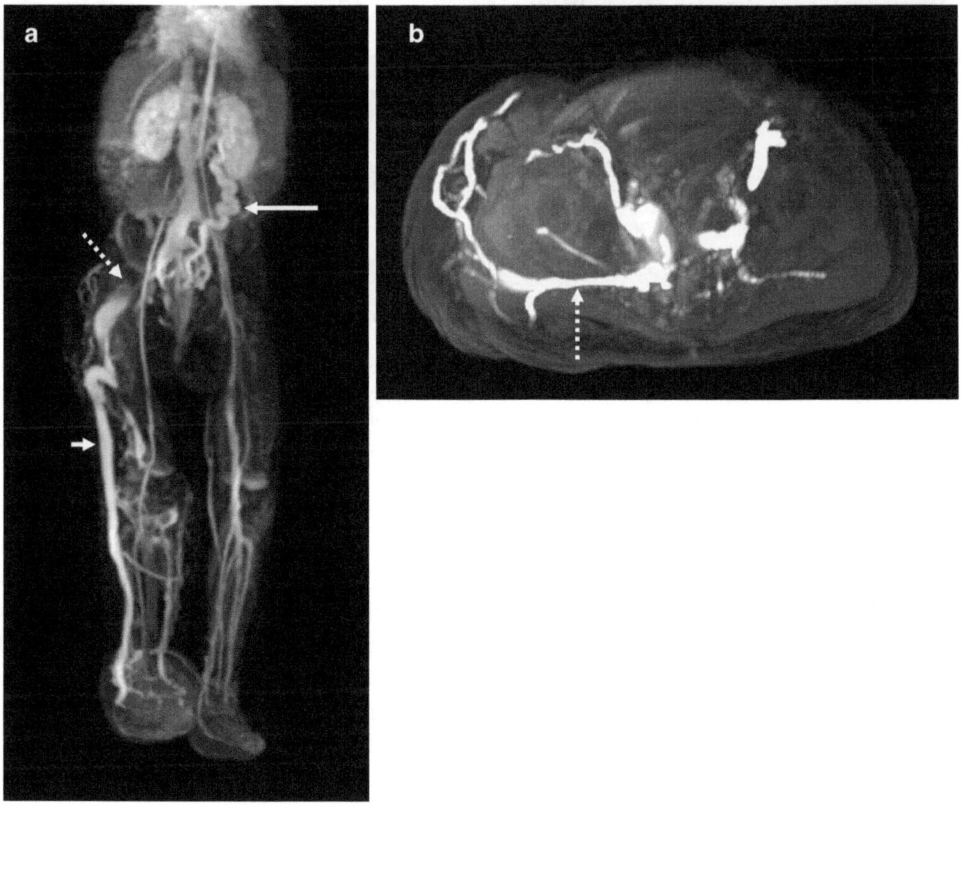

Fig. 20.12 One-year-old girl with Klippel-Trénaunay syndrome (same case as in Fig. 20.8). (**a**) MR venography demonstrating the lateral marginal vein of Servelle (short arrow) extending from the foot to the thigh, where it continues as the sciatic vein (dashed arrow), in association with a hypoplastic deep venous system. The left gonadal vein (long arrow) appears dilated and tortuous. (**b**) Axial maximum-intensity projection of non-contrast MR venography showing a persistent sciatic vein (dashed arrow) draining into the internal iliac vein

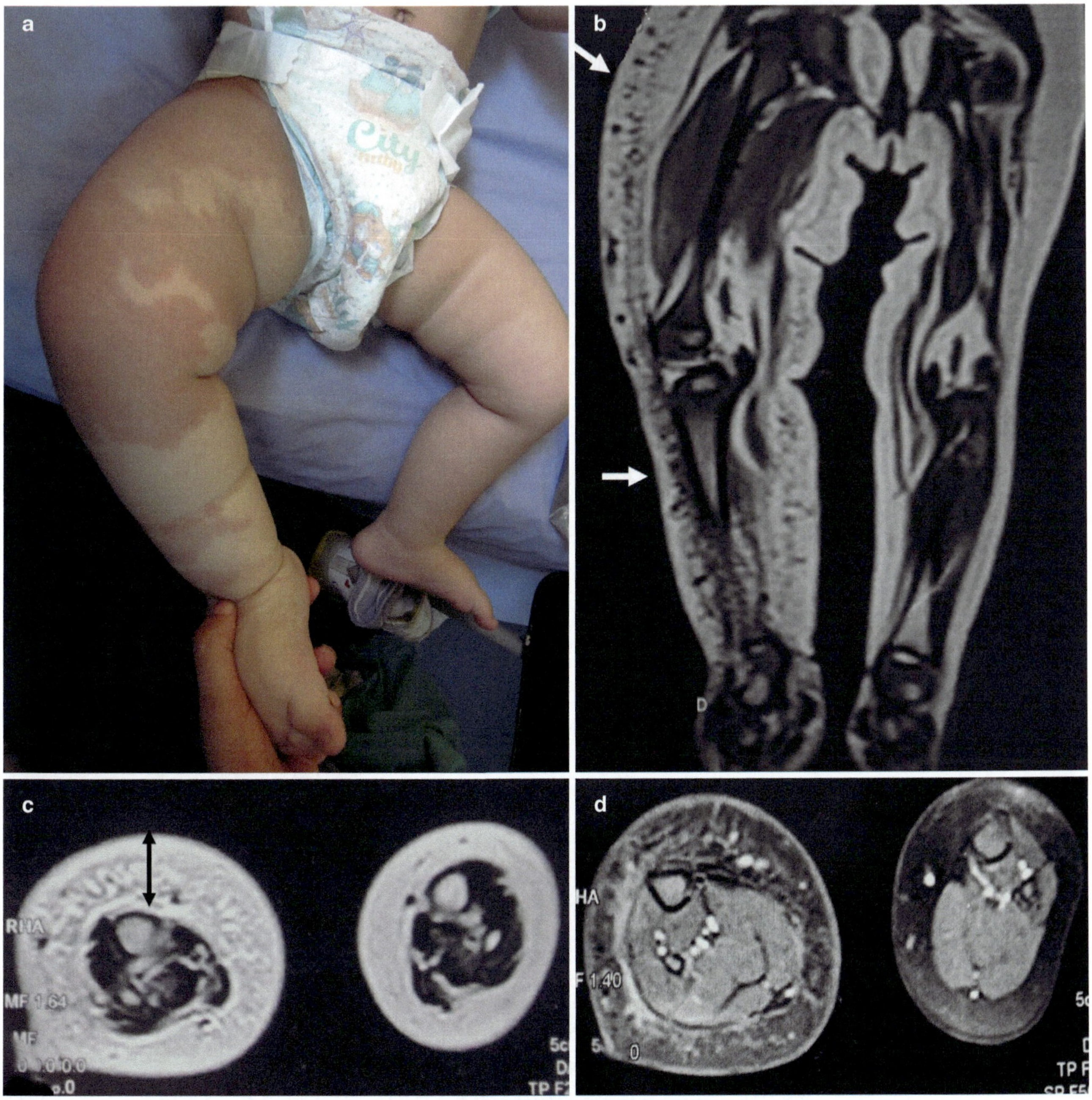

Fig. 20.13 One-year-old girl with Klippel-Trénaunay syndrome. (**a**) Clinical appearance showing overgrowth of the right lower extremity with a port-wine stain (capillary malformation). (**b**) Coronal T1-weighted MRI demonstrating soft tissue hypertrophy and subcutaneous stranding (arrows). (**c**) Axial T2-weighted image and (**d**) contrast-enhanced fat-suppressed T1-weighted MRI showing soft tissue hypertrophy mostly in the subcutaneous tissue (double arrowhead), with faint post-contrast enhancement in (**d**)

Diagnostic Evaluation

Diagnosis of KTS is mainly clinical, while investigations should focus on the extent of lesions, the status of the deep venous system, and confirming the absence of significant arteriovenous shunting [1, 2]. In addition to the common affection of the lower extremities, imaging should include the pelvis and retroperitoneum as well. Skeletal defects are assessed by plain radiographs. MRI best demonstrates the soft tissue component and lymphatic malformations (Fig. 20.14). The abnormal venous system in KTS requires dedicated studies such as MR venography (Fig. 20.12); CT venography provides excellent vascular mapping with three-dimensional reconstruction images but involves significant radiation (Fig. 20.7d). Direct contrast venography is usually performed at the time of endovascular treatment [2, 5].

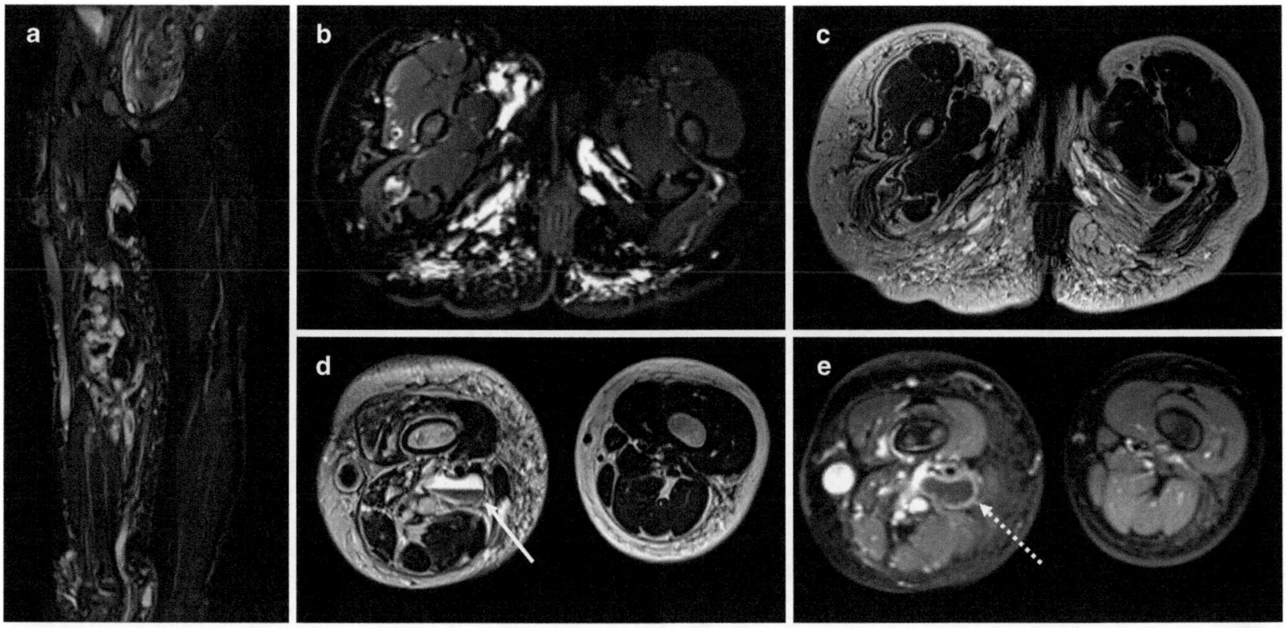

Fig. 20.14 One-year-old girl with Klippel-Trénaunay syndrome (same case as in Figs. 20.8 and 20.11). MRI demonstrates a trans-spatial abnormal signal extending through multiple tissue planes, involving the right lower limb and perineum. Findings are shown across different planes and sequences: (**a**) Coronal STIR image of the lower limb. (**b**, **c**) Axial STIR and axial T2-weighted images at the level of the anal canal. (**d**, **e**) Axial T2-weighted and contrast-enhanced T1-weighted images at the mid-thigh. Note the cystic lesion with fluid–fluid level (arrow) and marginal post-contrast enhancement (dashed arrow)

Non-operative Management

Compression therapy helps reduce limb circumference in cases of significant edema, though it does not affect soft tissue or bony overgrowth. This can be achieved using compression garments (either custom-made or ready-to-wear; Fig. 20.15) while elastic compression bandages offer a suitable alternative, particularly for younger children (Fig. 20.1b) [2].

Several medications may be used along the course of the disease, which depend on associated complications: antibiotics for superadded infection and cellulitis; anticoagulation for thromboembolic complications; and iron supplementation to treat anemia because of recurrent GI bleeding (VMs of the anorectum) or bleeding from skin lesions.

Recent advances in the genetics of the overgrowth syndromes have led to the discovery of new medications, sirolimus, which is one of the m-TOR inhibitors with promising results in the management of such complex cases) (Fig. 20.6) [5, 10].

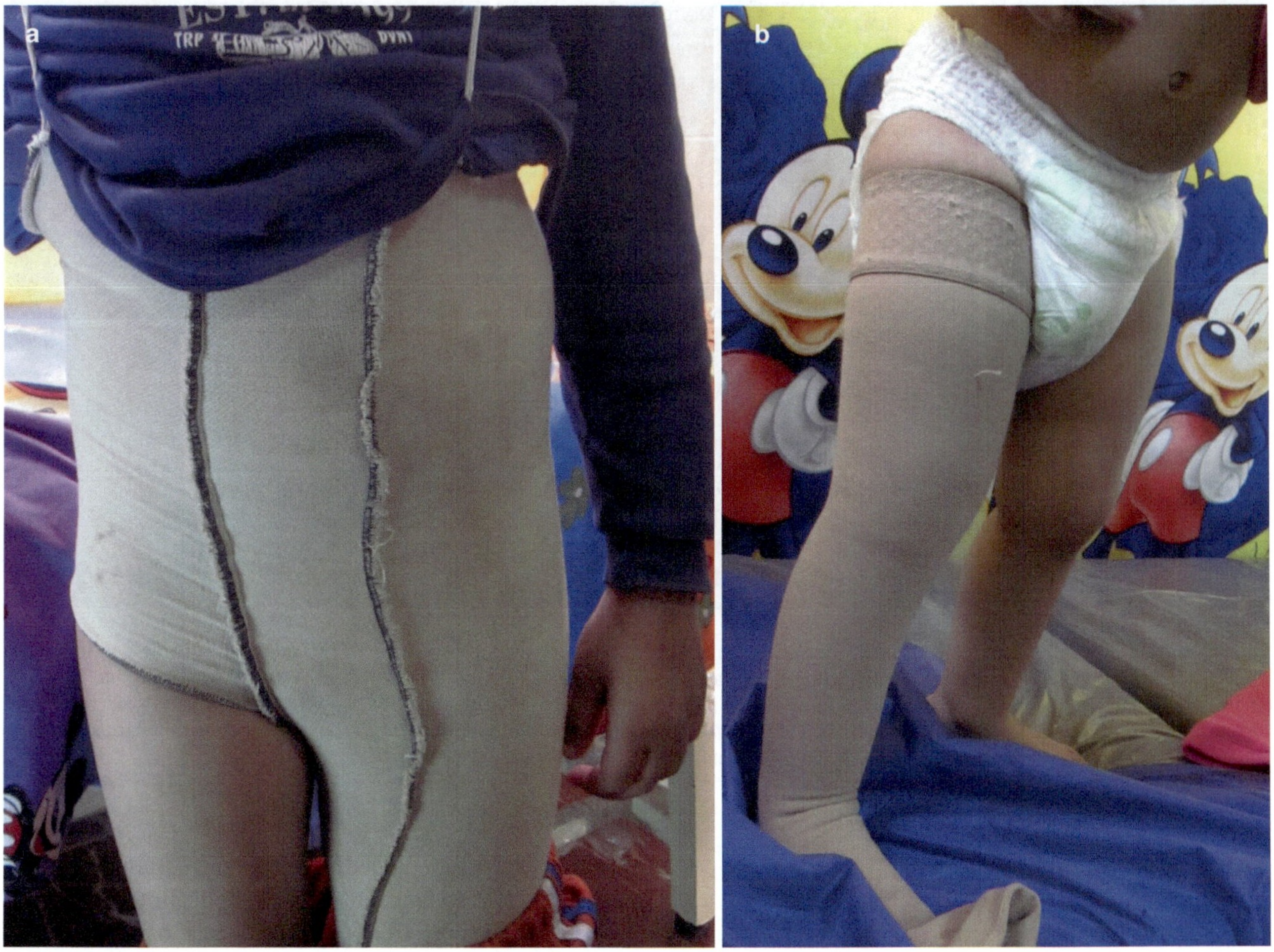

Fig. 20.15 Different forms of compression garments used by patients with Klippel-Trénaunay syndrome: (**a**) custom-made garment; (**b**) ready-to-wear garment

Interventional and Surgical Management

The abnormal superficial veins in KTS typically demonstrate stagnant flow and are consequently the major source of serious thromboembolic complications and pain. Traditionally, it was believed that the superficial venous system should not be removed if the deep venous system appeared insufficient. However, Alomari noted that veins are always present within the muscular compartment [1, 2]. Based on modern understanding, abnormal superficial veins should be treated, as they contribute to both patient discomfort and the risk of pulmonary embolism.

Macro-cystic LMs can be managed by sclerotherapy or surgical excision (see Chaps. 9 and 10). Abnormal dilated veins can be managed by sclerotherapy, surgical vascular procedures (vein stripping), or more recently endovenous laser ablation therapy [11]. Cutaneous lesions (CMs) can be managed by laser.

Orthopedic interventions are most effectively carried out by a specialized orthopedic surgeon who is part of a multidisciplinary vascular anomalies team, ensuring a comprehensive understanding of the underlying pathology. Managing limb length discrepancy necessitates early correction of the hemodynamic and metabolic factors contributing to bone abnormalities. A combined approach involving both orthopedic and vascular surgical procedures is widely recognized as the primary strategy for optimal outcomes [12].

Debulking Procedures Drawbacks include trading the bulk for a scar, inherent poor healing and wound complications, and the risk of neurovascular injury. However, recent reports have shown 80% patient satisfaction with debulking procedures in KTS [2].

References

1. Uller W, Fishman SJ, Alomari AI. Overgrowth syndromes with complex vascular anomalies. Semin Pediatr Surg. 2014;23:208–15.
2. Driscoll DJ, Gloviczki P. Combined slow-flow vascular malformation of the lower limb: Klippel- Trenaunay syndrome. In: Mulliken JB, Burrows PE, Fishman SJ, editors. Mulliken & Young's vascular anomalies. 2nd ed. Oxford University Press; 2013. p. 1027–40.
3. Laredo J, Lee BB. Hemolymphatic malformation: mixed form congenital vascular malformation. In: Kim YW, Lee BB, Yakes WF, Do YS, editors. Congenital vascular malformations. Berlin/Heidelberg: Springer-Verlag; 2017. p. 105–12.
4. Servelle M. Klippel and Trenaunay's syndrome. 768 operated cases. Ann Surg. 1985;201:365–73.
5. Tollefson MM. Klippel-Trenaunay Syndrome. In: Perkins JA, Balakrishnan K, editors. Evidence-based management of head and neck vascular anomalies. Springer Nature Switzerland; 2018. p. 273–80.
6. Das A, Mondal AK, Saha A, et al. Angiokeratoma circumscriptum neviforme: an entity, few and far between. Indian Dermatol Online J. 2014;5(4):472–4. https://doi.org/10.4103/2229-5178.142503.
7. ISSVA classification for vascular anomalies. https://www.issva.org/UserFiles/file/ISSVA-Classification-2018.pdf.
8. Alomari AI. Diversion venography—a modified technique in Klippel-Trenaunay syndrome: initial experience. J Vasc Interv Radiol. 2010;21(5):685–9.
9. Mattassi R. Management of deep vein aplasia, hypoplasia, and lateral marginal vein. In: Kim YW, Lee BB, Yakes WF, Do YS, editors. Congenital vascular malformations. Berlin/Heidelberg: Springer-Verlag; 2017. p. 291–6.
10. AbouZeid A, Alfrih A, Mohammad S, et al. Klippel-Trenaunay syndrome: a single-center experience with combined slow-flow vascular malformations. Egypt Pediatric Association Gaz. 2025;73:106. https://doi.org/10.1186/s43054-025-00455-7.
11. Maag BC, Towbin RB, Schaefer CM, Towbin AJ. Klippel-Trenaunay syndrome. Appl Radiol. 2024;5:10–3. https://doi.org/10.37549/AR-D-24-0014.
12. Hauert J, Loose DA. Orthopedic problems. In: Mattassi R, Loose D, Vaghi M, editors. Hemangiomas and vascular malformations. Milano: Springer; 2015. https://doi.org/10.1007/978-88-470-5673-2_43.

21 PIK3CA-Related Overgrowth Spectrum (PROS)

Introduction and Pathogenesis

The PIK3CA gene encodes p110α, a key subunit of the PI3-kinase enzyme that triggers signaling pathways regulating cell proliferation, survival, and growth. Acting downstream, mTOR1 promotes these effects through AKT phosphorylation [1]. Somatic mutations in PIK3CA have been associated with various vascular malformations. Specifically, postzygotic somatic activating mutations give rise to a wide range of developmental disorders collectively termed the PIK3CA-Related Overgrowth Spectrum (PROS) [2]. These mutations occur in two categories: oncogenic hotspot mutations and non-hotspot mutations [3].

The PIK3CA spectrum encompasses different phenotypic diseases—one of them is mainly vascular lesions, the second is non-vascular tissue overgrowth, and the third is a specific overgrowth of different tissues. The wide phenotypic spectrum, ranging from an isolated digit to diffuse multisystem involvement, is likely related to the type and timing of mutation development during embryogenesis [4].

Clinical Presentation

The clinical diagnostic criteria for PIK3CA-related overgrowth spectrum (PROS), as outlined by Keppler-Noreuil et al. [5], emphasize the presence of a somatic PIK3CA mutation along with congenital or early childhood onset of sporadic, mosaic overgrowth. In cases where a mutation cannot be identified, a presumptive diagnosis of PROS may still be considered if the clinical features are consistent. Diagnosis requires characteristic findings, either as part of a spectrum of features—including overgrowth of adipose, muscle, nerve, or skeletal tissue; vascular malformations (capillary, venous, lymphatic, or arteriovenous); epidermal nevi; or hemi-megalencephaly—or as isolated manifestations such as large lymphatic malformations, isolated macrodactyly or limb/hand/foot overgrowth, truncal adipose overgrowth, dysplastic megalencephaly with focal cortical dysplasia, epidermal nevus, seborrheic keratoses, or benign lichenoid keratoses. The condition is typically progressive, with potential complications such as scoliosis, disproportionate limb growth, central nervous system abnormalities (hydrocephalus, Chiari malformation, cerebellar tonsillar ectopia, megalencephaly, enlarged corpus callosum), regional lipomatous undergrowth with adjacent overgrowth, infiltrating lipomatosis, and risk of tumors such as Wilms tumor or ovarian cystadenoma [5, 6].

Characteristic features of PROS include asymmetric overgrowth affecting different body regions—most commonly the brain (Fig. 21.1), limbs (Fig. 21.2), trunk (Fig. 21.3), and

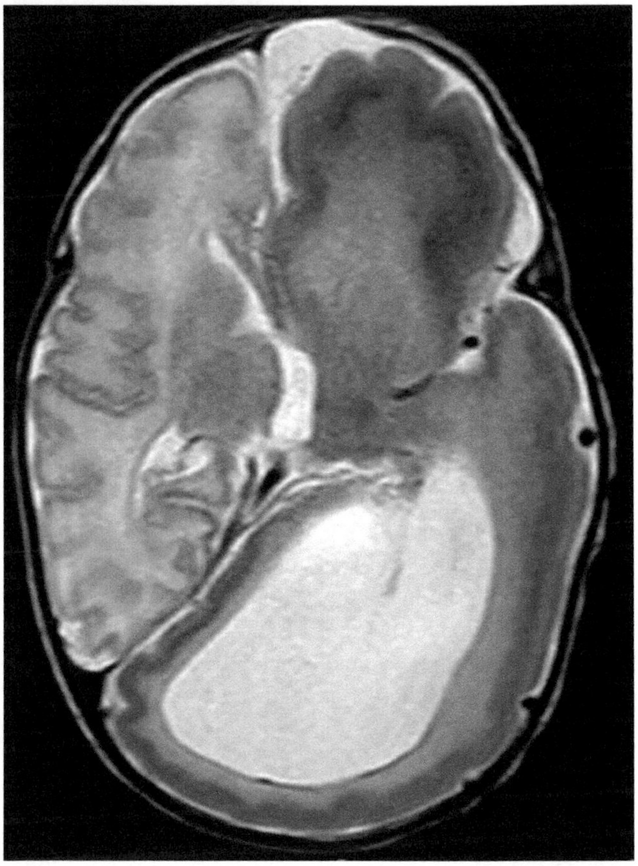

Fig. 21.1 MRI brain (axial T2-WI) demonstrating hemi-megalencephaly on the left side in a 3-month-old boy

A. A. AbouZeid et al., *Atlas of Pediatric Vascular Anomalies*, https://doi.org/10.1007/978-3-032-30866-5_21

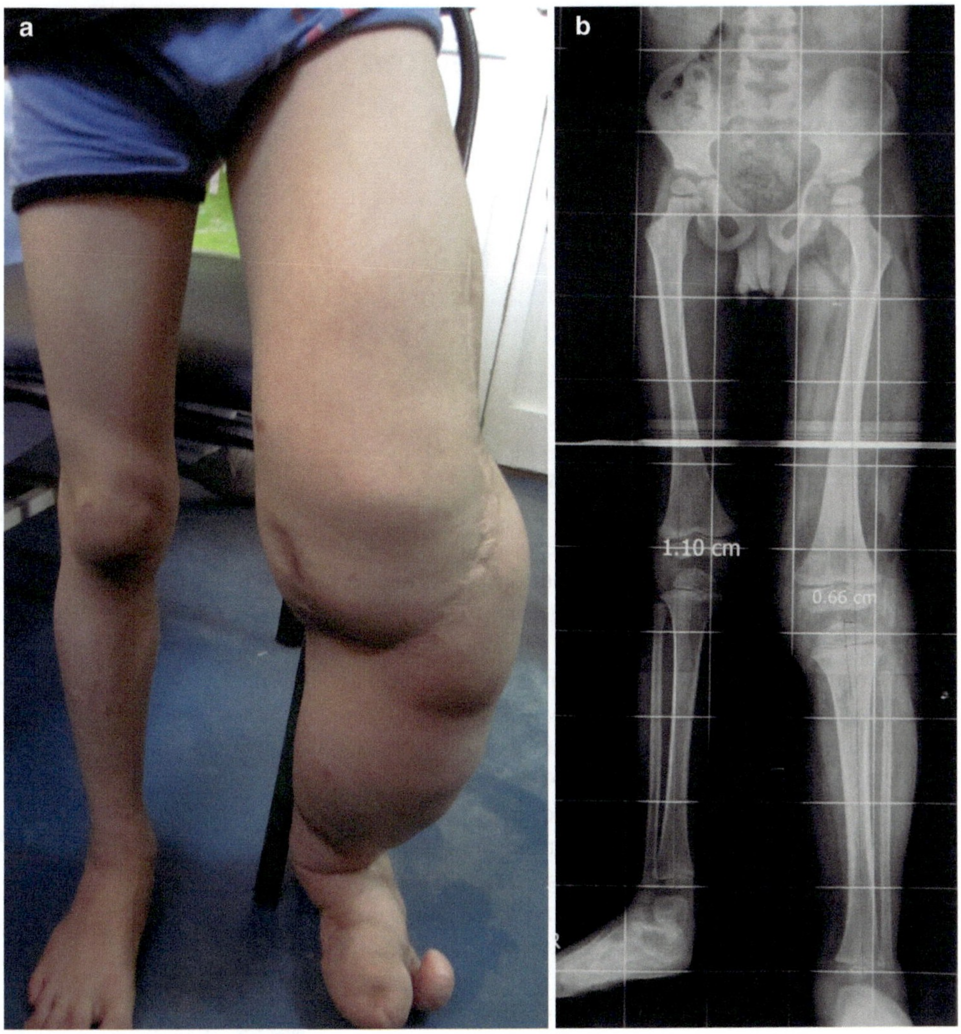

Fig. 21.2 Asymmetric or segmental overgrowth affecting left lower limb. (**a**) Clinical photograph. (**b**) Scanogram of the lower limb shows enlargement of the left lower limb with significant limb length discrepancy

face (Fig. 21.4)—and involving multiple tissue types such as nervous, vascular, lymphatic, skeletal, or adipose tissue. The condition is typically present at birth, and patients may also develop multiple lipomas, most frequently on the trunk, where they often infiltrate surrounding structures. In individuals with PIK3CA variants, limb anomalies are common, including leg-length discrepancy, sandal gap deformity (Fig. 21.5), and syndactyly (Fig. 21.6) [7]. The commonly encountered skin manifestations are epidermal nevi (Fig. 21.7), café-au-lait spots, seborrheic keratoses, hypo−/hyperpigmented areas [8].

Different vascular anomalies have been associated with PROS including capillary, lymphatic, venous, arteriovenous, and combined malformations. Capillary malformations may appear as demarcated dark red/purple patches of irregular shape, defined as "capillary malformation with geographic borders" (Fig. 21.8), or as reticulated patches with poorly defined edges (Fig. 21.9), called "reticulated capillary malformations" [8].

In 2021, Canaud et al. [9], defined three categories of PIK3CA-related conditions (Fig. 21.10): (A) PIK3CA-realted overgrowth spectrum disorders (PROS), characterized by overgrowth of the affected tissues; (B) exclusive vascular proliferation, named PIK3CA-related vascular malformations; (C) exclusive non-vascular proliferation, named PIK3CA-related non-vascular lesions [9].

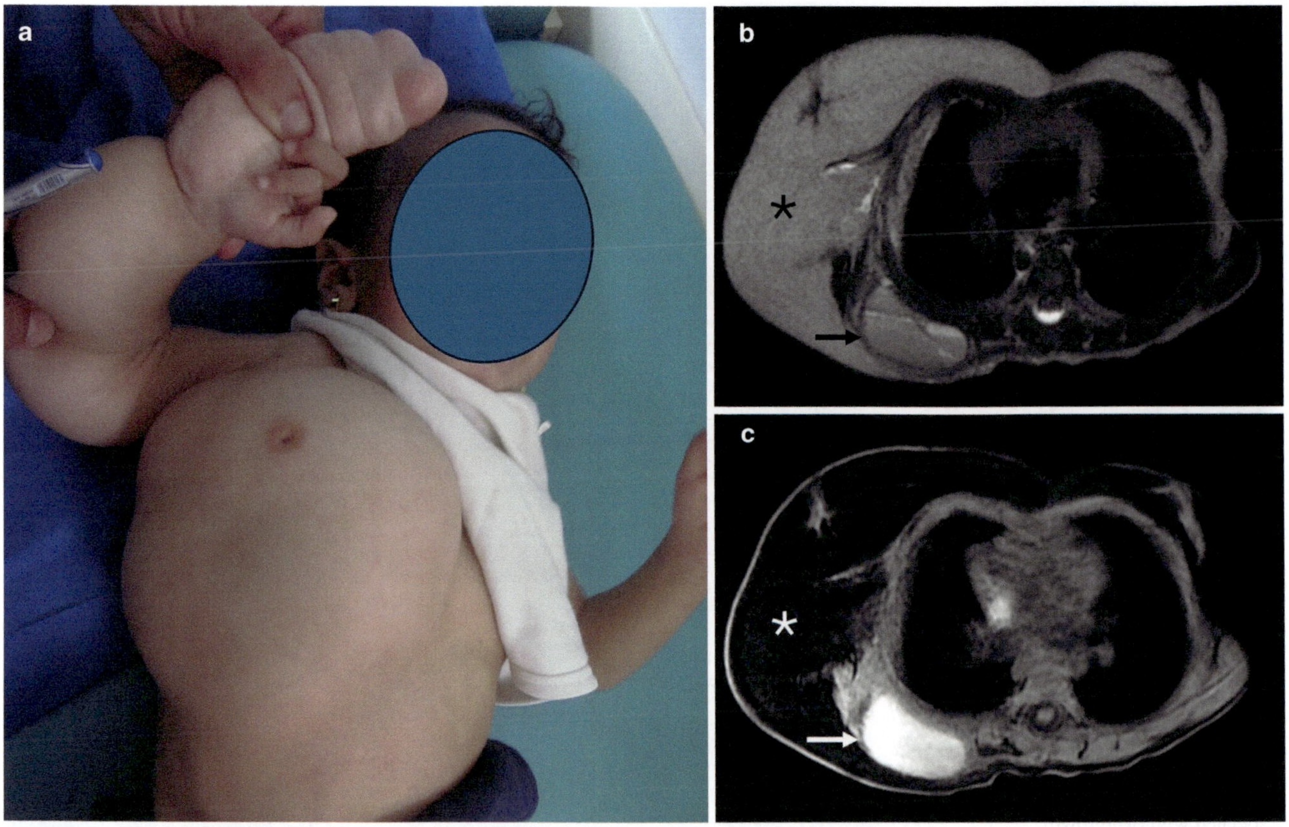

Fig. 21.3 (**a**) A 1-year-old girl presenting with asymmetric (segmental) lipomatous overgrowth involving the right upper limb and trunk. Note the hypertrophy and fusion of the little and index fingers on the affected right hand. (**b**, **c**) Axial MRI showing lipomatous overgrowth (*) that appears hyperintense on T2-weighted imaging (T2WI) and becomes hypointense following fat suppression (**c**). This is associated with a cystic component signifying the lymphatic malformation (arrow)

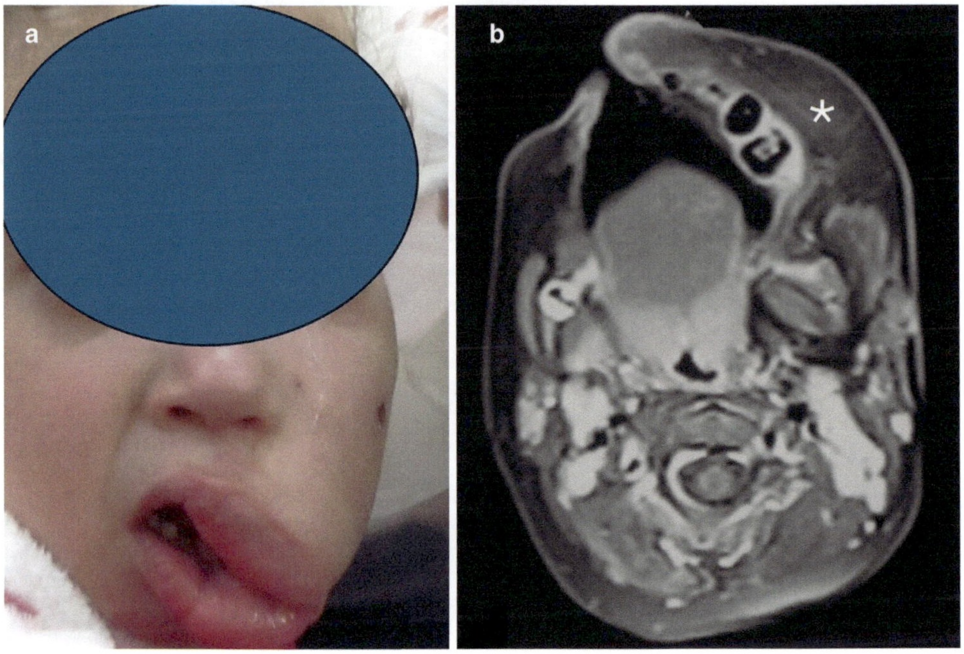

Fig. 21.4 Asymmetric or segmental facial overgrowth. (**a**) Clinical photograph. (**b**) Axial contrast-enhanced, fat-suppressed T1-weighted MRI image demonstrating lipomatous overgrowth (asterisk)

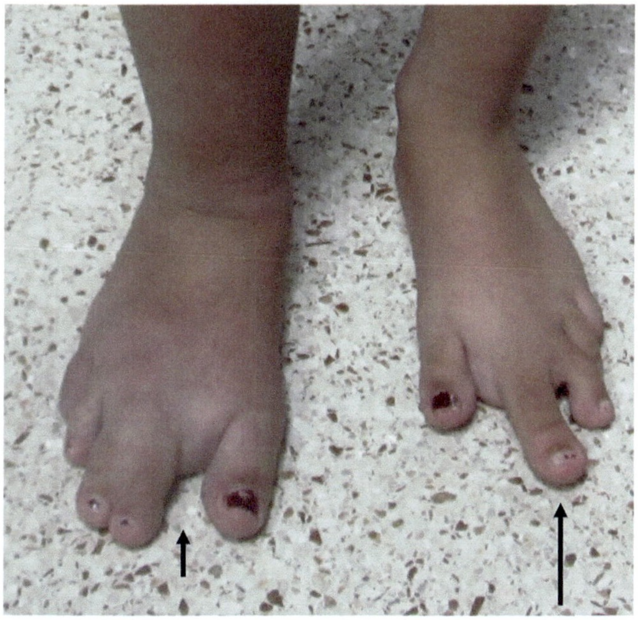

Fig. 21.5 Foot anomalies associating overgrowth syndromes: sandal gap deformity which is a wide first interdigital gap (short arrow), toe hypertrophy (long arrow), and syndactyly

Fig. 21.6 Limb anomalies associated with overgrowth syndromes involving the hands (**a**) and foot (**b**), showing syndactyly and asymmetric hypertrophy of the digits (fingers and toes)

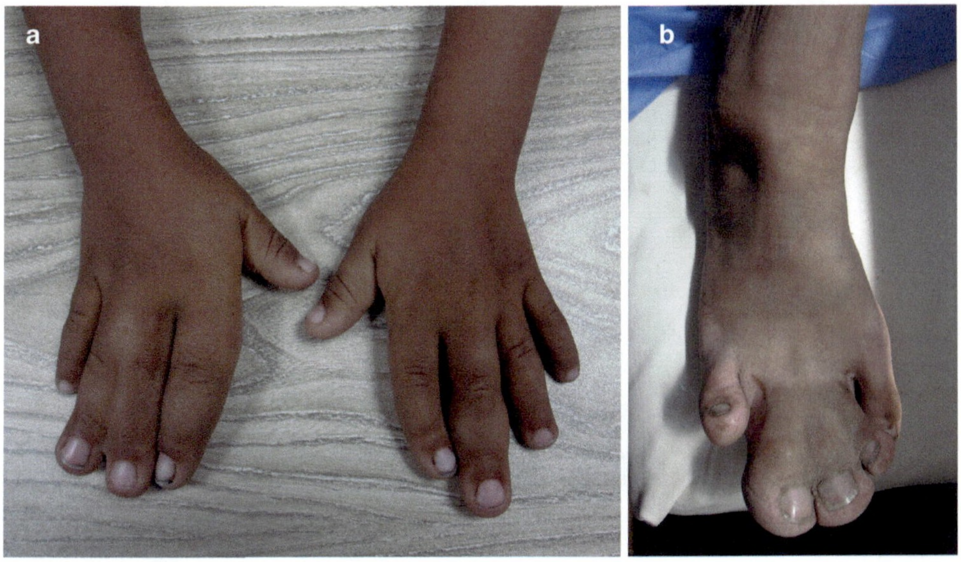

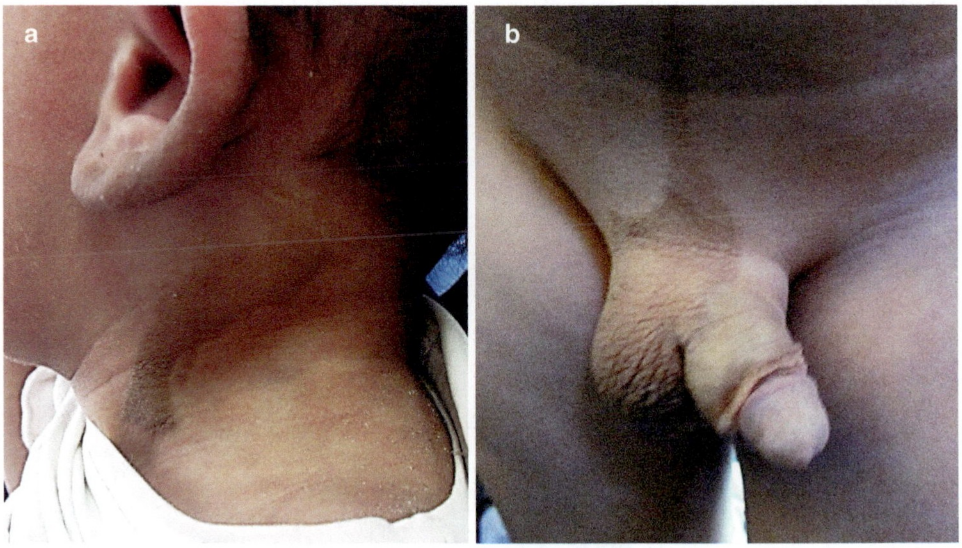

Fig. 21.7 Examples of linear epidermal nevus, typically presenting as linear or streak-like areas of thickened, rough, brownish skin. The lesions follow the lines of Blaschko, which correspond to patterns of embryonic skin cell migration

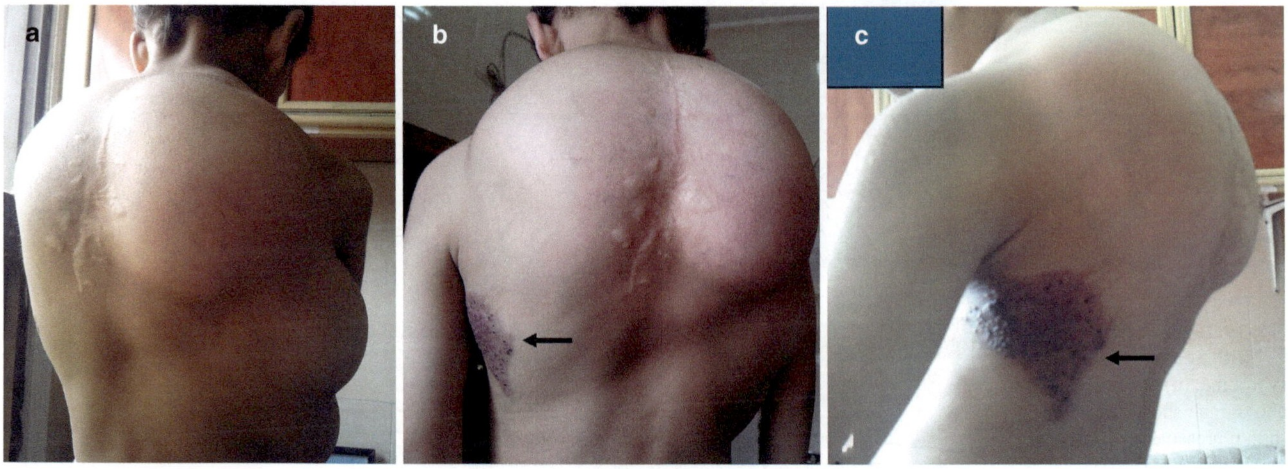

Fig. 21.8 Clinical manifestations of CLOVES syndrome in a patient with a confirmed PIK3CA mutation in tissue samples. (**a**–**c**) Asymmetric lipomatous overgrowth of the back and a geographic capillary malformation (arrow)

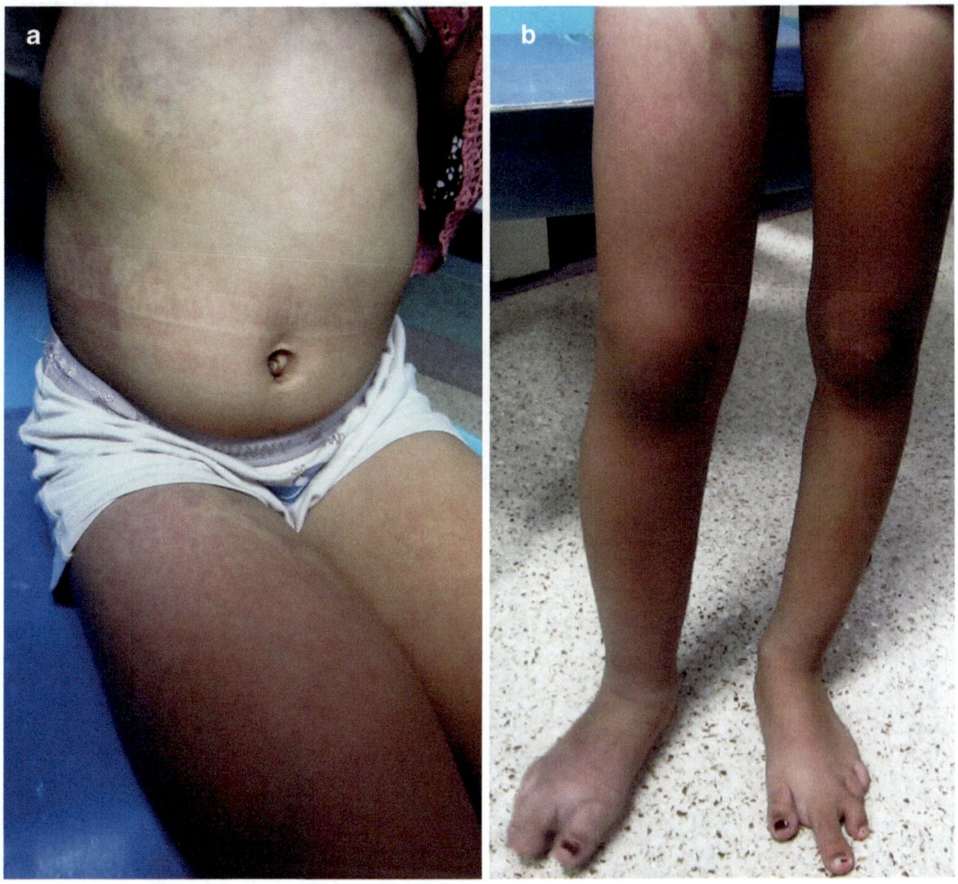

Fig. 21.9 Capillary malformation (CM) associating PIK3CA-related overgrowth spectrum (PROS) in a 7-year-old girl. (**a**) The CM involves the right lower limb and extends to the lower lateral trunk. (**b**) Note the discrepancy in limb growth

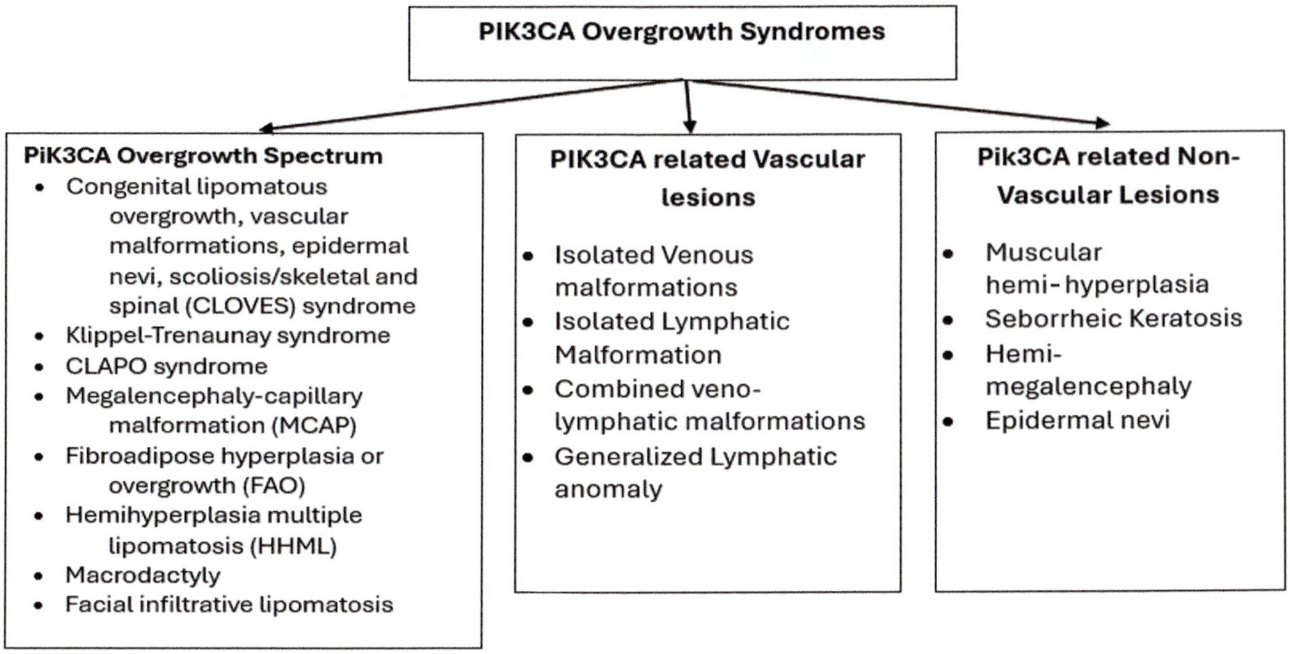

Fig. 21.10 The three categories of PIK3CA-related conditions

Syndromes Classified Under the Umbrella of PIK3CA-Related Overgrowth Spectrum (PROS)

- *CLOVES Syndrome (Congenital Lipomatous Overgrowth, Vascular Malformations, Epidermal Nevi, and Skeletal Abnormalities)*: CLOVES syndrome represents a severe phenotype within the PIK3CA-related overgrowth spectrum (PROS). It is characterized by asymmetric congenital overgrowth, complex vascular malformations, musculoskeletal deformities, and cutaneous lesions (Fig. 21.11). A hallmark feature of CLOVES syndrome is the extensive lipomatous overgrowth of the trunk (Fig. 21.12), which may infiltrate adjacent tissues (Fig. 21.11d) and contribute to scoliosis; in some cases, intraspinal extension has been reported [10]. The vascular malformations seen in CLOVES are typically combined, slow-flow lesions, although spinal arteriovenous malformations have occasionally been documented [11, 12]. Skeletal abnormalities, particularly scoliosis, are common and correlate with the extent and progression of the neighboring lipomatous mass [6]. Acral deformities include broad, spade-like hands (Fig. 21.13) with ulnar deviation of the digits and deep palmar or plantar furrows resulting from fatty tissue deposition. Epidermal nevi may also be present, often distributed in a blaschkoid pattern (Fig. 21.6).
- *Klippel-Trenaunay Syndrome (KTS)*: KTS is a complex vascular malformation marked by a combination of slow-flow vascular malformations (capillary, venous, and lymphatic) accompanied by abnormal tissue overgrowth. The disease affects the lower limbs in most cases. Venous malformations represent a hallmark in KTS, usually manifesting as dilated tortuous veins (refer to Chap. 20).
- *CLAPO Syndrome* (Capillary malformation of the lower lip, Lymphatic malformation of the face and neck, Asymmetry, and Partial/Generalized Overgrowth) is a rare disorder predominantly affecting the head and neck region. It is characterized by combined vascular malformations, primarily capillary and lymphatic, associated with segmental overgrowth.

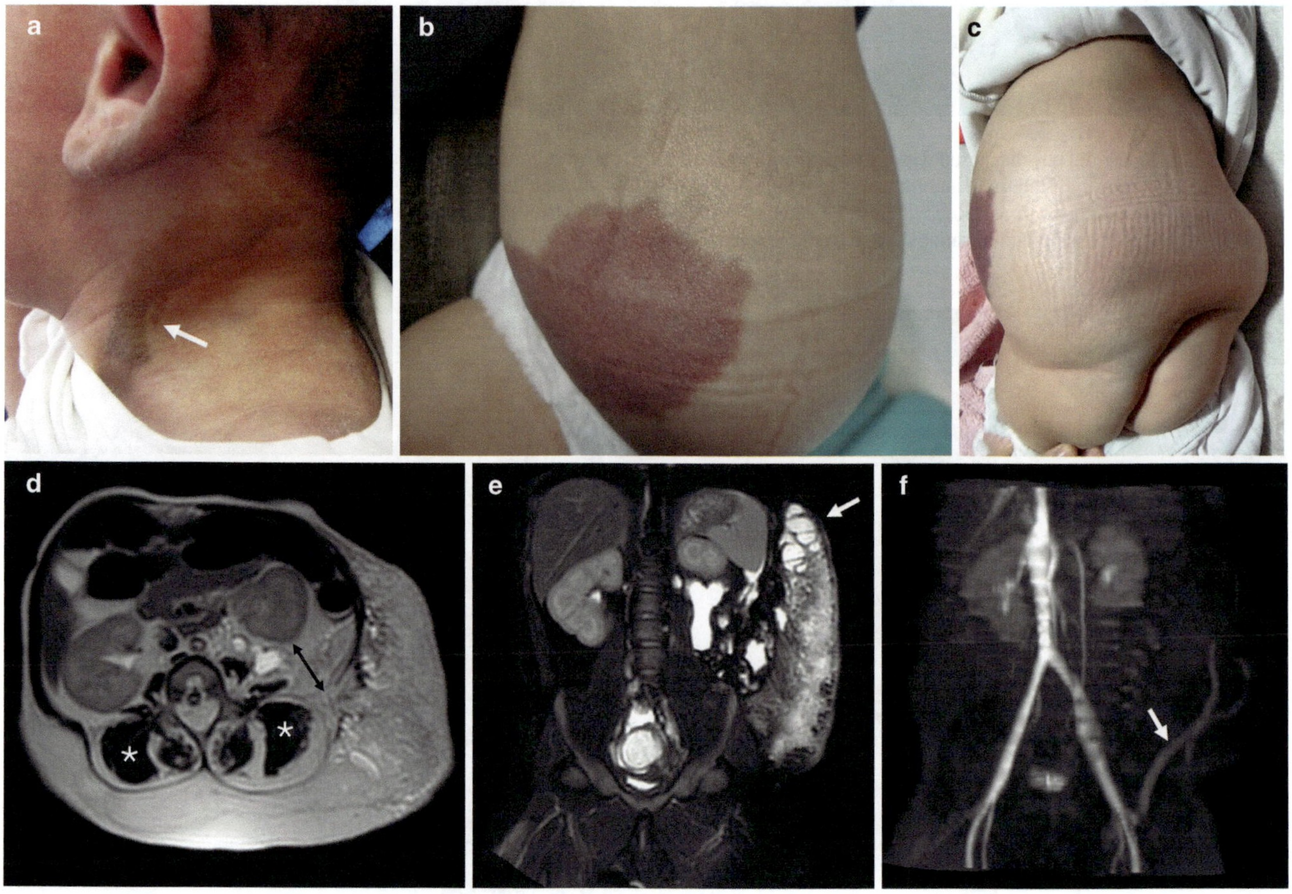

Fig. 21.11 A 4-month-old girl showing characteristic features of CLOVES syndrome. (**a**) Linear epidermal nevus (arrow). (**b, c**) Capillary malformation overlying truncal lipomatous overgrowth. (**d–f**) MRI study demonstrating the deep components of the lesion: (**d**) Axial T2-weighted image (T2WI) reveals deep extension of lipomatous overgrowth around the back muscles (asterisk) and into the retroperitoneum, displacing the left kidney anteriorly (double arrowhead line). (**f**) Non-contrast MR venography shows an associated anomalous vein (arrow) beneath the capillary malformation

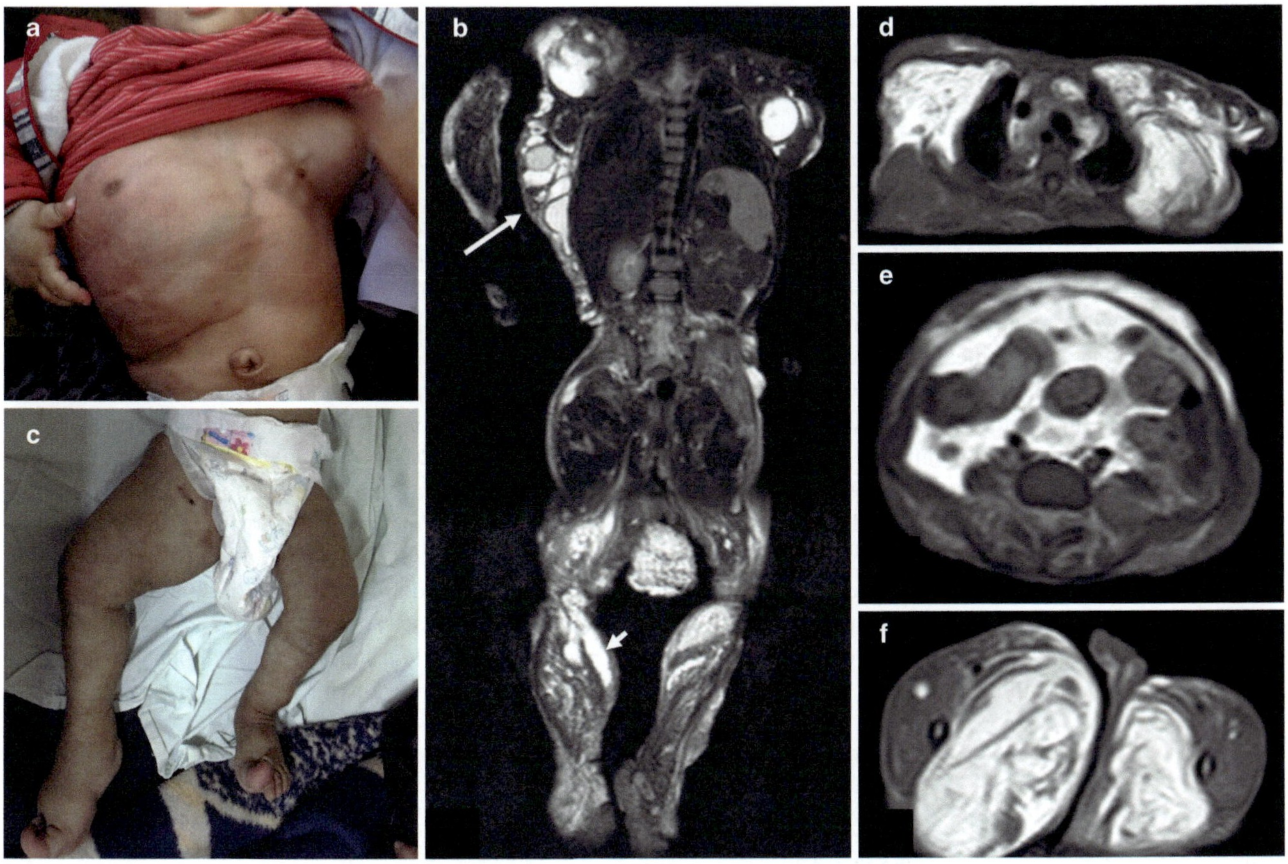

Fig. 21.12 A 1-year-old boy diagnosed with CLOVES syndrome. (**a**, **b**) Asymmetric overgrowth of the trunk and limbs. (**c**–**f**) Whole-body MRI demonstrates tissue overgrowth composed of fatty and vascular elements. (**c**) STIR sequence reveals multiple variable-sized cystic lesions consistent with lymphatic malformations (long arrow) and dilated veins with bright signal intensity (short arrow). (**d**–**f**) Axial T1-weighted images at the levels of the upper thorax (**d**), mid-abdomen (**e**), and upper thigh (**f**) show fatty overgrowth exhibiting bright signal intensity

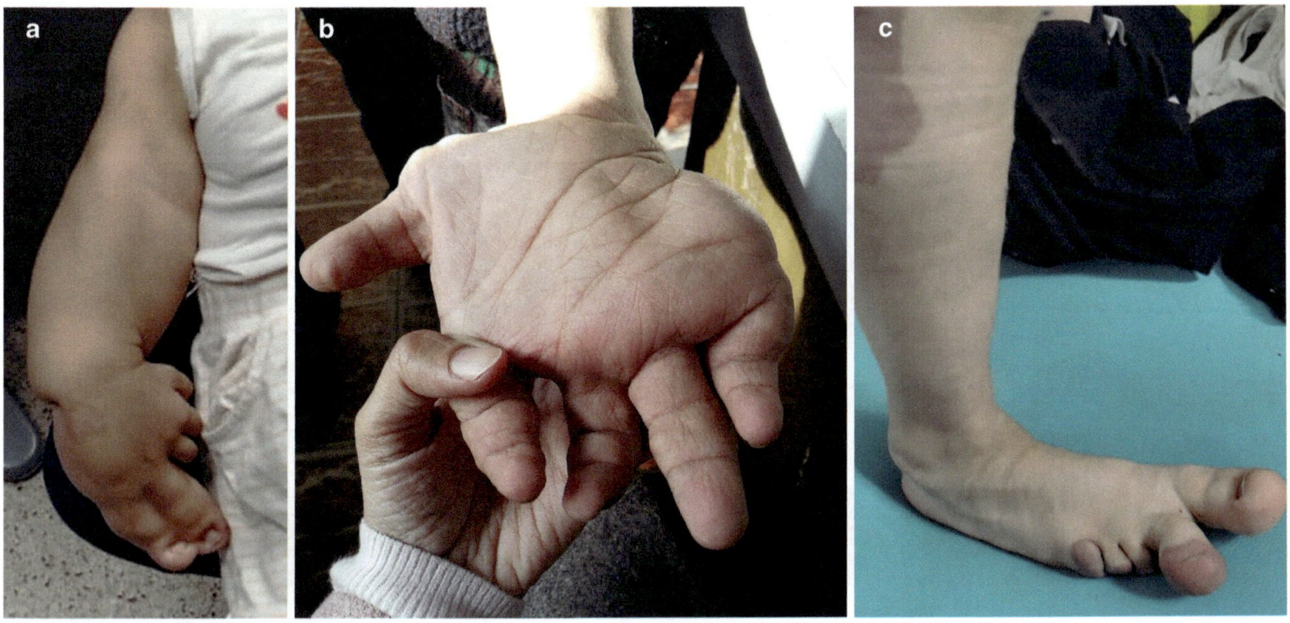

Fig. 21.13 Limb and skeletal manifestations in patients with PIK3CA-related overgrowth syndrome, showing (**a**) limb hypertrophy and syndactyly, (**b**) abnormal hand growth, and (**c**) asymmetric overgrowth of the toes

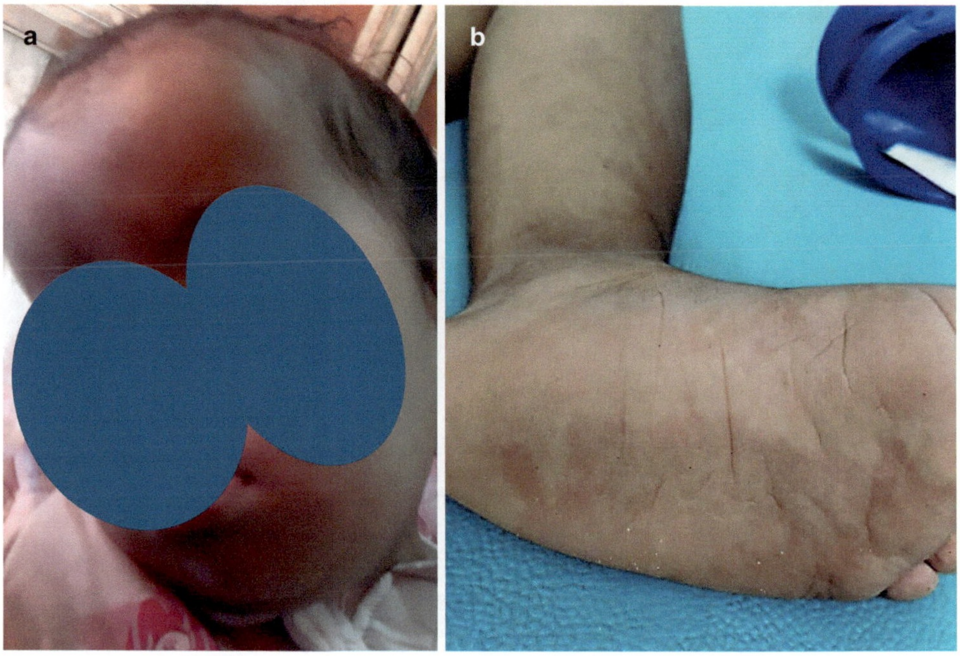

Fig. 21.14 Megalencephaly-capillary malformation, a subtype of the PIK3CA-related overgrowth spectrum (PROS), showing (**a**) a prominent forehead and (**b**) faint, reticulated capillary malformations

- *Megalencephaly–Capillary Malformation (MCAP) Syndrome*: Megalencephaly with associated neurologic manifestations is recognized as part of the PIK3CA-related overgrowth spectrum (PROS). Individuals with MCAP typically present with congenital or early postnatal megalencephaly, segmental body overgrowth, and reticulated or confluent capillary malformations (Fig. 21.14) [13]. Compared with other PIK3CA-related disorders, the PIK3CA variants identified in MCAP are frequently located at non-hotspot regions of the gene and are associated with less-activating mutations [14].
- *Diffuse capillary malformation with overgrowth (DCMO)*: DCMO is characterized by widespread capillary malformations that are typically pale pink, reticulated, and involve contiguous anatomical regions. Overgrowth of an extremity may occur, affecting soft tissue and/or bone, but it does not necessarily correspond to the location or extent of the capillary malformations. MRI imaging is generally unnecessary unless there are clinical signs suggesting a deeper vascular malformation. Unlike Klippel-Trénaunay syndrome (KTS), DCMO does not present with the same complications, apart from leg length discrepancy resulting from asymmetric overgrowth.
- *Fibroadipose hyperplasia or overgrowth (FAO)*: A condition characterized by progressive, segmental enlargement of subcutaneous, muscular, and visceral fibroadipose tissues, with skeletal overgrowth [15].
- *Facial infiltrative lipomatosis*: A benign but locally aggressive condition characterized by asymmetric hemifacial overgrowth and noticeable facial asymmetry [16].

Differential Diagnosis of PIK3CA-Related Overgrowth Spectrum (PROS)

It is important to consider other syndromes such as Proteus syndrome and PTEN Hamartoma Tumor Syndrome [5]. Proteus syndrome is associated with a somatic activating *AKT1* mutation [8]. PTEN Hamartoma Tumor Syndrome is associated with vascular anomalies and fat overgrowth [17]. In addition, there are overlapping clinical phenotypes with the mosaic RASopathies [18].

Another important differential diagnosis in neurofibromatosis type 1, *NF1*, which is a genetic tumor-predisposition syndrome caused by germline mutations in the *NF1* gene. The NF1 protein (neurofibromin) is a negative regulator of the RAS signaling pathway [19]. The presence of café au lait macules, and limb overgrowth due to plexiform neurofibroma [20], puts the disease in overlap manifestation due to PROS (Fig. 21.15).

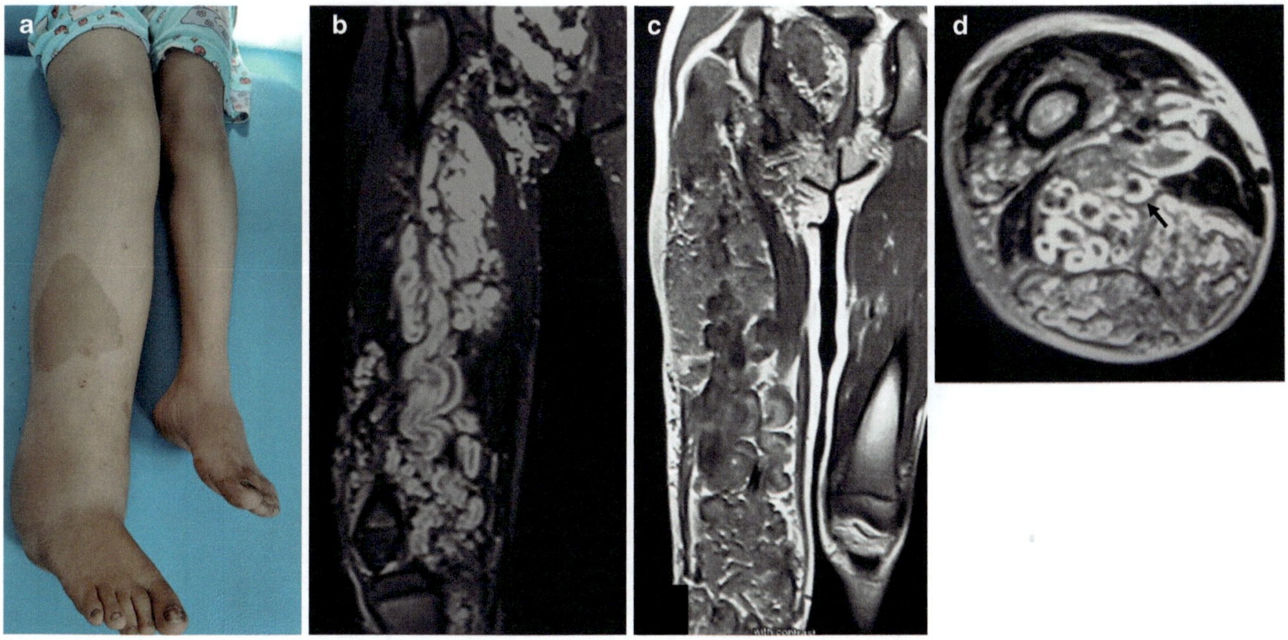

Fig. 21.15 A 5-year-old girl with right lower limb overgrowth secondary to massive plexiform neurofibromatosis. (**a**) Clinical image showing limb enlargement with multiple café-au-lait macules. (**b**–**d**) MRI demonstrates extensive plexiform neurofibromatosis with high signal intensity on T2 fat-suppressed sequence (**b**), intermediate signal intensity on T1-weighted image (**c**), and the characteristic "target sign" (arrow) on axial T2-weighted image (**d**)

Follow-Up of Patients with Overgrowth

Initial evaluation for patients with PROS should include thorough clinical examination and imaging assessment, aiming to develop a follow-up plan special for each individual based on involved tissues. The follow-up needs to include the anthropometric growth parameters, back examination for alignment, leg lengths, occipitofrontal circumference. Orthopedic evaluations are frequently needed for functional assessment need for corrective or adjustment of shoes. Neurodevelopmental and ocular evaluations are part of initial and follow-up evaluations [21].

The initial imaging modality is selected based on the anatomic regions involved. Magnetic resonance imaging (MRI), often complemented by magnetic resonance venography (MRV) and magnetic resonance angiography (MRA), is commonly employed to assess the extent of tissue involvement and to characterize vascular lesions. MRI of the brain and spine should be included when neurological manifestations are suspected based on clinical findings. Doppler ultrasonography is valuable for monitoring vascular anomalies, particularly to evaluate for venous thrombosis in cases of large venous malformations.

Several of the common mutations identified in PROS are hotspot variants, also found in cancer, theoretically suggesting an elevated risk of malignancy in affected individuals. Nevertheless, malignant transformation is rarely observed in clinical practice, with only isolated anecdotal reports and, therefore, no standardized cancer screening guidelines have been established for these patients.

Treatment Approaches

For successful treatment, multidisciplinary care is an essential part of effective approach. In the setting of lipomatous overgrowth, debulking surgery is considered to improve functional status and pain, while considering the best cosmetic outcome.

Orthopedic management of complications including scoliosis, macrodactyly, and leg length discrepancies is frequently needed. Neurosurgery might be considered in drug-resistant epilepsy and hydrocephalus. In cases of vascular malformations, sclerotherapy, laser therapy, and oral medications are the treatments of choice. The aim of the surgical procedure should be the morphological and functional improvement [22], while sclerotherapy is less invasive option [23]. Other therapeutic possibilities are skin lasers, endovascular lasers, manual lymphatic drainage, compression therapy, and cryotherapy [21].

Although there is risk of thrombosis, indication for anticoagulation is individualized in high-risk situations, especially with previous history of deep venous thrombosis [24].

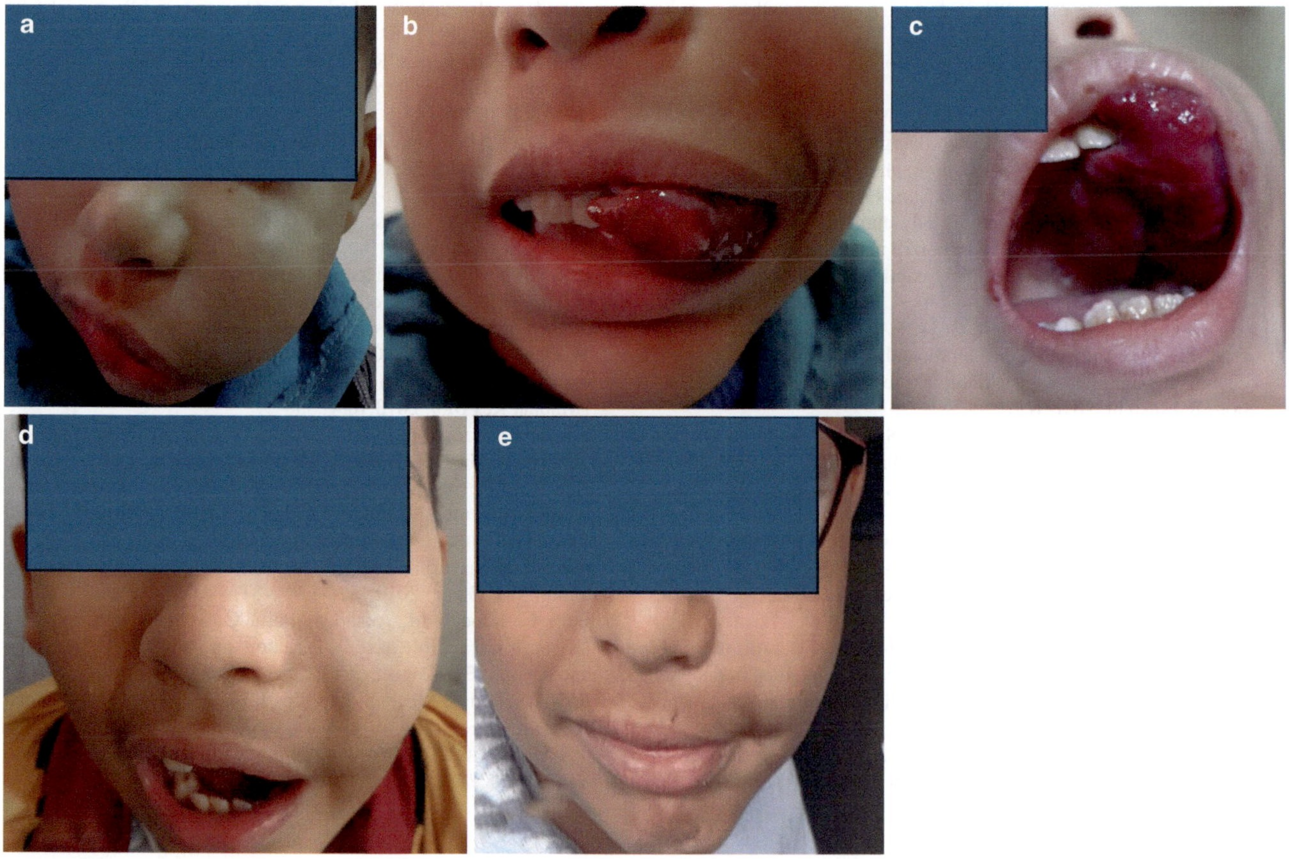

Fig. 21.16 Treatment response in a child with PROS harboring a somatic c.3203dup (Asn1068Tyrfs) hotspot mutation in PIK3CA. (**a**) Pre-treatment images showing left cheek overgrowth and periorbital swelling, with a mass protruding through the oral cavity (**b**, **c**). (**d**, **e**) Postoperative and post-Sirolimus therapy images demonstrating marked reduction in the size of the mass

Pharmacologic Treatment

Small-molecule inhibitors of PIK3CA pathway have been developed with the aim of treating activated pathways in cancer at different levels, with inhibitors of PI3K, AKT, and mTOR [25]. Alpelisib has been used with improvement in need for soft tissue and extremity bulk reduction, pain, enhanced quality of life, and functional abilities [26]. In the activation pathway, mTOR is downstream the PIK3CA, and mTOR inhibitors has been widely used in complicated vascular anomalies, fibroadipose hyperplasia, and PROS with good response (Fig. 21.16) especially in lymphatic malformations [1, 22].

References

1. Parker VER, Keppler-Noreuil KM, Faivre L, Luu M, Oden NL, De Silva L, et al. Safety and efficacy of low-dose sirolimus in the PIK3CA-related overgrowth spectrum. Genet Med. 2019;21(5):1189–98.
2. Hughes M, Hao M, Luu M. PIK3CA vascular overgrowth syndromes: an update. Curr Opin Pediatr. 2020;32(4):539–46.
3. Limaye N, Kangas J, Mendola A, Godfraind C, Schlögel MJ, Helaers R, et al. Somatic activating PIK3CA mutations cause venous malformation. Am J Hum Genet. 2015;97(6):914–21.
4. Kang HC, Baek ST, Song S, Gleeson JG. Clinical and genetic aspects of the segmental overgrowth Spectrum due to somatic mutations in PIK3CA. J Pediatr. 2015;167(5):957–62.
5. Keppler-Noreuil KM, Rios JJ, Parker VER, Semple RK, Lindhurst MJ, Sapp JC, et al. PIK3CA-related overgrowth spectrum (PROS): diagnostic and testing eligibility criteria, differential diagnosis, and evaluation. Am J Med Genet A. 2015;167A(2):287–95.
6. Keppler-Noreuil KM, Sapp JC, Lindhurst MJ, Parker VER, Blumhorst C, Darling T, et al. Clinical delineation and natural history of the PIK3CA-related overgrowth spectrum. Am J Med Genet A. 2014;164A(7):1713–33.
7. Carli D, De Pellegrin M, Franceschi L, Zinali F, Paonessa M, Spolaore S, et al. Evolution over time of leg length discrepancy in patients with syndromic and isolated lateralized overgrowth. J Pediatr. 2021;234:123–7.
8. Öztürk Durmaz E, Demircioğlu D, Yalınay Dikmen P, Alanay Y, Alanay A, Demirkesen C, et al. A review on cutaneous and musculoskeletal manifestations of CLOVES syndrome. Clin Cosmet Investig Dermatol. 2022;15:621–30.
9. Canaud G, Hammill AM, Adams D, Vikkula M, Keppler-Noreuil KM. A review of mechanisms of disease across PIK3CA-related disorders with vascular manifestations. Orphanet J Rare Dis. 2021;16(1):306.
10. Martinez-Lopez A, Blasco-Morente G, Perez-Lopez I, Herrera-Garcia JD, Luque-Valenzuela M, Sanchez-Cano D, et al. CLOVES

syndrome: review of a PIK3CA-related overgrowth spectrum (PROS). Clin Genet. 2017;91(1):14–21.
11. Bloom J, Upton J. CLOVES syndrome. J Hand Surg Am. 2013;38(12):2508–12.
12. Bertino F, Braithwaite KA, Hawkins CM, Gill AE, Briones MA, Swerdlin R, et al. Congenital limb overgrowth syndromes associated with vascular anomalies. Radiographics. 2019;39(2):491–515.
13. Wright DR, Frieden IJ, Orlow SJ, Shin HT, Chamlin S, Schaffer JV, et al. The misnomer "macrocephaly-cutis marmorata telangiectatica congenita syndrome": report of 12 new cases and support for revising the name to macrocephaly-capillary malformations. Arch Dermatol. 2009;145(3):287–93.
14. Mirzaa G, Timms AE, Conti V, Boyle EA, Girisha KM, Martin B, et al. PIK3CA-associated developmental disorders exhibit distinct classes of mutations with variable expression and tissue distribution. JCI Insight. 2016;1(9)
15. Lindhurst MJ, Parker VER, Payne F, Sapp JC, Rudge S, Harris J, et al. Mosaic overgrowth with fibroadipose hyperplasia is caused by somatic activating mutations in PIK3CA. Nat Genet. 2012;44(8):928–33.
16. Moreno SD, Liu RH, Robbins Q, Burkes J. Advances in the treatment of congenital infiltrating lipomatosis of the face: the role of PIK3CA mutations and microvascular reconstruction. J Craniofac Surg. 36(1):229–33.
17. Tan WH, Baris HN, Burrows PE, Robson CD, Alomari AI, Mulliken JB, et al. The spectrum of vascular anomalies in patients with PTEN mutations: implications for diagnosis and management. J Med Genet. 2007;44(9):594–602.
18. Al-Olabi L, Polubothu S, Dowsett K, Andrews KA, Stadnik P, Joseph AP, et al. Mosaic RAS/MAPK variants cause sporadic vascular malformations which respond to targeted therapy. J Clin Invest. 2018;128(11):5185.
19. Gutmann DH, Ferner RE, Listernick RH, Korf BR, Wolters PL, Johnson KJ. Neurofibromatosis type 1. Nat Rev Dis Primers. 2017;3(1):17004.
20. Uebelhoer M, Boon LM, Vikkula M. Vascular anomalies: from genetics toward models for therapeutic trials. Cold Spring Harb Perspect Med. 2012;2(8)
21. Gazzin A, Leoni C, Viscogliosi G, Borgini F, Perri L, Iacoviello M, et al. Work-up and treatment strategies for individuals with PIK3CA-related disorders: a consensus of experts from the Scientific Committee of the Italian Macrodactyly and PROS Association. Genes (Basel). 2023;14(12)
22. Wiegand S, Wichmann G, Dietz A. Treatment of lymphatic malformations with the mTOR inhibitor sirolimus: a systematic review. Lymphat Res Biol. 2018;16(4):330–9.
23. Snyder EJ, Sarma A, Borst AJ, Tekes A. Lymphatic anomalies in children: update on imaging diagnosis, genetics, and treatment. AJR Am J Roentgenol. 2022;218(6):1089–101.
24. Keppler-Noreuil KM, Lozier J, Oden N, Taneja A, Burton-Akright J, Sapp JC, et al. Thrombosis risk factors in PIK3CA-related overgrowth spectrum and proteus syndrome. Am J Med Genet C Semin Med Genet. 2019;181(4):571–81.
25. Belli C, Repetto M, Anand S, Porta C, Subbiah V, Curigliano G. The emerging role of PI3K inhibitors for solid tumour treatment and beyond. Br J Cancer. 2023;128(12):2150–62.
26. Raghavendran P, Albers SE, Phillips JD, Zarnegar-Lumley S, Borst AJ. Clinical response to PI3K-α inhibition in a cohort of children and adults with PIK3CA-related overgrowth Spectrum disorders. J Vasc Anom. 2022;3(1):e038.

GPSR Compliance

The European Union's (EU) General Product Safety Regulation (GPSR) is a set of rules that requires consumer products to be safe and our obligations to ensure this.

If you have any concerns about our products, you can contact us on ProductSafety@springernature.com

In case Publisher is established outside the EU, the EU authorized representative is:

Springer Nature Customer Service Center GmbH
Europaplatz 3
69115 Heidelberg, Germany

Batch number: 10731528

Printed by Printforce, the Netherlands